Comprehensive Textbook on Vitiligo

Comprehensive Textbook on Vitiligo

EDITOR IN CHIEF

Vineet Relhan, MD
Associate Professor
Department of Dermatology and Venereology
Maulana Azad Medical College
and
Lok Nayak Hospital
New Delhi, India

EDITORS

Vijay Kumar Garg, MD
Senior Professor and Head
Department of Dermatology
Santosh Medical College
Ghaziabad, Uttar Pradesh, India

Sneha Ghunawat, MD
Consultant Dermatologist
Columbia Asia Hospital
and
Meraki Skin Clinic
Gurugram, India

Khushbu Mahajan, MD
Consultant Dermatologist
Kubba Skin Clinic
and
Mahajan Skin Centre
Delhi, India

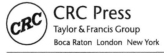

CRC Press
Taylor & Francis Group
Boca Raton London New York

CRC Press is an imprint of the
Taylor & Francis Group, an **informa** business

First edition published 2021
by CRC Press
6000 Broken Sound Parkway NW, Suite 300, Boca Raton, FL 33487-2742

and by CRC Press
2 Park Square, Milton Park, Abingdon, Oxon, OX14 4RN

© 2021 Taylor & Francis Group, LLC

CRC Press is an imprint of Taylor & Francis Group, LLC

Library of Congress Cataloging-in-Publication Data

Names: Relhan, Vineet, editor. | Garg, Vijay K. (Professor), editor. | Ghunawat, Sneha, editor. | Mahajan, Khushbu, editor.
Title: Comprehensive textbook on vitiligo / edited by Vineet Relhan, Vijay Kumar Garg, Sneha Ghunawat, Khushbu Mahajan.
Description: First edition. | Boca Raton, FL : CRC Press, 2020. | Includes bibliographical references and index. | Summary: "Vitiligo is a disorder having a significant impact in dark-skinned individuals. Along with the historical, cultural, and psychological aspects of the disease the multifactorial pathogenesis of this disorder are discussed in detail with special emphasis on the newer hypothesis proposed in the causation"-- Provided by publisher.
Identifiers: LCCN 2020015085 (print) | LCCN 2020015086 (ebook) | ISBN 9781138063594 (hardback) | ISBN 9781315112183 (ebook)
Subjects: MESH: Vitiligo--etiology | Vitiligo--drug therapy | Vitiligo--surgery
Classification: LCC RL790 (print) | LCC RL790 (ebook) | NLM WR 265 | DDC 616.5/5--dc23
LC record available at https://lccn.loc.gov/2020015085
LC ebook record available at https://lccn.loc.gov/2020015086

ISBN: 978-1-138-06359-4 (hbk)
ISBN: 978-0-367-54372-3 (pbk)
ISBN: 978-1-315-11218-3 (ebk)

Typeset in Minion Pro
by Nova Techset Private Limited, Bengaluru & Chennai, India

**Visit the Taylor & Francis Web site at
http://www.taylorandfrancis.com**

**and the CRC Press Web site at
http://www.crcpress.com**

CONTENTS

SECTION I
The Basics of Vitiligo

SECTION II
Clinical Profile of Vitiligo

SECTION III
Diagnosis and Assessment of Vitiligo

SECTION IV
Topical Treatment for Vitiligo

SECTION V
Systemic Treatment for Vitiligo

SECTION VI
Phototherapy and Lasers

SECTION VII
Other Therapies for Vitiligo

SECTION VIII
Surgical Treatment of Vitiligo

SECTION IX
Miscellaneous

If God wanted me to be black, I'd be black. If God wanted me to be white I'd be white.

But he chose for me to be both and original. So I guess that's the way I'm supposed to be.

Winnie Harlow

Vitiligo is a disorder with great psychological and social impact. It is referred to even in the great scriptures found all over the world. It is often considered a non-disease, a simple aesthetic problem. In spite of it stigmatizing the human race since ancient times, there have been many gaps in knowledge regarding the pathogenicity and therapeutics. One of the reasons for this has been the asymptomatic nature of the condition. With the evolvement of modern science, recent advances have been made in the medical and surgical treatments of the disease.

In the past, vitiligo has mostly been considered an autoimmune disorder by scientists. With recent molecular research theories, new dimensions have been added to its pathogenesis and treatment. It has always captured the interest of immunologists, biologists, and dermatologists around the world. The enigmatic nature of the disease has also garnered the interest of scientists and clinicians. This book was a dream project, as it is a comprehensive compilation of all aspects of the disease. It was our aim to highlight the links in the pathophysiology, clinical, and therapeutic aspects of the disease.

A great attempt has been made to fill in the missing gaps pertaining to the unsolved issues of the disease as well as to understand the scope of future research.

The book exhaustively deals with all aspects of vitiligo, including basic biology, pathogenesis, clinical variants, psychological impact, and treatment aspects, both medical and surgical. We have aimed to present a complete practical guide on the disease. The contributors are experts from across the globe and have graciously shared their experiences and wisdom in their respective topics. We hope that readers benefit by reading the book and incorporating these pearls of wisdom in their practices. Emphasis has been placed on the clinical and therapeutic aspects to help readers enhance their skills. Pictorial depictions help in better understanding of the surgical procedures.

We thank all our global experts for their contributions. The information is compiled and presented in a comprehensible and scientific manner. The book has materialized due to the hard work and collective efforts of the entire editorial team and the dedicated authors. The cooperation of the juniors, technical staff, and the patients, has been of utmost importance in this journey. We also thank Shivangi Pramanik (Commissioning Editor, Medical) and Himani Dwivedi (Editorial Assistant, Medical) of CRC Press/Taylor & Francis, for their assistance with the publication process.

We would like to acknowledge our mentors, colleagues, trainees, and patients who have been a source of knowledge and inspiration.

Vineet Relhan, MD, is Associate Professor in the Department of Dermatology, Maulana Azad Medical College and associated Lok Nayak Hospital, New Delhi. He has a keen interest in dermatosurgery and has been looking after the dermatosurgery operation theatre in the department since 18 years. His focus is on vitiligo and nail surgeries. He has guided many postgraduate dissertations in vitiligo surgery, including both tissue and cellular grafting. He has more than 18 years of teaching experience with UG and PG students. He is a recognized PG teacher at Delhi University and has many publications in national and international peer-reviewed journals. He has contributed seven chapters in various textbooks on dermatology. Dr. Relhan was President of the Indian Association of Dermatologists, Venereologists, and Leprologists (IADVL), Delhi State Branch, in 2017. He is the founding member and Treasurer of Nail Society of India and the Vice-President for the Geriatric Aesthetic Dermatology Society of India. He was the organizing secretary of the successful conference of Association of Cutaneous Surgeons of India held in 2019 at Delhi (India), which was attended by more than 1500 delegates.

He is a recipient of the National IADVL President Appreciation Award for 2015 and was awarded the Dr. K.C. Kandhari award by IADVL Delhi State Branch in 2019.

Vijay Kumar Garg, MD, Professor of Dermatology was the Head of Department of Dermatology and Venereology at Maulana Azad Medical College and Lok Nayak Hospital, Delhi (India). His climb has been studded with hard and tireless work for the specialty. In the process he has multiple contributions to his credit. He has been the President of IADVL, Delhi State Branch, and as Organizing Secretary he organized the 33rd National Conference of IADVL along with the 4th South Asian Regional Conference Dermatology Conference, attended by more than 5000 delegates, in February 2005. He has been actively involved in various IADVL activities as a central council member for more than 6 years. Dr. Garg has more than 32 years of UG and PG teaching experience, more than 180 indexed publications, and 12 books to his credit. He has been an examiner to various universities and served as an expert and advisor to various recruitment bodies. He retired from MAMC in May 2018. He is currently Professor and Head in the Department of Dermatology, Santosh Medical College, Ghaziabad, Uttar Pradesh, India.

Sneha Ghunawat, MD, completed her graduation and postgraduation at Maulana Azad Medical College, New Delhi. She was awarded the Prof. V.N. Sehgal Award (Gold Medal) during her postgraduation due to her outstanding performance. She has also been awarded a fellowship in lasers and aesthetics by the International Society of Dermatology under the guidance of Dr. Evangeline Handog in the Philippines. To pursue her interest in clinical dermatology, she underwent training in clinical dermatology at the National University of Health, Singapore. Dr. Ghunawat's areas of interest include clinical dermatology, lasers, and aesthetics. Her zeal for learning and knowledge has taken her to many national and international conferences as a speaker and has earned her many scholarships. She has many national and international publications in eminent journals and has authored many chapters in various textbooks. She has also pursued a course in trichology under IADVL.

Khushbu Mahajan, MD, is currently serving as Consultant Dermatologist at Kubba Skin Clinic and Mahajan Skin Centre, Delhi. She received her MBBS and MD in dermatology, venereology, and leprology from Maulana Azad Medical College (MAMC) and Lok Nayak Hospital, Delhi. She previously served as Senior Resident and Senior Research Associate at MAMC and Lok Nayak Hospital, and as Associate Professor at NDMC Medical College and Hindu Rao Hospital, Delhi. Dr. Mahajan is a recipient of the P.M. Varghese Award and Prof V.N. Sehgal Gold Medal (for Excellence in Dermatology) from MAMC. She has more than 25 publications and three books to her credit, has contributed chapters in numerous books, is a reviewer for the *International Journal of Dermatology* and *Indian Journal of Dermatology, Venereology and Leprology*, and has presented papers at numerous national and international conferences. Dr. Mahajan has also received travel awards and grants from a number of institutions, including IADVL, Women's Dermatologic Society, Indian Council of Medical Research, and Centre for Scientific and Industrial Research for presenting her research work at various international forums including the World Congress of Dermatology and American Academy of Dermatology. She has been invited as a speaker to numerous state- and national-level conference, and has been a part of organizing scientific committees for various conferences including Pigmentarycon 2016 and ACSICON 2019, and has conducted workshops on acne scar surgery, vitiligo surgery, and lasers.

CONTRIBUTORS

Pooja Agarwal
Department of Skin and Venereal Disease
Smt SCL General Hospital
Ahmedabad, India

Shilpi Agarwal
Consultant Dermatologist
Mumbai, India

Tasleem Arif
Ellahi Medicare Clinic
Kashmir, India

Karalikkattil T. Ashique
Amanza Skin Clinic (Amanza Health Care)
Perinthalmanna, Kerala, India

Safia Bashir
Department of Dermatology, Sexually Transmitted Diseases and
    Leprosy
Government Medical College Srinagar
Kashmir, J & K, India

Neetu Bhari
All India Institute of Medical Sciences
New Delhi, India

Ramesha Bhat M.
Father Muller Medical College
Kankanady, Mangalore, India

S.N. Bhattacharya
Department of Dermatology
University College of Medical Sciences and GTB Hospital
Dilshad Garden, New Delhi, India

Raffaele Dante Caposiena Caro
Università degli studi di Tor Vergata
Rome, Italy

Kavish Chauhan
DermaClinix
Delhi, India

Manju Daroach
Department of Dermatology, Venereology, and Leprology
PGIMER
Chandigarh, India

Surabhi Dayal
Department of Dermatology, Venereology and Leprology
Pandit B.D. Sharma University of Health Sciences
Rohtak, Haryana, India

Prachi Desai
Department of Dermatology
University Hospital of North Durham
County Durham and Darlington NHS Foundation Trust
Durham, United Kingdom

Sandipan Dhar
Department of Pediatric Dermatology
Institute of Child Health
Kolkata, West Bengal, India

Rachita Dhurat
LTMMC & LTMG Hospital
Mumbai, India

Biagio Didona
Istituto Dermopatico dell'Immacolata–IRCCS
Rome, Italy

Dario Didona
Istituto Dermopatico dell'Immacolata–IRCCS
Rome, Italy

Neha Dubey
Meraki Skin Clinic
Gurugram, India

İjlal Erturan
Faculty of Medicine
Department of Dermatology
Süleyman Demirel University
Isparta, Turkey

Emily Yiping Gan
KK Women's and Children's Hospital
Singapore

Shilpa Garg
Sir Ganga Ram Hospital
New Delhi, India

Sneha Ghunawat
Columbia Asia Hospital
and
Meraki Skin Clinic
Gurugram, India

Chander Grover
Department of Dermatology and Sexually Transmitted Diseases
University College of Medical Sciences and GTB Hospital
New Delhi, India

Sanjeev Gupta
MM Institute of Medical Sciences and Research
Mullana, Ambala, India

Somesh Gupta
Department of Dermatology and Venereology
All India Institute of Medical Science
New Delhi, India

Sunil K. Gupta
Department of Dermatology
Dayanand Medical College and Hospital
Ludhiana, India

Sanjeev Handa
Department of Dermatology, Venereology and Leprology
PGIMER
Chandigarh, India

Iffat Hassan
Department of Dermatology, Sexually Transmitted Diseases and
    Leprosy
Government Medical College Srinagar
Kashmir, J & K, India

Huma Jaffar
Department of Dermatology
University Medicine Cluster
National University Hospital
Kent Ridge, Singapore

Rubina Jassi
Lady Hardinge Medical College
New Delhi, India

Jyothi Jayaraman
Father Muller Medical College
Kankanady, Mangalore, India

Dilip Kachhawa
SN Medical College
Jodhpur, India

Feroze Kaliyadan
College of Medicine
King Faisal University
Hofuf, Saudi Arabia

Hemant Kumar Kar
Dr. Ram Manohar Lohia Hospital
New Delhi, India

Gayatri Karad
Skin Diseases Centre
Nashik, Maharashtra, India

Vandana Kataria
Department of Dermatology and Sexually Transmitted Diseases
Maulana Azad Medical College
and
Lok Nayak Hospital
New Delhi, India

Ishmeet Kaur
Department of Dermatology
NDMC Medical College and Hindu Rao Hospital
Delhi, India

Sandeep Kaur
Consultant Dermatologist
Ludhiana, India

Selma Korkmaz
Faculty of Medicine
Department of Dermatology
Süleyman Demirel University
Isparta, Turkey

Ambika Kumar
People Tree Hospital
Dasarahalli, Bengaluru, India

Neha Kumar
Grade III Dermatology
CGHS Safdarjung Hospital
New Delhi, India

Rajesh Kumar
Grant Medical College
Bombay Hospital
and
Breach Candy Hospital
Mumbai, India

Ravinder Kumar
Department of Zoology
Punjab University
Chandigarh, India

Rashmi Kumari
Department of Dermatology and Sexually Transmitted Diseases
Jawaharlal Institute of Postgraduate Medical Education and Research
Puducherry, India

Koushik Lahiri
WIZDERM
Apollo Gleneagles Hospitals
Kolkata, India

Bharat Bhushan Mahajan
Department of Dermatology
Government Medical College
Amritsar, India

Khushbu Mahajan
Kubba Skin Clinic
and
Mahajan Skin Centre
Delhi, India

Imran Majid
Cutis Institute of Dermatology
Srinagar, Kashmir, India

Vibhu Mehndiratta
Lady Hardinge Medical College
New Delhi, India

Madhulika Mhatre
Wockhardt Hospital
Mumbai, India

George Millington
Department of Dermatology
Norfolk and Norwich University Hospital
Norwich, England

Rachita Misri
Department of Dermatology
NDMC Medical College and Hindu Rao Hospital
Delhi, India

Debdeep Mitra
Base Hospital Delhi Cantt
New Delhi, India

Malathi Munisamy
Department of Dermatology and Sexually Transmitted Diseases
Jawaharlal Institute of Postgraduate Medical Education and
    Research
Puducherry, India

Venkataram Mysore
Venkat Center for Skin and Plastic Surgery
Bengaluru, India

Richa Nagpal
Department of Dermatology
Government Medical College
Amritsar, India

Anusha H. Pai
Derma-Care
Mangalore, India

Ganesh S. Pai
Derma-Care
Mangalore, India

Deepika Pandhi
Department of Dermatology and Sexually
    Transmitted Diseases
University College of Medical Sciences and GTB Hospital
University of Delhi
Delhi, India

Giovanni Paolino
Sapienza-Università di Roma
Rome, Italy

Davinder Parsad
Department of Dermatology
Post Graduate Institute of Medical
    Education and Research
Chandigarh, India

Naveed Pervaiz
Department of Zoology
Panjab University
Chandigarh, India

Mualla Polat
Faculty of Medicine
Department of Dermatology
Abant Izzet Baysal University
Bolu, Turkey

Swetalina Pradhan
Department of Dermatology and Venereology
All India Institute of Medical Sciences
Patna, India

Reddy R. Raghunatha
Roots Institute of Dermatological Sciences
Banaswadi, Bengaluru, India

Seema Rani
Department of Zoology
Hindu Girls' College
Sonepat, Haryana, India

Vineet Relhan
Department of Dermatology and Venereology
Maulana Azad Medical College
and
Lok Nayak Hospital
New Delhi, India

Revanta Saha
Venkat Center for Skin and Plastic Surgery
Bengaluru, India

Priyadarshini Sahu
Department of Dermatology, Venereology and Leprology
Pandit B.D. Sharma University of Health Sciences
Rohtak, Haryana, India

Thurakkal Salim
Cutis Institute of Dermatology
Calicut, Kerala, India

Rashmi Sarkar
Department of Dermatology
Lady Hardinge Medical College
New Delhi, India

A.S. Savitha
Sapthagiri Institute of Medical Sciences
Bengaluru, India

Bela J. Shah
Department of Dermatology, Venereology and Leprology
B.J. Medical College
Civil Hospital
Ahmedabad, India

B.M. Shashikumar
Mandya Institute of Medical Sciences
Mandya, Bengaluru, India

Sudhanshu Sharma
Department of Dermatology
SHKM, Government Medical College
Nuh, Mewat (Haryana), India

Manjunath Shenoy
Department of Dermatology
Yenepoya Medical College
Mangalore, India

Shweta Sethi
Department of Dermatology
Government Medical College
Amritsar, India

Archana Singal
Department of Dermatology and Sexually Transmitted Diseases
University College of Medical Sciences and GTB Hospital
New Delhi, India

Sanjay Singh
All India Institute of Medical Sciences
New Delhi, India

Aditi Manu Sobti
Department of Dermatology
University Medicine Cluster
National University Hospital
Kent Ridge, Singapore

Sahana M. Srinivas
Department of Pediatric Dermatology
Indira Gandhi Institute of Child Health
Bengaluru, Karnataka, India

Gurvinder P. Thami
Department of Dermatology and Venereology
Government Medical College and Hospital
Chandigarh, India

Devinder Mohan Thappa
Department of Dermatology and Sexually Transmitted Diseases
Jawaharlal Institute of Postgraduate Medical Education and
    Research
Puducherry, India

Shashank Tyagi
Department of Dermatology
Government Medical College
Amritsar, India

Christopher Tzermias
Intensive Quality Dermatology Care
Athens, Greece

Özge Uzun
Faculty of Medicine
Department of Pharmacology
Abant Izzet Baysal University
Bolu, Turkey

Gunjan Verma
Manipal Hospitals
Delhi, India

Anuja Yadav
Lady Hardinge Medical College
New Delhi, India

Sam Shiyao Yang
Yang and Yap Clinic and Surgery (Pte Ltd)
Singapore

Mehmet Yildirim
Faculty of Medicine
Department of Dermatology
Süleyman Demirel University
Isparta, Turkey

Vijay Zawar
Skin Diseases Centre
Nashik, Maharashtra, India

THE BASICS OF VITILIGO

Chapter 1

HISTORY AND CULTURAL ASPECTS OF VITILIGO

George Millington

CONTENTS

INTRODUCTION

In this chapter, the history of vitiligo until the end of the twentieth century is outlined, covering medical, scientific, and social aspects. Since records began, humans have considered why there might be variations in skin color and what might constitute the nature of those differences, but we still have only limited scientific insight into what causes natural variations in constitutional pigmentation and how that might be relevant to disorders such as vitiligo [1].

HISTORY OF VITILIGO

Vitiligo or some form of depigmentation has been mentioned in the texts of every major religion, with its first description dating back more than 4000 years to the earliest Indian and Egyptian texts [2]. An early record is in the Vedic books from India, where the sun god Bhagavantam developed pale spots after being gazed upon by his illegitimate son [2]. In one of the first textbooks of Ayurvedic medicine from India, the Charaka Samhita (100 AD), svitra ("whiteness") is recorded as a diagnosis [2]. Other early descriptions also are included in the Koran and Buddhist scripts [2]. Vitiligo, the "small blemish" (from the Latin *vitulum*) [2] was first described accurately more than 1500 years BC [1]. Another good description also exists in a collection of Japanese Shinto prayers, Amarakosa, dating from 1200 BC [2].

Leprosy is recorded as a pale swelling, distinct from vitiligo, in the Ebers Papyrus, an Egyptian collection of writings from 1500 to 3000 BC [2]. However, there is no such demarcation between the two diseases in either the Bible or in the first European description of the disease by Hippocrates [2]. This non-distinction continues in some communities in the world today, where vitiligo sufferers are sometimes avoided in the same age-old way as people with leprosy [2]. To his credit, Hippocrates was the first to report that vitiligo was easier to treat at the start of the illness, rather than when it had established itself as a chronic condition [2]. This is still a recognized feature of the condition [2]. Both ancient Egyptian and Indian writings depict psoralen-containing plants such as Ammi majus [2] and *Psoralea corylifolia* [2] being applied to pale macules and then exposed to sunlight, which is a forerunner of contemporary psoralen with ultraviolet A radiation (PUVA) [2]. There is some evidence of early attempts at treatment using traditional Chinese medicine [3] and other herbal remedies described by the eleventh century Persian physician Avicenna [4].

CULTURAL ASPECTS OF VITILIGO

The Military Order of St. Lazarus of Jerusalem originated in a leper hospital founded in the twelfth century by the Crusaders of the Latin Kingdom. It may be that the institution was an extension of the work of the much-better-known Order of St. John [5]. Those cared for by the Order of St. John were transient cases, but the lepers of St. Lazarus were initially isolated in permanent seclusion. It is highly likely that the so-called "lepers" suffered from other common hypopigmentary diseases too, including vitiligo [2,5]. In return they were regarded as brothers or sisters of the hospital that sheltered them, and they obeyed the common rule that united them with their religious guardians. Like many other religious orders in the Levant, the twin problems of endemic "leprosy" and other diseases and a shortage of warriors forced the Order to develop their own fighting force, probably in the thirteenth century. Uniquely, the disabled were armed and expected to fight [5]. How effective these "leper" knights were as troops is open to debate. All records available suggest that they were not very successful. For example, the Patriarch of Jerusalem stated that all the Knights of St. Lazarus were killed during the defeat at La Forbie in 1244 [5].

Not all societies appear to have discriminated against the hypopigmented. In the seventeenth century Yi dynasty in Korea, the medical textbook the *Dongui Bogam* describes the skin disorders of vitiligo, tinea versicolor, nevus depigmentosus, nevus anemicus, and albinism as a single hypopigmentary condition. Treatment is correspondingly also described as if for a single disease entity [2]. Socially too, the seventeenth century Koreans were tolerant of depigmentation cosmetically. A portrait of Chang Myeong Song, a high-ranking government official in the Yi dynasty, shows "vitiliginous" depigmentation of the face and neck. This suggests there was no confusion of this illness with leprosy in seventeenth century Korea; otherwise perhaps this portrait of a ruler would have been altered to disguise the affliction [2].

It is probable that ancient descriptions represent other ailments too, as prior to Willan's wide-ranging classification of skin diseases in the early nineteenth century there would have been no recognized system, in European medicine at least, of cataloging cutaneous disorders [2].

Prior to Willan, the French physician Claude-Nicolas Le Cat published a comprehensive volume on ethnic differences in skin pigmentation. In this book, he precisely detailed several cases of vitiligo that started in small areas and then progressed symmetrically over the hands and face [2]. He also described depigmentation following burns from boiling water in these individuals, thus illustrating the phenomenon of Köebnerization [2]. However, it is only in the past century that the term vitiligo vulgaris has been used to describe the disease process of acquired melanocyte destruction [2].

The end of the nineteenth century was a time of much advancement in the understanding of vitiligo. Moritz Kaposi in Vienna was one of the first to describe the histopathology, observing only a lack of pigment granules in the deep rete cells [2]. At around the same time, in Bergen, Gerhard Hansen observed the presence of small rods within "lepra cells" and thus established a clear pathogenesis for leprosy [2]. Pierre-Louis Alphée Cazenave, working in France, made the link between vitiligo and alopecia areata [2]. Both Neumann in Vienna [2] and Brocq [2] in Paris observed that episodes of emotional stress can lead to flare-ups of vitiligo. They also both noticed that none of the then-available treatments made much impact on the disease [2].

Research into the cause of vitiligo diverged into several paths over the course of the twentieth century. In the early twentieth century, the cause of vitiligo was first attributed to damage to peripheral nerves [2]. Lerner, in 1959, reported a patient with transverse myelitis whose vitiligo was limited to skin above the cord lesion [6]. He proposed that normal pigmentation resulted from a balance of the effects of melanocyte-stimulating hormone (MSH) secreted from the pituitary on darkening the skin and the release of a substance from the peripheral nerves which lightened them. This balance was therefore disrupted in vitiligo [6,7].

In 1940 it was observed that vitiligo clusters in families, which would favor a genetic component to the illness [2]. Subsequent research in the 1970s suggested that this inheritance was non-Mendelian [2].

In the late nineteenth century, Hopkins identified a yellow and a white pigment from the English Brimstone and Cabbage White butterflies, respectively [8]. By the 1920s these pigments were classified as pteridines and named according to their colors, xanthopterin and leucopterin [9]. In humans, L-tyrosine is the precursor for melanin. The pteridine 6R-L-erythro-5,6,7,8 tetrahydrobiopterin (6BH$_4$) is an essential electron donor in the hydroxylation of the aromatic amino acids, namely L-phenylalanine, L-tyrosine, and L-tryptophan [10]. Vitiligo has been associated with an overproduction of 6BH$_4$, which may explain the characteristic yellow/green or bluish fluorescence of the hypopigmented macules on Woods light examination, as distinct from other hypomelanoses [11]. Whether these observations are causal or a byproduct of vitiligo is unclear.

Destruction of melanocytes in vitiligo may, in fact, relate to accumulation of toxic metabolic byproducts. This could include free-radical formation from exogenous phenolic compounds [12]. Such a reaction could be more likely in the genetically susceptible [13]. Lerner proposed that this genetic tendency was based around deficiencies in protective mechanisms that eliminate toxic precursors or byproducts from the melanocyte, such as DOPA, dopachrome, and 5,6-dihydroxyindole [14]. It was then discovered that the outer membrane of the melanosome impeded the diffusion of such toxic products of melanin biosynthesis into the cytoplasm and nucleus. Either inherited or genetic defects in this membrane could theoretically result in death of melanocytes [15].

Perhaps the most convincing argument in the pathogenesis of vitiligo is the autoimmune hypothesis, which is built upon several observations. First, vitiligo is associated with disorders that are considered to have an autoimmune origin, including autoimmune thyroid disease [2], insulin-dependent diabetes mellitus [2], alopecia areata [2], pernicious anemia [2], Addison disease [2], and autoimmune polyendocrine syndromes [2]. Second, vitiligo is associated with typical major histocompatibility antigens seen in autoimmunity [16,17]. Third, several moderately effective therapies for vitiligo

rely on an immunosuppressive effect, including PUVA [18], topical corticosteroids [19], and topical cytotoxic drugs such as fluorouracil [20]. Finally, antibodies to melanocyte antigens are present in the circulation of many patients with the disease [21].

In the modern era, a number of systemic and topical treatments have been tried in vitiligo [22]. Systemic therapies tried with variable success include phenylalanine, antimalarials, khellin, levamisole, folic acid, and clofazimine [22]. Topical steroids and topical calcineurin inhibitors are reasonably effective in a proportion of cases [22]. The evidence for topical vitamin D derivatives, topical 5-fluorouracil, and pseudocatalase is less clear. In those individuals who have lost most of their natural color, application of monobenzone to the remaining pigmented areas may be a therapeutic option [22].

Vitiligo is a highly stressful condition [23] and frequently treatments are ineffective [2,22]. In this situation, it is very important to remember the role of cosmetic camouflage [22].

CONCLUSION

Despite scientific advances in the understanding of the pathogenesis of vitiligo, most treatments remain inadequate in terms of disease eradication. Also, the proof that, unlike leprosy, it is not an infectious disease, has not altered the stigma associated with vitiligo in some societies. We have much to learn from both the sociological and medical history of vitiligo if we are to make progress in improving both the research and management of this ancient disease in the modern world.

REFERENCES

1. Millington GWM, and Levell NJ. From genesis to gene sequencing: Historical progress in the understanding of skin color. *Int J Dermatol* 2007;46:103–5.

2. Millington GWM, and Levell NJ. Vitiligo: The historical curse of depigmentation. *Int J Dermatol* 2007;46:990–5.

3. Tan EK, Millington GWM, and Levell NJ. Acupuncture in dermatology: An historical perspective. *Int J Dermatol* 2009;48:648–52.

4. Pourmand M, Asgharzadeh M, Rashedi J, and Mahdavi Poor B. Vitiligo treatment in ancient Iranian Medicine. *Iran J Public Health* 2016;45:1100–1.

5. Marcombe D. *Leper Knights: The Order of St Lazarus of Jerusalem in England, c.1150–1544.* Boydell & Brewer, 2004.

6. Lerner AB. Vitiligo. *J Invest Derm* 1959;32:285.

7. Millington GWM. Proopiomelanocortin (POMC): The cutaneous roles of its melanocortin products and receptors. *Clin Exp Dermatol* 2006;31:407–12.

8. Hopkins FG. Note on a yellow pigment in butterflies. *Nature* 1889;40:335.

9. Wieland H, and Schöpf C. Über den gelben Flügelforbstorff des Citronen-falters (Gonepteryx rhemni). *Berichte de Deutschen Chemischen Gesellschaft* 1925;58:2178.

10. Ziegler I. Production of pteridines during hematopoiesis and T-lymphocyte proliferation: Potential participation in the control of cytokine signal transmission. *Med Res Rev* 1990;10:95–114.

11. Schallreuter KU, Wood JM, Pittelkow MR, Gutlich M, Lemke KR, Rodl W, Swanson NN, Hitzemann K, and Ziegler I. Regulation of melanin biosynthesis in the human epidermis by tetrahydrobiopterin. *Science* 1994;263:1444–6.

12. Bleehen SS, Pathak MA, Hori Y, and Fitzpatrick TB. Depigmentation of skin with 4-isopropylcatechol, mercaptoamines, and other compounds. *J Invest Dermatol* 1968;50:103–17.

13. Riley PA. Mechanism of pigment-cell toxicity produced by hydroxyanisole. *J Pathol* 1970;101:163–9.

14. Lerner AB. On the etiology of vitiligo and gray hair. *Am J Med* 1971;51:141–7.

15. Wick MM. l-Dopa methyl ester as a new antitumour agent. *Nature* 1977;269:512–3.

16. Foley LM, Lowe NJ, Misheloff E, and Tiwari JL. Association of HLA-DR4 with vitiligo. *J Am Acad Dermatol* 1983;8:39–40.

17. Dunston GM, and Halder RM. Vitiligo is associated with HLA-DR4 in black patients. A preliminary report. *Arch Dermatol* 1990;126:56–60.

18. Parrish JA, Fitzpatrick TB, Shea C, and Pathak MA. Photochemotherapy of vitiligo. Use of orally administered psoralens and a high-intensity long-wave ultraviolet light system. *Arch Dermatol* 1976;112:1531–4.

19. Kumari J. Vitiligo treated with topical clobetasol propionate. *Arch Dermatol* 1984;120:631–5.

20. Tsuji T, and Hamada T. Topically administered fluorouracil in vitiligo. *Arch Dermatol* 1983;119:722–7.

21. Naughton GK, Eisinger M, and Bystryn JC. Antibodies to normal human melanocytes in vitiligo. *J Exp Med* 1983;158:246–51.

22. Nordlund JJ. The medical treatment of vitiligo: An historical review. *Dermatol Clin* 2017;35:107–16.

23. Manolache L, Petrescu-Seceleanu D, and Benea V. Correlation of stressful events with onset of vitiligo in children. *J Eur Acad Dermatol Venereol* 2009;23:187–8.

Chapter 2

DEFINITION, EPIDEMIOLOGY, AND PREVALENCE

Ishmeet Kaur and Archana Singal

CONTENTS

DEFINITION

Vitiligo is an acquired disorder of pigmentation that manifests as circumscribed depigmented macules and patches, often associated with leukotrichia. It is usually progressive in nature, characterized by selective loss of melanocytes that can affect skin, mucous membranes, inner ear, and leptomeninges [1].

The Vitiligo European Task Force (VETF) defines vitiligo vulgaris/nonsegmental vitiligo as an acquired chronic pigmentation disorder characterized by white patches, often symmetrical, which usually increase in size with time, corresponding to a substantial loss of functioning epidermal and sometimes hair follicle melanocytes [2]. A similar definition had been proposed for segmental vitiligo, but with a unilateral distribution which may also follow a total or partial dermatomal pattern [2].

HISTORICAL ASPECTS

There are different opinions on the origin of the term vitiligo. The word *vitiligo* was first used by Celsus in his Latin medical literature called *De Medicina*. Some believe it to be derived from the Latin word *vituli*, which represents the appearance of the white glistening of the flesh of calves, while some suggest it is derived from the word *vitium*, which means blemish [3].

There are many references to vitiligo in ancient Indian literature as well. Vitiligo has also been identified in the ancient Vedic scripture of India called "Atharva Veda," where it was mentioned as the word *kilas* derived from the Sanskrit word *kil*, which means white spot. Vitiligo was also mentioned in an Indian medical compilation called Charaka Samhita as the term *svitra*, meaning spreading whiteness [3].

EPIDEMIOLOGY

AGE AND SEX

Vitiligo can present at any age but almost half of the cases present before the age of 20 years and about 70%–80% present before 30 years of age [4]. The average age of presentation is 22–24 years [5,6]. The prevalence has been found to increase with age. It has been seen that the bilateral form of vitiligo usually affects the older age group as compared to unilateral and segmental forms [7]. Although in most of the studies it affects men and women equally, some studies show that it may have a female preponderance, which is probably because of social stigma and cosmetic concerns making them seek more treatment [7,8]. The disease has been found to start earlier in the Indian population, with a mean age of presentation of 25 years in males and 20 years in females [5,9,10].

PREVALENCE

Vitiligo is the most common pigmentary disorder and affects approximately 0.5%–1% of the world's population. The highest incidence has been reported in India, followed by Mexico and Japan [11].

INDIA

India has a wide range of prevalence, varying from 0.46% to as high as 8.8%, with an average prevalence of 0.25%–2.5%. The highest prevalence has been seen in Gujarat and Rajasthan. In a large study conducted in Surat, the prevalence of vitiligo varied from 0.47% in the rural population to 1.78% in the urban population [8]. In a study conducted in Uttarakhand, the prevalence was found to be 2.64% [12], while in a study conducted in Calcutta, it was 0.46% [5]. In a retrospective analysis by Handa and Kaur, the prevalence found was 2.5%, with almost equal frequency of males and females [13]. This regional variation is probably due to the different ethnic backgrounds and sociocultural implications of the disease in different geographical areas [13].

FAMILY HISTORY

A positive family history is seen, ranging from 7%–36% of cases. Around 20% of the cases have at least one affected first-degree relative, which supports the involvement of genetic factors in the pathogenesis. The risk of development of vitiligo increases by 7- to 10-fold in first-degree family members like parents, siblings, and children [10]. In a study conducted by Das et al., the relative risk of vitiligo in parents, siblings, and children varied between 7.93–10.41, 10.77–11.04, and 19.21–20.07, respectively [5]. In a study conducted in Manipal, 20% of patients with vitiligo had positive family history. Out of these, 8.75% had first-degree relatives with vitiligo, 7.5% had second-degree relatives, and 3.5% had third-degree relatives [6]. The mode of inheritance is still unclear and is proposed to be polygenic with variable penetrance. Various studies have also found a positive association of vitiligo with HLA-DR4. Other HLA associations that have been found to be associated include HLA-DR1, DR7, A2, B13, B21, and Cw6 [10].

HOST FACTORS

Vitiligo occurs worldwide and does not show any significant racial or regional variation. However, a higher incidence is reported in populations with a darker skin type, which may be due to a greater color contrast and associated social stigma, due to which such patients tend to present early in the course of the disease. Further, it has been found to be associated with other autoimmune diseases and endocrinal disorders like thyroiditis and diabetes [14], as discussed in detail in later chapters. A positive correlation has also been found between vitiligo and population with the M blood group [15] and G6PD enzyme deficiency [16].

REFERENCES

1. Prasad D, Kumaran SM, and Sachidanand S. *IADVL Textbook of Dermatology. Depigmentary and Hypopigmentary Disorders*, 4th ed. Mumbai, India: Bhalani Publishers; 2016, pp. 1308–10.

2. Taïeb A, and Picardo M. VETF Members. The definition and assessment of vitiligo: A consensus report of the Vitiligo European Task Force. *Pigment Cell Res* 2007;20(1):27–35.

3. Kopera D. Historical aspects and definition of vitiligo. *Clin Dermatol* 1997;15(6):841–3.

4. Alzolibani AA, Al Robaee A, and Zedan K. Genetic epidemiology and heritability of vitiligo. Available from: https://cdn.intechopen.com/pdfs-wm/24967.pdf. (Accessed on 18th June 2017).

5. Das SK, Majumder PP, Chakrabotry R, Majumdar TK, and Haldar B. Studies on vitiligo. I. Epidemiological profile in Calcutta, India. *Genet Epidemiol* 1985;2:71–8.

6. Alkhateeb A, Fain PR, Thody A, Bennett DC, and Spritz RA. Epidemiology of vitiligo and associated autoimmune diseases in Caucasian probands and their families. *Pigment Cell Res* 2003;16(3):208–14.

7. Barona MI, Arrunátegui A, Falabella R, and Alzate A. An epidemiologic case-control study in a population with vitiligo. *J Am Acad Dermatol* 1995;33:621–5.

8. Shah H, Mehta A, and Astik B. Clinical and sociodemographic study of vitiligo. *Indian J Dermatol Venereol Leprol* 2008;74:701.

9. Singh S, and Pandey SS. Epidemiological profile of vitiligo in Northern India. *J Appl Pharmaceut Sci*. 2011;1:211–4.

10. Majumder PP. Genetics and Prevalence of Vitiligo Vulgaris. In: Hann SK, Nordlund JJ, and Lerner AB, eds. *Vitiligo: A Monograph on the Basic and Clinical Science*. Oxford, UK: Blackwell Science Ltd.; 2000, pp. 18–20.

11. Sehgal VN, and Srivastava G. Vitiligo: Compendium of clinico-epidemiological features. *Indian J Dermatol Venereol Leprol* 2007;73(3):149–56.

12. Agarwal S, Ojha A, and Gupta S. Profile of vitiligo in Kumaun region of Uttarakhand, India. *Indian J Dermatol Venereol Leprol* 2014;59:209.

13. Handa S, and Kaur I. Vitiligo: Clinical findings in 1436 patients. *J Dermatol* 1999;26:653–7.

14. Habib A, and Raza N. Clinical pattern of vitiligo. *J Coll Physicians Surg Pak* 2012;22:61–2.

15. Wasfi AI, Saha N, El Munshid HA, El Sheikh FS, and Ahmed MA. Genetic association in vitiligo: ABO, MNSs, Rhesus, KeII and Duffy blood groups. *Clin Genet* 1980;17(6):415–7.

16. Saha N, Ahmed MA, Wasfi AI, and El Munshid HA. Distribution of serum proteins, red cell enzymes and haemoglobins in vitiligo. *Hum Hered* 1982;32(1):46–8.

Chapter 3

VITILIGO
An Indian Scenario

Sunil K. Gupta and Sandeep Kaur

CONTENTS

INTRODUCTION

Vitiligo is a common melanocytopenic depigmentation disorder seen in India and worldwide in which destruction of melanocytes in the skin, mucous membranes, eyes, inner ear, leptomeninges, and hair bulbs occurs. It is characterized by depigmented milky white macules of variable sizes and shapes. Although it does not cause restriction of capacity to work or life expectancy, cosmetic disfigurement resulting from vitiligo can lead to psychosocial trauma for the patient and can have a significant impact on quality of life.

EPIDEMIOLOGY AND PREVALENCE

The worldwide incidence is 1% [1]. Gujarat and Rajasthan states have the highest prevalence, around 8.8% [2]. The prevalence in rest of India is 0.46%–8.8% [3]. Interestingly, the incidence of vitiligo appears to be higher in the Somavamsha Sahasrarjun Kshatriya community [4]. This wide variation in vitiligo prevalence can be attributed to the varying ethnic backgrounds of the study populations and differences in environmental conditions, as well as higher reporting of vitiligo in populations where an apparent color contrast and stigma attached to the condition may force patients to seek early consultation. Vitiligo patients account for 2.5% of dermatology outpatients as reported by Handa and Kaur [3], and 2.64% as reported by Agarwal et al. [5].

This disease has no predilection for either sex, as reported by Kar and others [6–8], although higher reporting among females may be due to the greater social consequences faced by women affected by this condition. It has been reported to occur from birth through the eighth decade of life [3,4,6]. Kar reported an incidence of 43.2% of cases in 0–20 years of age as compared to a low incidence of only 9.9% in individuals over 40 years of age. This may either be due to predisposition of younger ages to development of vitiligo or earlier reporting due to social stigma associated with the disease [6]. Moreover, young children are more vulnerable to recurrent infections, bowel upsets, and malnutrition, and thus are exposed to toxic, strong medication for these conditions [9]. The same age group is fond of fast food containing high levels of preservatives, additives, colorants, and antioxidants [9].

A positive family history has been reported in 27.3% of patients by Tawade et al. [4], 11.5% by Handa and Kaur [3], 10% by Sarin and Kumar [7], 6.6% by Kar [6], and 6.25% of cases by Behl et al. [8]. Out of 998 cases of vitiligo reported by Tawade et al. [4], 272 (27.3%) had one or more relative with vitiligo. Among these 207 (76.1%) cases had only one relative affected, whereas 65 (28%) cases had more than one relative with vitiligo. Handa and Kaur [3] found that first-degree relatives (parent/brother/sister/son/daughter) were affected in 85 (5.9%), and second-degree relatives (grandparent/maternal and/or paternal uncle or aunt) in 80 (5.6%) patients. Ten patients (0.7%) had more than one family member with the disease.

A positive family history favors the role of genetic factors in the pathogenesis of vitiligo. Vitiligo is thought to follow polygenic inheritance [10]. One hypothesis postulates that recessive alleles at multiple unlinked autosomal loci interact epistatically in the pathogenesis of vitiligo [11]. The mode of transmission is probably autosomal dominant with variable penetrance [12]. In the South Indian population, it was also found that the polymorphism of the angiotensin-converting enzyme (ACE) gene is capable of modulating cutaneous neurogenic inflammation and autoimmunity with the development of vitiligo [13]. Also, a positive family history is considered to be a poor prognostic factor in vitiligo.

Various factors such as trauma, burns, herpes zoster, etc. may initiate the onset of vitiligo in certain genetically predisposed individuals. Vitiligo shows a predilection for friction-prone sites. The legs seem to be the most frequently affected in the majority (50%) of cases. Hands, face, and bony prominences were the next most common sites, followed by feet, trunk, and neck [6].

CLINICAL FEATURES

With regard to site of onset, the face has been described as the most common site of onset in 22.9%, independent of the clinical type of vitiligo [3]. In Western literature, the extremities are the most commonly involved sites of onset. In a study by Agarwal et al. [5], the most common site of onset was the lower limbs, followed by the head and neck, upper limbs, trunk, genitalia, and mucosae.

The frequency of distribution of various subtypes of vitiligo varies in different studies. Among the various types, the circumscript variety was found to be the most common as reported by Kar [6]. Other

Table 3.1   An overview of the latest studies related to vitiligo published in Indian literature

Study	N	Sex	Onset <20 yrs	Family history	Type of vitiligo	Leukotrichia	Koebner phenomenon	Associations
Agarwal et al. [5] (2014)	762	F = M	57.25%	19%	Acrofacial (44.5%), *Vitiligo vulgaris* (30.5%), focal (12.6%), segmental (9.4%), mucosal (1.4%), mixed (0.4%), universal vitiligo (0.4%)	33.5%	26.3%	Thyroid disease (8.9%), diabetes (5.9%), atopic dermatitis (4.9%), alopecia areata (2.6%), psoriasis (1.9%, Down syndrome (0.4%)
Krupa Shankar et al. [14] (2012)	80	F = M	–	20%	Generalized (31.3%), segmental (30%), focal (18.8%), acrofacial (8.8%), mucosal (11.3%)	–	–	Hypothyroidism (11.3%), hypoacusis (10%), retinal abnormalities (8.8%), vitamin B_{12} deficiency (30%), hypothyroidism (11.3%), high absolute eosinophil count (16.3%), diabetes mellitus (8.8%)
Singh et al. [15] (2011)	200	F > M	43.5%	22%	*V. vulgaris* (45.5%), acrofacial (21.5%), focal (18.5%), segmental (11%), mucosal (2%), universal (1.5%)	9.5%	–	Thyroid disease (12%), diabetes (3%), alopecia areata (2%), hypertension (2%), rheumatoid arthritis (1%), psoriasis (0.5%)
Shah et al. [16] (2008)	365	F > M	54.51%	13.7%	*V. vulgaris* (64.9%), focal (18.6%), acrofacial (0.8%), mucosal (14.8%), segmental (1.4%), universal (8.2%)	9%	6%	Alopecia areata (0.55%), chronic urticaria (0.27%), premature canities (0.55%), diabetes mellitus (0.55%), hypertension (1.37%), hypothyroidism (0.27%), epilepsy (1%), deafness (1.37%)
Gopal et al. [17] (2007)	150	M > F	–	36%	Generalized vitiligo (48%), acrofacial (22.7%), focal (16%), segmental (13.3%)	–	7.4%	Anemia (20%), diabetes mellitus (16%), hypothyroidism (12%), alopecia areata (7.4%), poliosis (18%), premature graying of hair (6.6%), hypoacusis (20%), ocular abnormalities (16%)
Dave et al. [18] (2002)	199	M > F	–	7.5%	*V. vulgaris* (48.2%), acrofacial (34.7%), mucosal (10%), segmental (7%)	43.2%	16.6%	–
Kar PK [6] (2001)	120	F = M	43.2%	6.6%	Circumscript (46.6%), inflammatory (13.3%), segmental (10%), symmetrical (6%), linear (5%), universalis (1.6%), others (16.6%)	–	–	Diabetes mellitus (2.6%), giardiasis (12%), ascariasis (10%)
Handa and Kaur [3] 1999	1436	M > F	48.9%	11.5%	*V. vulgaris* (69.8%), focal vitiligo (14.9%), segmental (5.0%)	11.5%	5%	Atopic/nummular eczema (1.4%), bronchial asthma (0.7%), diabetes mellitus (0.6%), thyroid disease (0.5%), and alopecia (0.4%).
Tawade et al. [4] 1997	998	F > M	63.7%	27.3%	*V. vulgaris* (64.73%), acrofacial (13.73%), focal (8.42%), universalis (5.81%), segmental (5.71%), mucosal (1.6%)	–	–	Diabetes mellitus (1.6%), ascariasis (1.6%), premature canities (1.5%), giardiasis (0.8%), hypertension (0.5%), amebiasis (0.3%), psoriasis (0.2%), rheumatoid arthritis (0.1%), thyroid disease (0.1%)
Behl et al. [9] (1994)	1000	F = M	45.5%	23.1%	–	–	–	–

researchers have reported vitiligo vulgaris to be the most common type of presentation [3,4]. This indicates that the Indian population tends to have more extensive disease.

Koebner phenomenon was observed in 5.0% of the study population reported by Handa and Kaur [3] and 26.3% of cases by Agarwal et al. [5]. Leukotrichia was described in 11.5% of cases by Handa and Kaur [3] and 33.5% by Agarwal et al. [5]. The finding of leukotrichia is important because such cases are more likely to show poor response to medical treatment. Thus it is considered as a poor prognostic factor. Handa and Kaur also observed halo nevi in 2.0% of patients with vitiligo [3]. Spontaneous repigmentation can be seen in 19.5% of patients, mostly as perifollicular or marginal pigmentation [3].

Progressive vitiligo is characterized by an increase in size or number of lesions. Dave et al. reported progression of vitiligo in 76.9% of the patients in their study [18]. The clinical indicators significantly associated with progression include a positive family history ($p = 0.027$), Koebner phenomenon ($p = 0.036$), mucosal involvement ($p = 0.032$), and nonsegmental vitiligo ($p = 0.033$) [18]. The factors that have not been significantly associated with disease progression are longer duration, older age at onset, trichrome sign, and leukotrichia [18]. The prediction of disease progression at the outset helps the dermatologist to establish realistic treatment outcomes and individualize therapeutic options.

ASSOCIATIONS

No significant association has been recorded between vitiligo and smoking, alcohol, or diet [14]. Vitiligo may be associated with other autoimmune disorders such as diabetes mellitus, thyroid disease, alopecia areata, and pernicious anemia [3–6]. Association with conditions like amebiasis, giardiasis, and worm infestation is not understood and may simply reflect the high incidence of these conditions in India [4].

Gopal et al. reported various ocular abnormalities in patients with vitiligo (16%) in the form of uveitis, iris pigmentary abnormalities including hypopigmented patches on the iris, heterochromic iris, and retinal pigmentary abnormalities which were statistically significant ($c^2 = 7.39$, $P < 0.001$) [17]. Twenty-one (19.8%) patients with generalized vitiligo and three (9.8%) patients with localized vitiligo had ocular abnormalities, this difference being statistically significant ($c^2 = 3.89$, $P < 0.05$) [17].

Table 3.1 summarizes the characteristics of vitiligo seen in the Indian population.

REFERENCES

1. Wolff K, Goldsmith LA, Katz SI, Gilchrest BA, Paller AS, and Leffell DJ. *Fitzpatrick's Dermatology in General Medicine*, 7th edn. Vol. I. USA: McGraw Hill; 2007, pp. 616–21.

2. Dutta AK, Dutta PK, and Dhar S. Pigmentaiy disorders In: Valia RG ed., *IADVL Text Book and Atlas of Dermatology*. 2nd Edn. Bombay, India: Bhalani Publishing House; 2001, 607.

3. Handa S, and Kaur I. Vitiligo: Clinical findings in 1436 patients. *J Dermatol* 1999;26:653–7.

4. Tawade YV, Parakh AP, Bharatia PR et al. Vitiligo: A study of 998 cases attending KEM Hospital in Pune. *Indian J Dermatol Venereol Leprol* 1997;63:95–8.

5. Agarwal S, Ojha A, and Gupta S. Profile of vitiligo in Kumaun region of Uttarakhand, India. *Indian J Dermatol* 2014;59:209.

6. Kar PK. Vitiligo: A study of 120 cases. *Indian J Dermatol Venereol Leprol* 2001;67:302–4.

7. Sarin RC, and Kumar AS. A clinical study of vitiligo. *Indian J Dermatol Venereol Leprol* 1977;83:190–4.

8. Behl PN, Agarwal RS, and Singh G. Aetiological studies in vitiligo and therapeutic response to standard treatment. *Indian J Dermatol* 1961;6:101.

9. Behl PN, Kotia A, and Sawal P. Vitiligo: Age group-related trigger factors and morphological variants. *Indian J Dermatol Venereol Leprol* 1994;60:275–9.

10. Das SK, Majumder PP, Majumdar TK, and Haldar B. Studies on vitiligo. II. Familial aggregation and genetics. *Genet Epidemiol* 1985;2:255–62.

11. Majumder PP, Das SK, and Li CC. Genetic model for vitiligo. *Am J Hum Genet* 1988;43:119–25.

12. Ando I, Chi HI, Nakagawa H, and Otsuka F. Differences in clinical features and HLA antigens between familial and non-familial vitiligo of non-segmental type. *Br J Dermatol* 1993;129(4):408–10.

13. Deeba F, Jamil K, Syed R et al. Association of angiotensin converting enzyme gene I/D polymorphism with vitiligo in South Indian population. *Int J Med Med Sci* 2009;1:009–12.

14. Krupa Shankar DS, Shashikala K, and Madala R. Clinical patterns of vitiligo and its associated co-morbidities: A prospective controlled cross-sectional study in South India. *Indian Dermatol Online J* 2012;3:114–8.

15. Singh S, Usha, and Pandey SS. Epidemiological profile of vitiligo in Northern India. *J Appl Pharm Sci* 2011;01:211–4.

16. Shah H, Mehta A, and Astik B. Clinical and sociodemographic study of vitiligo. *Indian J Dermatol Venereol Leprol* 2008;74:701.

17. Gopal KV, Rama Rao GR, Kumar YH et al. Vitiligo: A part of a systemic autoimmune process. *Indian J Dermatol Venereol Leprol* 2007;73(3):162–5.

18. Dave S, Thappa DM, and DSouza M. Clinical predictors of outcome in vitiligo. *Indian J Dermatol Venereol Leprol* 2002;68:323–5.

Chapter 4

BASIC SCIENCE

Neha Kumar and S.N. Bhattacharya

CONTENTS

The fundamental factors governing the *visual impact* are as follows:

1. *Biochemical*: Melanin, heme, carotenoids

2. *Histological*
   - Anatomical variation
   - Race, ethnicity, and gender
   - Melanocytes (density, pattern of distribution, functioning)
   - Melanin type (eumelanin/pheomelanin)
   - Thickness of epidermis
   - Anatomical disposition of cutaneous vasculature
   - Degenerative deposits (lipofuscin)

3. *Physical*: Tyndall effect in the skin—melanin helps in significant reduction in transmission and scatters more by acting as a colloidal suspension in the skin, giving rise to the Tyndall effect. The relatively transparent stratum corneum scatters light minimally, whereas the deeper layers scatter more. The variations in light wavelength among colors affect this scattering, and the pigment situated in deeper layers appears blue (Mongolian spot, tattoos).

MELANIN SYNTHETIC PATHWAYS

The quantity and type of melanin produced, and its eventual distribution through the epidermis, affect the skin color. Understandably, the migration, differentiation, and maturation during melanoblast development are essential for eventual pigmentation.

RAPER–MASON PATHWAY

Tyrosine → (tyrosinase: hydroxylation and immediate oxidation) → Dopaquinone → (paired reduction) → DOPA and cyclo-DOPA → (spontaneous conversion) → Dopachrome → (loses carboxylic acid group) → 5,6-dihydroxyindole (DHI) → oxidizes and polymerizes → DHI-melanin (dense, high-molecular-weight complex) → two types—eumelanin (brown-black) and pheomelanin (yellow-red). Figure 4.1 depicts the melanin synthetic pathway. It is regulated physiologically, primarily through melanocortin 1 receptor (MC1R), and modulated by its ligands, melanocyte-stimulating hormone (MSH), and agouti-signaling protein (ASIP).

In 1980, Pawelek reported tyrosinase-related protein1 (TYRP1) and DOPAchrome tautomerase (DCT) produced in melanocytes, which prevented spontaneous decarboxylation of Dopachrome to DHI and led to production of more soluble and lighter colored carboxylated melanin, known as DHICA melanin [1].

Orlow et al. [2] demonstrated that three tyrosinase-related melanogenic enzymes are polymerized in a complex within melanocytes, which facilitates their physiological interactions.

CUTANEOUS MELANIN PIGMENTATION

The quantity of melanin and the degree of epidermal melanization are the most important determinants of skin color. Melanin synthesis occurs in the cytoplasmic organelle, "melanosomes" within the melanocyte. The entire process of epidermal melanization occurs in epidermal melanin units. The distribution of these units throughout the skin surface eventually determines the quantity and quality of melanization, which results in the baseline skin and hair color within an individual. At any given time, an individual's skin color has two components:

1. *Constitutive skin color*: Biological potentiality of epidermal melanin units, under the control of cellular genetic program, independent of UV exposure and other relevant factors (as given in Figure 4.2a).

2. *Facultative skin color*: Affected by UV exposure, hormones, nutrients, chemicals, environmental factors (as given in Figure 4.2b and Figures 4.3 through 4.5).

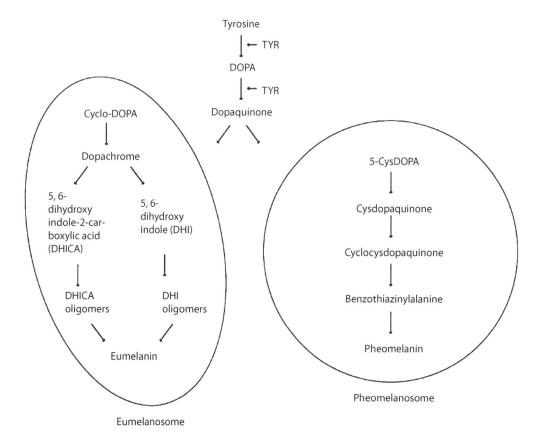

Figure 4.1   Melanin synthetic pathway.

GENETIC DETERMINANTS OF HUMAN SKIN PIGMENTATION (CONSTITUTIVE PIGMENTATION)

Human skin color is one of the most rapidly evolving traits, where closely related populations show large differences in average pigmentation levels. The interpopulation variation in pigmentation has been estimated to be 88%, compared to 10%–15% for arbitrarily selected genetic markers [3]. Variations that govern the pigmentary differences among populations are as follows:

1. *Cellular level*: More melanin, larger size, scattered distribution of melanosomes rather than being clustered is typical of darkly pigmented skin types as compared to light skin types [4].

2. *Biochemical level*: Multiple gene mutations involving the pigmentation pathways, including tyrosinase activity, encoded by TYR gene (rate-limiting enzyme in melanogenesis) [5].

Pigmentary genetic studies have been performed using candidate genes or admixture linkage in recently admixed populations (West African/European/Indigenous American populations) and genome-wide association studies for non-admixed populations.

Earlier evidence suggested that variations in six to eight genes (*SLC24A5, SLC45A2 [MATP], KITLG, OCA2, TYR*, and *ASIP*) underlie the skin color differences between European and West African populations [6]. Considering admixed population studies, at least 10 genes are now recognized to contribute to population-level differences [7]. The HapMap project discovered an amino acid substitution in human homolog (*SL24A5*Thr111*) as the single largest effect of any known gene on skin color differences between Europeans and West Africans. This mutation (and similarly *SLC45A2*) was found to

be fixed across most of Europe and is rare (approximately 2.5%) in East Asia, possibly resulting from substantial selective pressure [8].

In 2008, Ginger et al. [9] observed downregulation of melanin production by inserting *SLC24A5*Thr111* allele into DNA of cultured melanocytes. The following hypothesis was proposed:

- This mutation could change the pH of the trans-Golgi network, thereby modifying tyrosinase activity.
- Based on the timing of *SLC24A5* expression during cell proliferation, it could also modulate the trafficking of pre-melanosomes.

A few genes show selection in both East Asian and European population (e.g., *KITLG*); however, there is also evidence of independent evolution of light skin pigmentation in European (*SLC24A5* and *SLC45A2*) and East Asian populations, suggesting that the shared phenotype has not resulted from a shared ancestral mutation. These selective events mirror the migration trends of humans in Europe and Asia over the past 50,000 years. However, not all selective events were recent. The genetic variation at *EDN3* supports selection on pigmentation in common ancestors of humans prior to their racial divergence [10]. The various hypotheses to evolutionary pressures influencing skin pigmentation are [11]:

- Darker skin pigmentation evolved possibly more than once because it reduces photolysis of folic acid, which protects against neural tube defects and is essential for DNA replication, repair, and other functions.
- Adaptive benefit of lighter skin pigmentation (controversial). In a low-UVR environment, less dermal melanin allows for production of more vitamin D_3 (needed for normal skeletal, immune, and cardiovascular system development).

Despite the lack of clarity on the evolutionary pressures, it is clear that selection of genes involved in skin pigmentation is as strong as or stronger than genes determining immunity, reproduction,

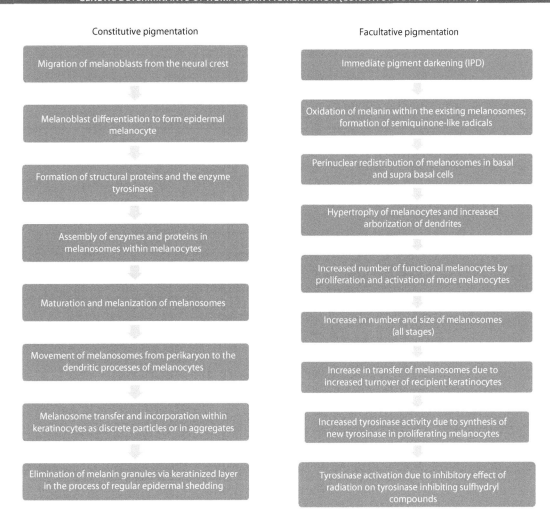

Constitutive pigmentation

Migration of melanoblasts from the neural crest

Melanoblast differentiation to form epidermal melanocyte

Formation of structural proteins and the enzyme tyrosinase

Assembly of enzymes and proteins in melanosomes within melanocytes

Maturation and melanization of melanosomes

Movement of melanosomes from perikaryon to the dendritic processes of melanocytes

Melanosome transfer and incorporation within keratinocytes as discrete particles or in aggregates

Elimination of melanin granules via keratinized layer in the process of regular epidermal shedding

Facultative pigmentation

Immediate pigment darkening (IPD)

Oxidation of melanin within the existing melanosomes; formation of semiquinone-like radicals

Perinuclear redistribution of melanosomes in basal and supra basal cells

Hypertrophy of melanocytes and increased arborization of dendrites

Increased number of functional melanocytes by proliferation and activation of more melanocytes

Increase in number and size of melanosomes (all stages)

Increase in transfer of melanosomes due to increased turnover of recipient keratinocytes

Increased tyrosinase activity due to synthesis of new tyrosinase in proliferating melanocytes

Tyrosinase activation due to inhibitory effect of radiation on tyrosinase inhibiting sulfhydryl compounds

Figure 4.2   The various steps involved in the biological events associated with both constitutive and facultative skin pigmentation.

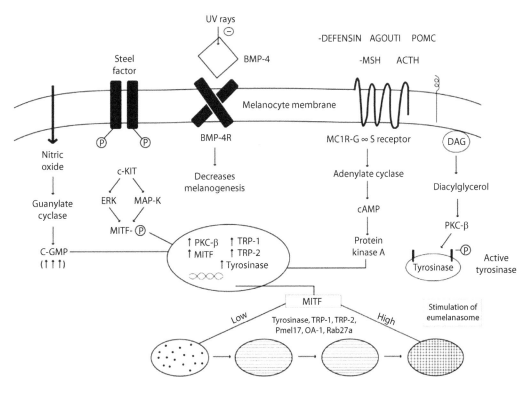

Figure 4.3   Signaling pathways in melanogenesis.

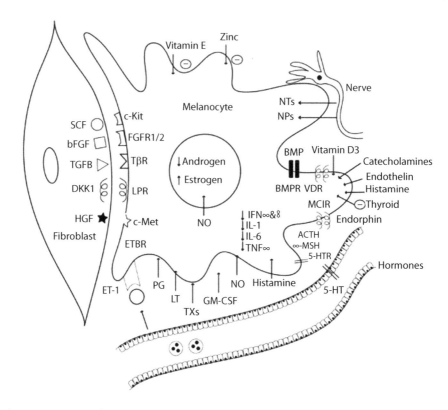

Figure 4.4   The role of hormones, growth factors, cytokines, and mediators in melanogenesis.

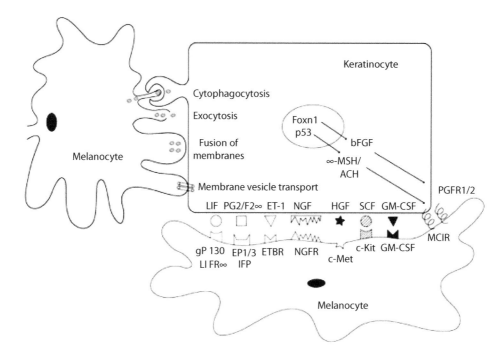

Figure 4.5   Keratinocyte-derived growth factors and melanosome transfer hypothesis.

and diet, all of which are essential to health [12–14]. Pigmentation genes are more than twice as likely to show evidence of selection as randomly selected genes in both Chinese and European populations [15]. To date, more than 25 pigmentation genes show evidence of selection on skin color, which dates back to before the emergence of first anatomically modern Homo sapiens (Figure 4.6).

REFERENCES

1. Korner AM, and Pawelek J. Dopachrome conversion: A possible control point in melanin biosynthesis. *J Invest Dermatol* 1980;75(2):192–5.

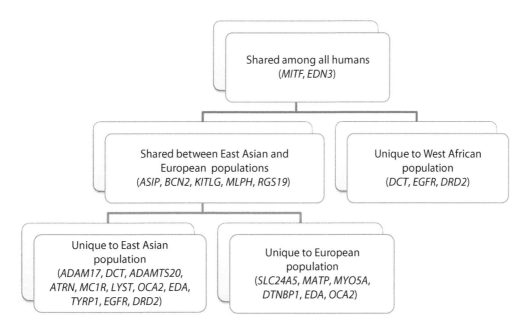

Figure 4.6   The evolutionary genetic architecture of skin pigmentation in three geographic types of human population.

2. Orlow SJ, Zhou BK, Chakraborty AK et al. High molecular weight forms of tyrosinase and the tyrosinase related proteins: Evidence for a melanogenic complex. *J Invest Dermatol* 1994;103:196–201.

3. Relethford JH. Apportionment of global human genetic diversity based on craniometrics and skin color. *Am J Phys Anthropol* 2002;118:393–8.

4. Sturm RA, Box NF, and Ramsay M. Human pigmentation genetics: The difference is only skin deep. *BioEssays* 1998;20:712–21.

5. Fuller BB, Spaulding DT, and Smith DR. Regulation of the catalytic activity of preexisting tyrosinase in Black and Caucasian human melanocyte cell cultures. *Exp Cell Res* 2001;262:197–208.

6. Sturm RA. Molecular genetics of human pigmentation diversity. *Hum Mol Gen* 2009;18:R9–17.

7. Parra EJ, Kittles RA, and Shriver MD. Implications of correlation between skin color and genetic ancestry for biomedical research. *Nat Genet* 2004;36:S54–60.

8. Norton HL, Kittles RA, Parra EJ et al. Genetic evidence for the convergent evolution of light skin in Europeans and East Asians. *Mol Biol Evol* 2007;24:710–22.

9. Ginger RS, Askew SE, Ogborne RM et al. SLC24A5 encodes a trans-Golgi network protein with potassium dependent sodium-calcium exchange activity the regulates human epidermal melanogenesis. *J Biol Chem* 2008;283:5486–95.

10. McAvoy B, Beleza S, and Shriver MD. The genetic architecture of normal variation in human pigmentation: An evolutionary perspective and model. *Hum Mol Genet* 2006;15(Spec 2):R176–81.

11. Jablonski NG, and Chaplin G. The evolution of human skin coloration. *J Hum Evol* 2000;39:57–106.

12. Lao O, de Gruijter JM, van Duijn K et al. Signatures of positive selection in genes associated with human skin pigmentation as revealed from analysis of single nucleotide polymorphisms. *Ann Hum Genet* 2006;71:354–69.

13. Voigt BF, Kudaravalli S, Wen X et al. A map of recent positive selection in human genome. *PLOS BIOL* 2006;4:e72.

14. Myles S, Somel M, Tang K et al. Identifying genes underlying human pigmentation differences among human populations. *Hum Genet* 2007;120:613–21.

15. Williamson SH, Hubisz MJ, Clark AG et al. Localizing recent adaptive evolution in the human genome. *PLOS GENET* 2007;3:e90.

TANNING (FACULTATIVE PIGMENTATION): MOLECULAR ASPECTS

Tanning is commonly described as increased melanization of the epidermis observed after exposure to UV rays, as an adaptive (facultative) response to protect against further UV damage [1].

Molecular basis of tanning:

- Increase in the number of cell surface receptors to MSH [2,3].
- Increase in the melanogenic response to MSH via increased protein levels and activity of tyrosinase [2,3].
- DNA restriction enzymes → stimulate melanin synthesis in cultured pigment cells by increasing MSH binding and melanogenic response to MSH. This implicated the role of UV-mediated DNA damage in the tanning response [4].
- Accelerating damaged DNA repair in the UV-irradiated pigment cells by T4 endonuclease also enhanced the melanization response.
- p53 activation (during DNA damage) led to increased read-out from transfected tyrosinase promoter, linked to a reporter gene. Therefore, p53 could directly or indirectly stimulate tyrosinase transcription [5].
- The key observation that UV action spectrum for tanning is virtually identical to that causing cyclobutane pyrimidine dimer (CPD) production, leading to suggestions that thymidine dinucleotide (TT) might serve as a molecular signal for increased melanogenesis (tanning) [1].

The mechanisms suggested for the role of CPD (TT) are as follows [6]:

- TT increased m-RNA and protein expression of tyrosinase as well as melanin content of cultured human and murine pigment cells.
- TT supplementation increased cell surface binding of MSH in cultured pigment cells, possibly by increased αMSH production and/or increased affinity/effecter activity for αMSH through MC1R.
- TT upregulated and activated p53 in a variety of cell types.

THE ROLE OF TELOMERE DISRUPTION

Telomeres are the terminal portions of all mammalian chromosomes, consisting of short tandem repeats of non-coding DNA sequence (e.g., TTAGGG). These are normally in the form of loop structures, concealing the tandem repeat in the proximal double strand.

Upon disruption by UV, the single-stranded TTAGGG is exposed [7] → activation of ataxia telangiectasia-related kinases → activation of p53 → apoptosis of treated cells [8]. This suggests that DNA damaging agents such as CPDs or influx of DNA repair proteins at the site of damage might also expose single-stranded TTAGGG repeats; hence, TTAGGG-containing DNA sequences might alone suffice as a cellular DNA damage signal to trigger tanning [9].

Interesting facts have been noted which highlighted telomeres as an ideal target for DNA damage [9,10]:

- TT dimers—one third of the repeat sequence is the favored substrate for CPDs.
- GGG—one half of the sequence is the substrate for almost all oxidative damage.
- AG/G residues—the favored site for formation of chemical adducts to DNA.
- Following UV irradiation, CPDs are seven times more frequent in telomeric DNA than in other portions of the genome.

TT (A PART OF THE TELOMERE REPEAT SEQUENCE) VS. FULL TELOMERE SEQUENCE: MELANOGENESIS STIMULATORS

Experiments demonstrated that an 11-base oligonucleotide GTTAGGGTTAG was indeed far more effective on a molar basis than TT in stimulating tanning of cultured pigment cells or of human skin supplemented ex vivo [9]. Telomere homolog oligonucleotides, termed T-oligos, act via multiple mechanisms including increased expression of tyrosinase and melanogenic gene products such as TRP1, Mart1, and gp100 [11].

TYROSINASE ACTIVATION

Tyrosinase is a phosphoprotein, activated upon phosphorylation (by protein kinase C-β [PKC-β]). The intramelanosomal portion of phosphorylated tyrosinase catalyzes the production of eumelanin. PKC-β, which is activated by diacylglycerol (DAG) generated from UV-irradiated cell membranes, is among the gene products transcriptionally upregulated following UV irradiation [12].

MELANOCYTE KERATINOCYTE INTERACTIONS IN TANNING

It is proven that tanning occurs to a far greater degree in intact skin or melanocyte–keratinocyte co-cultures than in pure individual cell cultures, supporting the role of keratinocyte-derived products

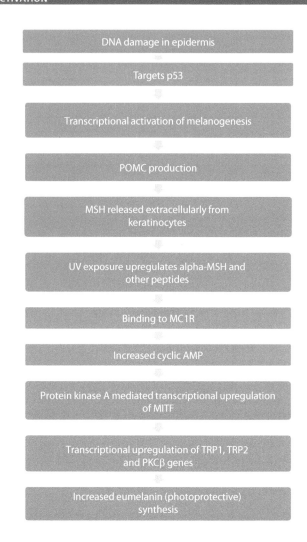

Figure 4.7   Steps in tanning. POMC, pro-opiomelanocortin; PKC, protein kinase C; MITF, microphthalmia inhibitory transcription factor.

in UV-induced tanning [13]. Keratinocyte-derived gene products which are upregulated by UVR act as paracrine factors to stimulate survival, melanogenesis, and/or melanin transfer by melanocytes, including induction via p53 and T-oligos [14]. MC1R ligand MSH, a cleavage product of pro-opiomelanocortin (POMC), is regulated in keratinocytes by p53 via a p53 consensus sequence in POMC gene promoter [15]. Figure 4.7 depicts the steps in tanning [14].

TANNING INCLUDES ENHANCED DNA REPAIR CAPACITY

As described previously, tanning is the human skin's protective response against acute and chronic UV damage. However, the increased epidermal melanin content associated with a "good tan" offers only a modest degree of photoprotection. A study performed by Halder and Bridgeman-Shah showed that excised, darkly pigmented epidermis covering intact viable skin reduces UV damage maximally to a factor of four (up to 400%), as compared to lightly pigmented epidermis [16].

CONCLUSION

In summary, UV-induced increase in epidermal melanin content (increased melanogenesis) is only one aspect of p53-mediated DNA

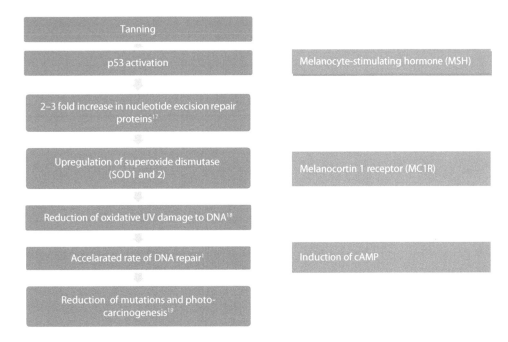

Figure 4.8   Flowchart depicting mechanism by which tanning enhances DNA repair.

damage response, which includes upregulation of DNA repair capacity as well as antioxidant defenses [17] (as shown in Figure 4.8). Recently, interest has grown in studying the major molecular variations that impact the tanning response in different populations. MC1R polymorphisms, splice variants, and variations in p53 and other DNA damage response genes are all being studied currently as possible factors influencing tanning response outcomes.

REFERENCES

1. Gilchrest BA. Molecular aspects of tanning. *J Invest Dermatol* 2011;131:E14–7.

2. Bolognia J, Murray M, and Pawelek J. UVB-induced melanogenesis may be mediated through the MSH receptor system. *J Invest Dermatol* 1989;92:651–6.

3. Chakraborty AK, Orlow SJ, Bolognia JL et al. Structural/functional relationships between internal and external MSH receptors: Modulation of Cloudman melanoma cells by UVB radiation. *J Cell Physiol* 1991;147:1–6.

4. Eller MS, Ostrom K, and Gilchrest BA. DNA damage enhances melanogenesis. *Proc Natl Acad Sci USA* 1996;93:1087–92.

5. Nylander K, Bourdon JC, Bray SE et al. Transcriptional activation of tyrosinase and TRP-1 by p53 links UV irradiation to the protective tanning response. *J Pathol* 2000;190:39–46.

6. Eller MS, Yaar M, and Gilchrest BA. DNA damage and melanogenesis. *Nature* 1994;372:413–4.

7. Karlseder J, Broccoli D, Dai Y et al. p53- and ATM-dependent apoptosis induced by telomeres lacking TRF2. *Science* 1999;283:1321–5.

8. Denchi EL, and de Lange T. Protection of telomeres through independent control of ATM and ATR by TRF2 and POT1. *Nature* 2007;448:1068–71.

9. Gilchrest BA, Eller MS, and Yaar M. Telomere-mediated effects on melanogenesis and skin aging. *J Invest Dermatol Symp Proc* 2009;14:25–31.

10. Rochette PJ, and Brash DE. Human telomeres are hypersensitive to UV-induced DNA damage and refractory to repair. *PLOS GENET* 2010;6:e1000926.

11. Puri N, Eller MS, Byers HR et al. Telomere-based DNA damage responses: A new approach to melanoma. *FASEB J* 2004;18:1373–81.

12. Park HY, Wu C, Yonemoto L et al. MITF mediates cAMP-induced protein kinase C-β expression in human melanocytes. *Biochem J* 2006;395:571–8.

13. Archambault M, Yaar M, and Gilchrest BA. Keratinocytes and fibroblasts in human skin equivalent model enhance melanocyte survival and melanin synthesis after ultraviolet irradiation. *J Invest Dermatol* 1995;104:859–67.

14. Park HY, Kosmadaki M, Yaar M et al. Cellular mechanisms regulating human melanogenesis. *Cell Mol Life Sci* 2009;66:1493–506.

15. Cui R, Widlund HR, Feige E et al. Central role of p53 in suntan response and pathologic hyperpigmentation. *Cell* 2007;128:853–64.

16. Halder RM, and Bridgeman-Shah S. Skin cancer in African Americans. *Cancer* 1995;75:667–73.

17. Eller MS, Asarch A, and Gilchrest BA. Photoprotection in human skin-a multifaceted SOS response. *Photochem Photobiol* 2008;84:339–49.

Chapter 5

ETIOPATHOGENESIS

Dario Didona, Biagio Didona, Giovanni Paolino, and Raffaele Dante Caposiena Caro

CONTENTS

GENETICS OF VITILIGO

The genetics of vitiligo is complex. Simple Mendelian genetics is not useful to explain the genetic basis of vitiligo. Incomplete penetrance, multiple susceptibility loci, and genetic heterogeneity characterize this autoimmune disease. Furthermore, vitiligo and other autoimmune diseases share several loci. Indeed, vitiligo is often associated with other autoimmune disorders, including type 1 diabetes, systemic lupus erythematosus, and Graves disease (Table 5.1) [1]. The first evidence about the genetic basis of vitiligo was reported by Addison in 1855, who described a patient with idiopathic adrenal insufficiency, generalized vitiligo, and pernicious anemia [1].

It has been reported that the relative risk of vitiligo for first-degree relatives is increased 7- to 10-fold [2]. However, the concordance of vitiligo in monozygotic twins is not extremely high (23%) [2]. Therefore, environmental factors also play an important role in developing vitiligo.

A large number of genes have been already studied, aiming to identify a link with vitiligo. Several methods have been used to conduct these studies [3]. On one hand, candidate gene association studies have been performed because they are simple to conduct. A commonly simple comparison of allele frequencies in cases and controls is used in this type of study. However, such studies are frequently subject to false positivity. Based on the results of candidate gene association studies, about 33 candidate genes linked to vitiligo have been described [4]. On the other hand, several genome-wide linkage studies have been conducted in the Caucasian and Chinese populations, discovering additional linkage signals on chromosomes 7, 8, 9, 11, 13, 17, 19, 22, and 1, 4, 6, 14, 22, respectively [1]. Such studies are useful to identify the position of a genetic marker inherited with a specific disease. However, genome-wide association studies are now considered the most useful study design in identifying genetic variants associated with complex diseases like vitiligo. Such studies have confirmed genetic associations of about 40 genes and loci with vitiligo [4,5].

HLA-associated genes, including HLA-A*02, HLA-DRB1*04, and HLA-DRB1*07 alleles, have been identified by several previous studies as being strongly linked to vitiligo [6,7]. In addition, genome-wide association studies found major association signals in the MHC on chromosome 6p21.3 in Caucasian and Chinese patients. Specifically, an important association signal has been

Table 5.1 Vitiligo risk genes shared with other autoimmune diseases

Autoimmune disease	Gene
Asthma; Crohn's disease; type I diabetes; multiple sclerosis	BACH2
Type I diabetes; rheumatoid arthritis; systemic lupus erythematosus; Graves disease	BTNL2
Type I diabetes; Graves disease	C1QTNF6
Type I diabetes; rheumatoid arthritis	CASP7
Inflammatory bowel disease	CCR6
Multiple sclerosis; systemic lupus erythematosus	CXCR5
Crohn's disease; Graves disease	FGFR1OP
Type I diabetes; Graves disease; multiple sclerosis; lupus	FIH1
Juvenile idiopathic arthritis; Behçet disease	GZMB
Systemic lupus erythematosus; rheumatoid arthritis	HLA region
Systemic lupus erythematosus; rheumatoid arthritis; type I diabetes	IL2RA
Alopecia areata; type I diabetes	KZF4
Rheumatoid arthritis	LPP
Systemic lupus erythematosus; rheumatoid arthritis	PTPN22
Type I diabetes; rheumatoid arthritis; lupus	SH2B3
Autoimmune thyroid disease	SLA
Autoimmune thyroid disease	SMOC2
Systemic lupus erythematosus	UBASH3A
Crohn's disease; inflammatory bowel disease	ZMIZ1

described in Caucasian patients in the class I gene region (primarily between HLA-A and HCG9) and in the class II gene region (principally between HLA-DRB1 and HLA-DQA1, in linkage disequilibrium with HLA-DRB1*04), while in Chinese patients the most important MHC association signal has been described in the class III gene region [1].

However, a few non-HLA genes, including lymphoid-specific protein tyrosine phosphatase nonreceptor type 22 (PTPN22), tyrosinase (TYR), and cytotoxic T-lymphocyte—associated protein 4 (CTLA4), have been reported as being associated with vitiligo [1].

The PTPN22 gene, located on the 1p13.3-p13.1 locus, has recently been demonstrated as an inherited risk factor for generalized vitiligo [8]. In addition, PTNPN22 gene, which is involved in regulating Cbl proto-oncogene (that encodes a RING finger E3 ubiquitin ligase) function in the T-cell receptor signaling pathway, has been found mutated in several autoimmune diseases, including type 1 diabetes, rheumatoid arthritis, systemic lupus erythematosus, and Graves disease. Moreover, it has been reported that the *PTPN22* R620W polymorphism was associated with generalized vitiligo in Caucasian patients. However, this association was not confirmed by a study carried out in generalized vitiligo patients from Gujarat in India [9], but it has been postulated that the R620W polymorphism is rare in non-Caucasian populations.

TYR encodes tyrosinase, a melanocytic enzyme that catalyzes the rate-limiting steps of melanin biosynthesis. In addition, *TYR* is a major autoantigen in generalized vitiligo. Tyrosinase epitopes are presented to the immune system on the surface of melanocytes and melanoma cells by HLA class I molecules, principally HLA-A*02 [5]. A specific association between the major (R; Arg) allele of the R402Q polymorphism (rs1126809) of *TYR* and generalized vitiligo has been reported [5]. Conversely, it has been highlighted that the minor (Q; Gln) allele of the *TYR* R402Q polymorphism was protective for generalized vitiligo [7].

CTLA4, located on chromosome 2q33, encodes a T-cell coreceptor regulating T-cell activation. It has been described as the first vitiligo non-MHC candidate gene association [7]. Moreover, it is associated with several autoimmune diseases that are epidemiologically associated with vitiligo. Indeed, *CTLA4* association was strongest in vitiligo patients who were also affected by another concomitant autoimmune disease. Although several authors have reported inconsistent results regarding the association between *CTLA4* and vitiligo, this association has received widespread independent confirmation, including by unbiased genome-wide association studies [7].

The X-box binding protein 1 (*XBP1*) gene, mapped on 22q12 locus, is related to the expression of MHC class II genes. Specifically, XBP1 protein has been described as transcription factor through recognition of the X2 promoter element of both HLA DR-α and HLA DP-β [2]. In addition, an elevation in the expression of a particular *XBP1* polymorphism (allele C of rs2269577) has recently been detected in lesional skin of vitiligo patients [2].

Thymic stromal lymphopoietin (*TSLP*) gene localized at chromosome 5q22.1 encodes thymic stromal lymphopoietin, which produces a cellular signal through a heterodimeric receptor complex composed of the thymic stromal lymphopoietin receptor and the IL-7R alpha chain [2]. This protein leads naive CD4+ T cells to produce Th2 response cytokines (IL-4, IL-5, IL-13, tumor necrosis factor-alpha [TNF-α]) and inhibits production of Th1 response cytokines (IL-10, IFN-γ). As a result, when deficiency of *TSLP* gene expression occurs, the dominance of Th1 response, which is involved in vitiligo development, is expected [7].

Forkhead box P3 (*FOXP3*) gene localized at Xp11.23 region encodes the protein scurfin. The gene plays a pivotal role in the development and function of CD25+CD4+ regulatory T cells. In addition, *FOXP3* gene mutations causes the IPEX (immunodysregulation polyendocrinopathy enteropathy X-linked) syndrome, characterized by an association of several autoimmune diseases, including diabetes mellitus type 1, thyroid autoimmune diseases, inflammatory bowel diseases, allergic diseases (e.g., atopic dermatitis, food allergies), and vitiligo [10].

In conclusion, approximately 36 convincing nonsegmental vitiligo susceptibility loci have been identified. The biggest association study included 33 candidate genes of generalized vitiligo. However, only *FOXP3*, *XBP1*, and *TSLP* showed an association with vitiligo. In contrast, genome-wide association studies revealed seven different regions of significant association with generalized vitiligo outside the MHC region. The latest conducted genome-wide association study led to identification of 13 so-far-unknown susceptibility genes.

ENVIRONMENTAL FACTORS IN VITILIGO

Vitiligo is a complex disease in which several factors play a role. Although the exact pathogenesis is not clear, it has been proposed that environmental factors could play an important role in developing vitiligo in genetically susceptible individuals. A precipitating factor could more easily promote cellular apoptosis in genetically susceptible individuals, whose melanocytes are more fragile than normal [11]. Involved precipitating factors include sunburn, pregnancy, stress, and exposure to cytotoxic compounds [12] (Table 5.2). All these precipitating factors share the ability to stimulate the production of melanin. Recently, provoking factors of vitiligo have been reported by using a questionnaire [12]. The authors reported that emotional stress (55.4%) was the most frequent precipitating factor, followed by sunburn (28.8%), mechanical factors (19.2%), and chemical factors (16.4%) [12]. It has frequently been reported that patients initially develop vitiligo at the site of skin trauma, often a massive sunburn [12]. It has been postulated that melanocytes might be more fragile in genetically susceptible individuals, leading to local melanocyte death, inflammation, and autoimmunity after trauma [11]. Recently, patients working in production or manufacturing more commonly reported that their workplace affected the development of vitiligo lesions, as compared with vitiligo patients who had other jobs. These results suggest that mechanical trauma might affect the development of vitiligo [12].

Some authors have thought that UV might induce melanocyte-specific genes, leading either to a direct cytotoxicity, produced by toxic melanin intermediates (auto-cytotoxic theory) [11,13], or to an affection of the REDOX-free state, producing reactive oxygen species (ROS)-induced cell damage (oxidative theory) [11,14]. It has been reported that during synthesis of melanin, specific quinones and indoles are produced as intermediates that could be themselves cytotoxic to melanocytes [14]. This intermediate toxic production in genetically susceptible individuals results above the threshold, inducing melanocyte death. The mechanism by which UV aggravates vitiligo has not been clearly discovered, but vitiligo patients have fragile melanocytes that are thought to be easily destroyed through apoptosis and necrosis after overexposure to UV. It has been reported that 28.8% of patients experienced aggravation of vitiligo after sunburn [11].

Table 5.2   Selected list of substances associated with contact/occupational vitiligo

Phenol/catechol derivatives
Hydroquinone
Monobenzyl ether of hydroquinone
Monomethyl ether of hydroquinone
Monoethyl ether of hydroquinone
Sulfhydryls
β-Mercaptoethylamine hydrochloride
Sulfanolic acid
Cystamine dihydrochloride
3-Mercaptopropylamine hydrochloride
Drugs
Chloroquine
Fluphenazine
Various
Mercurials
Benzyl alcohol
Arsenic
p-Phenylenediamine

It has been reported that aliphatic derivatives of phenols or other common compounds could promote the development of vitiligo in genetically susceptible individuals [15]. Vitiligo lesions have been described in people who are professionally exposed to several phenolic compounds [15]. The prolonged contact with these compounds could lead to free radical production, cytotoxicity, and melanocyte death. This kind of vitiligo has been named contact/occupational vitiligo [15]. Some authors have reported that several environmental chemicals showed a selective toxicity to melanocytes both in vitro and in vivo [16]. Most toxins are aromatic or aliphatic derivatives of phenols and catechols, which are added in bleaching creams. However, only some exposed individuals developed hypopigmentation. In addition, it has been reported that other chemicals precipitate vitiligo, such as sulfhydryls, systemic drugs, mercurials, and arsenic [15]. A contact/occupational vitiligo has been described in people working with rubber and industrial oils containing several chemicals, including phenolic antioxidants, phenolic germicidal detergents, and para-tertiary-butylphenol [15]. Some individuals develop vitiligo-like lesions in a short period of time, whereas others develop the lesions after several years of exposure [15]. These considerations confirm the role of genetic factors in developing vitiligo lesions in genetically susceptible individuals. However, the mode of action of these chemicals on the melanocyte is still not clear. Boissy and Manga investigated the activity of 4-tertiary-butylphenol (4-TBP), a common inducer of vitiligo, and found that melanocytes are more sensitive than keratinocytes to the cytotoxic effect of 4-TBP [15]. In addition, this cytotoxicity is enhanced by cytokines such as basic fibroblast growth factor and alpha-melanocyte–stimulating hormone. Moreover, 4-TBP it has been described as an inducer of apoptosis, leading to DNA fragmentation and membrane blebbing. Although how phenols and catechols could induce melanocytic apoptosis is still under debate, these chemicals are structurally similar to tyrosine, the most important substrate in the pathway for melanin synthesis. Therefore it has been postulated that derivatives of phenols and catechols could compete with tyrosine for hydroxylation by tyrosinase and interfere with melanin synthesis. Moreover, free radicals generated by the catalytic action of tyrosinase on these phenolic/catecholic derivatives could lead to apoptosis through peroxidation of membranes [14,15]. However, it has been excluded that tyrosinase could mediate the effect of 4-TBP and alter sensitivity of cells to catecholic compounds [15]. By contrast, Boissy and Manga demonstrated that tyrosinase-related protein-1 (Tyrp1), a melanocyte-specific enzyme, mediates the action of phenol/catechol derivatives on melanocytes, demonstrating that Tyrp1 appears to be overexpressed in a cultured line of vitiligo melanocytes [15].

Finally, a passive transfer of generalized vitiligo after bone marrow transplantation from donors with vitiligo has been reported [17].

AUTOIMMUNITY IN VITILIGO

The pathogenesis of vitiligo is still under debate, although the role of autoimmunity in vitiligo is clear. Nevertheless, autoimmune mechanisms interplay with several other factors, including genetics and environmental and oxidative stress (Figure 5.1). Both cell-mediated and humoral immunity are involved. We discuss next the main and most studied elements of the immune system involved in vitiligo.

KERATINOCYTES
The adrenergic metabolism, the production of soluble and membrane factors, is altered in vitiligo keratinocytes. A pivotal role is played by endothelin-1 (ET-1), which shows a paracrine effect on

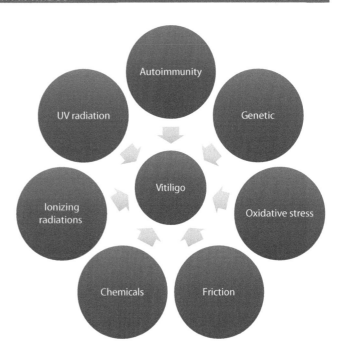

Figure 5.1   Interaction between immune system, genetic, and external risk factors in vitiligo.

melanocytes, reducing their survival and the production of pigment [11]. These findings are confirmed by the presence of significant difference in the haplotype frequencies of the ET-1 gene between vitiligo patients and healthy controls [11].

TNF-α is also involved in the pathogenesis of vitiligo [11]. A recent study found that keratinocytes in depigmented areas are more susceptible to TNF-α–mediated apoptosis compared to normally pigmented epidermis [11]. As a consequence of the keratinocyte apoptosis, there is a decrease in stem cell factor, leading also to melanocyte apoptosis.

LANGERHANS CELLS AND DERMAL DENDRITIC CELLS
Langerhans cells appear to be activated in depigmented skin based on their high HLA-DR expression. Furthermore, their location in the epidermis could lead to direct contact with melanocyte and cellular antigens [11]. Inflammatory CD11c+ dermal dendritic cells (DDCs) might also capture melanocyte antigens [18]. In addition, inflammatory DDCs may stimulate Th17 cell proliferation through their production of IL-23 [18].

It has been discovered that CD11c+ DDCs express perforin and granzyme B and exhibit cytotoxic activity against tumor cells. It is possible that, in addition to presenting melanocyte-specific self-antigens, CD11c+ dermal DDCs at the leading edge of vitiligo lesions are directly involved in the killing of melanocytes [18].

INFLAMMOSOME
Inflammasome is constitutive of the innate immune system and is responsible for regulating the immunological response to several stimuli. It consists mainly of a molecular pattern recognition receptor, an apoptosis-associated speck-like protein, which contains a caspase-recruitment domain adaptor protein, and a caspase-1 enzyme [19]. Recent reports identified single-nucleotide polymorphisms in the promoter and coding regions of NLR family pyrin domain containing 1 (Nlrp1) associated with vitiligo, vitiligo-associated autoimmune diseases, Addison disease, and type I diabetes [19]. Nlrp1 is highly expressed in T cells and Langerhans cells in the skin, explaining the potential role of mutant Nlrp1 in autoimmune diseases of the skin. This ultimately results in depigmentation in irregular patches of the skin and hair [19].

MELANOCYTES

Melanocytes play a pivotal role in the skin's immune system [11]. They may trigger NF-kB and/or mitogen-activated protein kinase—signaling pathways, thereby producing several proinflammatory cytokines and chemokines [11]. In addition, they secrete a wide range of immunological molecules, including inducible nitric oxide synthase (iNOS), inflammatory cytokines, and chemokines that affect keratinocytes, lymphocytes, fibroblasts, mast cells, and endothelial cells in the skin, as well as the same melanocytes [11]. It has been reported that stimulated human melanocytes release IL-8, which is a key inflammatory chemokine that allows the apoptosis of keratocytes and melanocytes [20].

CD8+, CD4+, AND CXCL10

Cutaneous biopsies from vitiligo show a T-lymphocyte CD8+/perforin+/granzyme+ infiltrate in the dermis and in the dermal—epidermal junction in apposition with dying melanocytes and melanocyte fragments [21]. Elevated levels of melanocyte-reactive CD8+ T cells have been detected in both blood and perilesional skin from vitiligo patients [21].

In vitro studies demonstrated an increased production of proinflammatory cytokines IL-6 and IL-8 by monocytes of patients with active vitiligo [11]. Other chemokines play a pivotal role in vitiligo as IFN-γ and IFN-γ–induced chemokines, including C-X-C motif chemokine ligand 10 (CXCL10), since they are widely expressed in the skin and blood of patients with vitiligo [21]. The activation of CXCL10 leads to the recruitment of autoreactive T cells that cause melanocytes destruction. Indeed, serum CXCL10 is usually higher in patients with vitiligo compared with healthy controls, and its level is associated with disease activity and is significantly decreased after successful treatment, suggesting it may be used as a biomarker to monitor the disease activity and treatment response [21].

T-REGULATORY CELLS

In most patients with vitiligo, the balance of cytotoxic/suppressor and helper/inducer T cells in peripheral blood is disturbed [11]. Moreover, in progressive disease, the CD4+/CD8+ ratio is decreased [21]. In addition, a dysfunction of T-regulatory cells (T-regs) has been observed, suggesting that T-regs are unable to control the immunological attack and destruction in vitiligo patients [21].

TH17

Recently, the role of Th17 cells has gained more attention in vitiligo, as immunohistochemical analysis showed Th17 cell infiltration in vitiligo skin samples in addition to CD8+ T cells [22]. Moreover, the influence of a Th17 cell-related cytokine environment (IL-17A, IL-1b, IL-6, and TNF-α) in local depigmentation in autoimmune vitiligo has been noted [22]. IL-17 has also been reported to be involved in augmented production of ROS, thereby implicating its role in oxidative stress-mediated cell damage [22]. These findings are particularly exciting in view of the increasing availability of biologic therapeutics that target the IL-17 axis [22].

IL-21 AND FOLLICULAR HELPER T CELLS

An elevated level of IL-21 has been reported in vitiligo patients, highlighting the involvement of a new subset of T cells called follicular helper T (Tfh) [22]. Tfh cells and IL-21 are believed to play a central role in B cell activation and results in the immune dysregulation that leads to autoimmunity [22]. In addition, IL-21 is crucial in the activation of CD8+ T cells.

JAK-STAT SIGNALING PATHWAY

The JAK-STAT signaling pathway is essential to transmit extracellular signals of several cytokines to the nucleus, including IL-12, IL-6, IL-17, IL-21, IL-23, and IFN-γ [22]. It mediates the biological activities of these cytokines and is essential for the development and regulation of immune responses. Dysregulation of the JAK-STAT pathway contributes to numerous autoimmune diseases, including vitiligo [22]. Four members of the JAK family have been described: JAK1, JAK2, JAK3, and tyrosine kinase 2. Among these, JAK1 and JAK2 are directly involved in IFN-γ signaling, which activates STAT1 and thus induces the transcription of IFN-γ–induced genes, including CXCL10, which through its receptor CXCR3 recruits more autoreactive T cells to the epidermis, resulting in widespread melanocyte destruction [22].

OXIDATIVE STRESS

Oxidative stress is one of the possible pathogenic events in vitiligo. The excess of ROS is caused by overproduction and/or inadequate antioxidant defense. ROS are reactive chemical species containing oxygen, including hydrogen peroxide (H_2O_2), superoxide anions, hydroxyl radicals, and singlet oxygen [23]. These are produced during multiple cellular processes. Environmental sources, including pollution and ionizing or UV radiation, lead to excessive ROS production. ROS may oxidize cell components, leading to melanocyte destruction and consequent depigmentation [23].

Superoxide dismutase (SOD) is a group of metalloenzymes that protects cells from the toxic effects of superoxide radicals. It converts the O_2^- anion to O_2 and H_2O_2. Several studies showed that SOD activity is higher in serum in the erythrocytes and in the skin of vitiligo patients [23]. However, other studies showed that SOD activity is lower in the serum and skin of vitiligo patients compared to healthy controls [24].

Glutathione peroxidase (GP) is the name of an enzyme family that turns H_2O_2 and other peroxides into water. The activity of GP in vitiligo is still controversial. Some authors reported a significant decrease in GP level in the serum of vitiligo patients [23]; others reported that GP activity in plasma, serum, and erythrocytes of vitiligo patients is increased compared to those in healthy controls [23].

Catalase (CAT) is another important endogenous antioxidant enzyme that prevents ROS damage by eliminating H_2O_2. CAT mutations play a pivotal role in affecting the enzyme activity. Several papers suggested an association between CAT polymorphism and the risk of vitiligo, although the results are controversial [23]. However, Casp et al. reported significant differences in CAT activity between vitiligo patients and controls [25]. In addition, Gavalas et al. highlighted that the CAT genotype was significantly overrepresented in vitiligo patients compared with controls [26].

Several nonenzymatic agents, such as vitamin A, vitamin E, and vitamin C, show an important antioxidant activity. However, their role in vitiligo is still under debate. Although it has been reported that the levels of vitamins E and A are normal in the plasma of vitiligo patients, some authors found lower levels of both vitamins E and C in the plasma of patients affected by vitiligo [23].

Melanin is produced from L-tyrosine by tyrosinase (TYR) [27]. The 5,6,7,8-tetrahydrobiopterin (6-BH4) is an essential cofactor for the synthesis of L-tyrosine from L-phenylalanine by phenylalanine hydroxylase (PAH) and for the hydroxylation of L-tyrosine to L-DOPA by tyrosine hydroxylase (TH) [27]. Schallreuter et al. reported that vitiligo patients had an increase in GTP-cyclohydrolase I (GTP-CH-I) activity, which led to an excessive synthesis of 6-BH4 [27]. Moreover, the influence of H_2O_2 on dihydropteridine reductase (DHPR), the last enzyme in the 6-BH4-recycling process, which is deactivated when H_2O_2 levels are greater than 30 μM, has been demonstrated [28]. In addition, higher levels of 6-BH4 are associated with an overproduction of norepinephrine, which directly

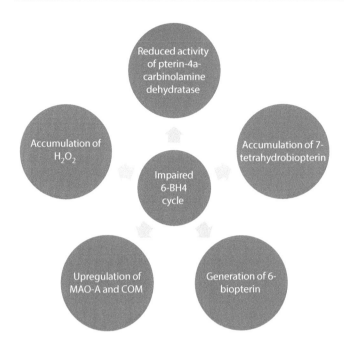

Figure 5.2 Impaired 5,6,7,8-tetrahydrobiopterin (6-BH4) cycle in vitiligo. COM, catechol-O-methyltransferase; MAO, monoamine oxidase-A.

stimulates the upregulation of both monoamine oxidase-A (MAO-A) and catechol-O-methyltransferase metabolic pathways in these patients [28]. Another consequence of the augmented levels of 6-BH4 and increased MAO-A activity in the epidermis of vitiligo patients is the accumulation of toxic levels of H_2O_2. Furthermore, it has been reported that DHPR activity is significantly decreased in patients with vitiligo [28].

The association between the overproduction and the compromised recycling of 6-BH4 leads to the following results [29] (Figure 5.2): (i) generation of 6-biopterin by oxidation reactions, which is cytotoxic to the melanocytes; (ii) an accumulation of 7-tetrahydrobiopterin (7-BH4) which is an inhibitor of PAH; (iii) reduced activity of pterin-4a-carbinolamine dehydratase, which dehydrates 4a-carbinolamine to quinonoid dihydropterin (qBH2); and (iv) accumulation of H_2O_2 due to an enhanced short circuit to qBH2. The H_2O_2 overproduction is also due to the thioredoxin reductase (TR) system, which is critical for redox regulation of protein function and reduction of 6-biopterin to qBH2. The TR inhibition by calcium may play an important role in etiology of vitiligo.

Finally, melanocytes and keratinocytes from perilesional vitiligo skin demonstrate ultrastructural abnormalities in their mitochondria [30]. The mitochondrial damage is related to an increase in ROS production. ROS may activate the cytosolic pro-apoptotic members of the B-cell lymphoma-2 family. They relocate to the mitochondrial surface and form the transmembrane pores [30]. In addition, they promote the release of many pro-apoptotic proteins [30].

AUTOPHAGY

Autophagy is a controlled self-digestion involved in many H_2 functions such as protein and organelle degradation [31]. Autophagy also protects cells against oxidative damage and innate pathogens. Furthermore, it is involved in antigen presentation as well as pathogen clearance and lymphocyte homeostasis. Three distinct types of autophagy have been identified: micro-autophagy, macro-autophagy, and chaperone-mediated autophagy (CMA) [31].

Both micro- and macro-autophagy are involved in engulfing large structures through both selective and nonselective mechanisms. On the other hand, CMA degrades only soluble proteins in a selective way [32]. In macro-autophagy, a multimembrane structure known as a phagophore engulfs the cytoplasmic organelles, producing a vesicular structure called an autophagosome. Subsequently, the autophagosome fuses with the lysosome, forming a single membrane structure called an autolysosome [31]. On the other hand, micro-autophagy is characterized by direct engulfing of organelles, involving a process of invaginating, protrusion, and/or septation of the lysosomal-limiting membrane [32]. Instead, CMA involves the 70 KDa heat shock-cognate protein and the lysosomal-associated membrane protein 2A receptor (LAMP2A) to transport specific cytosolic proteins, all characterized by pentapeptide sequence Lys-Phe-Gln-Arg-Gln, into lysosomes [32].

Autophagy plays an important role in cellular homeostasis, eliminating damaged organelles as well as aggregated intracellular proteins [33]. Autophagy is also involved in keratinocyte differentiation and melanocyte survival as well as in the pathogenesis of several autoimmune diseases, including systemic sclerosis and vitiligo [33]. However, the exact role of autophagy in vitiligo has not been completely elucidated. It has been reported that in both lesional and nonlesional skin of vitiligo patients, higher levels of ROS were observed. Furthermore, vitiligo melanocytes showed a major sensibility to ROS due to the intrinsic antioxidant defects [34]. This imbalance between the pro-oxidants and the antioxidant status may cause accumulation of oxidized and damaged proteins or organelles, leading to the destruction of melanocytes [34].

The increase in ROS generation and/or the reduction in the antioxidant activity exposes the cells to accumulation of irreversibly damaged proteins, lipids, nucleic acids, and carbohydrates [34]. Autophagy can be upregulated in response to oxidative stress. After exposure to H_2O_2, the number of both autophagosomes and autolysosomes is increased, suggesting that H_2O_2-induced oxidative stress can activate autophagy in normal melanocytes [34]. Moreover, in skin cells pretreated with chloroquine, a substance that blocks autophagic activity, an important increase of ROS and apoptosis H_2O_2-induced is observed [34]. However, vitiligo melanocytes demonstrated faint autophagic induction in response to H_2O_2-induced oxidative stress, higher levels of ROS, and increased apoptosis compared to healthy melanocytes [34]. This impaired autophagy is probably a consequence of an aberrant nuclear factor E2-related factor 2-nucleoporin p62 (Nrf2-p62)–signaling pathway [35] (Figure 5.3). Nrf2 and its downstream genes protect the cell against oxidative stress and chemical-induced cellular damage [34]. Furthermore, Nrf2 gene polymorphisms in the A^{-650} allele may be a risk factor

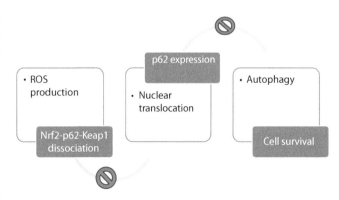

Figure 5.3 Nrf2-p62 pathway in vitiligo melanocytes. Nuclear factor E2-related factor 2-nucleoporin p62 (Nrf2-p62) does not dissociate from Kelch-like ECH-associated protein (Keap1) in vitiligo melanocytes, leading to aberrant activation of the Nrf2-p62 pathway that reduces the p62 expression, causing cell death.

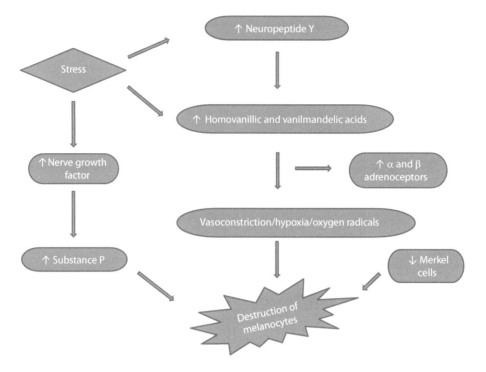

Figure 5.4   Role of neural hypothesis in the pathogenesis of vitiligo.

for vitiligo, suggesting that the Nrf2-associated antioxidant process plays an active role in the pathogenesis of vitiligo [35]. In addition, recent studies suggest that the Nrf2 pathway protects cells from several pro-oxidant stimuli via the induction of autophagy [35]. Indeed, knockdown cells for Nrf2 showed a significantly reduced level of autophagosomes induced by H_2O_2 [34].

NEURAL HYPOTHESIS

Several theories have been put forth to explain the destruction of melanocytes in vitiligo. The most important are the self-destructive, autoimmune, and neural hypotheses. In this chapter, we illustrate the neural hypothesis (Figure 5.4).

The basis of the neural hypothesis of vitiligo was first described by Lerner in 1959, who highlighted that segmental vitiligo follows the dermatome, although not exactly [36]. The author also reported in rabbit and mouse models that after a sympathectomy the color of the ipsilateral eye became lightened, demonstrating that tyrosinase activity was low in the iris, provoking cessation of melanin production [37].

Both peripheral nerve sheath and melanocytes arise from neural crest cells (NCC). These cells migrate from the neural tube to dorsolateral and ventral directions [38] (Figure 5.5). On the one hand, cells with only a dorsolateral trajectory are committed to melanocytic fate; on the other hand, cells with a ventral trajectory are committed to neuronal, glial/melanocyte, or endoneurial fibroblast fate [38]. It has been shown that SOX10+ NCCs fail to initiate the neuronogenesis, adopting a glial pathway to give rise to Schwann cells and melanocytes, highlighting the link between pigmentary disorders (as vitiligo) and neural cells [38]. Neuregulin 1 is an axon-derived growth factor which, when overexpressed, promotes glial fate and suppresses melanocytic activity [39]. Furthermore, melanocytes with the overexpression of embryo retinal epithelium can dedifferentiate back to their unpigmented glial progenitor [39].

One of the most important findings that stresses the pivotal role of the neural hypothesis in vitiligo is the role of the sympathetic nervous

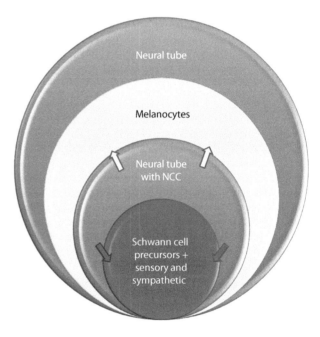

Figure 5.5   Migration of neural crest cells from the neural tube to dorsolateral and ventral directions. NCC, neural crest cells.

system. Wu et al. found an elevated α- and β-adrenoceptor response in vitiligo [40]. Neuropeptides and neuronal markers also play a pivotal role in the pathogenesis of vitiligo. It has been reported that neuropeptide Y (NPY) was usually increased in the marginal areas of vitiligo and was associated with a high presence of noradrenaline, leading to a local autoimmune effect [34]. Furthermore, precipitant factors such as stress significantly increase NPY, allowing the onset and activity of the disease [34]. Yehuda et al. performed a case-control study in military members with posttraumatic stress disorder and a healthy control group, finding that the NPY level was associated with symptom recovery, highlighting a protective role in stress exposure [41] (Figure 5.1).

Another key point in the neural hypothesis of vitiligo is the role of nerve growth factor (NGF). It has been found that NGF was increased in vitiligo and that stress upregulated NGF expression in hair follicles, increasing in the dorsal root ganglia substance P in neurons [34].

The catecholamine metabolite levels have been studied by Morrone et al., showing that homovanillic acid and vanilmandelic acid were higher in vitiligo patients. Furthermore, it was shown that these catecholamines were related to the activity of the disease since they led to vasoconstriction, hypoxia, and overproduction of oxygen radicals that destroy melanocytes [42]. Morrone et al. postulated that the level of circulating catecholamines and urinary metabolites grew also because of the stress due to the disease spreading [42]. As a result, the increased levels of catecholamines at skin autonomic nerves led to cytotoxic damage of melanocytes, either directly or indirectly through their metabolites [42].

Zinc alpha-2 glycoprotein (ZAG) is a glycoprotein secreted by several cells, including keratinocytes. ZAG shows immunomodulant activity because of its affinity to MHC-1. ZAG stimulates melanogenesis and maintains cell–cell adhesion through integrin-mediated adhesion. Therefore, its lack could cause reduced melanin production [43].

Pathologically, degenerative changes in dermal nerves and sweat glands have been reported in vitiligo patients [44]. In addition, thicker Schwann cell basement membranes have been found surrounding the nerve fibers when compared with healthy controls [44]. Furthermore, Bose found a reduction in Merkel cells, which was associated with a destruction of melanocytes [45].

REFERENCES

1. Shen C, Gao J, Sheng Y et al. Genetic susceptibility to vitiligo: GWAS approaches for identifying vitiligo susceptibility genes and loci. *Front Genet* 2016;7:3.

2. Czajkowski R, and Męcińska-Jundziłł K. Current aspects of vitiligo genetics. *Adv Dermatol Allergol* 2014;4:247–55.

3. Spritz RA. Six decades of vitiligo genetics: Genome-wide studies provide insights into autoimmune pathogenesis. *J Investig Dermatol* 2012;132:268–73.

4. Birlea SA, Jin Y, Bennett DC et al. Comprehensive association analysis of candidate genes for generalized vitiligo supports XBP1, FOXP3, and TSLP. *J Investig Dermatol* 2011;131:371–81.

5. Jin Y, Birlea SA, Fain PR et al. Genome-wide association study for vitiligo identifies susceptibility loci at 6q27 and the MHC. *Nat Genet* 2010;42:676–80.

6. Ramire LD, Marcos EVC, Godoy DAS, and de Souza-Santana FC. Association of class I and II HLA alleles and haplotypes with susceptibility to vitiligo: A study of patients with vitiligo from southeast Brazil. *Int J Dermatol* 2016;55:347–55.

7. Spritz RA, and Andersen GHL. Genetics of vitiligo. *Dermatol Clin* 2017;35:245–55.

8. Laberge GS, Bennet DC, Fain PR, and Spritz RA. PTPN22 is genetically associated with risk of generalized vitiligo, but CTLA4 is not. *J Investig Dermatol* 2008;128:1757–62.

9. Laddha NC, Dwivedi M, Shajil EM, Prajapati H, and Marfatia YS. Association of PTPN22 1858C/T polymorphism with vitiligo susceptibility in Gujarat population. *J Dermatol Sci* 2008;49:260–2.

10. Bennett CL, Christie J, Ramsdell F, Brunkow ME, Ferguson PJ, Whitesell L, Kelly TE, Saulsbury FT, Chance PF, and Ochs HD. The immune dysregulation, polyendocrinopathy, enteropathy, X-linked syndrome (IPEX) is caused by mutations of FOXP3. *Nat Genet* 2001;27:20–1.

11. Rashighi M, and Harris JE. Vitiligo pathogenesis and emerging treatments. *Dermatol Clin* 2017;35:257–65.

12. Kemp HH, Waterman EA, and Weetman AP. Autoimmune aspects of vitiligo. *Autoimmunity* 2001;34:65–77.

13. Sturm RA. Human pigmentation genes and their response to solar UV radiation. *Mutat Res* 1998;422:69–76.

14. Dell'Anna, ML, and Picardo M. A review and a new hypothesis for non-immunological pathogenetic mechanisms in vitiligo. *Pigment Cell Res* 2006;19:406–11.

15. Boissy RE, and Manga P. On the etiology of contact/occupational vitiligo. *Pigment Cell Res* 2004;17:208–14.

16. Cummings MP, and Nordlund JJ. Chemical leukoderma: Fact or fancy. *Am J Contact Dermatitis* 1995;6:122–7.

17. Alajlan A, Alfadley A, and Pedersen K-T. Transfer of vitiligo after allogeneic bone marrow transplantation. *J Am Acad Dermatol* 2002;46:606–10.

18. Zaba LC, Fuentes-Duculan J, Steinman RM, Krueger JG, and Lowes MA. Normal human dermis contains distinct populations of CD11c+BDCA-1+dendritic cells and CD163+FXIIIA+ macrophages. *J Clin Invest* 2007;117:2517–25.

19. de Sá DC, and Neto CF. Inflammasomes and dermatology. *An Bras Dermatol* 2016;91:566–78.

20. Hong Y, Song B, Chen H-D, and Gao X-H. Melanocytes and Skin Immunity. *J Investig Dermatol Simp Proc* 2015;17:37–9.

21. Manga P, Elbuluk N, and Orlow SJ. Recent advances in understanding vitiligo. *F1000 Res* 2016;5:2234.

22. Boniface K, Taïeb A, and Seneschal J. New insights into immune mechanisms of vitiligo. *G Ital Dermatol Venereol* 2016;151:44–54.

23. Ezzedine K, Eleftheriadou V, Whitton M, and van Geel N. Vitiligo. *Lancet* 2015;386:74–84.

24. Yildirim M, Baysal V, Inaloz HS, Kesici D, and Delibas N. The role of oxidants and antioxidants in generalized vitiligo. *J Dermatol* 2003;30:104–8.

25. Casp CB, She J-X, and Mccormack WT. Association of the catalase gene (CAT) with vitiligo susceptibility. *Pigment Cell Res* 2002;15:62–6.

26. Gavalasa NG, Akhtara S, Gawkrodgerb DJ, Watsona PF, Weetmana AP, and Kemp EH. Analysis of allelic variants in the catalase gene in patients with the skin depigmenting disorder vitiligo. *Biochem Biophys Res Commun* 2006; 345:1586–91.

27. Schallreuter KU, Wood JM, Pittelkow MR, Gütlich M, Lemke KR, Rödl W, Swanson NN, Hitzemann K, and Ziegler I. Regulation of melanin biosynthesis in the human epidermis by tetrahydrobiopterin. *Science* 1994;263:1444–6.

28. Hasse S, Gibbons NCJ, Rokos H, Marles LK, and Schallreuter KU. Perturbed 6-tetrahydrobiopterin recycling via decreased dihydropteridine reductase in vitiligo: More evidence for H2O2 stress. *J Investig Dermatol* 2004;122:307–13.

29. Iannella G, Antonio GA, Didona D, Didona B, Granata G, Manno A, Pasquariello B, and Magliulo G. Vitiligo: Pathogenesis, clinical variants and treatment approaches. *Autoimmun Rev* 2016;15:335–43.

30. Dell'Anna ML, Ottaviani M, Bellei B, Albanesi V, Cossarizza A, Rossi L, and Picardo M. Membrane lipid defects are responsible for the generation of reactive oxygen species in peripheral blood mononuclear cells from vitiligo patients. *J Cell Physiol* 2010;223:187–93.

31. Zhou X-J, and Zhang H. Autophagy in immunity: Implications in etiology of autoimmune/autoinflammatory diseases. *Autophagy* 2012;8:1286–99.

32. Nagar R. Autophagy: A brief overview in perspective of dermatology. *Indian J Dermatol Venereol Leprol* 2017;83:290–7.

33. Mizushima N, Levine B, Cuervo AM, and Klionsky DJ. Autophagy fights disease through cellular self-digestion. *Nature* 2008;451:1069–75.

34. Picardo M. Vitiligo: New insights. *Br J Dermatol* 2012;16:472–3.

35. He Y, Li S, Zhang W, Dai W, Cui T, Wang G, Gao T, and Li C. Dysregulated autophagy increased melanocyte sensitivity to H2O2-induced oxidative stress in vitiligo. *Sci Rep* 2017;7:42394.

36. Lerner AB. Vitiligo. *J Investig Dermatol* 1959;32:285–310.

37. Lerner AB, Shiohara T, Boissy RE, Jacobson KA, Lamoreux LM, and Moellmann GE. A mouse model for vitiligo. *J Investig Dermatol* 1986;87:299–304.

38. Ernfors P. Cellular origin and developmental mechanisms during the formation of skin melanocytes. *Exp Cell Res* 2010;316:1397–407.

39. Kaucká M, and Adameyko I. Non-canonical functions of the peripheral nerve. *Exp Cell Res* 2014;321:17–24.

40. Wu C-S, Yu H-S, Chang H-R, Yu C-L, Yu C-L, and Wu B-N. Cutaneous blood flow and adrenoceptor response increase in segmental-type vitiligo lesions. *J Dermatol Sci* 2000;23:53–62.

41. Yehuda R, Brand S, and Yang R-K. Plasma neuropeptide Y concentrations in combat exposed veterans: Relationship to trauma exposure, recovery from PTSD, and coping. *Biol Psychiatry* 2005;59:660–3.

42. Morrone A, Picardo M, de Luca C, Terminali O, Passi S, and Ippolito F. Catecholamines and vitiligo. *Pigm Cell Res* 1992;5:65–9.

43. Bagherani N. The newest hypothesis about vitiligo: Most of the suggested pathogeneses of vitiligo can be attributed to lack of one factor, zinc-alpha2-glycoprotein. *ISRN Dermatol* 2012;2012:405268.

44. Yadav AK, Singh P, and Khunger N. Clinicopathologic analysis of stable and unstable vitiligo: A study of 66 cases. *Am J Dermatopathol* 2016;38:608–13.

45. Bose SK. Probable mechanisms of loss of Merkel cells in completely depigmented skin of stable vitiligo. *J Dermatol* 1994;2:725–8.

CLINICAL PROFILE OF VITILIGO

Chapter 6

CLASSIFICATION OF VITILIGO

Vineet Relhan and Rubina Jassi

CONTENTS

INTRODUCTION

Vitiligo is a disorder of pigmentation which may involve skin, mucosa, or hair. Classification of vitiligo is essential to identify the clinical spectrum, severity, and prognosis, as well as management of the disease. With advancements in science, there has been a dynamic change in the classification of vitiligo. In this chapter, we discuss various landmarks in the classification of vitiligo that have been used in the past as well as the recent standard accepted classification. Most of the classifications of vitiligo classified it on a clinical basis; however, a few also classified vitiligo according to pathological, therapeutic, or surgical parameters.

EVOLUTION OF THE CLASSIFICATION OF VITILIGO

Jerret and Szabo, in 1958, classified vitiligo as absolute and partial (subtypes I and II, respectively) depending upon the complete or partial absence of melanocytes [1].

In 1959, Lerner classified vitiligo into three groups [2]:

1. Segmental, localized, partial, or focal vitiligo (dermatomal pattern)
2. Vitiligo vulgaris (generalized or over hands, face, axillae, and limbs)
3. Complete, total, or universal

In 1988, Koga and Tango described two forms of vitiligo as type A and type B, depending on the local response to physostigmine, mentioned next [3].

- *Type A Vitiligo*: Type A was nondermatomal vitiligo. These lesions had no response to physostigmine. This type was responsive to topical steroids, thereby supporting an autoimmune mechanism of pathogenesis.
- *Type B Vitiligo*: Type B was dermatomal vitiligo, associated with dysfunction of sympathetic nerves. Such lesions were nonresponsive to topical steroids but responded well to nialamide (irreversible monoamine oxidase inhibitor).

Behl et al., in 2003, classified vitiligo on the basis of clinical stage to assist the management of vitiligo on the basis of prognosis of the disease [4]. They classified vitiligo into progressive and quiescent stages. Progressive vitiligo (V1) included features like development of new lesions, increase in size of old lesions, and ill-defined borders of lesion(s), while quiescent vitiligo (V2) was characterized by non-appearance of new lesions, static lesions, well-defined lesions with hyperpigmented borders, and lesions decreasing in size or disappearing.

Later, in 2010, Taieb and Picardo classified vitiligo into four main types as nonsegmental vitiligo (NSV), segmental vitiligo (SV), mixed (NSV+SV), and unclassified, as described next [5].

1. Nonsegmental vitiligo (NSV): Focal, acrofacial, mucosal, generalized, universal
2. Segmental (SV): Focal, mucosal, uni-/bi-/multisegmental
3. Mixed (NSV+SV)
4. Unclassified: Mucosal (one site), multifocal nonsegmental

Based upon this classification, the most recent and accepted classification of vitiligo was given at the Vitiligo Global Issues Consensus Conference (VGICC) in 2012. They classified vitiligo in three major forms: Nonsegmental vitiligo, segmental vitiligo, and unclassified/undetermined vitiligo [6]. The description and the subtypes of each are mentioned next [6].

SEGMENTAL VITILIGO

SV is characterized by depigmented macules strictly involving one or more segments of the body. These lesions never cross the midline. Body hair involvement is more frequently seen with SV as compared to NSV. SV has a rapid and progressive onset, but only up to 6–24 months, following which further extension is rarely seen. SV can be uni-, bi-, or plurisegmental depending upon the number of lesions.

NONSEGMENTAL VITILIGO

NSV is characterized by depigmented macules that vary in size from a few to several centimeters in diameter. The macules may be present on both sides of body and tend to have symmetrical distribution. Body hair involvement is less likely to be seen in NSV compared to SV. NSV further includes the following variants of vitiligo:

a. *Acrofacial*: Limited to face, head, hands, and feet, characteristically over the distal fingers and facial orifices.
b. *Mucosal*: Involvement of either oral or genital mucosa or both. It may be associated with generalized vitiligo, but if present in isolation for 2 years or more, it is categorized under unclassified vitiligo.
c. *Generalized/Common*: Multiple depigmented macules and patches all over the body. Vitiligo lesions are usually symmetrical. Fingers, hands, and face are generally the initial sites, but depigmentation may extend to involve any part of the body.

d. *Universal:* The term *universalis* refers to the extent of the disease, involving up to 80%–90% body surface area. This is the most extensive form of vitiligo. However, a few specks of normal pigmentation can be seen. The hair follicles may be spared in this type.

e. *Mixed:* Coexistence of SV and NSV is termed *mixed vitiligo.* SV usually precedes NSV.

f. *Rare forms:* Vitiligo punctata, minor, and follicular vitiligo, have been listed under this category.

Descriptions of these variants are given next along with other rare variants not listed in the classification.

UNCLASSIFIED/UNDETERMINED VITILIGO

This includes two forms of vitiligo that do not fit into either SV or NSV. They are:

a. *Focal vitiligo:* Small, discrete, isolated patches of vitiligo which do not fit into SV or NSV classifications after at least 2 years of onset, but later may progress into either of the two forms.

b. *Mucosal vitiligo:* Isolated involvement of oral or genital mucosae without cutaneous involvement until 2 years of follow-up.

RARE VARIANTS OF VITILIGO

a. *Tri-, quadri-, pentachrome vitiligo* [7]: These lesions are classified according to the number of shades of pigmentation that surround the depigmented macule.

Trichrome vitiligo	Quadrichrome vitiligo	Pentachrome vitiligo
Presence of narrow/ broadband of intermediate pigmentation between central depigmentation and normal skin	Presence of four colors of pigmentation, usually seen in dark individuals	Presence of five sequential shades of pigmentation in the order white, tan, brown, blue gray, and normal skin color

b. *Inflammatory vitiligo* [7]: Presents in the form of erythematous lesions with raised borders, and the lesions are associated with an itching and burning sensation.

c. *Blue vitiligo* [8]: Occurrence of vitiligo lesions over areas of postinflammatory hypermelanosis. Such lesions have been observed in acquired immunodeficiency syndrome (AIDS) patients.

d. *Occupational/contact vitiligo:* A distinct entity precipitated by exposure to chemicals (aliphatic or aromatic derivatives of phenols and catechols) [9–12]. This depigmentation may be limited to the site of contact or may eventually progress to involve other body parts also, mimicking NSV [13]. However, contact vitiligo is not included in any of the classifications of vitiligo.

e. *Vitiligo punctata:* Presence of discrete, well-defined, sharply demarcated, punctate-sized (1–1.5 mm) macules over the body at any site [6].

f. *Vitiligo minor:* Partial defect of pigmentation [6], thereby presenting as hypochromic macules rather than depigmented macules. The term *hypopigmented vitiligo* may be used to denote vitiligo minor [14].

g. *Follicular vitiligo:* One of the rare entities in vitiligo, primarily targeting the hair follicle melanocytes. Leukotrichia can be seen in the vitiliginous and nonvitiliginous areas. Although NSV lesions are less likely to show leukotrichia, NSV is usually associated either before or after the onset of follicular vitiligo [15,16].

In addition to the clinical classifications, vitiligo can also be classified on the basis of surgical stability [6]:

a. *Stable:* Any vitiligo patient with 12 months of photographically assessed stability is considered suitable for surgical purposes.

b. *Unstable:* Patients with increased activity in the lesions in the past 12 months are surgically not acceptable.

REFERENCES

1. Jarrett A, and Szabo G. The pathological varieties of vitiligo and their response to treatment with meladinine. *J Dermatol* 1956;68:313–26.

2. Lerner AB. Vitiligo. *J Invest Dermatol* 1959;32:285–310.

3. Koga M, and Tango T. Clinical features and course of type A and type B vitiligo. *Br J Dermatol* 1988;118:223–8.

4. Behl PN, Aggarwal A, and Srivastava G. Vitiligo. In: Behl PN, and Srivastava G, eds. *Practice of Dermatology*, 9th ed. New Delhi: CBS Publishers; 2003, pp. 238–41.

5. Taieb A, and Picardo M. Epidemiology, definitions and classification. In: Picardo M, and Taieb A, eds. *Vitiligo.* Heidelberg: Springer Verlag; 2010, pp. 13–24.

6. Ezzedine K, Lim HW, Suzuki T et al. Revised classification/nomenclature of vitiligo and related issues: The Vitiligo Global Issues Consensus Conference. *Pigment Cell Melanoma Res* 2012;25(3):E1–E13.

7. Sehgal VN, and Srivastava G. Vitiligo: Compendium of clinico-epidemiological features. *Indian J Dermatol Venereol Leprol* 2007;73:149–56.

8. Ivker R, Goldaber M, and Buchness MR. Blue vitiligo. *J Am Acad Dermatol* 1994;30:829–31.

9. Lerner AB. On the etiology of vitiligo and gray hair. *Am J Med* 1971;51:141–7.

10. Boissy RE, and Nordlund JJ. Biology in vitiligo. In: Arndt K, LeBoit PE, Robinson JK, and Wintroub BU, eds. *Cutaneous Medicine and Surgery: An Integrated Program in Dermatology.* Philadelphia: W.B. Saunders Company; 1995, pp. 1210–8.

11. Boissy RE, and Manga P. On the etiology of contact/occupational vitiligo. *Pigment Cell Res* 2004;17:208–14.

12. Boissy RE. Vitiligo. In: Picardo M, and Taieb A, eds. *Occupational Vitiligo.* Heidelberg: Springer Verlag; 2010, pp. 175–80.

13. Cummings MP, and Nordlund JJ. Chemical leukoderma: Fact or fancy. *Am J Contact Dermatitis* 1995;6:122–7.

14. Ezzedine K, Mahe A, Van Geel N et al. Hypochromic vitiligo: Delineation of a new entity. *Br J Dermatol* 2015;172:716–21.

15. Ezzedine K, Amazan E, Séneschal J et al. Follicular vitiligo: A new form of vitiligo. *Pigment Cell Melanoma Res* 2012;25:527–9.

16. Gan EY, Carlo Andre M, and Pain C. Follicular vitiligo: A report of 8 cases. *J Am Acad Dermatol* 2016;74:1178–84.

Chapter 7

VITILIGO VULGARIS

Huma Jaffar and Aditi Manu Sobti

CONTENTS

DEFINITION

Vitiligo (*vit-ill-eye-go*) is an acquired idiopathic disorder specifically destroying the melanocytes (pigment-producing cells) that results in well-defined, depigmented, and cosmetically displeasing patches on the skin or mucous membrane. Vitiligo is classified according to the area of its distribution as localized, generalized, or universal [1]. Localized types of vitiligo include focal, segmental, and mucosal, while the generalized form encompasses acrofacial, vitiligo vulgaris, and mixed varieties. Involvement of more than 80% of the body is considered as universal vitiligo. The focus of this chapter is the clinical profile of vitiligo vulgaris, one of the most common varieties of vitiligo [2–4].

EPIDEMIOLOGY

Worldwide, the reported prevalence [5] of vitiligo ranges from 0.4% to 2.0%, with variations between regions. However, Gujarat in India is reported to have the highest prevalence (8.8%) in the world [6]. Vitiligo can affect all races with same frequency, but the contrast in skin color makes it more obvious in darker-skinned individuals. Vitiligo can affect both men and women equally, but being mainly a cosmetically disfiguring disease, women present more frequently, reflecting a greater incidence. It usually affects young individuals, beginning before the age of 20 years in about half of those afflicted and by the age of 40 years in 95% of patients [7]. The mean age of onset is usually lower in those with a strong family history, reflecting the genetic etiology [8].

CLINICAL FEATURES

The symptoms of vitiligo vulgaris are mainly related to the embarrassment they cause due to cosmetic disfigurement. The lesions are typically asymptomatic. However, a rare variant, inflammatory vitiligo, can be itchy [9].

Vitiligo is typically diagnosed by the clinical presentation. The classical clinical presentation of vitiligo vulgaris is hypo- or depigmented, discrete or coalescing, macules or patches, usually symmetrically distributed with convex borders that are surrounded by normal skin (Figure 7.1a–c). The hypopigmented macules are usually sharply demarcated but may be diffuse (Figure 7.2a). Woods lamp (which emits wavelength 320–450 nm with the peak at 365 nm) examination helps to sharply demarcate the depigmented borders (Figure 7.2b). The epidermis is normal in all respects except for loss of pigmentation. Depigmented epidermis showing signs of atrophy, injury, inflammation, or other processes is typically a manifestation of some other disorder affecting the skin [9].

Vitiligo vulgaris can occur on any part of the body. The sites of predilection for vitiligo vulgaris are the fingers and wrists, axillae and groin, and body orifices, such as the mouth, eyes (Figure 7.3), and genitals. It may present as single or multiple lesions coalescing to affect a large surface area of the skin. Vitiligo is often discovered insidiously during the summer or spring, when the surrounding normal skin tends to get darker due to tanning, making the contrast with lesional skin more obvious [10].

Koebner, or isomorphic, phenomenon is an interesting sign seen in vitiligo, where the lesions can develop at the site of trauma. This phenomenon can be hypothesized to be an explanation for lesions of vitiligo vulgaris affecting particular sites. In one study [11], an observation was made that younger individuals had a higher incidence of lesions on the lower extremities compared to older individuals, who had more lesions on the upper limbs. The authors attributed this distribution to the trauma effect: the lower extremities in the younger age group were more prone to injuries during outdoor play activities, while the hands and elbows of the older individuals might be traumatized with the pressure of elbows on desks or household activities involving the hands and wrists. For similar reasons, depigmentation in the beard and axillary areas in men and women, respectively, were commonly observed due to shaving-induced trauma.

Hair follicles can be affected by vitiligo vulgaris and may present as depigmented hairs called leukotrichia (Figure 7.4). Leukotrichia may serve as an important prognostic sign. When present, leukotrichia is associated with poor prognosis, indicating resistance to medical treatment. Presence of pigmented hairs when present in vitiliginous lesions is a predictor of good response to treatment, as evident in the form of perifollicular repigmentation (Figure 7.5a,b). The hair follicles being naturally rich in melanocytes may account for this repigmentation [12].

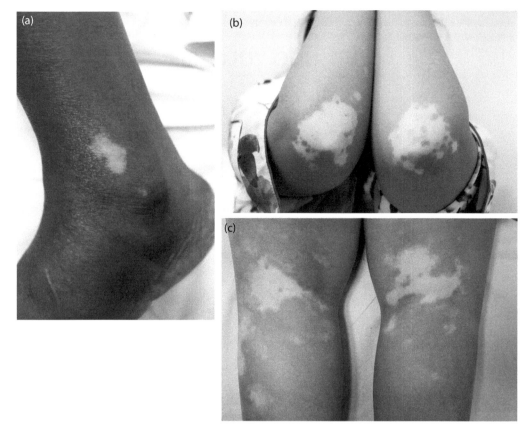

Figure 7.1 Depigmented vitiligo vulgaris: at left ankle (a); bilateral symmetrical lesions at elbows (b) and knees (c).

The color of vitiligo vulgaris ranges from hypo- to depigmented lesions, depending on the severity of loss of pigment. A few other colored variants are reported, including trichrome vitiligo, quadrichrome vitiligo, and pentachrome blue vitiligo. In trichrome vitiligo, a tan zone between normal and depigmented skin is seen (Figure 7.6). This tan zone shows a greater number of inflammatory cells, Langerhans cells, and melanophages than vitiliginous or normal skin. In addition, the number of melanocytes in the tan zone is greater than vitiliginous but lesser than the normal skin. Quadrichrome vitiligo has additional marginal or perifollicular hyperpigmentation. This perifollicular pigmentation is seen more in the darker skin types and in the areas of repigmentation. In addition to medium brown unaffected skin color, the colors include white, tan, dark brown, and black [13]. Pentachrome blue vitiligo has additional blue-gray macules due to the presence of melanin incontinence in dermal melanophages [14].

COURSE OF DISEASE

Vitiligo vulgaris usually begins insidiously. Some studies documented that severe sunburn, pregnancy, skin trauma, and/or emotional stress may precede its onset [15]. While it has a primarily progressive course, vitiligo vulgaris can wax and wane, arrest altogether, or, rarely, spontaneously resolve. One study [16] found progressive disease in 88.8% of patients, mostly related to positive family history. When vitiligo is progressing slowly, it can occur either as centrifugal expansion of current lesions and/or include appearance of new lesions.

Minor injuries to the skin can cause depigmentation at the site of injury, called Koebner phenomenon, as discussed earlier. Scratches,

abrasions, surgical scars, skin burns, or cosmetic procedures such as dermabrasion may spread the depigmentation [17].

Arrest of depigmentation, either spontaneous or induced, allows melanocytes to regenerate from pigmented hair follicles, a potential reservoir of melanocyte stem cells, and reproduce pigment, resulting in repigmentation of lesional skin [18].

VITILIGO AND SUN DAMAGE

Several studies have been conducted on the prevalence of sun damage in depigmented skin. Although the absence of photoprotective melanocytes in vitiligo should pose more sun damage, the incidence and degree of sun damage in observed studies is much less in vitiliginous depigmented skin. This discrepancy has been observed even in individuals who had intense exposure either to natural sunlight or with psoralen plus ultraviolet A (PUVA) treatment, a recognized carcinogen [19–23].

Vitiligo and skin cancer have an interesting relationship. There are reports of decreased risk of both melanoma and nonmelanoma skin cancer (NMSC) in vitiligo patients [24]. However, it is still unclear why the vitiliginous depigmented skin is resistant to malignant transformation, and this warrants further research.

Melanoma, one of the dangerous skin cancers of the pigment-producing epidermal melanocytes, for obvious reasons cannot arise in the depigmented skin of vitiligo. However, melanoma may arise in the normal surrounding skin. Furthermore, it has been demonstrated that the development of vitiligo in patients with metastatic melanoma may portend a favorable prognosis, possibly supporting the explanation for the theory of melanocyte destruction in vitiligo [25].

With regard to NMSC, only a few reports of developing such cancers (squamous cell cancer) on the vitiliginous skin exist [26].

(a)

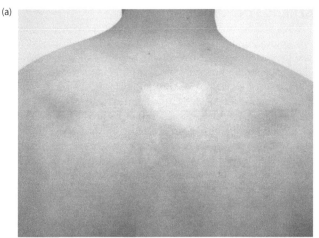

(b)

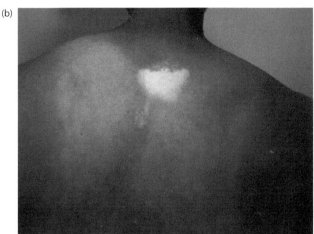

Figure 7.2 Sharply demarcated vitiligo vulgaris on the back, surrounded by a zone of hypopigmentation (a). Woods lamp accentuation of the vitiligo (b).

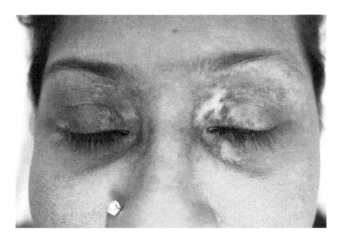

Figure 7.3 Vitiligo vulgaris predilection around eyes.

ASSOCIATIONS (TABLE 7.1)

AUTOIMMUNE DISORDERS

Vitiligo vulgaris is shown to involve an autoimmune destruction of melanocytes [17]. This autoimmune process can be seen manifesting concurrently as autoimmune diseases associated with vitiligo. The association is more commonly observed in

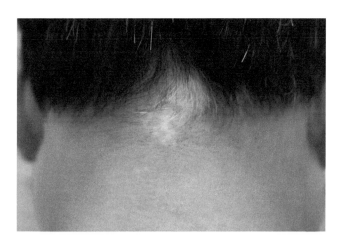

Figure 7.4 Leukotrichia (depigmented hairs); poor prognostic sign.

(a)

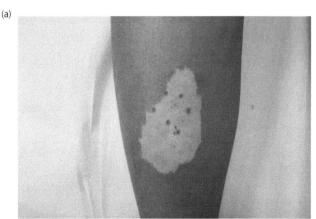

(b)

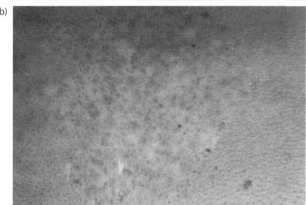

Figure 7.5 Perifollicular repigmentation on the right shin (a) and chest area (b).

generalized vitiligo vulgaris as compared to the segmental variety [8]. The strongest evidence is found with hypo- or hyperthyroid disease, ranging from 0.5% to 43% across various studies [27]. Diabetes and pernicious anemia are other common systemic associations.

In one controlled study, an increased incidence of the following autoantibodies in vitiligo patients has been reported: antinuclear (12.4%), antimicrosomal (7.1%), and anti-smooth muscle antibodies (25.7%) [28].

Vitiligo can occur in association with immune-related skin disorders like psoriasis, lichen planus, and alopecia areata. Coexistence of vitiligo, psoriasis, and lichen planus in the same individual has been reported [29,30].

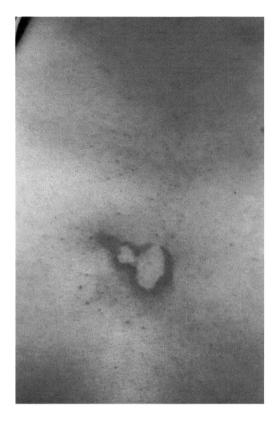

Figure 7.6 Trichrome vitiligo on the chest with a tan zone between the normal and depigmented skin.

Table 7.1 Associations of vitiligo

a. Autoimmune/immune disorders	
i. Systemic	Addison disease
	Autoimmune thyroid disease
	Diabetes mellitus
	Inflammatory bowel disease
	Multiple sclerosis
	Myasthenia gravis
	Pemphigus vulgaris
	Pernicious anemia
	Rheumatoid arthritis
	Systemic lupus erythematosus
	Alopecia areata
ii. Cutaneous	Atopic dermatitis
	Chronic urticaria
	Halo nevi
	Lichen planus
	Morphea
	Psoriasis
b. Genetic syndromes	
	APECED syndrome
	Kabuki syndrome
	MELAS syndrome
	Schmidt syndrome
	Vogt-Koyanagi-Harada disease
c. Others	
i. Systemic	Ocular anomalies
	Hearing loss
	Raised serum homocysteine levels
	Metabolic syndrome
	Sarcoidosis
ii. Cutaneous	Ichthyosis
	Twenty-nail dystrophy

GENETIC SYNDROMES

Vitiligo vulgaris may also be associated with a number of inherited syndromes. Autoimmune polyendocrinopathy candidiasis-ectodermal dysplasia (APECED) syndrome is associated (also called polyglandular autoimmune syndrome type 1 [PGA1]); it is a combination of Addison disease, hypoparathyroidism, ectodermal dysplasia, and/or chronic mucocutaneous candidiasis, and may also include alopecia areata, vitiligo, malabsorption syndrome, gonadal failure, pernicious anemia, chronic active hepatitis, corneal dystrophy, and enamel dystrophy [31]. Another similar syndrome, called Schmidt syndrome/polyglandular autoimmune syndrome type 2 (PGA2), also presents with polyglandular failure (Addison disease, hypothyroidism, and type I diabetes mellitus), occasional vitiligo, and/or hypogonadism [32].

Kabuki syndrome is a rare multiple malformation disorder characterized by developmental delay, distinct facial anomalies, congenital heart defects, limb and skeletal anomalies, and short stature. Associated autoimmune abnormalities are idiopathic thrombocytopenic purpura, hemolytic anemia, thyroiditis, and vitiligo [33].

A rare progressive neurodegenerative disorder, mitochondrial myopathy, encephalopathy, lactic acidosis, and stroke (MELAS) syndrome, presents with central nervous system abnormalities, neurosensory hearing loss, diabetes mellitus, and cardiomyopathy. One study found vitiligo in 11% (3/28) of MELAS patients [34].

Vogt-Koyanagi-Harada syndrome is a rare systemic T-cell—mediated disorder that can affect the melanocytes in all three sites mentioned previously, causing meningitis (nausea, vomiting, photophobia) from brain involvement, tinnitus and hearing loss from inner ear involvement, and eye pain, visual changes, and loss of vision from eye involvement. It can be associated with vitiligo (8%–100%) [35–37].

OTHERS

Since melanocytes are also present in the retina of eyes, and the middle ear, vitiligo may affect these organs. Up to 40% of patients with vitiligo may present with some form of ocular involvement in the form of choroidal anomalies, uveitis, iritis, and some degree of fundal pigment disturbance. Functional loss of melanocytes in the middle ear (stria vascularis) is reported to be associated with hearing loss in 20% of patients [9,17,38–41].

Homocysteine levels may represent a new biomarker of the extent of vitiligo. A study in Egypt in 2014 [42] proposed that elevation of serum homocysteine (Hcy) level might be a precipitating factor for vitiligo in predisposed individuals. Elevation in Hcy is associated with relative deficiencies of vitamin B_{12}, suggesting that aggressive supplementation with this vitamin may benefit vitiligo patients.

Recently, there has been growing evidence that vitiligo can also be related to systemic inflammatory disorders, such as obesity and the metabolic syndrome characterized by a combination of abdominal obesity, glucose intolerance, diabetes mellitus, dyslipidemia, and hypertension. This association is also blamed on homocysteine. Homocysteine is known to inhibit the enzyme tyrosinase that participates in melanin synthesis. It is also involved in cardiovascular risks in patients with metabolic syndrome. Thus, studies suggest that the presence of vitiligo is correlated with a family history of cardiovascular disease [43].

SOCIAL IMPACT

Vitiligo is a socially stigmatized discoloration of skin. This has been documented for centuries in the diverse ancient literature [44]. Vitiligo, a socially devastating condition, may lead to embarrassment and poor self-confidence with significant impact on the social, marital, educational, and mental health aspects of life. Studies of vitiligo patients using the Dermatology Life Quality Index (DLQI), the most widely used questionnaire to measure the impact of skin disease on life quality, have revealed these significant bearings. Quality of life can be affected over a wide range of scores (from 4.82 to 14.72). The worst DLQI scores in vitiligo patients were reported with the clinical variables including the involvement of exposed body parts, darker skin type, larger surface area, and poor response to treatment. The psychosocial affect was stated to be more common in women and children [45].

The prevalence of psychiatric morbidity (depressive episodes, adjustment disorders, and anxiety) was seen in 25% of patients with vitiligo. In some studies, the physical disfigurement caused by depigmented patches emphasized the importance of physical appearance in psychological adjustment [45].

CONCLUSION

Vitiligo vulgaris is a common form of vitiligo which runs a chronic course with progressive skin depigmentation and psychosocial impact. A better understanding of the disease and evaluation of psychosocial impact may help the treating physician to deal with patients in a holistic manner.

REFERENCES

1. Alikhan A, Felsten LM, Daly M, and Petronic-Rosic V. Vitiligo: A comprehensive overview. Part I. Introduction, epidemiology, quality of life, diagnosis, differential diagnosis, associations, histopathology, etiology, and work-up. *J Am Acad Dermatol* 2011;65:473–91.

2. Martis J, Bhat R, Nandakishore B, and Shetty J N. Clinical study of vitiligo. *Indian J Dermatol Venereol Leprol* 2002;68(2):92–3.

3. Shajil EM, Agrawal D, Vagadia K, Marfatia YS, and Begum R. Vitiligo: Clinical profiles in Vadodara, Gujarat. *Indian J Dermatol* 2006;51:100–4.

4. Shah H, Mehta A, and Astik B. Clinical and sociodemographic study of vitiligo. *Indian J Dermatol Venereol Leprol* 2008;74:701.

5. Silverberg NB. The epidemiology of vitiligo. *Curr Dermatol Rep* 2015;4(1):36–43.

6. Dwivedi M, Laddha NC, Shajil EM, Shah BJ, and Begum R. The ACE gene I/D polymorphism is not associated with generalized vitiligo susceptibility in Gujarat population. *Pigm Cell Melanoma Res* 2008;21:407–8.

7. Nordlund JJ, and Majumder PP. Recent investigations on vitiligo vulgaris *Dermatol Clin* 1997;15:69–78.

8. Zhang Z, Xu SX, Zhang FY et al. The analysis of genetics and associated autoimmune diseases in Chinese vitiligo patients. *Arch Dermatol Res* 2009;301:167–73.

9. Ortonne JP. Vitiligo and other disorders of hypopigmentation. In: Bolognia J, Jorizzo J, and Schaffer J, eds. *Dermatology*, 3rd ed. Philadelphia: Mosby Elsevier; 2008.

10. Kyriakis KP, Palamaras I, Tsele E, Michailides C, and Terzoudi S. Case detection rates of vitiligo by gender and age. *Indian J Dermatol* 2009;48:328–9.

11. Speeckaert, R, and van Geel N. Distribution patterns in generalized vitiligo. *J Eur Acad Dermatol Venereol* 2014;28:755–62.

12. Falabella R. Vitiligo and the melanocyte reservoir. *Indian J Dermatol* 2009;54(4):3–318.

13. Fargnoli MC, and Bolognia JL. Pentachrome vitiligo. *J Am Acad Dermatol* 1995;33(5):853–6.

14. Chandrashekar L. Dermatoscopy of blue vitiligo. *Clin Exp Dermatol* 2009;34:e125–6.

15. Mason CP, and Gawkrodger DJ. Vitiligo presentation in adults. *Clin Exp Dermatol* 2005;30:344–5.

16. Hann SK, Chun WH, and Park YK. Clinical characteristics of progressive vitiligo. *Int J Dermatol* 1997;36(5):353–5.

17. Halder RM, and Taliaferro SJ. Vitiligo. In: Wolff K, Goldsmith L, Katz S, Gilchrest B, Paller A, and Lefell D, eds. *Fitzpatrick's Dermatology in General Medicine*, 7th ed. New York: McGraw-Hill; 2008, pp. 616–22.

18. Richmond JM, and Harris JE. Vitiligo. In: Gaspari AA, Tyring SK, and Kaplan DH, eds. *Clinical and Basic Immunodermatology*. Switzerland: Springer International Publishing; 2017, pp. 511–26.

19. Abdullah AN, and Keczkes K. Cutaneous and ocular side-effects of PUVA photochemotherapy—A 10–year follow-up study [Review]. *Clin Exp Dermatol* 1989;14(6):421–4.

20. Schallreuter KU, Tobin DJ, and Panske A. Decreased photodamage and low incidence of non-melanoma skin cancer in 136 sun-exposed Caucasian patients with vitiligo. *Dermatology* 2002;204(3):194–201.

21. Calanchini-Postizzi E, and Frenk E. Long-term actinic damage in sun-exposed vitiligo and normally pigmented skin. *Dermatologica* 1987;174:266–71.

22. Wildfang IL, Jacobsen FK, and Thestrup-Pedersen K. PUVA treatment of vitiligo: A retrospective study of 59 patients. *Acta Derm Venereol* 1992;74(4):305–6.

23. Yashiro K, Nakagawa T, Takaiwa T, and Inai M. Actinic keratoses arising only on sun-exposed vitiligo skin. *Clin Exp Dermatol* 1999;24(3):199–201.

24. Teulings, HE, Overkamp, M, Ceylan, E, Nieuweboer-Krobotova L, Bos JD, Nijsten T, Wolkerstorfer AW, Luiten RM, and van der Veen JP. Decreased risk of melanoma and nonmelanoma skin cancer in patients with vitiligo: A survey among 1307 patients and their partners. *Br J Dermatol* 2013;168:162–71.

25. Nordlund JJ, Kirkwood J, Forget BM et al. Vitiligo in patients with metastatic melanoma: A good prognostic sign. *J Am Acad Dermatol* 1983;9:689–95.

26. Seo SL, and Kim IH. Squamous cell carcinoma in a patient with generalized vitiligo. *J Am Acad Dermatol* 2001;45(6):S227–S9.

27. Pagovich OE, Silverberg JI, Freilich E, and Silverberg NB. Thyroid abnormalities in pediatric patients with vitiligo in New York City. *Cutis* 2008;81:463–6.

28. Hann SK, Im S, Kim HI, Kim HS, Lee YJ, and Park YK. Increased incidence of antismooth muscle antibody in Korean vitiligo patients. *J Dermatol* 1993;20:679–83.

29. Chandrashekar L. Red in white sea sign. *J Eur Acad Dermatol Venereol* 2009;23:368.

30. Ujiie H, Sawamura D, and Shimizu H. Development of lichen planus and psoriasis on lesions of vitiligo vulgaris. *Clin Exp Dermatol* 2006;31(3):375–7.

31. Ahonen P, Myllarniemi S, Sipila I, and Perheentupa J. Clinical variation of autoimmune polyendocrinopathy-candidiasis ectodermal dystrophy (APECED) in a series of 68 patients. *N Engl J Med* 1990;322:1829–36.

32. Butler MG, Hodes ME, Conneally PM, Biegel AA, and Wright JC. Linkage analysis in a large kindred with autosomal dominant transmission of polyglandular autoimmune disease type II (Schmidt syndrome). *Am J Med Genet* 1984;18:61–5.

33. McGaughran J, Aftimos S, Jefferies C, and Winship I. Clinical phenotypes of nine cases of Kabuki syndrome from New Zealand. *Clin Dysmorphol* 2001;10:257–62.

34. Karvonen SL, Haapasaari KM, Kallioinen M, Oikarinen A, Hassinen IE, and Majamaa K. Increased prevalence of vitiligo, but no evidence of premature ageing, in the skin of patients with bp 3243 mutation in mitochondrial DNA in the mitochondrial encephalomyopathy, lactic acidosis and stroke-like episodes syndrome (MELAS). *Br J Dermatol* 1999;140:634–9.

35. Tsuruta D, Hamada T, Teramae H, Mito H, and Ishii M. Inflammatory vitiligo in Vogt-Koyanagi-Harada disease. *J Am Acad Dermatol* 2001;44:129–31.

36. Wong SS, Ng SK, and Lee HM. Vogt-Koyanagi-Harada disease: Extensive vitiligo with prodromal generalized erythroderma. *Dermatology* 1999;198:65–8.

37. Barnes L. Vitiligo and the Vogt-Koyanagi-Harada syndrome. *Dermatol Clin* 1988;6:229–39.

38. Flynn GE. Bilateral uveitis, poliosis, and vitiligo: With a hereditary factor. *Am J Ophthalmol* 1952;35:568–72.

39. Albert DM, Nordlund JJ, and Lerner AB. Ocular abnormalities occurring with vitiligo. *Ophthalmology* 1979;86:1145–60.

40. Albert DM, Sober AJ, and Fitzpatrick TB. Iritis in patients with cutaneous melanoma and vitiligo. *Arch Ophthalmol* 1978;96:2081–4.

41. Cowan CL Jr, Halder RM, Grimes PE, Chakrabarti SG, and Kenney JA Jr. Ocular disturbances in vitiligo. *J Am Acad Dermatol* 1986;15:17–24.

42. Sabry HH, Sabry JH, and Hashim HM. Serum levels of homocysteine, vitamin B12, and folic acid in vitiligo. *Egyptian J Dermatol Venereol [Serial Online]* 2014;34 [cited 2017 Jun 19]):65–9.

43. Ataş H, and Gönül M. Increased risk of metabolic syndrome in patients with vitiligo. *Balkan Med J* 2017;34(3):219–25.

44. Millington GWM, and Levell NJ. Vitiligo: The historical curse of depigmentation. *Int J Dermatol* 2007;46:990–5.

45. Pahwa P, Mehta M, Khaitan BK, Sharma VK, and Ramam M. The psychosocial impact of vitiligo in Indian patients. *Indian J Dermatol Venereol Leprol* 2013;79:679–85.

Chapter 8

SEGMENTAL VITILIGO

Pooja Agarwal

CONTENTS

INTRODUCTION

Vitiligo is defined as an idiopathic, well-circumscribed melanotic skin disorder characterized by milky white patches of variable size and shape. It affects 1%–2% of the world population [1]. Clinical vitiligo was first classified into two subtypes: nonsegmental vitiligo (NSV) and segmental vitiligo (SV) by Koga in 1977 [2]. Koga and Tango proposed that vitiligo in a nondermatomal distribution be referred to as Type A and vitiligo in a dermatomal distribution be Type B, the latter of which corresponds to what is known today as SV [3]. NSV accounts for 85%–95% of cases and usually presents with symmetrical lesions. By contrast, SV is characterized by certain features which include unilateral lesions with a dermatomal distribution and a tendency to occur at an earlier age than the nonsegmental form.

Recently, a consensus emerged that SV be classified separately from all other forms of vitiligo and that the term "vitiligo" be used as an umbrella term for all nonsegmental forms of vitiligo, including "mixed vitiligo," in which segmental and nonsegmental vitiligo are combined and which is considered a subgroup of vitiligo [4].

EPIDEMIOLOGY

SV constitutes 27.9% of all vitiligo cases [5]. The majority of SV cases occur in childhood and form the bulk of pediatric vitiligo cases. In children, the incidence of SV is 19%, as compared to 5% in adults [6].

PATHOGENESIS

The etiopathogenesis of SV remains unclear. However, several hypotheses have been proposed, including neuronal mechanisms and a mosaicism hypothesis [7–9].

This form of vitiligo is usually believed to be limited in nature, and secondary autoimmunity is not seen in the majority of cases. In clinical case reviews across the globe, children with SV do not report any thyroid disease or other autoimmune disease, whereas 10.7%–26% of children with generalized vitiligo may have discernible autoimmune abnormalities [10–13].

CLINICAL FEATURES

The typical lesion of SV is not significantly much different from that of NSV. Both may initially appear as focal or localized vitiligo, which involves a small area [14]. However, SV has a distinct natural history and unique clinical features. SV is characterized by early onset, rapid progression, and then a stable persistence. There are no specific precipitating factors [3,7,15]. Koebnerization is seen rarely in SV as opposed to nonsegmental disease.

The clinical pattern of the lesions is the most defining characteristic of SV, yet there is no consensus regarding it. Dermatomal pattern is believed to be the most common, and an area roughly related to the trigeminal dermatome is the most commonly affected. (Figure 8.1) [3,7,14]. Some authors have suggested SV to follow Blaschko's lines also [8,9,11]. However, specific patterns which do not follow dermatomal, blaschkoid, or acupuncture lines have been described on the face recently [16,17].

A common association of SV is the occurrence of white hair (i.e., poliosis, leukotrichia) in the lesional skin. This suggests that SV tends to involve the hair compartment sooner as compared to NSV, and hence has a poorer response to medical management [12].

Rarely, SV can cross the midline or occur in two contralateral segments [16].

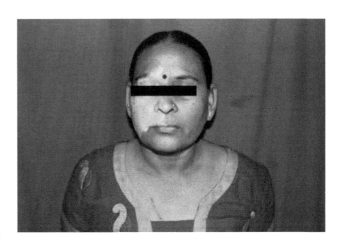

Figure 8.1   Segmental vitiligo in a 40-year-old female associated with leukotrichia of eyelashes.

Table 8.1 Differences between segmental and nonsegmental vitiligo

	Segmental vitiligo	Nonsegmental vitiligo
Age of onset	Often in childhood	Variable
Distribution	Unilateral/patterned	Bilateral, tendency toward symmetry
Leukotrichia	Very common	Variable
Progression	Rapid but limited progression	Chronic progressive course
Course	Predictable	Unpredictable
Associated abnormalities	Rare	Autoimmune disease may be seen
Family history	Usually absent	May be present
Medical therapy	Resistant to medical therapy	Variable result
Surgical therapy	Good response	Unpredictable results

Differentiating features between segmental and nonsegmental vitiligo are summarized in Table 8.1. It has been seen that in rare instances SV may progress into a generalized form, and that entity is called *mixed vitiligo* [18]. The coexistence of generalized and segmental vitiligo is seen in some patients and it may indicate that mixed vitiligo represents type 2 mosaicism of Happle [19–21]. It is observed that when both SV and NSV occur together, depigmentation and leukotrichia are more prominent in the segmental lesions than in the nonsegmental lesions. It has also been noted that in the same patient, segmental lesions do not respond as well to medical treatment as the focal lesions. This is in accordance with the theory that the segmental lesions of type 2 mosaicism are more severe than the nonsegmental type [19–21].

TREATMENT

Although medical treatment is often helpful in SV, complete repigmentation is almost always difficult to achieve. Facial lesions, shorter duration, and earlier initial response to therapy seem to be the favorable factors for medical therapy [22]. Medical management of SV is similar to nonsegmental lesions and includes the following:

- Topical corticosteroid may be tried as first-line therapy in SV. Potency of steroid seems to be the main factor in eliciting the response [23].
- Topical calcineurin inhibitors have shown good results because of their melanocyte-stimulating effect in addition to their immunomodulator action. They have the added advantage of fewer side effects than steroids [24,25].
- Narrowband ultraviolet B (NBUVB) and targeted phototherapy have shown inconsistent response in repigmentation in SV because of the depleted melanocyte reservoir in hair follicles.

A therapeutic trial of minimum 6 months may be given with topical therapy before declaring it as ineffective [25].

Patients with SV are considered to be good candidates for surgical treatment because of the stable and limited nature of the disease [26]. Surgical treatment should be considered as first-line therapy in patients with leukotrichia because medical management is bound to fail in these cases. Surgical treatments include [27]:

- Autologous epidermal grafting. This includes punch graft, Thiersch graft, blister graft, and full-thickness skin graft.
- Transplantation of melanocyte suspensions.
- Hair follicle transplantation. This is a novel procedure based on the concept of the presence of undifferentiated stem cells in the hair follicle. These cells form an excellent reservoir of melanocytes responsible for repigmentation. An additional advantage

of this procedure is the ease and minimal postoperative scarring [28].

PROGNOSIS AND COUNSELING

Vitiligo is one of those dermatological disorders where the psychological impact of disease causes more stress than the disease itself, so counseling of the patient and the family member forms a major part of the treatment. Since SV has a rapidly progressive course, it can cause great alarm to the patient as well as the guardian (in case of children). The limited nature of the disease and restriction of the depigmentation to a well-defined segment must be emphasized while counseling patients. Various therapeutic modalities and superior results of surgical intervention should be discussed in detail with each patient before starting any treatment.

REFERENCES

1. Shajil EM, Agrawal D, Vagadia K et al. Vitiligo: Clinical profiles in Vadodara, Gujarat. *Indian J Dermatol* 2006;51:100–4.
2. Koga M. Vitiligo: A new classification and therapy. *Br J Dermatol* 1977;97:255–61.
3. Koga M, and Tango T. Clinical features and course of type A and type B vitiligo. *Br J Dermatol* 1988;118:223–8.
4. Ezzedine K, Lim HW, Suzuki T et al. Revised classification/nomenclature of vitiligo and related issues: The Vitiligo Global Issues Consensus Conference. *Pigment Cell Melanoma Res* 2012 May;25(3):e1–13.
5. Handa S, Pandhi R, and Kaur I. Vitiligo: A retrospective comparative analysis of treatment modalities in 500 patients. *J Dermatol* 2001 Sep;28(9):461–6.
6. Halder RM, Grimes PE, Cowan CA et al. Childhood vitiligo. *J Am Acad Dermatol* 2003;20:207–10.
7. Hann SK, and Lee HJ. Segmental vitiligo: Clinical findings in 208 patients. *J Am Acad Dermatol* 1996;35:671–4.
8. Bolognia JL, Orlow SJ, and Glick SA. Lines of Blaschko. *J Am Acad Dermatol* 1994;32:157–90.
9. Taïeb A, Morice-Picard F, Jouary T et al. Segmental vitiligo as the possible expression of cutaneous somatic mosaicism: Implications for common nonsegmental vitiligo. *Pigment Cell Melanoma Res* 2008;21:646–52.
10. Pagovich OE, Silverberg JI, Freilich E et al. Thyroid abnormalities in pediatric patients with vitiligo in New York City. *Cutis* 2008;81:463–6.
11. Iacovelli P, Sinagra JL, Vidolin AP et al. Relevance of thyroiditis and of other autoimmune diseases in children with vitiligo. *Dermatology* 2005;210:26–30.
12. Prćić S, Djuran V, Katanić D et al. Vitiligo and thyroid dysfunction in children and adolescents. *Acta Dermatovenerol Croat* 2011;19:248–54.
13. Kakourou T, Kanaka-Gantenbein C, Papadopoulou A et al. Increased prevalence of chronic autoimmune (Hashimoto's) thyroiditis in children and adolescents with vitiligo. *J Am Acad Dermatol* 2005;53:220–3.
14. Taïeb A, and Picardo M. The definition and assessment of vitiligo: A consensus report of the Vitiligo European Task Force. *Pigment Cell Res* 2007;20:27–35.

15. Taïeb A, and Picardo M. Clinical practice. Vitiligo. *N Engl J Med* 2009;360:160–9.

16. Hann SK, Chang JH, Lee HS et al. The classification of segmental vitiligo on the face. *Yonsei Med J* 2000;41:209–12.

17. Kim DY, Oh SH, and Hann SK. Classification of segmental vitiligo on the face: Clues for prognosis. *Br J Dermatol* 2011;164:1004–9.

18. Ezzedine K, Gauthier Y, Leaute-Labreze C et al. Segmental vitiligo associated with generalized vitiligo (mixed vitiligo): A retrospective case series of 19 patients. *J Am Acad Dermatol* 2011;65(5):965–71.

19. Happle R. New aspects of cutaneous mosaicism. *J Dermatol* 2002;29:681–92.

20. Happle R. Segmental type 2 manifestation of autosome dominant skin diseases. Development of a new formal genetic concept. *Hautarzt* 2001;52:283–7.

21. Happle R. Superimposed segmental manifestations of polygenic skin disorders. *J Am Acad Dermatol* 2007;57:690–9.

22. Khalid M, and Mujtaba G. Response of segmental vitiligo to 0.05% clobetasol propionate cream. *Int J Dermatol* 1998;37:705–8.

23. Park J-H, and Lee D-L. Segmental Vitiligo. In: Park KKH, ed. *Vitiligo—Management and Therapy. InTech.* 2011. Available from: https://www.intechopen.com/books/vitiligo-management-and-therapy/segmental-vitiligo.

24. Shim W-H, Suh S-W, Jwa S-W et al. A pilot study of 1% pimecrolimus cream for the treatment of childhood segmental vitiligo. *Ann Dermatol* 2013;25(2).

25. Kathuria S, Khaitan BK, Ramam M et al. Segmental vitiligo: A randomized controlled trial to evaluate efficacy and safety of 0.1% tacrolimus ointment vs 0.05% fluticasone propionate cream. *Indian J Dermatol Venereol Leprol* 2012;78(1):68–73.

26. Falabella R, and Barona MI. Update on skin repigmentation therapies in vitiligo. *Pigment Cell Melanoma Res* 2009;22:42–65.

27. van Geel N, Ongenae K, and Naeyaert JM. Surgical techniques for vitiligo: A review. *Dermatology* 2001;202:162–6.

28. Na GY, Seo SK, and Choi SK. Single hair grafting for the treatment of vitiligo. *J Am Acad Dermatol* 1998;38:580–4.

Chapter 9

ACROFACIAL VITILIGO

Rajesh Kumar and Neetu Bhari

CONTENTS

INTRODUCTION

Vitiligo is a common acquired disorder of pigmentation characterized by depigmented macules in a localized or generalized distribution. Vitiligo is known to affect around 0.1%–2% of the population worldwide; in India, its prevalence is about 0.5%–2.5% (range: 0.46%–8.8%) [1]. Since there has been a lack of consensus regarding the nomenclature and classification used across the globe until now, a new classification system of vitiligo was proposed in 2012 by Vitiligo Global Issues Consensus Conference [2]. The major groups described in this classification are segmental and nonsegmental, of which nonsegmental vitiligo is a group comprising acrofacial, mucosal, generalized, universal, or mixed forms. Generalized and acrofacial are the most commonly reported patterns of vitiligo from India [3,4].

DEFINITION

Acrofacial vitiligo is classified as depigmented macules limited to the face, head, and distal extremities. It usually involves the perioral and periocular region over the face. Lesions in the genital areas are also included in the acrofacial group of vitiligo [5]. A recent study from China showed a significant association of mucosal vitiligo with lesions on the acrofacial areas and proposed that mucosal vitiligo is probably a special form of acrofacial vitiligo [6].

LIP-TIP VITILIGO

The form of acrofacial vitiligo which is limited to lips, tips of the fingers or toes, and the penile shaft is known as lip-tip vitiligo [7].

AGE OF ONSET AND DISTRIBUTION

The onset of vitiligo occurs in childhood or young adulthood, with a peak age at 10–30 years. Speeckaert and van Geel evaluated the association of age of onset and affected sites in 700 vitiligo patients [8]. Predominant involvement of the beard area in men and the periocular area in women was noted. An earlier age of onset, periocular vitiligo was observed when compared to the perioral area, and of lower extremities compared to upper extremities. Overall, acral area involvement is a marker of a long-lasting chronic disease.

FAMILY HISTORY

A familial association is rarer in acrofacial patterns compared to generalized vitiligo [9].

ASSOCIATION WITH AUTOIMMUNE DISEASES

Studies have shown an association of acrofacial vitiligo with autoimmune comorbidities such as thyroid disease and diabetes, though many studies have shown it to be less frequent than in generalized vitiligo [4]. Clinical and histological association with lichen sclerosus is reported [10].

PROGRESSION

Progression of acrofacial vitiligo to more severe forms or the generalized form is not predictable, and large prospective studies are required to evaluate this association.

DIAGNOSIS

Histological evaluation shows absence of melanocytes in the affected area, which differentiates it from the adjacent normal skin [11]. Other epidermal changes are nonspecific. Dermal findings can range from a mild-to-dense lichenoid band-like inflammatory infiltrate [12]. The reduction in functional melanocytes can also be confirmed by special stains such as Fontana-Masson, a stain for melanin, or dihydroxy-phenylalanine alanine for tyrosinase. Other useful immunohisto-chemical stains include HMB-45 (melanosome-associated cytoplasmic antigen), Mel-5 (70–80-kDa glycoprotein, pigmentation associated), NKI/beteb (l00-kDa melanosome-associated antigen), etc. [13].

TREATMENT

Acrofacial vitiligo is considered a comparatively treatment-resistant form of vitiligo. Various studies have shown a lower response of medical therapies in these cases; hence surgical options have more commonly been opted for in this variant of vitiligo.

PHARMACOLOGICAL TREATMENT

TOPICAL CORTICOSTEROID
Topical corticosteroid is the first-line treatment for acral pattern vitiligo. In a meta-analysis of nonsurgical repigmentation therapies in vitiligo, topical class 3 and 4 had the highest success rates (56% and 55%, respectively) [14]. Younger and darker-skin patients with head and neck involvement have shown a comparatively better response [15]. Caution is required in long-term use due to local adverse effects.

TOPICAL CALCINEURIN INHIBITORS
Topical calcineurin inhibitors such as tacrolimus 0.03%, 0.1% and pimecrolimus 0.1% are treatments of choice for lesions over the face, lips, and genitalia. In a comparative trial, they have shown similar efficacy to topical corticosteroids in acrofacial vitiligo [16]. Children have shown a better response over acrofacial areas compared to adults [17].

TOPICAL VITAMIN D$_3$
Recent studies have shown excellent efficacy and safety of topical vitamin D$_3$ analog in vitiligo. In a prospective case study of generalized (338), segmental (170), and localized (166) cases of vitiligo, topical vitamin D$_3$ therapy was significantly effective for the localized type. The treatment response rate was 21.1% for the generalized type, 29.0% for the segmental type, and 54.8% for the localized type [9].

PSORALEN AND ULTRAVIOLET A THERAPY
Topical psoralen and ultraviolet A (PUVA) therapy has been used in the localized form of vitiligo with good repigmentation. Combination with topical corticosteroids, calcineurin inhibitors, and vitamin D$_3$ analog has resulted in a better response compared to monotherapy [18].

NARROWBAND UVB
Narrowband UVB (NBUVB) is currently considered the treatment of choice for patients with moderate-to-severe vitiligo because of its good safety and efficacy profile. In a recent studies, the response rate noted with NBUVB was 46.3% for the generalized type, 20.3% for the segmental type, and 29.2% for the localized type [9]. Lee et al. proposed an early treatment of acrofacial vitiligo with phototherapy to induce complete repigmentation [19].

MONOCHROMATIC EXCIMER LIGHT
The effectiveness of a 308-nm monochromatic excimer light device (308-nm MEL) in vitiligo as a targeted phototherapy device has been recently described. In a randomized, multicentric, investigator-blinded study of 21 patients with localized symmetric vitiligo lesions predominantly on acral areas, 308-nm MEL showed a rapid and higher pigmentation score compared to NBUVB [20].

SURGICAL TREATMENT

PUNCH GRAFTING
Punch grafting is the easiest and most cost-effective surgical technique for localized lesions. Ohguchi et al. reviewed 644 cases of vitiligo in their prospective case study and observed that 1-mm minigraft was significantly effective for the segmental and localized types of vitiligo. The treatment response rate was 38.9% for the generalized type, 77.3% for the segmental type, and 73.3% for the localized type [9].

SUCTION BLISTER GRAFTING
This is an established technique for the treatment of resistant and stable vitiligo predominantly on acral areas. In a systematic review by Njoo et al. of 15 studies on epidermal blister grafting, a mean efficacy of 87% was noted with an excellent color match [21]. This technique has been successfully used in the management of eyelid and lip vitiligo as well [22,23].

SPLIT-THICKNESS SKIN GRAFTS
This procedure consists of grafting a very thin skin comprising the epidermis and upper papillary dermis onto the dermabraded patch of vitiligo. It has shown superior efficacy over blister grafting in the management of stable and treatment-resistant vitiligo [24].

AUTOLOGOUS NONCULTURED EPIDERMAL CELL SUSPENSION GRAFTING
This is a cellular transplantation technique which has the advantage of treating a large area with excellent color compatibility. In a recent study by Holla et al., 36 patients with 80 lesions over acral areas and joints were treated with noncultured epidermal cell suspension (NCECS) grafting; 51 regained >75% repigmentation and 23 regained 50%–75% repigmentation [25]. The lesions over distal fingers, toes, and the ankle joint had a poor response.

CONCLUSION

Acrofacial vitiligo is a distinct pattern of vitiligo which has specific prognostic properties; thus its detection and the formulation of an appropriate management and counseling strategy are essential.

REFERENCES

1. Sharma VK, Bhari N, and Manoj. KT. Vitiligo: Definition, incidence, etiology. In: Handog EB and Macarayo MJE, eds. *Melasma and Vitiligo in Brown Skin*, 1st ed. Springer (India) Pvt. Ltd; 2016. pp. 179–89.

2. Ezzedine K, Lim HW, Suzuki T et al. Revised classification/nomenclature of vitiligo and related issues: The Vitiligo Global Issues Consensus Conference. *Pigment Cell Melanoma Res* 2012;25:E1–13.

3. Handa S, and Dogra S. Epidemiology of childhood vitiligo: A study of 625 patients from North India. *Pediatr Dermatol* 2003;20:207–10.

4. Agarwal S, Ojha A, and Gupta S. Profile of vitiligo in Kumaun region of Uttarakhand India. *Indian J Dermatol* 2014;59:209.

5. Silva de Castro CC, do Nascimento LM, Olandoski M, and Mira MT. A pattern of association between clinical form of vitiligo and disease-related variables in a Brazilian population. *J Dermatol Sci* 2012;65:63–7.

6. Mchepange UO, Gao XH, Liu YY, Liu YB, Ma L, Zhang L, and Chen HD. Vitiligo in North-Eastern China: An association between mucosal and acrofacial lesions. *Acta Derm Venereol* 2010;90:136–40.

7. Sehgal VN, and Srivastava G. Vitiligo: Compendium of clinico-epidemiological features. *Indian J Dermatol Venereol Leprol* 2007 May-Jun;73(3):149–56.

8. Speeckaert R, and van Geel N. Distribution patterns in generalized vitiligo. *J Eur Acad Dermatol Venereol* 2014;28:755–62.

9. Ohguchi R, Kato H, Furuhashi T, Nakamura M, Nishida E, Watanabe S, Shintani Y, and Morita A. Risk factors and treatment responses in patients with vitiligo in Japan—A retrospective large-scale study. *Kaohsiung J Med Sci* 2015;31:260–4.

10. Attili VR, and Attili SK. Acral vitiligo and lichen sclerosus—association or a distinct pattern? A clinical and histopathological review of 15 cases. *Indian J Dermatol* 2015;60:519.

11. Kim YC, Kim YJ, Kang HY, Sohn S, and Lee ES. Histopathologic features in vitiligo. *Am J Dermatopathol* 2008;30:112–6.

12. Attili VR, and Attili SK. Lichenoid inflammation in vitiligo—A clinical and histopathologic review of 210 cases. *Int J Dermatol* 2008;47:663–9.

13. Le Poole IC, van den Wijngaard RM, Westerhof W, Dutrieux RP, and Das PK. Presence or absence of melanocytes in vitiligo lesions: An immunohistochemical investigation. *J Invest Dermatol* 1993;100:816–22.

14. Njoo MD, Spuls PI, Bos JD, Westerhof W, and Bossuyt PM. Nonsurgical repigmentation therapies in vitiligo. Meta-analysis of the literature. *Arch Dermatol* 1998;134:1532–40.

15. Cockayne SE, Messenger AG, and Gawkrodger DJ. Vitiligo treated with topical corticosteroids: Children with head and neck involvement respond well. *J Am Acad Dermatol* 2002;46:964–5.

16. Coskun B, Saral Y, and Turgut D. Topical 0.05% clobetasol propionate versus 1% pimecrolimus ointment in vitiligo. *Eur J Dermatol* 2005;15:88–91.

17. Udompataikul M, Boonsupthip P, and Siriwattanagate R. Effectiveness of 0.1% topical tacrolimus in adult and children patients with vitiligo. *J Dermatol* 2011;38:536–40.

18. Yoshida A, Takagi A, Ikejima A, Takenaka H, Fukai T, and Ikeda S. A retrospective study of 231 Japanese vitiligo patients with special reference to phototherapy. *Acta Dermatovenerol Croat* 2014;22:13–8.

19. Lee DY, Kim CR, and Lee JH. Recent onset vitiligo on acral areas treated with phototherapy: Need of early treatment. *Photodermatol Photoimmunol Photomed* 2010;26:266–8.

20. Casacci M, Thomas P, Pacifico A, Bonnevalle A, Paro Vidolin A, and Leone G. Comparison between 308-nm monochromatic excimer light and narrowband UVB phototherapy (311–313 nm) in the treatment of vitiligo—A multicentre controlled study. *J Eur Acad Dermatol Venereol* 2007;21:956–63.

21. Njoo MD, Westerhof W, Bos JD, and Bossuyt PM. A systematic review of autologous transplantation methods in vitiligo. *Arch Dermatol* 1998;134:1543–9.

22. Nanda S, Relhan V, Grover C, and Reddy BS. Suction blister epidermal grafting for management of eyelid vitiligo: Special considerations. *Dermatol Surg* 2006;32:387–91.

23. Babu A, Thappa DM, and Jaisankar TJ. Punch grafting versus suction blister epidermal grafting in the treatment of stable lip vitiligo. *Dermatol Surg* 2008;34:166–78.

24. Ozdemir M, Cetinkale O, Wolf R, Kotoğyan A, Mat C, Tüzün B, and Tüzün Y. Comparison of two surgical approaches for treating vitiligo: A preliminary study. *Int J Dermatol* 2002;41:135–8.

25. Holla AP, Sahni K, Kumar R, Parsad D, Kanwar A, and Mehta SD. Acral vitiligo and lesions over joints treated with non-cultured epidermal cell suspension transplantation. *Clin Exp Dermatol* 2013;38:332–7.

Chapter 10

MUCOSAL VITILIGO

A.S. Savitha, B.M. Shashikumar, and Reddy R. Raghunatha

CONTENTS

INTRODUCTION

Vitiligo is an autoimmune disease with destruction of melanocytes. As with the skin, the mucosa also exhibits pigmentation. Loss of normal pigmentation from the skin or the mucosa is a cause for psychological and social problems [1]. Both skin and mucosa are affected in vitiligo. Acrofacial vitiligo (AFV) is currently classified as a form of generalized vitiligo (GV) under nonsegmental vitiligo (NSV) [2]. AFV can be seen with either a limited involvement of the lips, tips of the fingers/toes, and penile shaft as the "lip-tip" form, or acral vitiligo (AV) in various stages of centripetal progression to the trunk [3]. In a study conducted at PGIMER, Chandigarh, the sites of onset in decreasing order of frequency were both lips simultaneously in 30.5%, lower lip in 25.4%, glans penis in 13.5%, prepuce and angles of mouth in 11.8% each, and labia minora in 1.6% of patients [4].

ORAL VITILIGO

The normal oral mucosal color is described as coral pink but, as with the gingiva, it exhibits an array of colors ranging from pale pink to coral pink in Caucasians and blue to brown-black in Asians and Africans [5]. Dark-skinned individuals are likely to have dark melanin pigmentation. The number of melanocytes in the mucosa corresponds numerically to that of skin; however, in the mucosa their activity is reduced. This may explain why oral vitiligo has long been considered uncommon [4]. Sometimes mucosal vitiligo can be the first indicator, which may manifest in unnoticeable sites. In a study by Nagarajan et al., 2% of patients presented with oral depigmentation as the only manifestation of vitiligo. Oral manifestations are far less often recognized, with occurrence most common in the lip (42%), followed by the palate, buccal mucosa, gingiva, and labial mucosa [6]. Besides the mucosal form of vitiligo, associated involvement of mucosae with other clinical variants (vulgaris or acrofacial) was seen in 17% of patients with late-onset vitiligo [7]. Patchy loss of pigment from the buccal mucosa, gingiva, and gum line is invariably observed in vitiligo [8]. Diascopy and Woods lamp examination may help detect clinically subtle macules of vitiligo [4].

Lip involvement can be of the following three types:

a. Commonly involves the vermilion border and spares the inner labial mucosa (Figure 10.1).

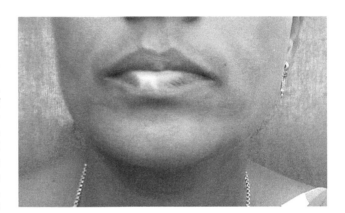

Figure 10.1   Lip vitiligo involving the vermilion border.

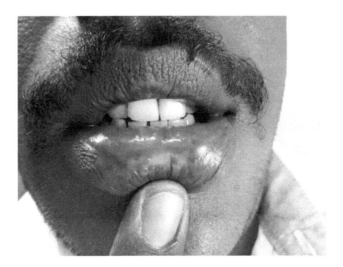

Figure 10.2   Involvement of the labial border only.

b. An inverse distribution which is sparing of vermilion, and band-like involvement of the labial mucosa [9] (Figure 10.2).

c. The lateral lower lip vitiligo type, which forms about 16% of all vitiligo patients [10]. It starts as a tiny dot at the lateral part of the lower lip and spreads medially as a linear streak along the vermilion border.

A study by Dutta and Mandal mentioned significant progression of vitiligo in patients with mucosal involvement, indicating that it could be a poor prognostic factor [11].

GENITAL VITILIGO

As with oral mucosa, involvement of the glans, vaginal, and anal mucosa is known. In a study of 5000 consecutive new male patients examined, 22 patients had vitiligo on the genitalia [12]. Involvement of vulval and vaginal mucosa is less often reported, probably due to non-examination of these areas routinely. Vitiligo occurring on non-exposed skin may be considered trivial but becomes complicated by psychological factors when it occurs on the genitals. Most patients and their sex partners ponder whether vitiligo on the penis is the consequence of a sexual act or a manifestation of a communicable disease [13]. Patients with genital involvement scored significantly worse on the VitiQoL than those without lesions in this area in a study by Morales-Sánchez et al. The prevalence of depression and anxiety was 34% and 60%, respectively [14]. Porter et al. studied the effect of vitiligo on sexual relationships and found that embarrassment during sexual acts was especially frequent for men with vitiligo [15].

DIFFERENTIAL DIAGNOSIS

ORAL LESIONS

- Submucosal fibrosis
- Depigmentation of palate due to reverse smoking
- Postinflammatory depigmentation, e.g., herpes simplex infections—this has to be differentiated from the isomorphic phenomenon in vitiligo induced by herpes simplex infections

GENITAL LESIONS

- Lichen sclerosus atrophicus—histopathology helps to differentiate these

MANAGEMENT

Management of mucosal vitiligo is a therapeutic challenge. With a medical line of management and photochemotherapy, melanocyte gets stimulated and migrates from the hair follicle reservoir, and from the periphery as well. Since mucosa is devoid of hair follicles, the repigmentation from the follicular reservoir cannot be achieved, hence the difficulty with the medical line of management. If mucosal involvement is part of generalized vitiligo, the disease has to be managed with medical management with or without photochemotherapy to achieve both stability and maximum possible repigmentation. Surgical management becomes essential in the majority of cases of mucosal vitiligo, especially over the lips, due to visibility and the enormous stigma associated with it, and in genital mucosa due to embarrassment during sexual acts harming sexual relationships. Many procedures and methods (Table 10.1) have been described and performed with success to recruit melanocytes into the depigmented areas in the form of tissue and cellular grafts. Even though cellular grafts have replaced tissue grafts over other body sites, they are still relevant with fairly good cosmetic results over the lips and other mucosa.

Table 10.1 Surgical procedures for management of mucosal vitiligo

A. Tissue grafting techniques
1. Miniature punch grafting (MPG)
2. Suction blister epidermal grafts (SBEG)
3. Mucosal advancement flap (new technique described by the authors)
B. Cellular grafts
1. Noncultured epidermal cell suspension (ECS)
2. Noncultured hair follicle cell suspension
3. Cultured melanocytic grafts
C. Other methods
1. Surgical excision and primary closure
2. Micropigmentation or tattooing

REFERENCES

1. Srivathsa SH. Case reports: Oral vitiligo. *Br Dent J* 2015;218:507.
2. Picardo M, and Taieb A. Epidemiology, definitions and classification. In: Picardo M, and Taieb A, eds. *Vitiligo*. Berlin, Heidelberg: Springer-Verlag; 2010, pp. 13–25.
3. Attili VR, and Attili SK. Segmental and generalized vitiligo: Both forms demonstrate inflammatory histopathological features and clinical mosaicism. *Indian J Dermatol* 2013;58:433–8.
4. Prasad D. Mucosal vitiligo. In: Picardo M, and Taieb A, eds. *Vitiligo*. Berlin, Heidelberg: Springer-Verlag; 2010, pp. 57–9.
5. Ponnaiyan D, Jagadeesan V, Perumal G, and Amarnath A. Correlating skin color with gingival pigmentation patterns in South Indians: A cross sectional study. *Oral Health Dent Manag* 2014;13:132–6.
6. Nagarajan A, Masthan MK, Sankar LS, Narayanasamy AB, and Elumalai R. Oral manifestations of vitiligo. *Indian J Dermatol* 2015;60(1):103.
7. Dogra S, Parsad D, Handa S, and Kanwar AJ. Late onset vitiligo: A study of 182 patients. *Int J Dermatol* 2005;44:193–6.
8. Dummet CO. The oral tissues in vitiligo. *Oral Surg Oral Med Oral Pathol* 1959;12:1073–9.
9. Chitole VR. Overgrafting for leukoderma of the lower lip: A new application of an already established method. *Ann Plast Surg* 1991;26:289–90.
10. Sahoo A, Singh PC, Patnaik S, Singh N, and Srichandran N. Vitiligo lateral lower lip. *Indian J Dermatol* 2002;47:15–7.
11. Dutta AK, and Mandal SB. Clinical study of 650 vitiligo cases and their classification. *Indian J Dermatol* 14:103–15.
12. Gaffoor PM. Depigmentation of male genitalia. *Cutis* 34:492–4.
13. Gupta S. Surgical management of vitiligo of eyelids and genitals: Special issues. In: Gupta S, Olsson MJ, Kanwar AJ, Ortonne J-P, eds. *Surgical Management of Vitiligo*. Singapore: Blackwell Publishing; 220–3.
14. Morales-Sánchez MA, Vargas-Salinas M, Peralta-Pedrero ML, Olguín-García MG, and Jurado-Santa CF. Impact of vitiligo on quality of life. *Actas Dermosifiliogr.* 2017;108(7):637–42.
15. Porter J, Beuf A, Lerner A et al. The effect of vitiligo on sexual relationships. *J Am Acad Dermatol* 1990;22:221–2.

Chapter 11

LEUKOTRICHIA IN VITILIGO

Ramesha Bhat M. and Jyothi Jayaraman

CONTENTS

INTRODUCTION

Leukotrichia is the graying of hair which is usually associated with vitiligo. Some authors use the term synonymously with "poliosis" [1]. Poliosis has been described classically in association with vitiligo in Alezzandrini syndrome and Vogt-Kayanagi-Harada syndrome.

Leukotrichia makes a vitiligo lesion appear more obvious, especially when it persists even after repigmentation of the skin lesion. Repigmentation by photochemotherapy is usually difficult in such cases because of a deficient melanocyte reservoir [2].

INCIDENCE

Leukotrichia is seen in approximately 48.6% of patients with segmental vitiligo [3]. In patients with mixed vitiligo, the appearance of leukotrichia at an early stage in segmental vitiligo may be an indicator of developing generalized skin lesions and progression into mixed vitiligo [4]. Incidence of leukotrichia on hairy areas was found to be between 11.5% and 44% in a study conducted on 1436 Indian patients with vitiligo [5]. A higher incidence was noted in elderly patients among the cases of late-onset vitiligo [6]. The scalp and eyebrows are frequently associated with leukotrichia. Also, premature graying of hair is seen in some patients with vitiligo.

FOLLICULAR MELANOGENESIS AND PATHOGENESIS OF LEUKOTRICHIA

Follicular melanocytes originate in the neural crest and migrate to the dermis and epidermis. Recruitment of neural crest cells is regulated by microphthalmia transcription factor (Mitf) and paired box transcription factor 3 (Pax3), which stimulate enzymes related to melanin synthesis. Migration of melanoblasts is controlled by endothelin B receptor type B and c-KIT oncogene receptor. Mutation of these is responsible for leukotrichia in piebaldism [7].

Melanoblasts migrate to the developing hair follicle, proliferate, and synthesize melanin, which occurs synchronously with the hair cycle. Binding of α-melanocyte-stimulating hormone (α-MSH) to

melanocortin type 1 receptor (MC1R) increases transcriptional activity of Mitf and thereby synthesis of melanogenic enzymes (tyrosinase, Trp 1 and 2) [7].

In the early and mid-anagen phase, maximum proliferation of hair follicle melanocytes is seen. This phase has been shown to depend on stem cell factor ligand (SCF) signaling [7]. During the catagen phase, melanogenic activity abruptly ceases. In the telogen phase, melanocytes do not express tyrosinase or Trp1 and do not proliferate. [7]

There are two types of melanocytes in the hair follicles: amelanotic melanocytes, which lack pigmentary granules, and melanotic melanocytes with pigment granules, which impart color to the skin and hair. Amelanotic melanocytes are usually present in the outer root sheath of the hair bulb and the middle and lower portions of the hair follicle, while the upper portion of the hair bulb and hair follicle contain melanotic melanocytes [8]. There exists a reservoir of melanocyte stem cells in the bulge region of the hair follicle. These cells differentiate into melanocytes in the hair matrix. Certain factors such as Pax3 and Mitf maintain the balance between stem cell population and differentiated melanocytes [8]. Leukotrichia in vitiligo occurs due to destruction or loss of follicular melanocytes. It has been observed that loss of melanocyte stem cells precedes the loss of differentiated melanocytes. Leukotrichia or gray hair associated with aging sheds some light on the dynamic interactions between hair cycle and pigmentation of hair. The tight coupling of hair follicle melanogenesis to the hair growth cycle differentiates follicular melanogenesis from the continuous melanogenesis in the epidermis. Pigment dilution results primarily from a reduction in tyrosinase activity within hair bulbar melanocytes. Suboptimal melanocyte—cortical keratinocyte interactions and defective migration of melanocytes from a reservoir in the upper outer root sheath to the pigment-permitting microenvironment close to the follicular papilla of the hair bulb can disrupt normal function of the pigmentary unit. Parallel dysregulation of antioxidant mechanisms or pro/anti-apoptotic factors are also likely to occur within the cells [8].

CLINICAL FEATURES

Leukotrichia is generally seen in segmental vitiligo (SV), which indicates that the condition is resistant to medical treatment and requires epidermal graft [9]. Contrary to SV, in nonsegmental vitiligo (NSV) body hairs are usually spared and remain pigmented, although hair depigmentation may occur with disease progression. It is also seen

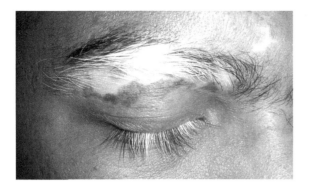

Figure 11.1 Leukotichia seen in association with vitiligo on hair-bearing area, in this case the eyebrow. (Image courtesy of Dr. Ashique KT, Consultant Dermatologist, KIMS *Al Shifa* Super Speciality Hospital, Perinthalmanna, Kerala, India.)

in vitiligo universalis and when vitiligo occurs on hair-bearing areas such as the scalp and eyebrows (Figure 11.1). There have been case reports of vitiligo with primary follicular involvement, and this entity has been named "follicular vitiligo" [10]. It manifests as marked generalized hair whitening with normal interfollicular pigmentation initially which may progress to form depigmented skin lesions of vitiligo. In contrast, in cases of NSV, leukotrichia usually is a late feature, often indicating poor prognosis of the disease. These cases show an unusual preferential involvement of follicular melanocytes as compared to the interfollicular epidermal melanocytes. In vitiligo lesions of these cases, it has been observed that melanocytes and their precursors, besides being absent in the basal epidermis, may also be absent in the hair follicle, clinically corresponding to depigmented vitiliginous skin and leukotrichia. On a microscopic level, follicular melanocytes are believed to be the primary target in follicular vitiligo. One plausible hypothesis in follicular vitiligo is that, in a patient genetically predisposed to vitiligo, accumulated cellular damage caused by increased oxidative stress occurs in follicular melanocytes, which leads to collapse of the immune privilege of the hair follicle and thereby activation of the immune response against a particular follicular melanocyte antigen. It appears that follicular vitiligo is a bridge between vitiligo vulgaris and alopecia areata. Presence of increased recruitment of mast cells and CD+8 T lymphocytes in lesional skin as well as peribulbar area is common to both the diseases [10].

TREATMENT MODALITIES IN REPIGMENTATION OF LEUKOTRICHIA

Vitiligo patches are often associated with leukotrichia, which usually remains even after complete repigmentation of the patches, which makes the treatment a therapeutic challenge.

Tyrosinase-positive melanocytes are only observed in black hair follicles; melanocytes still exist in the white hair follicles, although they are fewer in number than those in black hair follicles. These findings suggest that some amount of melanocyte reservoir exists even within the vitiligo lesions showing leukotrichia [8]. During repigmentation, many melanocytes were noted in the hair follicle with larger bodies and longer branching dendrites. Hair follicle split DOPA staining has shown no active melanocytes in vitiliginous skin, while many DOPA-positive (active) melanocytes in various stages of repigmentation were noticed in outer root sheath and orifices of hair follicles as well as nearby epidermis, suggesting that during the process of repigmentation, maturation and migration of follicular melanocytes to the epidermis take place [11]. Phototherapy can induce the formation of various chemical mediators and growth factors which could

stimulate epidermal melanocytes and stimulate the proliferation and migration of inactive melanocytes in the outer root sheaths of hair follicles present in the depigmented lesions. Hypertrophic melanocytes have been shown to occur in both the middle and deep portions of the hair follicles in the center of islands of repigmentation and also in the epidermis of the expanding repigmenting border. Mitosis of melanocytes was absent in these areas. An ultrastructural study showed that the melanocytes of repigmented areas were hyperactive. The melanosomes were larger than those of surrounding healthy skin, although the mode of packaging was unaltered. These observations suggest that melanocytes repigmenting vitiliginous skin under the influence of oral photochemotherapy are derived from a melanocytic reservoir localized in the hair follicles [11,12].

THEORIES OF REPIGMENTATION IN VITILIGO AND LEUKOTRICHIA

ANTEGRADE MIGRATION OF AMELANOTIC MELANOCYTES

Staricco observed in the 1950s that when a stimulus like dermabrasion or UV exposure is applied to vitiliginous skin, the amelanotic melanocytes from the outer root sheath cells divide, become DOPA positive and functionally active, and migrate to the epidermis. These cells do not produce melanin under normal conditions [8,12].

ANTEGRADE MIGRATION FROM MELANOCYTE RESERVOIR IN THE HAIR BULB

Differentiation of melanocyte stem cells occurs during the catagen and telogen phases. They undergo mitosis and redifferentiate in the hair bulb during the anagen phase of the hair cycle and migrate to the epidermis in a similar fashion to that explained in the preceding text [8,13].

RETROGRADE MIGRATION OF MELANOCYTES

Repigmentation of leukotrichia was noted to occur a few weeks or months after the skin lesions of vitiligo. It was postulated that this occurs as a result of retrograde migration of melanocytes from the repigmented epidermis to the area of leukotrichia and hence a delayed repigmentation of the white hair [8,14]. Despite complete repigmentation of vitiligo patches, leukotrichia often persists. The reason for the inadequate or incomplete melanin transfer is not known.

Various medical and surgical options for treatment of leukotrichia include psoralen with ultraviolet A (PUVA), oral Isoprinosine, intralesional placental extract, epidermal blister grafting with PUVA, surgical excision Thiersch grafting with PUVA and transplantation of epidermal blister bearing melanocytes, in vitro cultured epidermal grafting, minigrafting, chemical epilation followed by epidermal grafts, and electroepilation followed by Choi single-hair transplantation [8,15].

Intralesional injection of placental extract probably helps restore the melanogenic activity in the infundibulum and hair bulb of melanocytes of white hairs. It contains factors to stimulate melanocyte growth as well as motility [15].

Surgical repigmentation of hair is based on migration of melanocytes from the epidermis to the hair follicles. In vitro cultured epidermal grafts were first used by Falabella et al. in 1989 with in vitro cultured epidermal grafts bearing melanocytes [8]. A combination of epidermal skin grafting and PUVA was successfully tried by Hann et al. in treatment of leukotrichia [16].

In epidermal blister grafting and PUVA therapy, after preoperative removal of hair, blisters are created using cryotherapy with liquid nitrogen within 24 hours. The recipient site is prepared using LASER abrasion or suction blister. The roof of the blister is used as a graft from the donor site. One week after the procedure, the patient is given PUVA therapy to enable repigmentation [8]. Thin split-thickness skin grafting (STSG) can be combined with PUVA therapy. In this procedure, the recipient site is prepared by dermabrasion under local anesthesia. Particular care is taken to create a uniform, deeper plane of abrasion in cases of vitiligo with leukotrichia. Preoperative hair removal is not necessary. The preferred donor site for the graft is the medial aspect of the arm. The harvested graft is secured on the recipient site using silk sutures and sterile antiseptic, and pressure dressing is applied and kept for 6–7 days. Chemical epilation with thioglycolic acid salts has been attempted to dissolve the hair shafts in the epidermal grafts in hair-bearing areas where poor graft take-up has been observed. Repigmentation of hair may take a few months and improve over next few years [8].

Minigrafts used in the treatment of vitiligo have been shown to improve leukotrichia as early as within 10–16 weeks. However, STSG has been found to be more successful in repigmentation as compared to minigrafts.

Cosmetic results are better over eyebrows as compared to other hair-bearing areas such as scalp, beard, and mustache. There may also be a role for hair transplantation in the treatment of leukotrichia in resistant cases. Follicular unit transplant was first introduced to repigment vitiligo patches in 1998. A study by Parul et al. revealed that 23.9% of cases of leukotrichia showed improvement after follicular unit grafting. Though the appearance of pigment is delayed as compared to the other modalities, the color match is much more acceptable than that with other methods. This method can be easily applied to a small area of vitiligo. It can be performed in the eyelash area or at an angle of the mouth where performing other surgical methods, such as epidermal grafts or minigrafts, are difficult [17].

Periodic follow-up of patients following treatment as well as further studies are needed to explore the various surgical and medical options for treatment of leukotrichia, as it has been not addressed well in the current literature.

SUMMARY
Leukotrichia in vitiligo is more commonly seen in the segmental type and in anatomical sites such as eyebrows and scalp. It may also act as an indicator for development of generalized skin lesions in mixed vitiligo. It appears to make the skin lesions more obvious, causing significant distress to the patient. As leukotrichia tends to persist even after treatment of the vitiligo skin lesions, it warrants surgical treatment in most cases. Phototherapy plays a role when the reservoir of amelanotic melanocytes is activated, proliferates, and migrates to the epidermis to cause repigmentation. Surgical treatments such as epidermal grafts are based on making use of the epidermal melanocytes from the normal-appearing donor site. The unsightly appearance of white hairs in a vitiligo skin lesion makes it look more obvious, and active management is needed for optimal overall cosmetic results.

REFERENCES

1. Halder RM, and Taliaferro SJ. Vitiligo. In: Wolff K, Goldsmith LA, Kastz SI, Gilchrest BA, Paller AS, and Leffell DJ, eds. *Fitzpatrick's Dermatology in General Medicine*, 7th ed. New York: McGraw-Hill; 2008, p. 619.

2. Kim C-Y, Yoon T-J, and Kim T-H. Epidermal grafting after chemical epilation in the treatment of vitiligo. *Dermatol Surg.* 2001;27(10):855–6.

3. Hann SK, and Lee HJ. Segmental vitiligo: Clinical findings in 208 patients. *J Am Acad Dermatol* 1996;35:671–4.

4. Ezzedine K, Diallo A, Léauté-Labrèze C, Séneschal J, Prey S, and Ballanger F. Halo nevi and leukotrichia are strong predictors of the passage to mixed vitiligo in a subgroup of segmental vitiligo. *Br J Dermatol.* 2012;166(3):539–44.

5. Handa S, and Kaur I. Vitiligo: The loss of pigment in skin, hair and eyes. *J Dermatol* 1978;5:1–8.

6. Dogra S, Prasad D, Handa S, and Kanwar AJ. Late onset vitiligo: A study of 182 patients. *Int J Dermatol* 2005;44: 193–6.

7. Cotsarelis G, and Botchkarev V. Biology of hair follicles. In: Wolff K, Goldsmith LA, Kastz SI, Gilchrest BA, Paller AS, and Leffell DJ, eds. *Fitzpatrick's Dermatology in General Medicine*, 7th ed. New York: McGraw-Hill; 2008, pp. 747–9.

8. Agarwal K, and Agarwal A. Surgical management of leukotrichia. In: Gupta S, Olsson MJ, Kanwar AJ, and Ortonne JP, eds. *Surgical Management of Vitiligo*, 1st ed. India: Blackwell Publishing; 2007, pp. 229–37.

9. Lee DY, Park JH, Lee JH, Yang JM, and Lee ES. Is segmental vitiligo always associated with leukotrichia? Examination with a digital portable microscope. *Int J Dermatol* 2009;48: 1262.

10. Gan EY, Muriel CA, Pain C, Goussot JF, Alain T, Seneschal J, and Ezzedine K. Follicular vitiligo: A report of 8 cases. *J Am Acad Dermatol* 2016;74:1178–84.

11. Cui J, Shen LY, and Wang GC. Role of hair follicles in the repigmentation of vitiligo. *J Invest Dermatol.* 1991 Sep;97(3):410–6.

12. Starricco RG. Amelanotic melanocytes in the outer sheath of the human hair follicle and their role in the repigmentation of regenerated epidermis. *Ann NY Acad Sci* 1963;100:239–55.

13. Ortonne JP, Schmitt D, and Thovolet J. PUVA-induced repigmentation of vitiligo: Scanning electron microscopy of hair follicles. *J Invest Dermatol* 1980;74:40–2.

14. Horikawa T, Norris DA, Yohn JJ, Zekman T, Travers JB, and Morelli JG. Melanocyte mitogens induce both melanocyte chemokinesis and chemotaxis. *J Invest Dermatol* 1995;104: 256–9.

15. Bose SK. Is there any treatment of leukotrichia in stable vitiligo? *J Dermatol* 1997; 24: 615–7.

16. Hann SK, IM S, Park YK, and Hur W. Repigmentation of leukotrichia in epidermal grafting and systemic psoralen plus UV-A. *Arch Dermatol* 1992;128:998–9.

17. Thakur P, Sacchidanand S, Nataraj HV, and Savitha AS. A study of hair follicular transplantation as a treatment option for vitiligo. *J Cutan Aesthet Surg* 2015;8:211–7.

Chapter 12

OTHER SUBTYPES AND VARIANTS OF VITILIGO

Sam Shiyao Yang and Emily Yiping Gan

CONTENTS

INTRODUCTION

In the latest revised Vitiligo Global Issues Consensus Conference (VGICC) classification of vitiligo, the condition has been broadly divided into nonsegmental vitiligo (NSV) and segmental vitiligo (SV) [1]. However, there are a few conditions which fit into the general clinical spectrum of vitiligo but are difficult to strictly classify into either NSV or SV. These remain unclassified and include vitiligo punctata, vitiligo minor (hypochromic vitiligo), and follicular vitiligo.

This chapter highlights the clinical characteristics of pre-vitiligo and the unclassified subtypes of vitiligo and explores other morphological variants of vitiligo which may be present in a patient who has classic NSV or SV, namely trichrome/quadrichrome/pentachrome vitiligo, confetti-like depigmentation of vitiligo, inflammatory vitiligo, linear vitiligo, and blue vitiligo.

PRE-VITILIGO

Vitiligo is a disease that involves a progressive loss of melanocytes. In pre-vitiligo or early vitiligo, the skin has not fully depigmented but has lost part of its color, resulting in hypopigmentation. Over time, full depigmentation occurs and the clinical diagnosis of vitiligo becomes more apparent (Figures 12.1 and 12.2). Interestingly, some authors have described how vitiligo depigments in two specific clinical patterns—"marginal hypopigmentation," which may correspond to trichrome vitiligo, and "perifollicular depigmentation" [2]. Reflectance confocal microscopy studies have confirmed the presence of melanin in this early stage of vitiligo [3]. On a cellular level, T-cell infiltration drives the active spread at the margins of nonsegmental and segmental vitiligo, and the innate immune response also plays a key role in the progression of disease via increased production of interferon-alpha [4,5].

UNCLASSIFIED SUBTYPES OF VITILIGO

VITILIGO PUNCTATA (GUTTATE VITILIGO)

This unusual and uncommon form of vitiligo presents as discrete, hypopigmented-to-achromic macules, normally 2–4 mm in size, which are accentuated under Woods lamp examination [6]. They

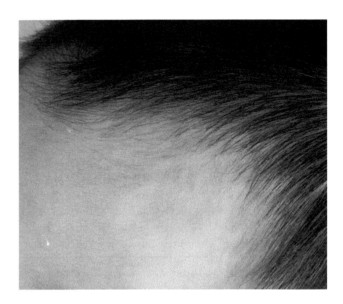

Figure 12.1 A discrete patch of hypopigmentation is initially seen in this patient over the left forehead. (Courtesy of National Skin Centre, Singapore.)

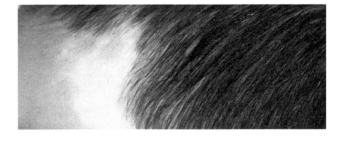

Figure 12.2 This same patch as seen in Figure 12.1 subsequently becomes fully depigmented 7 months later. (Courtesy of National Skin Centre, Singapore.)

tend to be located primarily on sun-exposed sites, such as the upper chest or extremities (Figure 12.3).

In a study of 13 patients, Falabella et al. documented numerous punctate hypopigmented and achromic spots developing following psoralens with natural sunlight (PUVAsol) therapy for vitiligo. Histologically, there was a reduction of melanocytes and melanin, but usually not a complete absence [7]. The authors hypothesized this

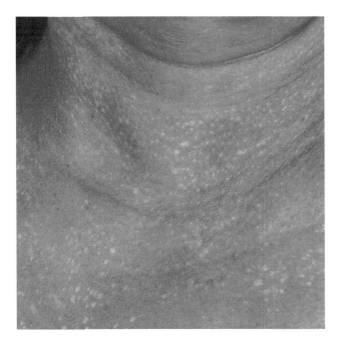

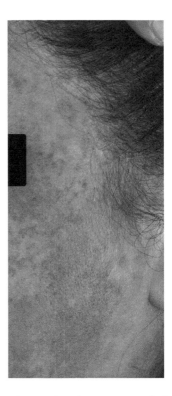

Figure 12.3 Discrete hypo- and depigmented macules are seen over the neck and chest of an patient. (Courtesy of National Skin Centre, Singapore.)

Figure 12.4 Hypopigmented patches are seen on the left side of the face of this patient. (Courtesy of National Skin Centre, Singapore.)

to be a unique subtype of vitiligo but also postulated that the phototoxic effect of phototherapy could have contributed to its onset [7]. In a more recent case report, Arunprasath et al. described a 40-year-old Indian female who presented with multiple depigmented macules on the right shoulder without any prior treatment. Histopathological examination of one of the lesions confirmed an absence of basal melanocytes, consistent with vitiligo [8].

Although rare, guttate vitiligo remains an important differential for lesions presenting as guttate hypomelanosis or leukoderma. It should be excluded before diagnosing conditions like idiopathic guttate hypomelanosis (IGH), arsenical keratosis, guttate leukoderma of Darier disease, or tuberous sclerosis and clear cell papulosis.

IGH can sometimes be difficult to differentiate clinically from guttate vitiligo. The former is characterized by multiple, discrete, round-to-oval macules that are found on the sun-exposed extensor surfaces of the forearms and lower limbs. Patients with IGH, however, tend to be older, usually more than 50 years old, and the lesions of IGH are typically found on a background of photoaged skin, which demonstrates other features of dermatoheliosis and solar elastosis, unlike in guttate vitiligo. Another distinguishing feature is that in IGH, the macules are classically porcelain-white, whereas in guttate vitiligo, the progression of color loss from hypopigmentation to full achromia may be observed [9].

HYPOCHROMIC VITILIGO

Hypochromic vitiligo or vitiligo minor is a rare condition so far reported only in dark-skinned individuals of skin types V and VI [10]. This terminology reflects the partial pigmentary defect, as the lesions are hypopigmented. Melanocytes in this condition are reduced in number but not completely lost. It has also been linked to autoimmunity, where 21% of patients have been reported to have a comorbid autoimmune disease [10].

Clinically, hypopigmented macules are typically present over the face and trunk, in a seborrheic distribution, although lesions may also be present in non-seborrheic areas (Figure 12.4).

Although hypopigmented patches are known to occur in common vitiligo, these are usually transiently hypopigmented at the onset or

present when vitiligo is unstable and spreading. The striking difference that makes this subtype stand out from common vitiligo is that these lesions remain stable over time, with no signs of obvious inflammation, no associated leukotrichia, and an absence of fluorescence on Woods lamp examination. The presence of associated isolated achromic macules in rare cases is, however, supportive of this being a subtype of vitiligo. Differential diagnoses of this condition include pityriasis alba, postinflammatory hypopigmentation, and hypopigmented mycosis fungoides [11].

In Ezzedine et al.'s initial study of 24 patients, where this entity was first described and proposed, the reported patients had an absence of or poor response to conventional vitiligo treatment. As this entity is still relatively new, further studies are needed to better delineate its features [10].

FOLLICULAR VITILIGO

This is a new subtype of vitiligo which involves the hair follicle melanocytic reservoir and demonstrates an unusual preference for follicular melanocytes. Patients with follicular vitiligo present primarily with whitening of their body and scalp hairs (Figure 12.5), and in certain cases, leukotrichia precedes cutaneous depigmentation (Figure 12.6) [12]. This is unlike classical vitiligo, where cutaneous depigmentation is the predominant clinical feature and hairs are usually spared. In progressive classical vitiligo, as skin pigment is depleted, hairs in the depigmented region may lose their color as well (Figures 12.5 and 12.6).

The pathogenesis of follicular vitiligo is still unclear. It is believed that in the setting of genetically predisposed individuals, melanocyte-intrinsic abnormalities coupled with accumulated oxidative stress result in cellular damage, loss of the hair follicle immune privilege, immune activation, and exposure of a unique follicular melanocyte antigen leading to loss of hair pigmentation. In this condition, melanocytes are absent in the hair follicle, whereas in classical vitiligo without leukotrichia, melanocytes are not completely absent from the follicular unit [13,14]. The follicular melanocytes therefore seem to be the preferentially targeted cell population here,

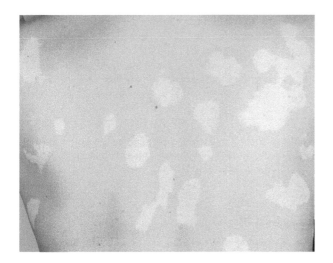

Figures 12.5 A patient with follicular vitiligo, which started with rapid depigmentation of the scalp hair over a few months. This was followed by development of depigmented patches on the scalp, trunk, and limbs. Figure shows numerous depigmented patches on her back, which developed after the onset of widespread scalp poliosis. (Courtesy of National Skin Centre, Singapore.)

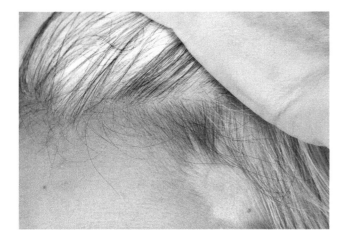

Figure 12.6 Same patient of follicular vitiligo showing poliosis, with white hairs originating from both normally pigmented and depigmented skin. (Courtesy of National Skin Centre, Singapore.)

rather than the epidermal melanocytes. It is likely that the epidermal and follicular melanocytes demonstrate different antigenic profiles, and so represent two separate reserves of slightly differing melanocytes, thereby explaining how this subtype of vitiligo arises.

In patients with follicular vitiligo, the absence of follicular melanocytes and their precursors unfortunately confers a poorer prognosis and treatment response [12].

MORPHOLOGICAL VARIANTS OF VITILIGO

TRICHROME/QUADRICHROME/PENTACHROME VITILIGO

Lesions of *trichrome vitiligo* contain three subtly different shades of white. This term was first coined by Fitzpatrick in the 1960s. The center is completely depigmented and achromic, followed by a zone of intermediate hypopigmentation, which is then surrounded by unaffected and clearly demarcated normal skin in the periphery. Over a period ranging from weeks to months, this lesion eventually evolves

into a classical fully depigmented vitiliginous macule. The presence of an intermediary or transitional zone between affected and normal skin suggests a centrifugal spread of hypomelanosis. This intermediate layer is also sometimes referred to as the "intermediate tan zone," while the entire pattern has also been referred to as "cockade-like" [6]. A cockade is an oval-shaped symbol of distinctive colors normally worn on a hat.

Of note, trichrome vitiligo tends to be found in photoprotected areas such as the trunk, abdomen, back, and buttocks. It is postulated that the lack of sun exposure and the lower melanocyte density on the trunk, as compared to the face, contribute to a slower rate of vitiligo spread, thereby allowing the characteristics of trichrome vitiligo to manifest (Figure 12.7). Histologically, lesions of trichrome vitiligo are characterized by the presence of an inflammatory infiltrate and vacuolar degeneration of the basal layer, which is especially accentuated around the melanocytes [15].

When a fourth color is observed, the lesions have been termed *quadrichrome vitiligo*. In such patients, this is a sign of improvement, where the additional brown color is present due to perifollicular or marginal repigmentation.

Interestingly, *pentachrome vitiligo* has been described, where there are five shades of colors, namely white, tan, medium brown (unaffected skin), dark brown, and black. Fargnoli and Bolognia described a 12-year-old girl with type VI skin who had pentachrome vitiligo [16]. She presented with areas of complete depigmentation over the face, trunk, and extremities, as well as hypopigmented tan macules and patches between depigmented areas and normal medium brown skin. Strikingly, this patient also had dark brown areas over the buttocks, toes, and fingers, and patches of black skin in the intragluteal folds and elbows. Histologically, the areas of depigmentation demonstrated complete loss of melanin while the hypopigmented tan areas had a corresponding decreased amount of epidermal melanin and fewer melanocytes. In the most hyperpigmented macules, there

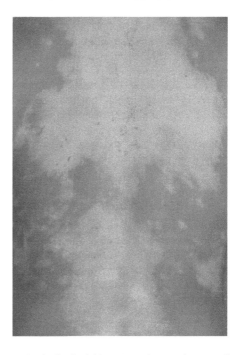

Figure 12.7 On the back of this patient, there are large confluent hypo- and depigmented patches, some of which demonstrate the trichrome vitiligo pattern, where there is complete depigmentation centrally, followed by a transitional zone of light brown hypopigmentation that is surrounded by normal skin. On closer inspection, confetti-like depigmented macules can also be seen along the borders of several patches. (Courtesy of National Skin Centre, Singapore.)

was an increase in number of melanocytes as well as an increase in epidermal melanin content. Sparse lymphocytic infiltrate and melanophages were observed in the biopsies taken from both hypo- and hyperpigmented areas [16]. This patient subsequently progressed into widespread spontaneous depigmentation within 1 year of presentation. What remains unusual about this case is the presence of markedly hyperpigmented areas with increased melanocytes, a feature that still remains unexplained.

CONFETTI-LIKE DEPIGMENTATION OF VITILIGO

This is defined by numerous 1- to 5-mm guttate depigmented macules, clustered in groups in a non-follicular pattern. The nonuniformity in size of the macules, from being pinpoint to several millimeters in diameter, explains the name "confetti-like." Of note, these macules are usually found at the borders of existing vitiliginous lesions (Figure 12.7), are best appreciated with Woods lamp examination and tend to involve the acral areas, arms, and face. Early pilot studies indicate that this may constitute a sign of active and spreading inflammation and may herald rapidly progressive disease [17].

Histologically, a lymphocytic infiltrate can be seen at the dermo–epidermal junction together with a lack of melanocytes. The presence of this feature also indicates a greater likelihood of rapidly progressive disease [18].

Few other conditions mimic this pattern of confetti-like hypopigmentation. Chemical leukoderma is a close differential, and a detailed history of chemical exposure is required. This pattern of hypopigmentation may also arise separately as a result of phototherapy or after repeated pigment laser treatment for melasma [19]. In the former, cumulative exposure to either PUVA (psoralens with UVA) or UVB is thought to cause direct cellular damage to the melanocytes [20].

INFLAMMATORY VITILIGO

Inflammatory vitiligo with raised borders (IVRB) is a variant that presents with a pruritic, raised erythematous border at the periphery of the depigmented patch, sometimes accompanied by scaling. Koebnerization has been reported with this rare variant, which can occur at any age and without gender predilection [21]. The lesions tend to involve extensive body surface areas and are generally considered progressive and unstable. Of note, concomitant inflammatory and clinically non-inflammatory patches may occur in the same patient [22]. Within the spectrum of inflammatory vitiligo, Lee et al. have also described a 61-year-old patient with thin, pink, scaly plaques as well as serpiginous lesions with fine scale, a variant they have termed figurate and papulosquamous vitiligo [23].

Mycosis fungoides is an important differential which cannot be missed, as this condition can sometimes present with hypopigmented lesions which have an inflammatory edge [24].

Histologically, a biopsy from the inflammatory border shows psoriasiform hyperplasia and parakeratosis, corresponding to the scaling seen clinically [21]. There is a mononuclear inflammatory infiltrate located perivascularly and often in a lichenoid pattern, with reports of degeneration of melanocytes and basal keratinocytes [25]. Immunohistochemistry of the inflammatory infiltrate has revealed CD8 cells and sparse CD4 cells [26,27].

This entity lends support to the theory that vitiligo is an inflammatory disorder. In fact, depigmentation in vitiligo has been observed to pass through two stages in patients with skin of color. In stage 1, the initial affected area may be urticarial or have a dermatitis-like morphology with underlying erythema. This subsequently fades into a milky or chalk-white color and becomes well demarcated from surrounding normal skin as it enters stage 2 [28]. Histologically, stage 1 frequently

demonstrates an inflammatory infiltrate, especially in the marginal areas, and these inflammatory cells gather in small foci surrounding melanocytes. In some cases, the inflammatory response may be large enough, resulting in extensive spongiosis and keratinocyte degeneration. This corresponds to the varied inflammatory clinical morphologies seen in stage 1. In stage 2, the inflammatory infiltrate is less common and, when present, much less intense as compared to stage 1.

In patients with inflammatory vitiligo, treatment with topical corticosteroids and calcineurin inhibitors leads to improvement of the erythema at the border, albeit without repigmentation. Early and aggressive treatment with oral corticosteroids and phototherapy is more likely to result in cessation of disease activity and improvement with repigmentation [29].

LINEAR VITILIGO

Linear vitiliginous patches are known to occur. Most commonly, they present as linear achromic lesions that match previously excoriated areas. This likely reflects an underlying Koebner or isomorphic phenomenon [30].

In addition, within the spectrum of phenotypes of segmental vitiligo, linear or bandlike unilateral lesions are often described. In some of these patients, the lesions have been described to roughly fit within known Blaschko lines [31]. Schallreuter et al. reported a 38-year-old woman with linear depigmented streaks and lines over the upper extremities and left leg, which followed the lines of Blaschko. She later developed depigmented macules and patches over her face and lips [32].

However, this Blaschko linear distribution is not common, and van Geel et al. have described how segmental vitiligo lesions follow a distinct pattern which does not entirely correspond to other unilateral or band-shaped dermatoses. Yet, clear clinical overlap has been observed between segmental vitiligo and some mosaic dermatoses of melanocyte origin such as segmental lentiginosis, thereby lending support to the role of somatic mosaicism in at least some cases of segmental vitiligo [33].

BLUE VITILIGO

This is a rare phenomenon first described in 1995 in an HIV-positive black man with vitiligo over his forearms and calves, for which he was treated with PUVA phototherapy. He was concurrently receiving zidovudine for HIV and bleomycin for Kaposi sarcoma. His depigmentation was initially progressive and reported to be blue in the areas of rapid progression. This blue color was postulated to be caused by the development of vitiligo in skin that was previously affected by postinflammatory hyperpigmentation secondary to phototherapy, and it was believed that the Tyndall effect resulted in an unusual scatter of short-wavelength visible light and hence the blue appearance [34].

Hamzavi et al. also reported a case of blue vitiligo in a 47-year-old Filipino man of Fitzpatrick skin type V who had a 2-year history of vitiligo. He underwent a split-body clinical trial, where one side was treated with narrowband UVB phototherapy while the other side remained covered up. Blue-gray patches were noted within the treated areas of vitiligo on his trunk and legs. Histologically, there was an absence of epidermal melanocytes and the presence of dermal melanophages [35].

In a more recent report published in 2009, Chandrashekar described a 23-year-old woman of Indian origin who presented with depigmented macules over her right forearm, the dorsum of her hands, and the right areola. Over the right forearm, the lesion had four zones of color: brown, blue, hypopigmentation, and complete depigmentation. Dermatoscopy showed blue dots of dermal melanin in an area without epidermal melanin. In this case, the author postulated that the postinflammatory hyperpigmentation could have been secondary to acute photosensitivity in the early stages of vitiligo when epidermal melanin was still present. This dermal melanin subsequently became clinically obvious as blue vitiligo when the progression of disease activity resulted in a loss of epidermal melanin [36].

CONCLUSION

This chapter summarizes the lesser known subtypes and morphological variants of vitiligo. It is important for dermatologists to recognize these variants, as early diagnosis and initiation of treatment would result in a better prognosis as well as reduced patient anxiety.

REFERENCES

1. Ezzedine K, Lim HW, Suzuki T et al. Vitiligo Global Issue Consensus Conference Panelists. Revised classification/nomenclature of vitiligo and related issues: The Vitiligo Global Issues Consensus Conference. *Pigment Cell Melanoma Res* 2012;25:1–13.

2. Menchini G, Comacchi C, Cappugi P, and Torchia D. Depigmentation patterns of nonsegmental vitiligo: A prospective study of macromorphologic changes in lesions. *Am J Clin Dermatol* 2013;14:55–9.

3. Lai LG, and Xu AE. In vivo reflectance confocal microscopy imaging of vitiligo, nevus depigmentosus and nevus anemicus. *Skin Res Technol* 2011;17:404–10.

4. Shin J, Kang HY, Kim KH, Park CJ, Oh SH, Lee SC, Lee S, Choi GS, and Han SK. Involvement of T cells in early evolving segmental vitiligo. *Clin Exp Dermatol* 2016;41:671–4.

5. Bertolotti A, Boniface K, Vergier B, Mossalayi D, Taieb A, Ezzedine K, and Seneschal J. Type I interferon signature in the initiation of the immune response in vitiligo. *Pigment Cell Melanoma Res* 2014;27:398–407.

6. Ortonne J, and Passeron T. Vitiligo and other disorders of hypopigmentation. In: Ortonne J, Bolognia J, Jorizzo J, and Rapini R, eds. *Dermatology*, 3rd ed. Spain: Elsevier; 2008, pp. 1023–1049.

7. Falabella R, Escobar CE, Carrascal E, and Arroyave JA. Leukoderma punctate. *J Am Acad Dermatol* 1988;18:485–94.

8. Arunprasath P, Reji S, and Srivenkateswaran K. Vitiligo ponctue. *The Clinical Picture* 2015;2:103.

9. Juntongjin P, and Laosakul K. Idiopathic guttate hypomelanosis: A review of its etiology, pathogenesis, findings, and treatments. *Am J Clin Dermatol* 2016;17:403–11.

10. Ezzedine K, Mahé A, van Geel N et al. Hypochromic vitiligo: Delineation of a new entity. *Brit J Dermatol* 2015;172:716–21.

11. Sharma VK. Hypochromic vitiligo: A perspective. *Brit J Dermatol* 2015;172:561–2.

12. Gan EY, Cario-André M, Pain C, Goussot JF, Taieb A, Seneschal J, and Ezzedine K. Follicular vitiligo: A report of 8 cases. *J Am Acad Dermatol* 2016;74:1178–84.

13. Ezzedine K, Amazan E, Séneschal J, Cario-André M, Léauté-Labrèze C, Vergier B, Boralevi F, and Taieb A. Follicular vitiligo: A new form of vitiligo. *Pigment Cell Melanoma Res* 2012;25:527–9.

14. Seleit I, Bakry OA, Abdou AG, and Dawoud NM. Immunohistochemical evaluation of vitiliginous hair follicle melanocyte reservoir: Is it retained? *J Eur Acad Dermatol Venereol* 2015;29:444–51.

15. Hann SK, Kim YS, Yoo JH, and Chun YS. Clinical and histopathological characteristics of trichrome vitiligo. *J Am Acad Dermatol* 2000;42:589–96.

16. Fargnoli MC, and Bolognia JL. Pentachrome vilitigo. *J Am Acad Dermatol* 1995;33:853–6.

17. Menchini G, Comacchi C, Cappugi P, and Torchia D. Depigmentation patterns of nonsegmental vitiligo. *Am J Clin Dermatol* 2014;14:55–9.

18. Sosa JJ, Currimbhoy SD, Ukoha U, Sirignano S, O'Leary R, Vandergriff T, Hynan LS, and Pandya AG. Confetti-like depigmentation: A potential sign of rapidly progressing vitiligo. *J Am Acad Dermatol* 2015;73:272–5.

19. Wong Y, Lee SS, and Goh CL. Hypopigmentation induced by frequent low-fluence, large-spot-size QS Nd:YAG laser treatments. *Ann Dermatol* 2015;27:751–5.

20. Bhatnagar A, Kanwar AJ, Parsad D, Narang T, and De D. Confetti-like hypopigmentation: A rare complication of common phototherapeutic modality. *J Eur Acad Dermatol Venereol* 2007;21:1253–302.

21. Verma SB. Inflammatory vitiligo with raised borders and psoriasiform histopathology. *Dermatol Online J* 2005;11:13.

22. Ezzedine K, Seneschal J, Attili R, and Taieb A. *Vitiligo*. Berlin Heidelberg: Springer; 2010.

23. Lee D, Lazova R, and Bolognia JL. A figurate papulosquamous variant of vitiligo. *Dermatology* 2000;200:270–4.

24. Soro LA, Gust AJ, and Purcell SM. Inflammatory vitiligo versus hypopigmented mycosis fungoides in a 58-year-old Indian female. *Indian Dermatol Online J* 2013;4:3121–5.

25. Tsuboi H, Yonemoto K, and Katsuoka K. Vitiligo with inflammatory raised borders with hepatitis C virus infection. *J Dermatol* 2006;33:577–8.

26. Sugita K, Izu K, and Tokura Y. Vitiligo with inflammatory raised borders, associated with atopic dermatitis. *Clin Exp Dermatol* 2006;31:80–2.

27. Tsuruta D, Hamada T, Teramae H, Mito H, and Ishii M. Inflammatory vitiligo in Vogt-Koyanagi-Harada disease. *J Am Acad Dermatol* 2001;44:129–31.

28. Sharquie KE, Mehenna SH, Naji AA, and Al-Azzawi H. Inflammatory changes in vitiligo Stage I and II depigmentation. *Am J Dermatopathol* 2004;26:108–12.

29. Gunasekera N, Murphy GF, and Sheth VM. Repigmentation of extensive inflammatory vitiligo with raised borders using early and aggressive treatment. *Dermatology* 2015;230:11–5.

30. Dupre A, and Christol B. Cockade-like vitiligo and linear vitiligo a variant of Fitzpatrick's trichrome vitiligo. *Arch Dermatol Res* 1978;28:197–203.

31. van Geel N, De Lille S, Vandenhaute S, Gauthier Y, Mollet I, Brochez L, and Lambert J. Different phenotypes of segmental vitiligo based on a clinical observational study. *J Eur Acad Dermatol Venereol* 2011;25:673–8.

32. Schallreuter KU, Krüger C, Rokos H, Hasse S, Zothner C, and Panske A. Basic research confirms coexistence of acquired Blaschkolinear vitiligo and acrofacial vitiligo. *Arch Dermatol Res* 2007;299:225–30.

33. van Geel N, Speeckaert R, Melsens E, Toelle SP, Speeckaert M, De Schepper S, Lambert J, and Brochez L. The distribution pattern of segmental vitiligo: Clues for somatic mosaicism. *Br J Dermatol* 2013;168:56–64.

34. Ivker R, Goldaber M, Buchness MR. Blue vitiligo. *J Am Acad Dermatol* 1994;30:829–31.

35. Hamzavi I, Shiff N, Martinka M, Huang Z, McLean D, Zeng H, and Lui H. Spectroscopic assessment of dermal melanin using blue vitiligo as an *in vivo* model. *Photodermatol Photoimmunol Photomed* 2006;22:46–51.

36. Chandrashekar L. Dermatoscopy of blue vitiligo. *Clin Exp Dermatol* 2009;34:125–6.

Chapter 13

VITILIGO AND ASSOCIATED COMORBIDITIES

Vibhu Mehndiratta and Anuja Yadav

CONTENTS

INTRODUCTION

Vitiligo is an acquired, progressive cutaneous achromia resulting from progressive loss of melanocytes with a complex etiopathogenesis that involves a polygenic inheritance and multiple etiological factors. It is stated that vitiligo affects 0.5%–1% of the world's population and can involve any age, the majority of cases beginning between the second and third decade [1]. It is clinically characterized by variously sized or shaped, single or multiple patches of milk-white color that may show hyperpigmented borders and a tendency to enlarge peripherally [2]. Vitiligo has been classified into two major forms: segmental vitiligo (typically unilateral maculae in a segmental/band-shaped distribution) and nonsegmental vitiligo (bilateral maculae, often distributed in an acrofacial pattern or scattered symmetrically over the entire body).

ASSOCIATED DISEASES

Vitiligo is associated with other autoimmune diseases (Table 13.1). "Autoimmunity" is held responsible for vitiligo, as there is evidence in the form of a higher prevalence of vitiligo in different autoimmune diseases with the presence of organ-specific antibodies in affected patients [3]. The autoimmune hypothesis of vitiligo is strongly supported by its frequent association (20%–30%) with autoimmune disease and/or with one or more organ and non-organ-specific autoantibodies (up to 50% in some studies) [4]. Among autoimmune diseases, the strongest association is with thyroid disease. Older age, later age of onset, and longer duration of vitiligo may play a role in the development of comorbid autoimmune diseases. Other autoimmune diseases reported in patients with vitiligo vary depending on the population studied; these include alopecia areata, Addison disease, autoimmune gastritis, inflammatory bowel disease (IBD), pernicious anemia, psoriasis, rheumatoid arthritis, systemic lupus erythematosus (SLE), and type 1 diabetes mellitus (T1DM). First-degree relatives of patients with vitiligo have a higher frequency of vitiligo and the aforementioned autoimmune diseases than that in the general population [5]. In addition, those with at least one comorbid disease were slightly more likely to have a greater body surface area (BSA) affected [5].

THYROID DYSFUNCTION

Thyroid functional disorders and autoimmune thyroid diseases have been reported in association with vitiligo, and it seems that the incidence of clinical and subclinical thyroid involvement is more common in vitiligo patients than healthy subjects [6]. Vitiligo frequently precedes the thyroid involvement; thus, screening vitiligo patients for thyroid function and thyroid antibody seems plausible [7]. Moreover, increased risk of autoimmune/endocrine diseases was shown in first- and second-degree relatives of vitiligo patients with positive organ-specific antibodies [8]. Hashimoto thyroiditis and Graves disease are the most important and prevalent autoimmune thyroid diseases associated with vitiligo. Elevated levels of anti-TPO are seen in more than 90% of cases of Hashimoto thyroiditis and about 75% of Graves disease cases. This figure is only 10% in healthy people, although it may reach 30% in the elderly [9,10].

PERNICIOUS ANEMIA

Ishida (1954) showed that many subjects with vitiligo secrete less gastric acid than normal; other studies revealed that achlorhydria was present in a significant number [11]. A close clinical relationship between pernicious anemia and vitiligo has since been established. In 1955 study done by Allison and Curtis along with Dawber found that 9% of patients with pernicious anemia have vitiligo [2]. There is also a case reported of a patient with vitiligo and carcinoma of the body of the stomach [2]. This has not previously been described, but in view of the association of vitiligo with achlorhydria and pernicious anemia, an association with carcinoma of the stomach might almost be predicted. Further work will be necessary to confirm this finding.

ADDISON DISEASE

Addison (1855) demonstrated one patient with predominant hyperpigmentation but also many areas of typical vitiligo [2]. The frequency of coincidence of vitiligo and Addison disease and autoimmune chronic gastritis has been reported from 0.6% to 50% in different studies [12].

DIABETES

In 1959, Lerner gave description of two cases about the occurrence of vitiligo with diabetes as first reference [2]. In 1968, Cunliffe et al. demonstrated a high incidence of diabetes in the family members of subjects with vitiligo [2]. A study of about 512 mature-onset diabetics done by Dawber in 1968 found that 25 patients have concomitant vitiligo [2]. The clinical association of "juvenile" diabetes and vitiligo has not so far been proven [2]. Vitiligo occurs more commonly in type 1 diabetes mellitus. A few recent studies have shown its increased occurrence in type 2 diabetes mellitus [13]. In a study, vitiligo was seen in 12% of type 2 diabetic patients, and in the age- and sex-matched controls it was 6% [12]. In another study by Afkhami-Ardekani et al. [14] in Iran, vitiligo was seen in 4.9% of type 2 diabetics where the prevalence of vitiligo in the general population was 0.6%. In a study by Vijayasingam et al. [15], the prevalence of vitiligo in similar subjects was 3.3% [15].

Table 13.1   Diseases associated with vitiligo

1. Thyroid disease (hyperthyroidism and hypothyroidism)
2. Pernicious anemia
3. Addison disease
4. Diabetes
5. Alopecia areata
6. Halo nevi
7. Primary biliary cirrhosis
8. Localized scleroderma (morphea)
9. Lichen planus
10. Atopic dermatitis
11. Psoriasis
12. Lupus erythematosus
13. Chronic mucocutaneous candidiasis
14. Inflammatory bowel disease
15. Malignant melanoma
16. Vogt-Koyanagi-Harada syndrome

ALOPECIA AREATA

Alopecia areata and vitiligo are common skin disorders that are known to coexist in an individual [16]. However, strict anatomical colocalization of vitiligo and alopecia areata has been very rarely reported in the literature [16].

Although the exact antigen is not known, it is widely accepted that alopecia areata and vitiligo are autoimmune diseases with cell-mediated immunity against hair follicle melanocytes, keratinocytes, and dermal papilla cells. Alopecia areata and vitiligo have been found to be associated with various other autoimmune cutaneous disorders such as lichen planus, psoriasis, Sjögren syndrome, and lupus erythematosus.

The prevalence of alopecia areata and vitiligo in the general population ranges from 0.1% to 3%, but there is a huge inconsistency regarding the prevalence of autoimmune diseases with alopecia areata. In a few studies on vitiligo, a very high association rate of almost 12.5% was noted, whereas other studies reported an association rate as low as 0.3% [16]. To our knowledge, only seven cases of colocalization have been reported so far in the world literature [16].

HALO NEVI

The association between vitiligo and halo nevi is well established. Several reports have documented the onset of vitiligo at the same time or shortly after the appearance of a halo nevus and, in a recent study, halo nevi were present in 31.1% of all vitiligo patients [1]. Halo nevus (HN), also known as Sutton's nevus or leukoderma centrifugum acquisitum, is a benign, mostly acquired, melanocytic nevus surrounded by a halo of depigmentation [17]. HN may be single, or multiple HN may be observed. The main localization of HN is the trunk [18]. Family history is mostly negative, but in some cases of HN, vitiligo, atopic dermatitis, or autoimmune disorders, mainly Hashimoto thyroiditis, have been reported in relatives. Some authors suggest that even if the exact etiology of halo phenomenon and vitiligo remains uncertain, a common immunologically-mediated response to pigmented cells might be considered [19].

PRIMARY BILIARY CIRRHOSIS

Although primary biliary cirrhosis, a well-characterized autoimmune disorder of the liver, is frequently associated with other autoimmune diseases, to date only one case has been described in association with vitiligo [20]. As primary biliary cirrhosis may be present at subclinical levels for a long time, antimitochondrial

antibodies can be studied as sensitive and specific markers of this disease in order to look for occult primary biliary cirrhosis [21].

LOCALIZED SCLERODERMA

Localized scleroderma (LS), or morphea, is characterized by sclerosis of the skin, and in some cases underlying tissue autoimmune phenomena such as vitiligo and Hashimoto thyroiditis associated with LS have been reported, suggesting the possible autoimmune basis of morphea. LS associated with vitiligo and another autoimmune phenomena like Hashimoto thyroiditis and autoimmune thrombocytopenic purpura has been rarely reported to occur simultaneously, with evidence of improvement to treatment with systemic steroids [22,23]. Some studies have also indicated an association of autoimmune diseases and an increased frequency of serum autoantibodies with morphea [24]. In the literature, it has been raised that this association is more than coincidence, and it suggests an autoimmune basis for these conditions [25].

LICHEN PLANUS

A number of cases describing associations between lichen planus (LP) and vitiligo have been reported. LP lesions have been described as confined to vitiliginous areas alone or even affecting both normal and vitiliginous skin [26,27]. It has been said to be more severe on sun-exposed vitiliginous areas, less so on sun-exposed normally pigmented skin, and the least severe on covered areas [28]. In most cases, vitiligo is described as the precursor disease, but concomitant onset and progression of both conditions has also been noted.

ATOPIC DERMATITIS

A history of atopic disease may be helpful to predict which patients with vitiligo will experience progression to extensive disease. There are several possible explanations for the association of vitiligo involving a BSA of at least 76% and itching or burning with atopic diseases. The proinflammatory state of AD may predispose toward melanocyte destruction, while scratching of pruritic atopic dermatitis (AD) lesions may koebnerize vitiligo. Alternatively, there may be a common genetic mutation(s) that predisposes to both AD and vitiligo. One such example might be vitamin D receptor polymorphisms that are associated with generalized vitiligo and severe AD [29]. Little is known about the atopic comorbidities associated with vitiligo. The co-occurrence of AD together with either vitiligo or alopecia areata (AA) may have important clinical ramifications, with potentially different phenotypes, prognosis, and/or response to therapy. It has been hypothesized that AD is increased in patients with vitiligo [30].

PSORIASIS

Anatomical cohabitation of psoriasis and vitiligo has been reported [31]. It is not suprising to see an association of vitiligo and psoriasis, as they affect 1%–3% of the population normally [32]. Cohabitation of two disorders that possess a prominent immunological component in their pathogenesis may offer a clue as to their causation.

LUPUS ERYTHEMATOSUS

Coexistence of SLE and vitiligo has been infrequently reported [33]. However, cases of vitiligo coexisting with discoid lupus erythematosus (DLE) have been much rarer. It has been observed that the autoimmune disorders are significantly elevated in vitiligo probands. A genetic explanation for the association between lupus erythematosus and vitiligo has recently been attempted. In a study of 16 European families, Nath et al. [34]. found that the SLVe1 gene on chromosome 17 may explain the relationship between SLE and vitiligo. Rahner et al. [35] related various mutS homolog 6 gene mutations (present in hereditary nonpolyposis colorectal cancer) with the presence of both autoimmune processes.

CHRONIC MUCOCUTANEOUS CANDIDIASIS

Previous reports have documented the fact that some patients with mucocutaneous candidiasis and vitiligo have a complement-fixing anti-pigment-cell factor in their serum. A study done by Nordlund et al. [36] suggested that these anti-pigment-cell factors, which are most probably antibodies, are not cytotoxic for pigment cells and thus not the cause of vitiligo. The association of vitiligo and anti-pigment-cell factors with the syndrome of mucocutaneous candidiasis implicates the immune system as a causal factor of vitiligo [36].

INFLAMMATORY BOWEL DISEASE

In inflammatory bowel diseases, ulcerative colitis (UC) is the one most frequently associated with selective IgA deficiency. It is also possible to encounter a series of autoimmune diseases, such as vitiligo and/or psoriasis. Some authors consider that vitiligo pathogenesis associated with IBD is autoimmune or, in other cases, genetic. The incidence of vitiligo in the general population is 0.3%, compared to 1.1% among UC patients. The association of inflammatory bowel pathology with IgA deficiency and vitiligo can be considered a rare case in medical practice [37].

MELANOMA

Areas of depigmentation sometimes develop in patients with melanoma [1]. These may be local or distant.

VOGT-KOYANAGI-HARADA SYNDROME

Vitiligo with uveitis, central nervous system involvement, and premature graying of the hair occurs in the Vogt-Koyanagi-Harada syndrome.

REFERENCES

1. Geel NV, and Speeckaert R. In: Burns T, Breathnach S, Cox N, and Griffiths C, eds. *Rook's Textbook of Dermatology*, Vol 3, 9th ed. 88. Oxford: Blackwell Science; 2016, pp. 34–35.

2. Dawber RPR. Clinical associations of vitiligo. *Postgrad Med J* 1970;46:276–7.

3. Bleehen SS. Disorders of skin color. In: Burns T, Breathnach S, Cox N, and Griffiths C, eds. *Rook's Textbook of Dermatology*, 7th ed. 39. Oxford: Blackwell Science; 2004, pp. 53–7.

4. Nordlund JJ, and Lemer AB. Vitiligo: It is important. *Arch Dermatol* 1982;118:5–8, 3.

5. Gill L, Zarbo A, Isedeh P, Jacobsen G, Lim HW, and Hamzavi I. Comorbid autoimmune diseases in patients with vitiligo: A cross-sectional study. *J Am Acad Dermatol* 2016;74:295–301.

6. Hegedus L, Heidenheim M, Gervil M, Hjalgrim H, and Hoier-Madsen M. High frequency of thyroid dysfunction in patients with vitiligo. *Acta Derm Venereol* 1994;74:120–3.

7. Shong YK, and Kim JA. Vitiligo in autoimmune thyroid disease. *Thyroidology* 1991;3:89–91.

8. Grimes PE, Halder RM, Jones C, Chakrabarti SG, Enterline J, Minus HR, and Kenney JA Jr. Autoantibodies and their clinical significance in a black vitiligo population. *Arch Dermatol* 1983;119:300–3.

9. Ai J, Leonhardt MJ, and Heymann RW. Autoimmune thyroid diseases. Etiology, pathogenesis, and dermatologic manifestations. *Am Acad Dermatol* 2003;48:641–59.

10. Braverman L, and Uitger RD, eds. *Werner and Ingbar's the Thyroid: A Fundamental and Clinical Text*, 9th ed. NewYork: Lippincott Williams and Wilkins; 2005, p. 363.

11. Ishida K. Studies on gastric acidity in various skin diseases. *Japanese J Dermatol Venerol* 1954;64:145.

12. Shahmoradi Z, Najafian J, Naeini, FF, and Fahimipour F. Vitiligo and autoantibodies of celiac disease. *Int J Prev Med* 2013;4:200–3.

13. Raveendra L, Hemavathi RN, and Rajgopal S. A study of vitiligo in type 2 diabetic patients. *Indian J Dermatol* 2017; 62:168–70.

14. Afkhami-Ardekani M, Ghadiri-Anari A, Ebrahimzadeh-Ardakani M, and Zaji N. Prevalence of vitiligo among type 2 diabetic patients in an Iranian population. *Int J Dermatol* 2014;53:956–8.

15. Vijayasingam SM, Thai AC, and Chan HL. Non-infective skin associations of diabetes mellitus. *Ann Acad Med Singapore* 1988;17:526–35.

16. Krishnaram AS, Saigal A, and Adityan B. Alopecia areata–vitiligo overlap syndrome: An emerging clinical variant. *Indian J Dermatol Venereol Leprol* 2013;79:535–37.

17. Geel NV, and Speeckaert R. In: Burns T, Breathnach S, Cox N, and Griffiths C, eds. *Rook's Textbook of Dermatology*, Vol 3, 9th ed. 88. Oxford: Blackwell Science; 2016, pp. 40–41.

18. Kolm I, Di Stefani A, Zalaudek I et al. Dermoscopy pattern of halo nevi. *Arch Dermatol* 2006;142:1627–32.

19. Stierman SC, Tierney EP, and Shwayder TA. Halo congenital nevocellular nevi associated with extralesional vitiligo: A case series with review of the literature. *Pediatr Dermatol* 2009;6:414–24.

20. Enat R, and Gilhar A. Vitiligo and primary biliary cirrhosis. *Am J Gastroenterol* 1984;79:804–5.

21. Munoz LE, Thomas TTC, Sheuer PJ et al. Is mitochondrial antibody diagnostic of primary biliary cirrhosis? *Gut* 1981;22:136–40.

22. Dervis E, Acbay O, Barut G, Karaoglu A, and Ersoy L. Association of vitiligo, morphea, and Hashimoto's thyroiditis. *Int J Dermatol* 2004;43:236–7.

23. Bonifati C, Impara G, Morrone A, Pietrangeli A, and Carducci M. Simultaneous occurrence of linear scleroderma and homolateral segmental vitíligo. *J Eur Acad Dermatol Venereol* 2006;20(1):63–5.

24. Harrington CI, and Dunsmore IR. An investigation into the incidence of autoimmune disorders in patients with localized morphoea. *Br J Dermatol* 1989;120:645–8.

25. Soylu S, Gül U, Gönül M, Kiliç A, Cakmak SK, and Demiriz M. An uncommon presentation of the co-existence of morphea and vitiligo in a patient with chronic hepatitis B virus infection: Is there a possible association with autoimmunity? *Am J Clin Dermatol* 2009;10:336–8.

26. Ujiie H, Sawamura D, and Shimizu H. Development of lichen planus and psoriasis on lesions of vitiligo vulgaris. *Clin Exper Dermatol* 2006;5:690–9.

27. Oktay FG, Mansur AT, and Ayding IE. Colocalization of vitiligo and lichen planus on scrotal skin: A finding contrary to the actinic damage theory. *Dermatology* 2006;212:390–2.

28. Baghestani S, Moosavi A, and Eftekhari T. Familial colocalization of lichen planus and vitiligo on sun exposed areas. *Ann Dermatol* 2013;25:223–5.

29. Heine G, Hoefer N, Franke A et al. Association of vitamin D receptor gene polymorphisms with severe atopic dermatitis in adults. *Br J Dermatol* 2013;168(4):855–8.

30. Mohan GC, and Silverberg JI. Association of vitiligo and alopecia areata with atopic dermatitis. *JAMA Dermatol* 2015;151(5):522–8.

31. De Moragas JM, and Winkelmann RK. Psoriasis and vitiligo. *Int J Dermatol* 1970;101:235–7.

32. Nordlund JJ. Vitiligo. In: Thiers and Dobson, eds. *Pathogenesis of Skin Disease*. New York: Churchill Livingstone; 1986, pp. 99–127.

33. Callen JP. Discoid lupus erythematosus in a patient with vitiligo and autoimmune thyroiditis. *Int J Dermatol.* 1984;23: 203–4.

34. Nath SK, Kelly JA, Namjou B et al. Evidence for a susceptibility gene, SLEV1, on chromosome 17p13 in families with vitiligo-related systemic lupus erythematosus. *Am J Hum Genet* 2001;69:1401–6.

35. Rahner N, Höeler G, Höegenauer C et al. Compound heterozygosity for two MSH6 mutations in a patient with early onset colorectal cancer, vitiligo and systemic lupus erythematosus. *Am J Med Genet A* 2008;146:1314–9.

36. Nordlund JJ, Howanitz N, Bystryn JC, Forget BM, and Lerne AB. Anti-pigment-cell factor and mucocutaneous candidiasis. *Arch Dermatol* 1981;117(11):705–8.

37. Naumcieff I, Burlea M, Diaconescu S et al. Ulcerative colitis associated with vitiligo and IgA deficiency in a young girl. *Arch Clin Cases* 2017;4(1):41–6.

Chapter 14

REPIGMENTATION IN VITILIGO

Bharat Bhushan Mahajan and Richa Nagpal

CONTENTS

INTRODUCTION

Vitiligo is a common pigmentary disorder of great sociomedical importance, especially in India. The incidence of vitiligo in India is about 3%, as compared to 1% of the world population [1]. It is defined as a circumscribed, acquired, idiopathic depigmentation of skin and hair, often familial, and characterized microscopically by total absence of melanocytes. Melanocytes are pigment-producing cells that originate from dorsal portions of the closing neural tube in vertebrate embryos. Progenitor melanoblasts migrate dorsolaterally between the mesodermal and ectodermal layers to reach their final destination in the hair follicles as well as in the skin, choroid, cochlea, ciliary body, and iris, and this whole process of migration is under tight control by various signaling molecules like Wnt, endothelin-3, stem cell factor (SCF) and c-Kit ligands. Melanocytes should be present in appropriate numbers in order to get normal pigmentation or repigmentation under stimulation with diverse therapies in cases of vitiligo.

BIOCHEMISTRY OF MELANOGENESIS

The major function of melanocytes is to synthesize melanin within specialized organelles called melanosomes and to transfer melanosomes to neighboring keratinocytes to provide protection against UV radiation. Two types of melanin are synthesized within melanosomes: eumelanin and pheomelanin. Eumelanin is dark, brown-black, and insoluble, whereas pheomelanin is light red-yellow, sulfur containing, and soluble. Melanins are indole derivatives of DOPA and are formed in melanosomes through a series of oxidative steps (Figure 14.1). The synthesis of both types of melanin involves a rate-limiting catalytic step in which tyrosine is oxidized by enzyme tyrosinase to L-DOPA, a reaction known as the Raper–Mason pathway. L-DOPA is further oxidized to dopaquinone.

EUMELANIN FORMATION

Dopaquinone is a highly reactive intermediate, and in the absence of sulfhydryl compounds it forms cyclodopa. The redox exchange between cyclodopa and dopaquinone then gives rise to the red intermediate Dopachrome and DOPA. Dopachrome then rearranges to 5,6-dihydroxyindole (DHI) and to a lesser extent to

5,6-dihydroxyindole carboxylic acid (DHICA). Finally, these two compounds are oxidized and polymerized to produce eumelanins.

PHEOMELANIN FORMATION

In contrast to eumelanins, pheomelanins contain sulfur in addition to nitrogen. and are formed from cysteinyldopa. Further oxidation of the thiol adducts leads to the formation of pheomelanin via benzothiazine intermediates.

MECHANISM OF REPIGMENTATION IN VITILIGO [2]

Repigmentation in vitiligo arises from three main sources:

a. The hair follicle unit

b. Unaffected melanocytes within areas of depigmented epidermis

c. Melanocytes located at the edge of vitiligo lesions

The main repigmentation patterns observed in vitiligo (Figure 14.2) are [3]:

a. Perifollicular

b. Marginal

c. Diffuse

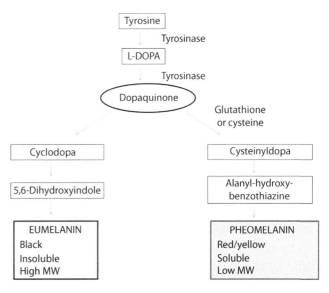

Figure 14.1 Pathway of melanogenesis.

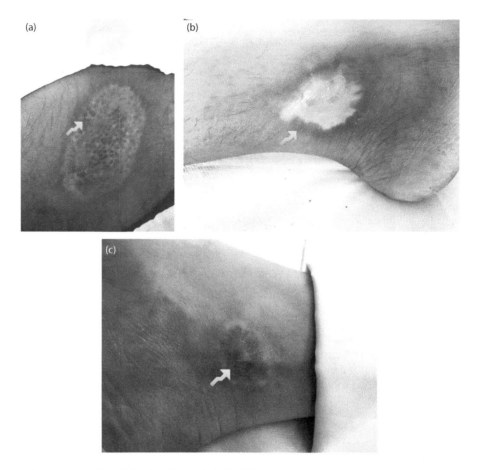

Figure 14.2   Types of repigmentation: (a) perifollicular, (b) marginal, (c) diffuse.

ROLE OF THE HAIR FOLLICLE UNIT (THE MELANOCYTE RESERVOIR)

The human hair follicle is a specialized skin appendage arising from epithelial–mesenchymal interactions beginning around the third month of embryonic development with the formation of the dermal papilla; further proliferation and differentiation of more than 20 different types of cells overlying the papilla initiate the hair follicle structure. The mature hair follicle consists of a morphologically permanent upper segment and a lower segment that remodels during hair cycling. In the bulbar region, multiple dendritic, tyrosinase-positive, large differentiated melanocytes located within the hair matrix provide melanin for hair shaft pigmentation. All the anatomical structures such as outer root sheath, sebaceous gland, infundibulum, and bulb bear the melanocyte reservoir and constitute the pigmentary hair follicle unit. (Figure 14.3).

The role of stem cells and the niche in repigmentation in vitiligo cannot be underestimated. Mammalian stem cells are divided into two categories: (i) stem cells that may differentiate into all of the specialized embryonic tissues, and (ii) stem cells that are present in adult tissues, are capable of regenerating, and maintain the normal tissue turnover and repair by providing new specialized and differentiated cells; these cells must be immature, slow cycling, self-maintaining, and fully competent to regenerate progeny [4–6]. Tissue-specific stem cells are usually found in a specialized environment within specific organs called the niche that provides important signals to guide their function [4] and are assumed to share two important characteristics:

a. The ability for indefinite self-renewal; some stem cells remain in the niche and others become a lineage-restricted transient amplifying cell or progenitor cell that leaves the niche and undergoes several limited cycles of proliferation before transforming into differentiated cells [7].

b. The capacity to differentiate into multi-specialized cell lineages of the specific tissue [6].

As mentioned, it is assumed that stem cells are maintained in a specific environment known as the niche. The bulge region of the hair follicle, defined as the portion of the outer root sheath of the hair follicle at the insertion site of the arrector pili muscle, constitutes currently the best characterized site of epidermal stem cell populations.

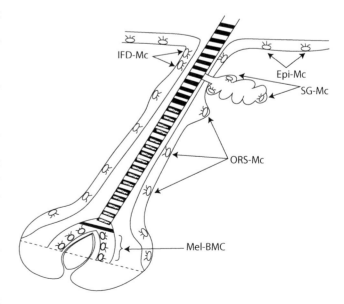

Figure 14.3   Melanocyte reservoir in hair follicle unit. Epi-Mc, epidermal melanocyte; IFD-Mc, infundibular melanocyte; ORS-Mc, outer root sheath melanocyte, Mel-BMc, melanotic bulb melanocyte.

In addition, there is evidence of other stem cells located in the interfollicular epidermis, that is, the portion of the epidermis located between the orifices of hair follicles [4].

Through immunohistological staining techniques and quantitative histomorphometry, the bulge region was found as a site of relative immune privilege, protecting the hair follicle epithelial stem cell reservoir from autoaggressive immune attacks [8], a finding that would not be surprising if occurring in pigment stem cells as well, and would constitute a possible explanation for the presence of pigmented hairs in vitiligo lesions.

FOLLICULAR MELANOGENESIS

Hair pigmentation is provided by very active follicular melanocytes located above the dermal papilla [9]. Synthesis and transfer of melanin granules are regulated by a group of enzymes, structural and regulatory proteins, transporters, and receptors and their ligands, acting on all development stages and cells of the hair follicle [10]. Follicular melanogenesis is tightly coupled to the anagen stage of the hair cycle, becoming switched off during catagen and remaining absent through telogen. During each hair cycle, at the point from the anagen to catagen, melanocytes in the hair bulb matrix undergo apoptosis, and their reconstitution occurs just when the next anagen phase begins, a sequence that is possible because of stem cells at the bulge that activate and induce melanocyte proliferation and migration; this cycle repeats itself producing melanin granules for hair shaft pigmentation.

ROLE OF UNAFFECTED MELANOCYTES

Even though hair follicles are absent in palmar skin, its repigmentation following NB-UVB or PUVA in vitiligo [11] raises the question on immature melanocyte precursors or stem cells remaining in vitiliginous lesions; in fact, a population of cells with molecular characteristics of stem cells and transient amplifying cells related to keratinocytes has been demonstrated at the tips of deep rete ridges in the interfollicular skin of breast, palms, and soles [12–14]; the possibility of similar stem cells related to melanocytes residing in any area of the skin which could act as a reservoir for such areas cannot be excluded, and the possible design of future therapeutic interventions at this level should not be underestimated.

Repigmentation arises mostly from hair follicle units wherever hair is available, but unaffected melanocytes may be present in vitiligo areas even many years after depigmentation takes place [15].

ROLE OF MELANOCYTES LOCATED AT THE EDGE OF VITILIGO LESIONS

The proliferation of melanocytes has been shown to be regulated by the tissue environment, particularly keratinocytes [16]. The keratinocytes produce several factors, such as stem cell factor [17], basic fibroblast growth factor (bFGF) [18], endothelins (ETs) [19], α-melanocyte-stimulating hormone (α-MSH), and adrenocorticotrophic hormone (ACTH) [20].

Histamine has been found to induce proliferation and migration of normal melanocytes and keratinocytes through the H2 receptor [21].

SPECIAL FACTORS REGULATING REPIGMENTATION

Two important factors are needed, cytokines and UV light, described here.

CYTOKINES

During in vitro stimulation of pigment cells, several cytokines have been observed to have different effects:

a. PGD2, LTB4, LTC4, LTD4, LTE4, thromboxane B_2, and HETE produce increased dendricity, edema, higher levels of tyrosinase, and immunoreactive b-locus [22,23];

b. Other cytokines including transforming growth factor alpha, basic fibroblast growth factor (bFGF), stem cell factor (SCF) and endothelin-1 (ET-1), increase melanocyte migration [24,25]; some of these cytokines (LTB4, LTC4, ET-1, EGF) are involved in both functions.

In addition, the SCF/KIT pathway plays a critical role in the control of normal human melanocyte homeostasis [26]. It is conceivable that in the future, cytokines may be used to induce melanocyte migration and stimulate repigmentation [27].

UV LIGHT

Both UVA and NB-UVB are potent melanocyte stimulants for repigmentation; sunlight overexposure with the full UV spectrum may induce marked pigmentation with diffuse skin darkening that depends on the intensity of UV light exposure.

Ultraviolet radiation produces two effects on vitiliginous skin:

a. Immunosuppression: To stop melanocyte destruction after UVB irradiation, T-regulatory (suppressor) cell activity is induced and released; IL10 may be important for the differentiation and activation of T-regulatory cells having suppressor autoimmune activity [28]. A higher suppressive effect has also been observed with narrowband NB-UVB on systemic immune responses [29]. In addition, sera from patients after PUVA contain higher levels of bFGF, SCF, and hepatocyte growth factor, which may induce regrowth of melanocytes [30].

b. Stimulation of growth factors: These molecules may be activated with UVR; this has been shown with UVR, as the number of residual melanocytes increases probably by enhancing melanocyte growth factors such as bFGF and ET-1 [16,31].

SIGNIFICANCE OF LEUKOTRICHIA

The presence of pigmented hairs in vitiliginous skin is a good prognostic sign for vitiligo recovery, speaking in favor of an intact melanocyte reservoir [32]. Nevertheless, after a number of years, in very active vitiligo vulgaris, melanocytes may become gradually destroyed, leading to leukotrichia, although this is not correlated with disease activity [33]. As leukotrichia represents melanocyte reservoir exhaustion, repigmentation of depigmented skin in vitiligo by medical therapies is very unlikely, and melanocyte transplantation may be the best therapy for depigmented skin [34].

Though repigmentation in vitiligo is a complex process, deep understanding of the mechanism of melanogenesis will ensure a new era in the management of vitiligo.

REFERENCES

1. Lerner AB. Vitiligo. *J Invest Dermatol* 1959;32:285–310.

2. Falabella R, and Barona MI. Update on skin repigmentation therapies in vitiligo. *Pigment Cell Melanoma Res* 2009;22:42–65.

3. Parsad D, Pandhi R, Dogra S, and Kumar B. Clinical study of repigmentation patterns with different treatment modalities

and their correlation with speed and stability of repigmentation in 352 vitiliginous patches. *J Am Acad Dermatol* 2004;50:63–7.

4. Abbas O, and Mahalingam M. Epidermal stem cells: Practical perspectives and potential uses. *Br J Dermatol* 2009;161:228–36.

5. Tiede S, Kloepper JE, Bodò E Tiwari S, Kruse C, and Paus R. Hair follicle stem cells: Walking the maze. *Eur J Cell Biol* 2007;86:355–76.

6. Li L, and Xie T. Stem cell niche: Structure and function. *Annu Rev Cell Dev Biol* 2005;21:605–31.

7. Lechler T, and Fuchs E. Asymmetric cell divisions promote stratification and differentiation of mammalian skin. *Nature* 2005;437:275–80.

8. Meyer KC, Klatte JE, Dinh HV et al. Evidence that the bulge region is a site of relative immune privilege in human hair follicles. *Br J Dermatol* 2008;159:1077–85.

9. Bernard BA. The biology of hair follicle. *J Soc Biol* 2005;199:343–8.

10. Nishimura EK, Jordan SA, Oshima H et al. Dominant role of the niche in melanocyte stem-cell fate determination. *Nature* 2002;416:854–60.

11. Davids LM, du Toit E, Kidson SH, and Todd G. A rare repigmentation pattern in a vitiligo patient: A clue to an epidermal stem-cell reservoir of melanocytes? *Clin Exp Dermatol* 2009;34:246–8.

12. Webb A, Li A, and Kaur P. Location and phenotype of human adult keratinocyte stem cells of the skin. *Differentiation* 2004;72:387–95.

13. Kaur P. Interfollicular epidermal stem cells: Identification, challenges, potential. *J Invest Dermatol* 2006;126:1450–8.

14. Tani H, Morris RJ, and Kaur P. Enrichment for murine keratinocyte stem cells based on cell surface phenotype. *Proc Natl Acad Sci U S A* 2000;97:10960–5.

15. Tobin DJ, Swanson NN, Pittelkow MR, Peters EM, and Schallreuter KU. Melanocytes are not absent in lesional skin of long duration vitiligo. *J Pathol* 2000;191:407–16.

16. Hirobe T. Role of keratinocyte-derived factors involved in regulating the proliferation and differentiation of mammalian epidermal melanocytes. *Pigment Cell Res* 2005;18:2–12.

17. Grabbe J, Welker P, Dippel E, and Czarnetzki BM. Stem cell factor, a novel cutaneous growth factor for mast cells and melanocytes. *Arch Dermatol Res* 1994;287:78–84.

18. Halaban R, Ghosh S, and Baird A. bFGF is the putative natural growth factor for human melanocytes. *In Vitro Cell Dev Biol* 1987;23:47–52.

19. Yada Y, Higuchi K, and Imokawa G. Effects of endothelins on signal transduction and proliferation in human melanocytes. *J Biol Chem* 1991;266:18352–7.

20. Schauer E, Trautinger F, Köck A et al. Proopiomelanocortin-derived peptides are synthesized and released by human keratinocytes. *J Clin Invest* 1994;93:2258–62.

21. Kim NY, Jeon S, Lee HJ, and Lee AY. Impaired PI3K/Akt activation-mediated NFkB inactivation under elevated TNF-a is more vulnerable to apoptosis in vitiliginous keratinocytes. *J Invest Dermatol* 2007;127:2612–7.

22. Tomita Y, Maeda K, and Tagami H. Melanocyte-stimulating properties of arachidonic acid metabolites: Possible role in postinflammatory pigmentation. *Pigment Cell Res* 1992;5:357–61.

23. Tomita Y, Iwamoto M, Masuda T, and Tagami H. Stimulatory effect of prostaglandin E2 on the configuration of normal human melanocytes in-vitro. *J Invest Dermatol* 1987;89:299–301.

24. Morelli JG, Kincannon J, Yohn JJ, Zekman T, Weston WL, and Norris DA. Leukotriene C4 and TGF-alpha are stimulators of human melanocyte migration *in vitro*. *J Invest Dermatol*.1992;98:290–5.

25. Horikawa T, Norris DA, Yohn JJ, Zekman T, Travers JB, and Morelli JG. Melanocyte mitogens induce both melanocyte chemokinesis and chemotaxis. *J Invest Dermatol* 1995;104:256–9.

26. Grichnik JM, Burch JA, Burchette J, and Shea CR. The SCF/KIT pathway plays a critical role in the control of normal human melanocyte homeostasis. *J Invest Dermatol* 1998;111:233–8.

27. Fitzpatrick TB. Mechanisms of phototherapy of vitiligo. *Arch Dermatol* 1997;133:1591.

28. Ponsonby AL, Lucas RM, and van der Mei IA. UVR, vitamin D and three autoimmune diseases-multiple sclerosis, type 1 diabetes, rheumatoid arthritis. *Photochem Photobiol* 2005;81:1267–75.

29. El-Ghorr AA, and Norval M. Biological effects of narrowband (311 nm TL01) UVB irradiation: A review. *J Photochem Photobiol* 1997;38:99–106.

30. Wu CS, Lan CC, Wang LF, Chen GS, Wu CS, and Yu HS. Effects of psoralen plus ultraviolet A irradiation on cultured epidermal cells *in vitro* and patients with vitiligo *in vivo*. *Br J Dermatol* 2007;156:122–9.

31. Abdel-Naser MB, El-Khateeb EA, Sallam TH, and Habib MA. Endothelin-1 is significantly elevated in plasma of patients with vitiligo treated with psoralen plus ultraviolet A. *Clin Exp Dermatol* 2006;31:571–5.

32. Nordlund JJ. The loss of melanocytes from the epidermis: The mechanism for depigmentation in vitiligo vulgaris. In: Hann SK, and Nordlund JJ, eds. *Vitiligo*. Oxford: Blackwell Science; 2000, pp. 7–12.

33. Hann SK, Chun WH, and Park YK. Clinical characteristics of progressive vitiligo. *Int J Dermatol* 1997;36:353–5.

34. Gupta S, Narang T, Olsson MJ, and Ortone JP. Surgical management of vitiligo and other leukodermas: Evidence-based practice guidelines. In: Gupta S, Olsson MJ, Kanwar A, and Ortonne JP, eds. *Surgical Management of Vitiligo*. Malden, MA: Blackwell Publishing; 2007, pp. 69–79.

SPECIAL GROUPS
Vitiligo and Pregnancy

Chander Grover and Prachi Desai

CONTENTS

INTRODUCTION

Vitiligo is an acquired, multifactorial autoimmune disorder of pigmentation characterized by circumscribed, depigmented macules and patches. Although its precise pathogenesis is not known, there are various hypotheses explaining its development. The most accepted theory is the autoimmune hypothesis based on an altered humoral or innate immune response leading to melanocyte destruction in the affected skin. Vitiligo is frequently associated with other autoimmune disorders, among which the most common is thyroid disorder.

Keeping the pathogenesis in mind, one would be prompted to assume an altered disease course during pregnancy as well as possible bad obstetric outcomes [1]. However, these issues have been a subject of very limited research. The present chapter summarizes evidence regarding vitiligo and pregnancy, especially with regard to the effect these conditions are likely to have on each other, in both the short and long term. As with other autoimmune disorders, the course of vitiligo in pregnancy is seen to be variably affected.

PREGNANCY AND VITILIGO: COMMON CONCERNS

Genetic factors are believed to play an important role in vitiligo pathogenesis. Many patients with vitiligo have a family history for it, and vitiligo is more common in first-degree relatives. Children of vitiligo-affected parents are more likely to develop the condition during the course of a lifetime. Notwithstanding limited evidence, vitiligo is considered hereditary [2]. Hence, it is only natural that parents-to-be are concerned about their newborn being at risk and need answers to their queries. Vitiligo is also known to be associated with various autoimmune disorders like oculocutaneous albinism, autoimmune polyendocrinopathy syndrome, congenital sensorineural hearing loss, etc.; these being additional worries for the parents.

In addition, vitiligo is a chronic disease, and most patients are on long-term therapy, either topical or systemic. It is natural that patients would be worried about the safety of these drugs during pregnancy. The treating physician needs to make an informed and judicious decision regarding introduction, continuation, or withdrawal of various treatments during pregnancy or lactation. While topical therapy (for limited disease) may be considered safe, the potential for drugs to affect morphogenesis and to cross the placental barrier needs to be taken into account. The pregnant woman is likely to consult both dermatologists as well as her obstetrician for this. The safety of drug therapy during lactation is also important, as even topical therapy in lactating females should be chosen carefully. As the individual response to disease and to the treatment is highly variable, management needs to be individualized, keeping all concerns in mind.

EFFECT OF PREGNANCY ON VITILIGO

It has been reported that pregnancy can act as a trigger for first-time onset of vitiligo. Such an entity has been described as "gravidic vitiligo." Existing disease can also be aggravated during pregnancy. Previous reports and case studies have shown development as well as worsening of vitiligo with pregnancy; alternatively, termination of pregnancy (including incidents of abortion) has been shown to trigger or worsen the disease. The precise reason for this is not understood. It has been postulated that a decrease in estrogen and progesterone levels may precipitate vitiligo in susceptible candidates [3,4].

In pregnant patients, frequent sites for appearance of lesions are the breast and abdomen. This is probably a colocalization with striae gravidarum, and it has been suggested that Koebner phenomenon could be at work. A history of preceding precipitating factors like trauma (physical or emotional), illness, pregnancy, etc. can be found in 11%–76% of patients. Since such stressors in life occur commonly, it is difficult to prove that they might cause or precipitate vitiligo [2].

Suggestions were made that although there is a distinct lack of studies analyzing this situation, whatever limited work is available shows that pregnancy has no consistent effect on the occurrence or course of vitiligo. In a study of 62 vitiligo patients who went on to become pregnant, it was reported that most did not observe any change in the degree of depigmentation during or immediately after pregnancy. In 7% of the patients, an increase in vitiligo severity was seen, whereas in 3% there was a reduction, with overall postpartum extension being recorded in 31% [3]. Another descriptive cross-sectional study of 57 patients by Dellatorre et al. observed that vitiligo remained stable in 66.66% of pregnancies, with improvement in 12.28% of these. This study also contradicted the popular notion that pregnancy can act as a triggering factor for vitiligo, since it showed an average time lapse of 23.73 years between the first gestation and the onset of vitiligo. Interestingly, it was noted that the course of vitiligo was stable in all subsequent pregnancies except in one patient who consistently showed a worsening in pattern with subsequent pregnancies. Future prospective studies can help resolve these issues [5].

In a recent survey-based study by Webb et al., it was reported that 75% of the 24 patients included were stable or showed improvement in vitiligo during pregnancy, suggesting a possible protective effect. The authors speculated that the protective effect could be multifactorial, as both immunological alterations and physiological changes in pregnancy could contribute. Serum cortisol levels are increased during the second and third trimesters. A positive feedback loop with increased progesterone levels could lead to increased levels of IL-10, an anti-inflammatory regulator, causing an overall suppression of maternal adaptive immunity resulting in positive stabilization of vitiligo activity. Interestingly, 20.8% of patients also showed a worsening of vitiligo during pregnancy, the reason for which could be the physiological/immunological changes in pregnancy or cessation of ongoing medications [6].

Thus, our present understanding shows that pregnancy may have a variable effect on the prognosis of vitiligo. Despite this unpredictable progression of the disease, a pregnant woman should be informed about the small chance of worsening of the disease activity and ensure compliance of the prescribed treatment, if any.

EFFECT OF VITILIGO ON PREGNANCY

Not only can pregnancy affect the course of vitiligo, the opposite could also happen. With vitiligo being an autoimmune disease, speculations exist it may produce poor obstetric outcomes, including recurrent abortions. Horev et al. carried out a retrospective data analysis of 79 pregnant women with vitiligo. They reported no significant differences with respect to obstetric risk factors, labor characteristics, complications, or birth outcome when compared to the normal population. It was suggested that pregnancy in patients with vitiligo could be managed on similar lines as the general obstetric population. Although the study had a larger sample size, the retrospective design was a significant limitation. Also details like type and severity of vitiligo, or medications used before and during pregnancy were not taken into account. Further well-designed studies are required to confirm these results [1].

MANAGEMENT OF VITILIGO DURING PREGNANCY

Being a chronic disorder requiring long-term therapy and possible therapy with immune-suppressive drugs, vitiligo during pregnancy must be managed prudently. It can be safely said that vitiligo should be treated conservatively during pregnancy. It is wiser to defer systemic treatments until after delivery.

DURING PREGNANCY

- Systemic corticosteroids (Pregnancy Category C drugs) may be used only and only if benefits far outweigh the risks during pregnancy. However, even these should be avoided in the first trimester. Prednisone, a nonfluorinated corticosteroid, should be the preferred choice because of the limited passage across the placenta. Clinicians recommend prolonged use limited to 7.5 mg/day and avoidance of doses >20 mg/day since systemic steroids can result in premature delivery, premature rupture of membranes, intrauterine growth retardation, and other side effects [7,8].

Table 15.1.1 Summary of various treatment options of use in pregnant patients

Treatment options	Name	Pregnancy category
Topical therapy	Corticosteroids	C
	Calcineurin inhibitors	C
	Vitamin D_3 analogs	C
Systemic therapy	Corticosteroids	C, avoid in 1st trimester
	Cyclosporin	C
	Methotrexate	X
	Azathioprine	D
	Mycophenolate mofetil (MMF)	D
Light-based therapy	Phototherapy (NBUVB)	–, Safe in pregnancy
	Photochemotherapy	C, avoid
	Excimer laser	–, Safe in pregnancy

- Phototherapy given as narrowband ultraviolet B (NBUVB) is considered a safe option in pregnancy. However, high doses of heat should be avoided. Since folic acid levels have been seen to decrease in patients on NBUVB, pregnant women should be supplemented with folic acid [8,9].
- Excimer laser has also been reported to be safe for use during pregnancy [9].

Various treatment options and their safety in pregnancy are summarized in Table 15.1.1.

POSTPARTUM
Topical treatments are relatively safe during parturition except for the use of Class 1 corticosteroid and calcineurin inhibitors over the nipple area. These should be used with caution. Systemic corticosteroids may also be considered during parturition if required, but the duration of administration should be kept at less than 3 weeks [8].

CONCLUSION

Prognosis of vitiligo in pregnancy is equivocal, with recent evidence negating the prior belief of pregnancy acting as a trigger or aggravating the disease. Similarly, no poor obstetric outcomes have been reported in pregnant women with vitiligo, unlike some other autoimmune conditions. Management of vitiligo in pregnancy should be largely conservative.

REFERENCES

1. Horev A, Weintraub AY, Sergienko R, Wiznitzer A, Halevy S, and Sheiner E. Pregnancy outcome in women with vitiligo. *Int J Dermatol* 2011:50(9):1083–5.

2. Hann KS, and Nordlund JJ. eds. Clinical features of generalized vitiligo. In: *Vitiligo: A Monograph on the Basic and Clinical Science.* 1st ed. Oxford, London: Blackwell Science Ltd.; 2000, pp. 35–49.

3. Ortonne J-P. In: Mosher DB, and Fitzpatrick TB, eds. *Vitiligo and Other Hypomelanoses of Hair and Skin - Topics in Dermatology.* New York and London: Plenum Medical Book Company; 1983.

4. Ankur H, and Gupta AS. Vitiligo in pregnancy. *JPGO* 2014;1(4). Available at: http://www.jpgo.org/2014/04/vitiligo-in-pregnancy.html.

5. Delatorre G, Oliveira C, Chaves TP et al. A study of the prognosis of vitiligo during pregnancy. *Surg Cosmet Dermatol* 2013;5(3):37–9.

6. Webb KC, Lyon S, Nardone B, West DP, and Kundu RV. Influence of pregnancy on vitiligo activity. *J Clin Aesthet Dermatol* 2016;9(12);21–5.

7. Lahiri K, Chatterjee M, and Sarkar R. *Pigmentary Disorders: A Comprehensive Compendium*, 1st ed. Jaypee Brothers Medical Publishers Ltd.; 2014, p. 209.

8. Kishan Kumar YH, Rao GR, Gopal KV, Shanti G, and Rao KV. Evaluation of narrow-band UVB phototherapy in 150 patients with vitiligo. *Indian J Dermatol Venereol Leprol* 2009;75(2):162–6.

9. Murase JE, Heller MM, and Butler DC. Safety of dermatologic medications in pregnancy and lactation: Part 1. Pregnancy. *J Am Acad Dermatol* 2014;70(3):401.e1–14.

SPECIAL GROUPS
Pediatric Vitiligo

Sandipan Dhar and Sahana M. Srinivas

CONTENTS

INTRODUCTION

Childhood vitiligo is an acquired pigmentary autoimmune disorder caused by total destruction of melanocytes and clinically manifested by hypomelanosis of the skin and hair [1,2]. Vitiligo is a cosmetically disfiguring disease associated with a great deal of stigma. Parents are very anxious and psychologically affected, as it affects the quality of life in children, especially teenagers. Childhood vitiligo differs from adult vitiligo as it has distinct epidemiological and clinical features and is strongly associated with family history and other autoimmune disorders [3].

EPIDEMIOLOGY

Childhood vitiligo may present in the neonatal period, infancy, early childhood, or adolescence. It is seen in all age groups, races, and geographical regions of the world. Worldwide prevalence of vitiligo is 0.4%–2%, with 50% of cases beginning in childhood [4]. In a recent study of vitiligo in all age groups, 35.2% cases were seen in children. Among them, 56.7% were girls, and 47.4% of children presented with vitiligo between the ages of 4–8 years [2]. Half to one-third of childhood vitiligo manifests by 20 years, with a mean age of onset between 4 and 5 years [5,6]. In a North Indian study of vitiligo, 23.4% of patients were children. Among them, 33.6% were in the age group of 0–6 years and 66.4% in the age group of 6–12 years [6]. Most of the studies show a female preponderance, except a few studies where an equal sex ratio has been documented [5,7,8]. Positive family history in childhood vitiligo is seen in 11%–46% in various studies [2,9]. The onset of vitiligo in children is earlier if there is a family history of vitiligo or other autoimmune disorders.

CLASSIFICATION OF CHILDHOOD VITILIGO

Childhood vitiligo can be classified into segmental and nonsegmental vitiligo (Table 15.2.1) [2]. Segmental vitiligo presents in a dermatomal pattern (zosteriform pattern). Localized vitiligo is classified into focal, acral (limited to distal extremities), acrofacial (acral with facial lesions), lip-tip, and mucosal vitiligo (oral/genital mucosa). Vitiligo vulgaris presents with multiple depigmented macules all over the body, whereas extensive or near total depigmentation (greater than 75%) of skin implies universal vitiligo. Based on the stability, vitiligo can be classified into stable and unstable vitiligo. Though the concept of stable vitiligo is still elusive, it is characterized by no new lesions, no progression of existing lesions, and absence of Koebner phenomenon in the past year [2].

Various studies have shown that the most common clinical type of vitiligo in children is vitiligo vulgaris, followed by focal and segmental vitiligo [2,7]. Incidence of acrofacial and mucosal vitiligo is lower in many studies. Universal vitiligo is rarely seen in children as compared to adults. The incidence of mucosal vitiligo varies from 0.6% to 13.8% in many studies [7].

CLINICAL FEATURES

Vitiligo presents as asymptomatic, well- to ill-defined depigmented ivory-white macules with distinct margins in a segmental or a nonsegmental distribution. Typical lesions may present as millimeters to centimeters, with geographic borders. Perifollicular pigmentation and islets of normal-to-increased pigmentation can be seen in a depigmented macule. Both Indian and Western studies have

Table 15.2.1   Classification of vitiligo based on morphology and distribution

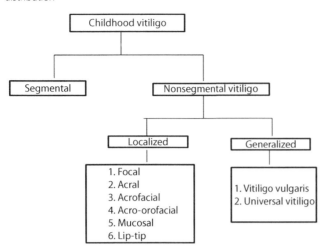

documented increased incidence of vitiligo in female children [2,3]. Vitiligo can present at any site on the body, including mucosa and hair.

CONGENITAL VITILIGO

Vitiligo presenting at birth is very rare. There are a few cases of congenital vitiligo reported in literature [10]. In an epidemiological study of 541 Chinese children, only 8 had vitiligo at birth [11]. The concept of congenital vitiligo is still controversial. In utero–onset vitiligo has been possibly attributed to placental transfer of maternal antibodies, immune attack in utero in genetically predisposed individuals, and genetic polymorphism with gene-to-gene interactions. Most of these cases reported in literature have male preponderance and acral distribution [10].

NONSEGMENTAL VITILIGO

Nonsegmental vitiligo accounts for 80% of all cases. Nonsegmental vitiligo occurs at any site of body in a more or less symmetrical pattern, but the most common initial sites of occurrence are the face, neck, and lower limbs, followed by the trunk and upper limbs (Figure 15.2.1) [12]. Periocular vitiligo is seen more in children than adults, and it is usually self-resolving (Figure 15.2.2). Childhood vitiligo may start as the localized type and eventually evolve into generalized forms [13]. Mucosal vitiligo in children may occur rarely as an isolated manifestation, but usually manifests as a part of generalized vitiligo (Figure 15.2.3). Vitiligo patches can be made visible by tanning of the surrounding skin.

SEGMENTAL VITILIGO

Segmental vitiligo represents one-fifth to one-third of all vitiligo cases in children. The prevalence of segmental vitiligo in various studies ranged from 4.6% to 32.5% [2,3,12]. Studies have shown the trigeminal segment to be the most common dermatome, followed by thoracic, cervical, lumbar, and sacral [14]. Segmental vitiligo presents as unilateral lesions that do not cross the midline and generally follow the lines of Blaschko. Progression of lesions is seen more in nonsegmental than segmental vitiligo.

LEUKOTRICHIA

Leukotrichia is seen in 3.7%–25% of childhood vitiligo cases [12]. Localized hair follicles of scalp can be involved, leading to poliosis, and this is more commonly seen in segmental vitiligo (Figure 15.2.4). Poliosis has been observed in 55.55% of children with vitiligo [9]. Scalp leukotrichia is a common finding in children with family history of vitiligo and other autoimmune disorders. Premature graying

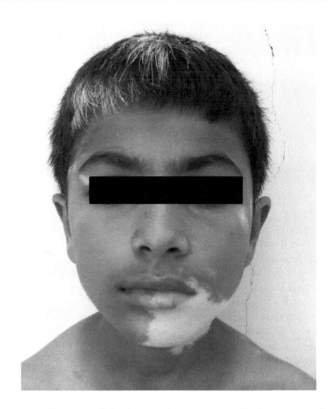

Figure 15.2.1   Multiple depigmented macules on the face along with leukotrichia.

was found to be more common among first- and second-degree relatives of children with vitiligo. In a study by Jaisankar et al., 4.4% of vitiligo children had premature graying of hair [15]. Some children manifest with total depigmentation of scalp hair, eyebrows, and eyelashes. Poliosis has also been reported to occur in nevus depigmentosus and needs to be differentiated from vitiligo [16].

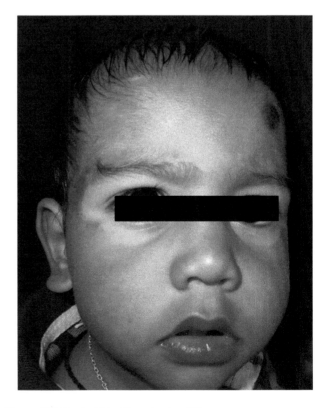

Figure 15.2.2   A child with periocular vitiligo.

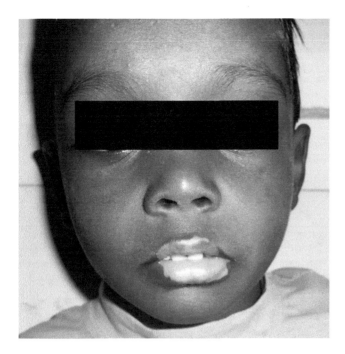

Figure 15.2.3   Vitiligo involving lip mucosa.

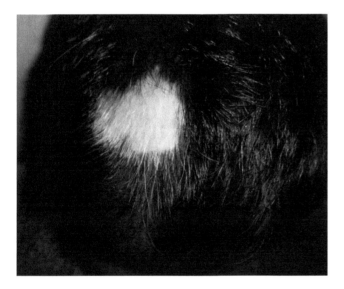

Figure 15.2.4   Scalp vitiligo with poliosis.

KOEBNER PHENOMENON

Koebner phenomenon has been documented more commonly in non-segmental vitiligo [3]. Sometimes children present with initial vitiligo lesions on knees, elbows, shins, arms, and hands due to Koebner phenomenon, as children are known to have trauma on these areas due to play activities. Koebner phenomenon indicates disease activity. Koebner phenomenon had varied incidence, ranging from 11.3% in a Handa and Dogra study [7] to 21% in a Sheth et al. study [12].

OTHER RARE FORMS

Trichrome vitiligo (depigmented area surrounded by hypopigmented zone which is separated from normal skin by a thin hyperpigmented rim); quadrichrome vitiligo (with marginal perifollicular hyperpigmentation) is not commonly seen in children. Rarely, peanut-sized depigmented macules, called punctate vitiligo, may be present on any site of the body [17]. Vitiligo minor is a rare, recently reported form, characterized by hypopigmented macules distributed mainly on the face and back [18]. Another rare form of vitiligo described in the literature is follicular vitiligo, which primarily involves the follicular reservoir of melanocytes with depigmentation of body hair and, rarely, depigmented macules [19].

ASSOCIATED DISORDERS

ASSOCIATED SKIN DISORDERS

Childhood vitiligo has been associated with atopic dermatitis, alopecia areata, halo nevi, and, rarely, with morphea, psoriasis, premature canities, pemphigus vulgaris, and lichen planus [20]. Halo nevi are more frequently associated with childhood vitiligo than adult vitiligo. Published studies have shown the prevalence of halo nevi ranging from 2.5% to 34% in cases of pediatric vitiligo. Halo nevi have been documented in 12% of cases of segmental vitiligo and 20% of cases of nonsegmental vitiligo [14].

ASSOCIATED AUTOIMMUNE DISORDERS

Vitiligo has been associated with several endocrinopathies and autoimmune disorders, including alopecia areata, diabetes mellitus, pernicious anemia, systemic lupus erythematosus, Addison disease, thyroid disorders, psoriasis, rheumatoid arthritis, Down syndrome, inflammatory bowel disease, and autoimmune polyglandular syndrome [2,3,12]. The most common autoimmune disorder associated with vitiligo is thyroiditis. Studies have shown vitiligo-associated autoimmune disorders to be seen more commonly in nonsegmental vitiligo. Indian studies have documented the prevalence of autoimmune disorders to be as low as 1.3% and as high as 17% [7,12]. The prevalence of thyroid disorders in childhood vitiligo varies from 0% to 25% in various studies [2]. Among thyroid dysfunction, hypothyroidism was more common than hyperthyroidism. Many authors have suggested that routine screening of the thyroid is necessary in children with vitiligo as early detection of autoimmune thyroiditis can prevent growth abnormalities. In the majority of cases, vitiligo precedes development of thyroid dysfunction, but rarely does the presence of thyroid autoantibodies precede the development of vitiligo. Antinuclear antibodies have been found to be increased in children with vitiligo in few studies, but many studies have not documented this finding [2]. Rarely, antigastric parietal cell antibodies have been documented in children with vitiligo [2]. Although studies have shown childhood vitiligo to be associated with various autoimmune disorders, there is lack of data to comment on whether these associations predispose to early onset or increased severity in children.

ASSOCIATED HEREDITARY SYNDROMES

Vitiligo has been associated with rare syndromes like Vogt-Koyanagi-Harada syndrome and Alezzandrini syndrome. Vogt-Koyanagi-Harada syndrome is characterized by uveitis, aseptic meningitis, dysacusia, alopecia, poliosis, and vitiligo. Alezzandrini syndrome is a constellation of segmental vitiligo, poliosis, ipsilateral uveitis, and partial hearing loss. In both conditions, vitiligo starts in late childhood or adolescence and is resistant to treatment [21].

PSYCHOLOGICAL EFFECTS OF VITILIGO

There are no validated studies regarding the psychological effect of vitiligo in children. In children, the quality of life is not affected, but altered, and this depends on age, extent of vitiligo lesions, course of the disease, and color of skin. An online parental questionnaire-based study in children aged 0–17 years showed that vitiligo lesions were not bothersome in 4.1% of teenagers, 45.6% in 0–6 years, and 50% in 7–14 years. The most bothersome sites of vitiligo lesions for children and parents were the face (25.6% and 37.4%, respectively) and legs (26.2% and 26.2%, respectively). An affected body surface area more than 25% was associated with self-consciousness, difficulty in friendships and schoolwork, and facing teasing and bullying among their peer group [22]. Teenagers seem to be affected more in the pediatric age group.

COURSE OF THE DISEASE

There is a lack of studies regarding the natural history and course of childhood vitiligo. Complete repigmentation is unusual in nonsegmental vitiligo, but the rate of spontaneous repigmentation is greater in children than adults. Repigmentation may be diffuse, marginal, or perifollicular. Studies have shown that progression of the disease was higher in nonsegmental vitiligo (23.29%) than segmental vitiligo (5.56%) [14]. In the author's experience, childhood vitiligo has a better prognosis than adult vitiligo. Progression and recurrence of the lesion is less common in children. Instability is seen more in children with autoimmune disorders. Periocular vitiligo has a good prognosis and resolves spontaneously. Stable vitiligo is less commonly seen in children and requires a surgical mode of therapy like miniature skin grafting [23,24].

DIAGNOSIS AND DIFFERENTIAL DIAGNOSIS

Diagnosis of vitiligo is based on clinical appearance. The classical presence of depigmented macules, repigmented macules within the depigmented macules, characteristic distribution, poliosis, leukotrichia, and Koebner phenomenon points to the diagnosis of vitiligo. Investigations are not required to confirm vitiligo, however in cases where there is doubt, Woods lamp examination can be performed. Woods lamp examination shows accentuation of the vitiligo lesions. Differential diagnosis of childhood vitiligo is summarized in Table 15.2.2 [2,13,17,25]. Children with nonsegmental vitiligo can be routinely screened for diabetes and thyroid abnormalities to rule out associated autoimmune disorders, especially if there is an alteration in normal growth velocity [2]. Annual assessment of thyroid function is recommended. T3, T4, and TSH levels, antithyroglobulin antibody, and antithyroperoxidase antibody (anti-TPO) can be done to rule out autoimmune thyroiditis. Other tests that can be done are complete blood count and fasting blood sugar. Screening for other autoantibodies to rule out lupus, rheumatoid arthritis, and inflammatory bowel disease can be performed only if symptoms are present [26].

COUNSELING ASPECTS IN PEDIATRIC VITILIGO

Counseling plays an important role in childhood vitiligo. Parents should be questioned and counseled about the impact of the disease on the child's personal development and the family. Older children should be evaluated for their perceptions regarding the disease, cosmetic disfigurement, and their interactions with peer groups. Parents should be counseled about the risk of developing vitiligo in first-degree relatives, twins, or in siblings, and the associated autoimmune disorders. Parents and children should be informed

about the course of the disease and the available treatment options. In childhood vitiligo it is important to inform parents about spontaneous repigmentation.

Table 15.2.2 Differential diagnoses of childhood vitiligo

Disorder	Characteristic features
Segmental vitiligo	
Pigmentary mosaicism (Hypomelanosis of ito, nevus depigmentosus)	Hypopigmented, *linear streaks and whorls along the lines of Blaschko*, margins are indistinct or serrated and may be associated with extracutaneous abnormalities
Congenital vitiligo	
Nevus anemicus	Pale white lesion with *indistinct border*, diascopy test: becomes unnoticeable as merges with surrounding skin
Ash leaf spots	Hypopigmented macules with *lanceolate shape*
Piebaldism	Depigmented macules from *birth*, areas of normal skin, *white forelock*
Waardenburg syndrome	Depigmented macules from *birth*, *white forelock*, *heterochromia of irises*, dystopia canthorum, sensorineural deafness
Oculocutaneous albinism	Diffuse depigmentation all over the body, involves *skin*, *hair*, *eyes*
Acquired vitiligo	
Pityriasis alba	*Ill-defined* hypopigmented macules with *fine scaling* on face, upper arm
Tinea versicolor	*Well-defined* hypopigmented macules with *fine scaling* on trunk
Postinflammatory hypopigmentation	*Preceding skin lesions* resolving with hypopigmentation
Leprosy	Hypopigmented macule with *decreased or loss of sensation, peripheral nerves enlarged*
Polymorphic light eruption	*Hypopigmented*, scaly macules, plaques on the *exposed part* of body
Seborrheic dermatitis	Ill-defined hypopigmented macules, *greasy scales* on the face involving *nasolabial fold*, *postauricular region*, chest
Lichen sclerosus et atrophicus	Multiple well-defined hypopigmented to *ivory-white atrophic* macules
Contact depigmentation	Hypopigmented-to-depigmented macules on the *area of contact*
Topical steroid abuse	Hypopigmented *atrophic macules, telangiectasia*

REFERENCES

1. Kanwar AJ, Dhar S, and Kaur S. Vitiligo in children. *Indian J Dermatol* 1993;38:47–52.

2. Palit A, and Inamdar AC. Childhood vitiligo. *Indian J Dermatol Venereol Leprol* 2012;78:30–41.

3. Agarwal S, Gupta S, Ojha A, and Sinha R. Childhood vitiligo: Clinicoepidemiologic profile of 268 children from the Kumaun region of Uttarkhand. *India Pediatr Dermatol* 2012;30:348–63.

4. Spritz RA. Shared genetic relationships underlying generalized vitiligo and autoimmune thyroid disease. *Thyroid* 2010;20:745–54.

5. Kanwar AJ, and Kumaran MS. Childhood vitiligo: Treatment paradigms. *Indian J Dermatol* 2012;57:466–74.

6. Sehgal VN, and Srivastava G. Vitiligo: Compendium of clinic-epidemiological features. *Indian J Dermatol Venereol Leprol* 2007;73:149–56.

7. Handa S, and Dogra S. Epidemiology of childhood vitiligo: A study of 625 patients from North India. *Pediatr Dermatol* 2003;20:207–10.

8. Lin X, Tang LY, Fu WW, and Kang KF. Childhood vitiligo in China: Clinical profile and immunological finding in 620 cases. *Am J Clin Dermatol* 2011;12:277–81.

9. Prcic S, Djuran V, Mikov A, and Mikov I. Vitiligo in children. *Pediatr Dermatol* 2007;24:666.

10. Kambhampati BN, Sawatkar GV, Kumaran MS, and Prasad D. Congenital vitiligo: A case report. *J Cut Med Surg* 2016; 20:354–5.

11. Hu Z, Liu JB, Ma SS et al. Profile of childhood vitiligo in China: An analysis of 541 patients. *Pediatr Dermatol* 2006;23:114–6.

12. Sheth PK, Sacchidanad S, and Asha GS. Clinico-epidemiological profile of childhood vitiligo. *Indian J Paediatr Dermatol* 2015;16:23–8.

13. Silverberg NB. Pediatric vitiligo. *Pediatr Clin N Am* 2014; 61:347–66.

14. Mazereeuw-Hautier J, Bezio S, Mahe E et al. Segmental and nonsegmental childhood vitiligo has distinct clinical characteristics: A prospective observational study. *J Am Acad Dermatol* 2010;62:945–9.

15. Mazereeuw-Hautier J, and Harper J. Vitiligo. In: Harper J, Orange A, and Prose N, eds. *Textbook of Pediatric Dermatology*, 2nd Ed. Oxford: Blackwell Publishing Ltd; 2006, pp. 1041–56.

16. Dhar S, Kanwar AJ, and Ghosh S. Leucotrichia in naevus depigmentosus. *Pediatr Dermatol* 1993;10:188–90.

17. Ezzedine K, and Silverberg N. A practical approach to the diagnosis and treatment of vitiligo in children. *Pediatrics* 2016;138:e20154126.

18. Ezzedine K, Mahe A, Van Geel N et al. Hypochromic vitiligo: Delineation of a new entity. *Br J Dermatol* 2015;172:716–21.

19. Ezzedine K, Amazan E, Seneschal J et al. Follicular vitiligo: A new form of vitiligo. *Pigment Cell Melanoma Res* 2012;25:527–29.

20. Dhar S, and Kanwar AJ. Colocalization of vitiligo and alopecia areata. *Pediatr Dermatol* 1993;11:85–6.

21. Paller AS, and Mancini AJ. Disorders of pigmentation. In: Paller AS, and Mancini AJ, eds. *Hurwitz Clinical Pediatric Dermatology*, 3rd ed. Philadelphia: Elsevier Saunders; 2006, pp. 265–305.

22. Silverberg JI, and Silverberg NB. Quality of life impairment in children and adolescents with vitiligo. *Pediatric Dermatol* 2014;3:309–18.

23. Malakar S, and Dhar S. Treatment of stable and recalcitrant vitiligo by autologous miniature punch grafting: A prospective study with 1000 patients. *Dermatology* 1999;198:133–9.

24. Kanwar AJ, Dhar S, and Dawn G. Oral minipulse therapy in vitiligo. *Dermatology* 1995;190:251–2.

25. Dhar S, Kanwar AJ, and Kaur S. Naevus depigmentosus in India: Experience with 50 patients. *Pediatr Dermatol* 1993;10:299–300.

26. Kakourou T, Kanaka-Gantenbein C, Papadopoulou A et al. Increased prevalence of chronic autoimmune (Hashimoto's) thyroiditis in children and adolescents with vitiligo. *J Am Acad Dermatol* 2005;53:220–3.

SPECIAL GROUPS
Vitiligo and Immunodeficiency

Chander Grover and Prachi Desai

CONTENTS

INTRODUCTION

For a long time, a paradoxical coexistence of autoimmunity and immunodeficiency in patients has interested scientists and physicians. By definition, an immune deficiency is a decreased ability of the immune system to fight infection. Conversely, autoimmunity is an increased response of the immune system to itself. These seemingly opposite conditions represent immune system dysfunctions. It is well known that combined or T-cell deficiencies are mainly associated with immunodeficiency, whereas autoimmune disorders are predominantly CD8 T-cell driven. Vitiligo is an autoimmune disease in which such a relationship can be seen [1,2].

PATHOPHYSIOLOGY

It has been proposed that the pathophysiology of autoimmune diseases, including vitiligo, may be linked to immunodeficiency. The existence of mechanisms of central immune tolerance prevents the persistence of autoreactive immune cells in later life. Even if a few autoreactive cells escape deletion within the thymus, these cells lose reactivity peripherally by various mechanisms. A loss of this tolerance could lead to onset of autoimmunity in patients with preexisting immunodeficiency. Other than this, dysfunction or aberration of mechanisms of apoptosis, proliferation signaling pathways, immune-mediated clearance, or innate cellular immunity could also contribute to autoimmunity in patients with immunodeficiency [3].

It has been hypothesized that cell-mediated immunity plays a crucial role in the pathogenesis of vitiligo. Autoreactive T cells predominantly infiltrate the lesional skin, evidenced by a strong association of vitiligo with humal leucocyte antigen (HLA), mostly major histocompatibility complex (MHC) Class II molecules. There is an increased CD8/CD4 ratio in lesional skin. Apart from this, Treg CD4 cells, which play a crucial role in the tolerance to self-antigens, are virtually absent in the lesional skin [4]. However, the overall relationship of vitiligo with immunodeficiency is not yet fully understood.

Associations of vitiligo with individual disorders of immunodeficiency are listed in Table 15.3.1. The details are discussed next.

Table 15.3.1 Immunodeficiency disorders associated with vitiligo

Primary immunodeficiency	Secondary/other causes of immunodeficiency
Common variable immunodeficiency	Human immunodeficiency virus infection
Ataxia telangiectasia	Idiopathic T-cell lymphocytopenia
Nijmegen breakage syndrome	Protein-losing enteropathy
IPEX syndrome	Nephrotic syndrome
Omenn syndrome	Hematological malignancies
Selective IgA deficiency	

IMMUNODEFICIENCY DISEASES ASSOCIATED WITH VITILIGO

PRIMARY IMMUNODEFICIENCY

Primary immunodeficiency diseases include numerous sporadic and genetic diseases characterized by an increased susceptibility to infections. These have varied clinical presentations, and there may be a paradoxical increase in autoimmune associations, including vitiligo. The underlying mechanisms are poorly understood; however, it is proposed that the genetic defect responsible for immunodeficiency could itself contribute to an abnormal development of T- and B-cell lines, which in turn predispose the patient to autoimmune phenomena. Important disorders in this category associated with vitiligo include the following.

COMMON VARIABLE IMMUNODEFICIENCY

Common variable immunodeficiency (CVID) is the most common primary immunodeficiency reported [3]. It is a heterogeneous disorder of unclear inheritance associated with a loss of memory and isotype-switched B cells as well as a varied T-cell phenotype. Autoimmune diseases have been reported in up to 25% of patients with CVID. The important ones include various cytopenias such as autoimmune thrombocytopenic purpura (frequently), and other disorders including rheumatoid arthritis, vasculitis, alopecia areata, and vitiligo [3].

AUTOIMMUNE POLYENDOCRINOPATHY-CANDIDIASIS-ECTODERMAL DYSTROPHY SYNDROME

Autoimmune polyendocrinopathy-candidiasis-ectodermal dystrophy (APECED) syndrome is a rare autosomal recessive disease characterized classically by a triad of hypothyroidism, primary adrenocortical insufficiency, and chronic mucocutaneous candidiasis. According to the diagnostic criteria proposed by Husebye et al., the minor components include vitiligo, alopecia areata, chronic diarrhea, keratitis, periodic rash with fever, severe constipation, autoimmune hepatitis, and enamel hypoplasia. Vitiligo has been reported in up to one-third of these patients and generally forms a part of the initial manifestations of the disease; however, it is less commonly found than alopecia areata, another autoimmune condition. Vitiligo tends to be extensive in these patients [4,5].

COMPLEMENT DEFICIENCY

Autoimmune associations with complement deficiency syndromes have been speculated based on various theories and in vitro studies. The heterozygous C4 complement deficiency has been linked to an increased risk of development of vitiligo as compared to the normal population. This could be due to complement-activating antimelanocyte antibodies, which cause a direct destruction of melanocytes by complement components. Other than this, patients with classical complement deficiencies also have an increased risk of developing systemic lupus erythematosus (SLE) [1,6].

SECONDARY IMMUNODEFICIENCY
HUMAN IMMUNODEFICIENCY VIRUS INFECTION

Human immunodeficiency virus (HIV) infection is one of the leading causes of CD4 T-cell depletion leading to an acquired form of immunodeficiency. Acquired immunodeficiency syndrome (AIDS) is the resultant symptom complex which can be staged on the basis of the clinical manifestations and presence of opportunistic infections. There are a few reports of vitiligo being associated with HIV infection. Although the overall incidence of vitiligo in the setting of HIV has been reported to be 0.2%–1.8% [7], it has been speculated that the coexistence might be more than just a chance association. Other autoimmune phenomena associated with HIV include AIDS-related complex (ARC)-associated thrombocytopenia. It is speculated that the HIV virus, various opportunistic infections, or dysimmunity could trigger vitiligo due to a paradoxical increase in the autoimmune manifestations. The possible proposed mechanisms include [8] the following:

- A direct viral infection of the melanocytes could be responsible for their destruction, as HIV is known to infect neural crest cells, including astrocytes and dendrocytes.
- A nonspecific polyclonal B-cell activation could result in production of melanocyte-specific autoantibodies.
- There could be a role of cellular cytotoxicity against melanocytes.
- There could be a T-cell infection leading to an imbalance of helper, suppressor, and cytotoxic cells, further precipitating melanocyte destruction.
- A molecular mimicry could exist between HIV antigens and HLA antigens, thus leading to melanocyte destruction.
- A combination of the aforementioned mechanisms could be responsible.

The clinical presentations of vitiligo in HIV-infected patients can be variable in terms of disease history, immune status, and treatment taken. Ezzedine et al. observed three possible situations with such a co-occurrence [1]. It could be that the presence of vitiligo could reveal immunosuppression. An improvement could occur in vitiligo during the course of immunodeficiency. The presentation of vitiligo could undergo modification with institution of antiretroviral therapy and/or immune restoration. This could be in the form of inflammatory signs, described as punctate advanced erythematous margins of vitiligo patches. Premature canities have been commonly seen in patients with HIV as they progress through AIDS, and this could be related to vitiligo [9].

UV IRRADIATION AND VITILIGO

UV irradiation has a variable effect on various autoimmune phenomena. Excessive UV rays may trigger autoimmunity, as is seen in SLE, while at the same time, UVB phototherapy has a definite role in the management of vitiligo. UV sensitization is a phenomenon not so well established in vitiligo, even though reports of sunburn-induced depigmentation exist. This may be considered as an extension of Koebner phenomenon. On the other hand, UV suppresses autoreactive T cells and increases IL-10, leading to regulation of Treg activity, which leads to an improvement in vitiliginous patches [1].

CONCLUSION

The coexistence of immunodeficiencies and vitiligo, although seemingly paradoxical, has been reported often. However, the link is poorly understood. T-cell and combined deficiencies can be associated with vitiligo. The role of B-cell and innate immunity deficiencies like complement disorders is not well described. In suspect cases, especially with generalized/widespread vitiligo, underlying T-cell immunosuppression and HIV infection should be investigated.

Since the research in this area is usually condition-specific and has been carried out by researchers in different fields, it has been hard to synthesize a comprehensive body of knowledge on this subject. It is important to understand the link better, which could help us further our knowledge.

REFERENCES

1. Ezzedine K, Lepreux S, and Taïeb A. Vitiligo and Immunodeficiencies. In: Picardo M, and Taïeb A, eds. *Vitiligo*. Springer; 2010, pp. 123–6.

2. Gerstmann L. Immune Deficiency. A Complicated Relationship. IG Living. 2009. http://www.igliving.com/magazine/articles/IGL_2009-06_AR_ImmuneDeficiency-and-Autoimmune-Disease-A-Complicated-Relationship.pdf

3. Todoric K, Koontz JB, Mattox D, and Tarrant TK. Autoimmunity in immunodeficiency. *Curr Allergy Asthma Rep* 2013;13(4):361–70.

4. Husebye ES, Perheentupa J, Rautemaa R, and Kämpe O. Clinical manifestations and management of patients with autoimmune polyendocrine syndrome type 1. *J Intern Med* 2009;265(5):514–29.

5. Collins SM, Dominguez M, Ilmarinen T, Costigan C, and Irvine AD. Dermatological manifestations of autoimmune polyendocrinopathy-candidiasis-ectodermal dystrophy syndrome. *Br J Dermatol* 2006;154(6):1088–93.

6. Sleasman JW. The association between immunodeficiency and the development of autoimmune disease. *Advance Dental Res* 1996;10:57–61.

7. Zhang Y, Cai Y, Shi M et al. The prevalence of vitiligo: A meta-analysis. *PLOS ONE*. 2016;11(9):e0163806.

8. Duvic M, Rapini R, Hoots WK, and Mansell PW. Human immunodeficiency virus-associated vitiligo: Expression of autoimmunity with immunodeficiency? *J Am Acad Dermatol* 1987;17(4):656–62.

9. Antony FC, and Marsden RA. Vitiligo in association with human immunodeficiency virus infection. *J Eur Acad Dermatol Venereol* 2003;17(4):456–8.

SPECIAL GROUPS
Vitiligo Onset in Late Age

Chander Grover and Prachi Desai

CONTENTS

INTRODUCTION

Vitiligo, a common acquired pigmentary disease, is known to occur more commonly in the younger age group. Up to 50% of the patients will develop lesions of vitiligo before 20 years of age. However, there is a subset of patients with an onset much later in life. The reasons for this have not been extensively explored. It could be that an overall increased life expectancy has led to an increased recognition of its occurrence, but there could be other factors at play. In addition, with late-onset disease there are more apprehensions in the patient's mind, including concerns about prognosis and management [1].

LATE-ONSET VITILIGO

Aging is associated with immunosenescence, seen as a documented decrease in immune response to specific antigens. However, there is a paradoxical increase in the incidence of autoimmune diseases in the aged population, probably owing to a decreased clearance of accumulated protein antigens. This observation could explain the pathogenesis of late-onset vitiligo. At the same time, aging is also associated with melanocyte senescence, leading to a decrease in the number of melanocytes on photo-exposed as well as photoprotected skin. This decrease is approximately 10%–20% over a decade. Whether this factor contributes to late-onset vitiligo is, however, unclear [1].

A study in the Romanian population indicated that the age of onset of vitiligo is mostly determined by environmental factors. The authors suggested that although the susceptibility for developing vitiligo is determined by genetic factors, the onset of the disease depends on environmental factors, which trigger the disease in susceptible individuals. Another model suggested two possible modes of inheritance of vitiligo: vitiligo of early onset is inherited in a dominant fashion with incomplete inheritance, whereas individuals predisposed to develop late-onset vitiligo seem to have a recessive inheritance [3].

EPIDEMIOLOGY

The exact cutoff for identifying vitiligo of late-onset type has not been defined. The identified limits have varied across reports. Late-onset vitiligo has been defined by diffrent authors variably with age of onset varying from 30 years, 40 years, and 50 years respectively in different studies [1–3].

No sex predilection has been reported in late-onset vitiligo. In a retrospective study of 182 patients by Dogra et al., there were 47.8% males and 52.2% females with the mean age of onset being 55 ± 2.3 years [2]. In a cross-sectional study by Esfandiarpour and Farajzadeh, there were 54 late-onset patients and 771 early-onset patients evaluated; 48.1% were females and 51.9% males. The mean age of onset in this group was 56.57 ± 7.05 years [4]. Both studies reported an incidence of around 6.5% of cases with late-onset vitiligo disease. Al-Mutairi and Al-Sebeih noted similar sex distribution; however, in their study, 68.02% patients had an onset between 40 and 50 years of age.

CLINICAL CHARACTERISTICS

Almost all vitiligo variants have been described in late-onset disease. Dogra et al. [2] found vitiligo vulgaris to be the most common presentation (83.5%), followed by focal vitiligo (3%), mucosal vitiligo (2.2%), and vitiligo universalis (0.5%). Mucosal involvement was noted in 17% of patients, with oral mucosa being maximally involved (71%). Associated leukotrichia was seen in 47.3% of sufferers. Head and neck were the most common early sites of involvement. Family history of vitiligo was present in almost 16% of these patients, in 11.5% first-degree relatives were affected, and in 4.4% second-degree relatives were affected. However, these studies had limitations, including a retrospective study design.

Esfandiarpour and Farajzadeh [4] reported vitiligo vulgaris to be the most common clinical type, affecting 59.3% of patients, followed by acrofacial, focal, universal, and segmental types. As compared

Table 15.4.1 Comparison of the clinical features of late-onset vitiligo among various studies conducted on the subject

Clinical features	Dogra et al. [1] (n = 182)	Esfandiarpour and Farajzadeh [4] (n = 54)	Al-Mutairi and Al-Sebeih [3] (n = 197)
Mean age of onset (y)	55 ± 2.3 yrs	56.57 ± 7.05 yrs	–
Age cutoff (y)	50	50	40
Geographical area	India	Iran	Kuwait
Females	52.2%	48.1%	51.77%
Males	47.8%	51.9%	48.22%
Family history	15.9%	27.8%	16.75%
Presence of Koebner phenomenon	14.8%	79.8%	16.75%
Leukotrichia	47.3%	77.8%	44.6%
Clinical types			
Generalized	83.5%	59.3%	71.57%
Acrofacial	3.8%	20.4%	3.04%
Localized	5.5%	13%	20.81%
Segmental	4.4%	3.7%	1.01%
Universal	0.5%	3.7%	2.03%
Pure mucosal	2.2%	0%	1.52%

to early-onset vitiligo, universal and localized types were found to be more commonly present in late-onset disease. Mucosal involvement was noted in a higher proportion (59.3%) of patients than the early-onset group (47%). Limbs were the most common first sites of involvement. A family history of vitiligo was found in 27.8% of patients, but no statistically significant differences were seen in comparison with the early-onset group. This study had an advantage of including the early-onset group; however, the patients were not followed up, which could have yielded more data.

In the study by Al-Mutairi and Al-Sebeih, vitiligo vulgaris was found to be the most common presentation followed by focal, acrofacial, universal, mucosal, and segmental types. Upper limb was the most common first site to be involved. Family history was noted in 16.75% patients. They also noted that 89.9% of the patients had 5%–20% of body surface area involved, and vitiligo was stable in 71.57% of patients.

Table 15.4.1 summarizes a comparative evaluation of these three different studies done on late-onset vitiligo. The differences observed could be due to racial or genetic variations between the study populations, or even the environmental factors unique to those areas and populations, as these studies were conducted in diverse groups. It was also noted by Kanwar et al. that late-onset vitiligo is more commonly associated with non-autoimmune conditions, a positive family history, and leukotrichia as compared to early-onset vitiligo [5].

ASSOCIATIONS

Vitiligo, being an autoimmune disorder, is commonly associated with an increased incidence of other autoimmune conditions. Dogra et al. reported this in up to 21.4% of the patients. Insulin-dependent diabetes mellitus, thyroid disease, and rheumatoid arthritis have been the observed associations, in decreasing order of frequency. Esfandiarpour and Farajzadeh reported up to 18.5% of patients being affected by other autoimmune diseases as compared to 23.1% as seen in the early-onset patients. Diabetes, followed by hypothyroidism, was the commonly observed association. The prevalence of diabetes (11%) was notably higher than in the general population (8.7%). This needs to be confirmed by further studies. Al-Multairi and Al-Sebeih reported that 39.59% of the patients had autoimmune/endocrine conditions; this was substantially higher than in other studies. They saw diabetes mellitus, autoimmune thyroid disease, rheumatoid arthritis,

pernicious anemia, and Addison disease in their study patients. Audiological abnormalities were found in 22.37% as compared to general population, but the results were not statistically significant. Lazzeri et al. noted in a retrospective analysis that adult-onset vitiligo was more commonly associated with autoimmune thyroid disease and thyroid nodules. Hence, they recommended ruling out thyroid associations in adult-onset vitiligo [1–4,6].

MANAGEMENT

Although management of vitiligo in those with adult-onset disease is largely on similar lines to early-onset disease, a few subtle differences are noteworthy. Halder and Chappell [7] opined that vitiligo in elderly patients has a slow progression and responds poorly to treatment, hence a more conservative approach can be followed. Topical corticosteroids, topical calcineurin inhibitors, calcipotriol, and narrowband UVB phototherapy are valid treatment options in the elderly. PUVA and systemic steroids need to be used cautiously, if at all, because of associated comorbidities. As the majority of these patients tend to have a stable disease, surgical approaches may be considered. However, this should be done after weighing the risk:benefit ratio [1].

CONCLUSION

Late-onset vitiligo is a relatively underexplored topic in the literature. Due to an increase in life expectancy and increased awareness, late-onset vitiligo is being increasingly recognized. Its potential to cause low self-esteem and depression cannot be underestimated. It is crucial for clinicians to recognize, prognosticate, and manage such cases well. It is also important to look for any associated autoimmune conditions.

REFERENCES

1. Parasad D, and De D. Late-onset vitiligo. In: Picardo M, and Taïeb A, eds. *Vitiligo*. Springer; 2010, pp. 123–6.

2. Dogra S, Parsad D, Handa S, and Kanwar AJ. Late onset vitiligo: A study of 182 patients. *Int J Dermatol* 2005;44(3):193–6.

3. Al-Mutairi N, and Al-Sebeih KH. Late onset vitiligo and audiological abnormalities: Is there any association? *Indian J Dermatol Venereol Leprosy* 2011;77:571–6.

4. Esfandiarpour I, and Farajzadeh S. Clinical characteristics of late-onset vitiligo in an Iranian population. *Dermatol Sin* 2012;30:43–6.

5. Kanwar AJ, Mahajan R, and Parasad D. Effect of age at onset on disease characteristics in vitiligo. *J Cutan Med Surg* 2013;17:253–8.

6. Lazzeri L, Colucci R, Cammi A, Dragoni F, and Moretti S. Adult onset vitiligo: Multivariate analysis suggests the need for a thyroid screening. *Bio Med Res Int* 2016;2016:8065765.

7. Halder RM, and Chappell JL. Vitiligo update. *Semin Cutan Med Surg.* 2009;28(2):86–92.

DIAGNOSIS AND ASSESSMENT OF VITILIGO

Chapter 16

DIFFERENTIAL DIAGNOSIS

Hemant Kumar Kar and Gunjan Verma

CONTENTS

INTRODUCTION

Vitiligo is an acquired chronic pigmentation disorder characterized by white patches, which usually increase in size over time, corresponding to a substantial loss of functional epidermal and sometimes hair follicle melanocytes. The presence of a family history for vitiligo, presence of Koebner phenomenon, leukotrichia, and associated autoimmune disorders such as thyroid disease are typical data by medical history that can support the diagnosis. Vitiligo can be diagnosed because of its acquired and progressive nature and also by its chalk-white color. Hypomelanoses of the skin encompass a wide spectrum of congenital and acquired alterations in melanin pigmentation. These diseases can be localized or universal. The pathobiology of cutaneous hypomelanosis is heterogeneous and includes defects in melanoblast migration from the neural crest to the epidermis, alterations in melanogenesis and melanin transfer to keratinocytes, and destruction of pigment cells by autoimmune and inflammatory processes. Importantly, some congenital forms of universal hypomelanosis are associated with involvement of internal organs (e.g., Hermansky-Pudlack or Chédiak-Higashi syndrome) and require interdisciplinary patient management. In this chapter, hypomelanotic (Figure 16.1a) or depigmentary disorders that may be confused with vitiligo (Figure 16.1b) are discussed.

DIFFERENTIAL DIAGNOSIS

HALO NEVI

Vitiligo and halo nevi are both pigmentary disorders of the skin characterized by the acquired loss of functional epidermal melanocytes manifesting as white macules and patches. The lesions are characterized by a pigmented nevus with a surrounding depigmented zone. Halo nevi are usually multiple, occurring more frequently on the trunk and present among teenagers. The central nevus part gradually loses its pigmentation and disappears, making the whole patch depigmented uniformly, resembling a vitiligo patch.

The cellular mechanism and biochemical changes that result in the appearance of these two types of achromic lesions are still uncertain, and the relationship between vitiligo and halo nevi has been in dispute, but these two disorders can both be seen in the same patient, making it difficult to diagnose the two conditions (Figure 16.2).

The infiltrate contains many cytotoxic T cells and may represent immunologically induced rejection. The peripheral blood has been shown to contain activated adhesive lymphocytes that disappear when the lesion is excised. Patients also demonstrate antibodies to melanocytes. Electron microscopic (EM) analyses in studies have found different morphologic alterations in mitochondria from perilesional vitiligo skin and from perilesional halo nevus skin, reflecting heterogeneous backgrounds between the two diseases, revealing that vitiligo and halo nevus may have separate pathogenic mechanisms [1].

NEVUS DEPIGMENTOSUS

In contrast to what the name suggests, nevus depigmentosus (ND) presents itself as a hypopigmentation rather than a depigmentation, an important factor in distinguishing it from vitiligo. It can be sometimes confused with segmental vitiligo (Figures 16.3 and 16.4). Other factors discriminating ND from vitiligo are the absence of a marked sensitivity to sun exposure and the potential for slightly tanning. There are three subtypes within the group of the ND:

a. Isolated form (solitary and well-defined lesions).

b. Segmental form (unilateral, band-shaped lesions, sometimes blaschkoid distribution).

c. Systematized from (extensive whorls and streaks of hypopigmentation following the lines of Blaschko [hypomelanosis of Ito or pigmentary mosaicism]) [2]. In ND, there is decrease in transfer of melanosomes to keratinocytes.

Woods lamp examination can aid in diagnosis. Figure 16.1a gives an account of the disorder, and an approach to a patient of hypomelanotic lesion.

Newer technologies are helpful in distinguishing the two conditions. In vivo reflectance confocal microscopy (RCM), a noninvasive technique for real-time en face imaging of the superficial layers of the skin down to the superficial dermis, with cellular level resolution close to conventional histopathology, can be used as an auxiliary tool to distinguish between the two [3]. The Mexameter is an objective skin color-measuring device and has been reported to provide a reproducible and sensitive means of quantifying small skin color differences between nevus depigmentosus and vitiligo [4].

NEVUS ANEMICUS

Nevus anemicus also presents as a depigmented lesion, a common mimicker of vitiligo, especially in children. The underlying mechanism is an aberrant, hypersensitive response to catecholamines resulting in pallor of the skin. Hence it has been called a pharmacological nevus. The lesion is well defined and has an irregular border. When the skin in these lesions is rubbed, no red coloring is observed as there is no vasodilatation possible. Nevus anemicus on diascopy merges with the surrounding skin and is not accentuated. Woods light does not accentuate it, as it lacks any underlying pigmentary abnormality

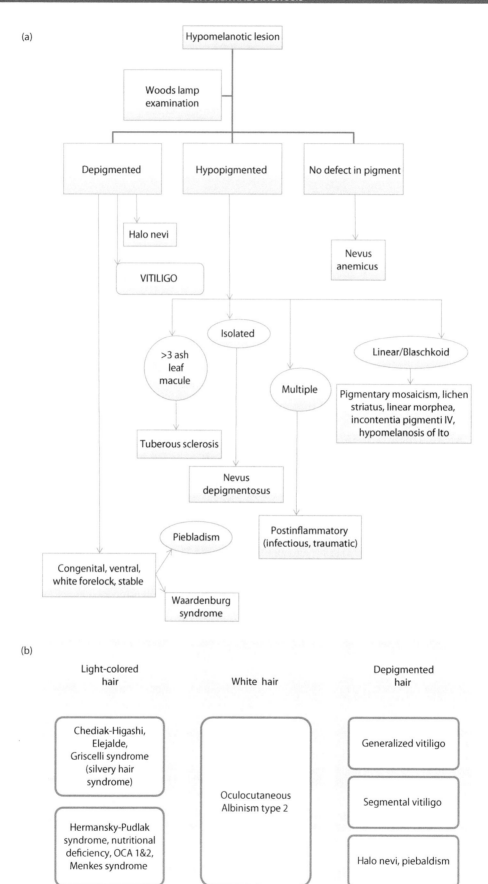

Figure 16.1 (a) Differential diagnosis of vitiligo (based on site). (b) Differential diagnosis of a patient of "depigmented or light-colored hair."

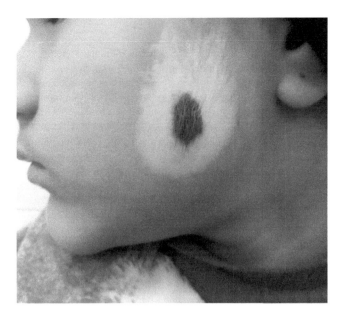

Figure 16.2 Halo nevi in a child (differential diagnosis of vitiligo).

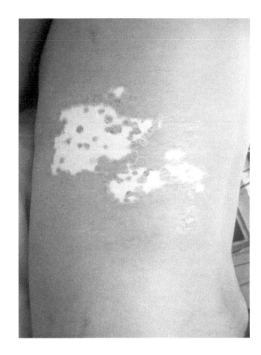

Figure 16.4 A case of segmental vitiligo.

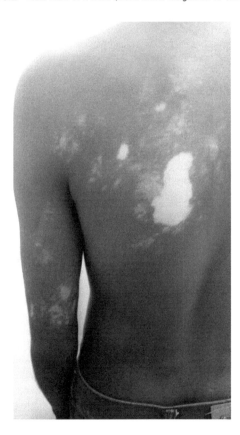

Figure 16.3 A case of nevus depigmentosus.

(Figure 16.1), and because of locally increased vascular reactivity to catecholamines, this simple bedside test can easily help the clinician to differentiate between the two nevi anemici that may occur on the neck and trunk of young children with neurofibromatosis when other features have not yet developed. It can also be observed in tuberous sclerosis (TSC) or as one component of phacomatosis pigmentovascularis.

INHERITED OR GENETICALLY INDUCED HYPOMELANOSIS (USUALLY PRESENT AT BIRTH)

PIEBALDISM

Piebaldism is a rare autosomal dominant disorder with an underlying defect of the tyrosine kinase transmembrane receptor on melanocytes, leading to impaired embryonic migration and survival of melanocytes in the skin. It results from a mutation in the *c-kit* proto-oncogene, mapped to the proximal long arm of chromosome 4 (4q12) or from deletions in the *SLUG* gene, which is a zinc finger neural crest transcription factor. Recently reported cases of piebaldism, which are milder or more severe than genetically expected, indicate that other factors (e.g., a modifier gene of *MC1R*) influence skin and hair color [5]. Piebaldism is clinically characterized by congenital extensive, symmetrically distributed depigmentation mainly on the forehead, front of the thorax, and extremities [5]. The extent of the lesions is variable, ranging from only a midfrontal poliosis or white forelock (present in 80%–90% of patients) and minimal areas of depigmentation to depigmentation of almost the entire body and hair (Figure 16.1b). Sometimes in the early age group and in initial stages it is hard to differentiate between piebaldism and segmental vitiligo having leukotrichia. However, a normal area of skin in between depigmented skin is the hallmark sign of piebaldism.

WAARDENBURG SYNDROME

Vitiligo should be differentiated from Waardenburg syndrome, which is also an autosomal dominant disorder with a similar clinical presentation. It is associated with heterochromia iridis, dystopia canthorum, congenital deafness, and occasionally a congenital megacolon (Hirschsprung disease). Waardenburg syndrome is an expression of a neurocristopathy, involving not only the melanocytes in the skin but also those at the level of the eyes, hair, cochlea, and meninges. Four subtypes have been identified. Piebaldism is comparable to these depigmented macules. However, the predominantly ventral distribution of the lesions, congenital character, stable course, white forelock, and the presence of hyperpigmented maculae within the areas of depigmentation are suggestive for piebaldism [6].

TUBEROUS SCLEROSIS

Ash leaf macules, a diagnostic feature of TSC, present as hypomelanotic skin lesions and first appear usually at birth or during infancy and are present in more than 90% of patients with TSC (Figure 16.5). These present as hypopigmented off-white-colored macules 1–3 cm in size, predominantly over the trunk and buttocks. Their shape may vary; classical lesions are ovoid or leaf-shaped, hence their name. Lesional leukotrichia and poliosis have been

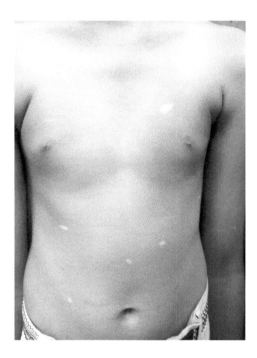

Figure 16.5   Ash leaf macule in tuberous sclerosis patient.

described [7]. In fair-skinned individuals, ash leaf macules can be made prominent by Woods light examination. Differentiation of an isolated ash leaf macule from vitiligo sometimes becomes difficult clinically as both can present as irregular round or polygonal macules, both can be segmental in distribution, and leukotrichia is a feature of both. Histopathologically, the number of melanocytes in ash leaf macules can be normal or decreased. Ultrastructurally on EM there is reduction in number, size, and melanization of melanosomes in ash leaf macule, which forms aggregates within keratinocytes [8]. However, in resource-poor settings where EM is not easily available, one has to rely on identification of other features of TSC and cutaneous as well as systemic findings to help in making the final diagnosis.

PIGMENTARY MOSAICISM (HYPOMELANOSIS OF ITO)

Hypomelanosis of Ito (HI) presents as bizarre whorled areas of depigmentation along Blaschko lines. HI, or incontinentia pigmenti achromians, is a rare neurocutaneous syndrome first described by Ito in 1952 as a purely cutaneous disease with skin hypopigmentation. Current theory suggests that hypomelanosis of Ito is a nonspecific manifestation of chromosomal mosaicism; however, chromosomal alteration have not been demonstrated in every case of HI. The clinical manifestations of HI are variable, but the most remarkable clinical markers are distinct patterns of skin involvement along the lines of Blaschko consisting of hypopigmented bizarre macular zones or spots with irregular borders, whorls, patches, or linear white streaks with various patterns of distribution and color that frequently appear on the trunk, occasionally on the extremities, and seldom on the face and scalp, with sparing of the palms, soles, and mucous membranes. Histopathologically, there is a decreased number and size of melanosomes in the basal layer of the epidermis. Other manifestations include patchy alopecia and nail abnormalities including ridging, dystrophy, and absence of nails. Dental abnormalities include increased tooth spacing and abnormal number, size, and shape. Craniofacial abnormalities include macrocephaly, low-set ears, small nose, and orbital hypertelorism. A wide variation of neurologic involvement is reported in HI, including developmental delay (40%–60%), epilepsy with early onset in life (11.5%–50%), and autistic behavior [9].

PROGRESSIVE MACULAR HYPOMELANOSIS

Progressive macular hypomelanosis (PMH) is a common skin disorder that is often misdiagnosed. Various authors have written about similar skin disorders, referring to them by different names, but the common consensus is that all these similar disorders are part of the same entity. PMH is characterized by ill-defined nummular, non-scaly hypopigmented spots on the trunk, often confluent in and around the midline, and rarely extending to the proximal extremities and neck/head region. There is no itch, pain, or preceding inflammation. PMH is characterized histologically by diminished pigment in the epidermis and a normal-looking dermis [10]. Electron microscopy shows a shift from large melanosomes in normal-looking skin to small aggregated, membrane-bound melanosomes in hypopigmented skin. PMH should be differentiated from other disorders with hypopigmentation on the trunk such as pityriasis versicolor. Although common, particularly in Fitzpatrick skin types IV–VI, this condition is frequently misdiagnosed and treated inadequately with antifungals or topical steroids, resulting in patient frustration. The exact pathogenesis of progressive macular hypomelanosis is unknown; however, recent studies suggest hypopigmentation results from decreased melanin formation and altered melanosome distribution in response to *Propionibacterium acnes* bacteria. While there are no well-established or consistently effective therapies for progressive macular hypomelanosis, the newer advances in understanding of its pathogenesis urge consideration of alternative treatment strategies such as topical and systemic antimicrobial therapy.

SECONDARY HYPOMELANOSIS
POSTINFLAMMATORY HYPOMELANOSIS

a. *Pityriasis alba*: Pityriasis alba is another common dermatosis characterized by hypopigmentation, presenting with pale-white, well- to moderately defined, very slightly scaling plaques. A relationship with sun exposure, xerosis cutis, and atopy has been suggested. This disease is usually reported in children between 6 and 16 years old, with lesions typically occurring in the face and upper arms. On histological examination, a normal presence of melanocytes and melanin is seen.

b. *Lichen sclerosus et atrophicus*: Lichen sclerosus et atrophicus (LSA) is a chronic inflammatory dermatosis with anogenital and extragenital presentations. Extragenital lichen sclerosus is most common on the neck, shoulders, and upper trunk. Typical findings are white opalescent papules that may cluster and progressively result in parchment-like skin. LSA occurs mostly in the anogenital area (83%–98%), and sometimes extragenital sites (15%–20%). Extragenital LSA is relatively common on the neck, shoulder, and upper trunk, is generally asymptomatic, but can occasionally be pruritic [11]. When it occurs in genitalia it can be confused with mucosal vitiligo (Figure 16.6).

c. *Morphea*: Morphea is a condition with an unpredictable natural history. Clinical activity usually persists for 3–5 years, but new lesions can develop even after longer periods of time. Lesions undergo different clinical stages [12]. First there is an initial inflammatory stage in which lesions are erythematous to violaceous, edematous, and warm to the touch. Then it becomes whiter and sclerotic with a characteristic violaceous ring. As the resultant damage is manifested, the plaques become white and sclerotic with postinflammatory hyper/hypopigmentation. The collagen deposition destroys adnexal structures such as hair follicles and glands. Concurrent LSA and morphea lesions can present as atrophic porcelain-like papules overlying sclerotic plaques.

d. *Lichen striatus*: Lichen striatus is an asymptomatic linear dermatosis that occurs mostly in children and has been reported to follow the lines of Blaschko. The primary lesions (small, flat,

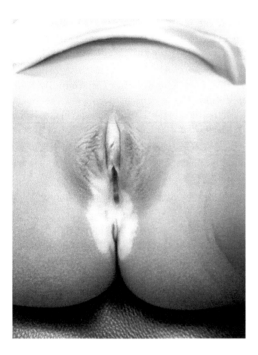

Figure 16.6   Mucosal vitiligo in child.

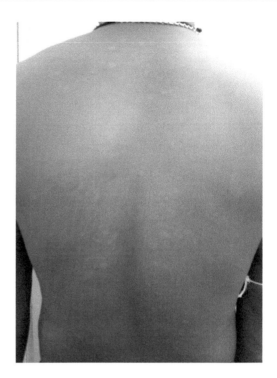

Figure 16.7   Hypopigmented macules present in a patient of post-kala-azar dermal leishmaniasis.

skin-colored to pink papules) can disappear spontaneously after several months or years, often leaving a linear macular hypopigmentation (postinflammatory).

POSTTRAUMATIC HYPOMELANOSIS
After a burn injury, a scar may heal with hypo- or depigmentation. Chemical leukoderma is a known term developed due to footwear- or bindi-induced allergic contact dermatitis presenting with hypo- or depigmentation. In one study, a boy developed hypopigmentation at the site of an adhesive pad for continuous electrocardiography monitoring during general anesthesia for dental rehabilitation [13]. All these can pose diagnostic difficulty in vitiligo.

POST-INFECTIOUS HYPOMELANOSIS
PITYRIASIS VERSICOLOR
Pityriasis versicolor, caused by yeasts of the *Malassezia* genus, is one of the most common yeast infections associated with pigmentary changes. Well-demarcated fine, scaly hyper- or hypopigmented macules/patches are commonly found on neck, upper back, arm, and chest areas on clinical examination. As most *Malassezia* species are lipid dependent, pityriasis versicolor is commonly seen in adolescence, associated with a high sebaceous activity in the skin. The clinical picture is often suggestive enough to establish the diagnosis, though it is confirmed microscopically. A yellow-green fluorescence may be observed on examination of affected areas with Woods light.

LEPROSY
Leprosy can present as hypopigmented macules or patches in indeterminate, tuberculoid, or borderline leprosy. It presents as discolored patches of skin, usually flat, that may be numb and look faded (lighter than the surrounding skin). Signs and symptoms due to damage to the cutaneous/peripheral nerves are:

- Numbness/anesthesia of patches or distal parts of limbs
- Muscle weakness or paralysis (especially in the hands and feet)
- Enlarged nerves (especially those around the elbow and knee and in the sides of the neck)
- Slit skin smear examination for AFB and skin biopsy confirm the diagnosis

POST-KALA-AZAR DERMAL LEISHMANIASIS
In post-kala-azar dermal leishmaniasis (PKDL), hypopigmented macules appear on the trunk and limbs, rarely on the face (Figure 16.7). In addition, there may be erythematous papules and nodules on the face, less commonly elsewhere. There may be facial erythema in butterfly distribution. LD bodies are present in skin biopsy.

ERUPTIVE HYPOMELANOSIS
A few cases have been reported in the literature of eruptive hypomelanosis, in which a child presents as paraviral exanthem which heals with hypomelanoses. It can be confused with vitiligo as it presents with hypopigmentation [14].

MISCELLANEOUS CONDITIONS
CUTANEOUS LYMPHOMA
Cutaneous T-cell lymphoma (CTCL) may present as diffuse hypopigmentation which may mimic vitiligo in the initial stage. Hypopigmented mycosis fungoides (HMF) is a rare variant of CTCL that often manifests in younger patients with darker skin types in a centripetal distribution (Figure 16.8). The average age of diagnosis is often around 14 years. The diagnosis is often missed due to its low incidence and lack of clinical suspicion. Misdiagnosis and failure to obtain biopsies can lead to a long latency period from onset of hypopigmented patches to diagnosis and treatment [15]. HMF has a clinically benign course and responds well to therapy; however, relapse is common. In order to correctly diagnose it, histopathological examination along with clinical examination is useful. Generalized lymphadenopathy, blood picture with hypopigmentation all over the body in an individual should raise a suspicious of CTCL. Both vitiligo and CTCL show a predominance of CD8+ T cells in tissue samples and hence the differentiation between the two diseases on clinical, histopathological, and even immunohistochemical grounds may be difficult. The findings, epidermotropism, hydropic degeneration of basal cells, partial loss of pigment, preservation of some melanocytes, presence of lymphocytes within the papillary dermis, increased density of the dermal infiltrate, and wiry fibrosis of the papillary dermal collagen are detected with a

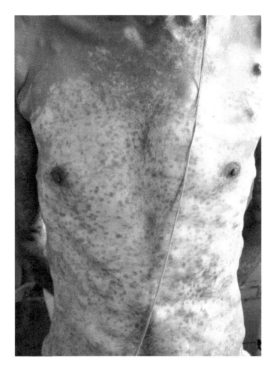

Figure 16.8 A patient of cutaneous T-cell lymphoma presented with multiple subcutaneous swelling with depigmentation of skin (differential diagnosis of vitiligo vulgaris).

significantly higher incidence in hypopigmented MF rather than in vitiligo. On the other hand, focal thickening of the basement membrane, complete loss of pigmentation, total absence of melanocytes, as well as absence or sparseness of lymphocytes in the dermal papillae, were seen much more frequently in vitiligo [16].

PITYRIASIS LICHENOIDES ET VARIOLIFORMIS ACUTA

A case of pityriasis lichenoides et varioliformis acuta (PLEVA) healing with hypopigmentation has been reported [17].

REFERENCES

1. Ding GZ, Zhao WE, Li X, Gong QL, and Lu Y. A comparative study of mitochondrial ultrastructure in melanocytes from perilesional vitiligo skin and perilesional halo nevi skin. *Arch Dermatol Res* 2015 Apr;307(3):281–9.

2. Di Lernia V. Segmental nevus depigmentosus: Analysis of 20 patients. *Pediatr Dermatol* 1999;16:349–53.

3. Pan ZY, Yan F, Zhang ZH, Zhang QA, Xiang LH, and Zheng ZZ. In vivo reflectance confocal microscopy for the differential diagnosis between vitiligo and nevus depigmentosus. *Int J Dermatol* 2011 Jun;50(6):740–5.

4. Park ES, Na JI, Kim SO, Huh CH, Youn SW, and Park KC. Application of a pigment measuring device--Mexameter--for the differential diagnosis of vitiligo and nevus depigmentosus. *Skin Res Technol* 2006 Nov;12(4):298–302.

5. van Geel N, Speeckaert M, Chevolet I, De Schepper S, Lapeere H, Boone B, and Speeckaert R. Hypomelanoses in Children. *J Cutan Aesthet Surg* 2013 Apr-Jun;6(2):65–72.

6. Oiso N, Fukai K, Kawada A, and Suzuki T. Piebaldism. *J Dermatol* 2013 May;40(5):330–5.

7. Apibal Y, Reakatanan W, and Chunharas A. Poliosis as the first clue of tuberous sclerosis. *Pediatr Dermatol* 2008;2013:486–7.

8. Jindal R, Jain A, Gupta A, and Shirazi N. Ash-leaf spots or naevus depigmentosus: A diagnostic challenge. *BMJ Case Rep* 2013;2013:bcr2012007008.

9. Kentab AY, Hassan HH, Hamad MH, and Alhumidi A. The neurologic aspects of hypomelanosis of Ito: Case report and review of the literature. *Sudan J Paediatr* 2014;14(2):61–70.

10. Relyveld GN, Menke HE, and Westerhof W. Progressive macular hypomelanosis: An overview. *Am J Clin Dermatol* 2007;8(1):13–9.

11. Ganesan L, Parmar H, Das JK, and Gangopadhyay A. Extragenital lichen sclerosus et atrophicus. *Indian J Dermatol* 2015;60:420.

12. Fett N, and Werth VP. Update on morphea: Part I. *J Am Acad Dermatol* 2011;64:231–42.

13. Tripi PA, Parthasarathy SN, and Honda K. ECG electrode induced hypopigmentation. *Middle East J Anaesthesiol* 2016 Jun;23(5):577–9.

14. Chuh A, Bharatia P, and Zawar V. Eruptive hypomelanosis in a young child as a paraviral exanthem. *Pediatr Dermatol* 2016 Jan-Feb;33(1):e38–9.

15. Tolkachjov SN, and Comfere NI. Hypopigmented mycosis fungoides: A clinical mimicker of vitiligo. *J Drugs Dermatol* 2015 Feb;14(2):193–4.

16. El-Darouti MA, Marzouk SA, Azzam O, Fawzi MM, Abdel-Halim MR, Zayed AA, and Leheta TM. Vitiligo vs. hypopigmented mycosis fungoides (histopathological and immunohistochemical study, univariate analysis). *Eur J Dermatol* 2006 Jan-Feb;16(1):17–22.

17. Ellerbroek V, and Hamm H. Pityriasis lichenoides et varioliformis acuta: Remission with hypopigmentation. *J Pediatr* 2016 Sep;176:211.

Chapter 17

NONINVASIVE TESTS

Hemant Kumar Kar and Gunjan Verma

CONTENTS

DERMOSCOPY

The loss of epidermal melanin in vitiligo lesions produces a window through which the light-induced autofluorescence of dermal collagen can be seen, resulting in the bright blue-white glow [1]. Dermoscopy scores over routine histopathology in the diagnosis of evolving lesions of vitiligo can obviate the need for a skin biopsy in doubtful cases.

Dermoscopy can be performed using a video dermoscope with built-in white light, polarized light, and ultraviolet (UV) light sources. Polarized light is used to study changes in the pigmentary network, while the UV source highlights the presence of a white glow in the lesion.

The most common dermoscopic features of guttate vitiligo include a well-demarcated, dense/glowing white area and perifollicular hyperpigmentation (which is more frequently seen in repigmenting or progressing lesions than in stable lesions) [2].

Dermoscopy is helpful in distinguishing other hypopigmented lesions. Dermoscopy of achromic/hypochromic lesions of pityriasis versicolor usually shows a fairly well demarcated white area with fine scales that are commonly localized in the skin furrows [3]. Dermoscopic examination of idiopathic guttate hypomelanosis may show multiple small areas coalescing into irregular/polycyclic macules, with several white shades and both well- and ill-defined edges, surrounded by patchy hyperpigmented network ("cloudy sky-like" pattern), while postinflammatory hypopigmentation often presents with some dermoscopic findings typical of the original lesions (e.g., the star-like arrangement in prurigo nodularis).

The utility of dermoscopy in the diagnosis of vitiligo is now well established. Chuh and Zawar noted a pattern of depigmentation with residual reservoirs of perifollicular pigment signifying focally active or repigmenting vitiligo [4]. Meng et al. studied 176 patients with various types of depigmentation, of whom 97 had vitiligo. They observed residual perifollicular pigmentation in 57 (91.9%) of 62 patients with progressing vitiligo and 22 (62.9%) of 35 with stable vitiligo [5]. However, residual perifollicular pigmentation was absent in the 79 patients with non-vitiligo depigmentation. The presence of telangiectasia, early reservoirs of pigmentation, and perilesional hyperpigmentation were related to the stage of vitiligo and treatment history of patients [6]. Various dermoscopic findings are associated with stability and repigmentation of vitiligo. These include marginal and perifollicular hyperpigmentation, reticular pigmentation, and marginal reticular pigmentation. Reduced pigmentary network, absent pigmentary network, reversed pigmentary network, perifollicular hyperpigmentation, and perilesional hyperpigmentation are seen in the evolving vitiligo lesions.

A white or depigmented net-like pattern with pigmentation in between has been termed *reversed pigmentary network*. However, reversed pigmentary network is a well-known finding in dermoscopy of melanoma and melanocytic nevus, in which it is described as reticular light areas with dark holes in the network [7].

WOODS LAMP EXAMINATION

The Woods lamp emits long-wave UV radiation (UVR), also called black light, generated by a high pressure mercury arc fitted with a compound filter made of barium silicate with 9% nickel oxide, the "Woods filter." This filter is opaque to all light rays except a band between 320 and 400 nm with a peak at 365 nm. Fluorescence of tissues occurs when Woods (UV) light is absorbed and radiation of a longer wavelength, usually visible light, is emitted. The output of Woods lamp is generally low (<1 mw/cm^2). The fluorescence of normal skin is very faint or absent and is mainly due to constituents of elastin, aromatic amino acids, and precursors or products of melanin [1,8].

The use of a Woods lamp does not require great skill. However, some practical points should be kept in mind to avoid misinterpretation of results.

- Ideally, the lamp should be allowed to warm up for about 1 minute.
- The examination room should be perfectly dark, preferably a windowless room or a room with black occlusive shades.
- The examiner should get dark-adapted in order to see the contrast clearly.
- The light source should be 4–5 inches from the lesion.
- Washing the area before subjecting it to Woods lamp examination should be avoided since it may yield false negative results due to dilution of the pigment.
- Topical medicaments, lint, and soap residues should be wiped off from the site to be examined, since these may fluoresce under Woods light. Common sources of error are bluish or purplish fluorescence produced by ointments containing petrolatum, green fluorescence by salicylic acid–containing medicaments, and light reflected from the examiner's white coat, producing light blue fluorescence.

Hypopigmentation in fair-skinned persons can be very difficult to discern. In hypopigmented or depigmented lesions there is less or no epidermal melanin. Consequently, there is a window through which the light-induced autofluorescence of dermal collagen can be seen. Due to the abrupt cutoff in the visible emission from lesional skin, the margins of hypopigmented or depigmented spots appear sharper under Woods light. The lesions appear bright blue-white due to autofluorescence. Woods lamp is therefore helpful in making a diagnosis of vitiligo, and particularly differentiating it from pityriasis alba, leprosy, and postinflammatory hypopigmentation or for identifying evolving lesions in a fair-skinned person. It is similarly useful in demonstrating evolving lesions of chemical leukoderma, leukoderma associated with melanoma, the ash leaf macules of tuberous sclerosis, and hypomelanosis, especially in the fair skinned. Woods lamp can also help to differentiate nevus depigmentosus from nevus anemicus; the latter does not show accentuation with Woods light. Follicular repigmentation following oral photochemotherapy can also be demonstrated earliest by the use of Woods light.

Recently, one study has found use of a Woods lamp as a UV light source to improve the speed and quality of suction blister harvesting [10].

The Woods lamp can also be used for targeted phototherapy in patients with vitiligo [11].

ULTRAVIOLET LIGHT PHOTOGRAPHY

UV light photography works on the principle that UV rays are more selectively absorbed than visible light by melanin in the epidermis. The UV radiation penetrates the epidermis, where it is attenuated by melanin; upon entering the dermis, it stimulates fluorescence emission by collagen bundles. Part of the emitted fluorescence is directed toward the surface of the skin, but it is attenuated by hemoglobin in the capillaries and by epidermal melanin. The results of Woods light examination can be recorded with UV photography. Woods lamp enhances the contrast between skin with little or no pigment and skin with excessive quantities of melanin.

DIFFUSE REFLECTANCE SPECTROSCOPY

Diffuse reflectance spectroscopy (DRS) has been used for more than 50 years to objectively measure skin pigmentation. This technique is based on different approaches to the analysis of light reflected by the skin [12].

When light impinges on the skin, approximately 4%–8% of the incident radiation is reflected off of the surface. Most of the incident light is attenuated by skin chromophores; that is, melanin, oxyhemoglobin, and deoxyhemoglobin. Oxyhemoglobin and deoxyhemoglobin absorb light specifically between 540 and 575 nm. Melanin heavily absorbs all wavelengths but demonstrates a monotonic increase toward shorter wavelengths [13]. DRS provides quantitative information about hemoglobin and melanin levels. In addition, it offers promise for analyzing and evaluating human skin in vivo in a rapid and noninvasive way, and the information obtained with DRS is potentially useful in the assessment and diagnosis of numerous pathologic conditions. The quality of pigmentation upon treatment cannot be assessed with clinical scoring systems. Spectroscopy is a useful tool for assessing the pigmentation quality [13].

COLORIMETRY-BASED IMAGE ANALYSIS

REFLECTANCE TRISTIMULUS CIE COLORIMETRY EVALUATION

Several studies have shown that the tristimulus colorimeter can be useful in the quantitative evaluation of UV-induced erythema, pigmentation, and disease severity. It is authorized by the Commission Internationale de l'Eclairage (CIE) and is regarded as the standard for colorimetry in industrial fields [14]. Tristimulus analysis converts intensity versus wavelength data (i.e., spectral information) into three numbers that indicate how the color of an object appears to a human observer.

REFLECTANCE CONFOCAL MICROSCOPY

Reflectance confocal microscopy (RCM) consists of a light source, a condenser, an objective lense, and a detector. Its light source is a near-infrared wavelength laser beam, which illuminates a specific point within the skin. Reflected light is collected through a pinhole in the detector. The illuminated spot is then scanned horizontally, producing black-and-white images from the epidermis to the upper reticular dermis with an imaging depth of up to 250–300 μm. To visualize a larger area, a two-dimensional sequence of images is captured and stitched in a software program to create a mosaic that displays up to 8 × 8 mm of tissue. Highly reflective skin components, including melanin, collagen, and keratin, appear bright (white) in RCM images.

The principle behind RCM lies in fact that melanin gives the strongest endogenous contrast in human skin when it is present in abnormal amounts in the skin. In vitiligo lesions, normal dermal papillary rings disappeared and no bright keratinocytes could be detected in the epidermis [9].

Kang et al. reported that RCM could be used to identify characteristic features of vitiligo and repigmented skin during treatment. These findings suggest that RCM could be used in the therapeutic monitoring and evaluation of vitiligo's evolution [1].

SUMMARY

The extent of vitiligo can be evaluated using the rule of nine, and the progression of the disease can be analyzed using a Woods lamp. For routine clinical exams, serial digital photographs can be used to monitor a patient's response to vitiligo treatment. The ideal scoring system must take into account patient perception. DRS gives information about skin pigmentation, and RCM offers great potential for the noninvasive assessment of pigmentary lesions. It will be necessary to establish an ideal, meaningful, and reproducible method that is objective, noninvasive, easy to use, and able to assess both morphometric and colorimetric changes during vitiligo treatment in the clinic and in clinical trials.

REFERENCES

1. Gupta LK, and Singhi MK. Wood's lamp. *Indian J Dermatol Venereol Leprol* 2004;70:131–5.

2. Errichetti E, and Stinco G. Dermoscopy in general dermatology: A practical overview. *Dermatol Ther (Heidelb)* 2016 Dec;6(4):471–507.

3. Thatte SS, and Khopkar US. The utility of dermoscopy in the diagnosis of evolving lesions of vitiligo. *Indian J Dermatol Venereol Leprol* 2014;80:505–8.

4. Chuh AA, and Zawar V. Demonstration of residual perifollicular pigmentation in localized vitiligo-a reverse and novel application of digital epiluminescence dermoscopy. *Comput Med Imaging Graph* 2004;28:213–7.

5. Meng R, Zhao G, Cai RK, Xiao M, and Jiang Z. Application of polarized light dermoscopy in the early diagnosis of vitiligo and its differential diagnosis from other depigmented diseases. *Chinese J Dermatol* 2009;42:810–3.

6. Chandrashekhar L. Dermoscopy: A tool to assess stability in Vitiligo. In: Khopkar U, ed. *Dermoscopy and Trichoscopy in Diseases of the Brown Skin: Atlas and Short Text*. New Delhi, India: Jaypee Brothers Medical Publishers; 2012, pp. 112–3.

7. Baak PY, Hofmann-Wellenhof R, and Massone C. Three cases of reverse pigment network on dermatoscopy with three distinctive histopathologic diagnoses. *Dermatol Surg* 2013;39:818–20.

8. Asawanoda P, and Taylor RC. Wood's light in dermatology. *Int J Dermatol* 1999;38:801–7.

9. Kang HY, Bahadoran P, and Ortonne JP. Reflectance confocal microscopy for pigmentary disorders. *Exp Dermatol* 2010;19:233–9.

10. Kaliyadan F, Venkitakrishnan S, and Manoj J. Use of a Wood's lamp as a ultra-violet light source to improve the speed and quality of suction blister harvesting. *Indian J Dermatol Venereol Leprol* 2010;76:429–31.

11. Kaliyadan F, and Ashique KT. Optimizing the efficacy of targeted phototherapy by marking early vitiligo lesions after visualizing under a Wood's lamp. *J Am Acad Dermatol* 2014 Sep;71(3):e69.

12. Marchesini R, Brambilla M, Clemente C et al. In vivo spectrophotometric evaluation of neoplastic and non-neoplastic skin pigmented lesions. I. Reflectance measurements. *Photochem Photobiol* 1991;53:77–84.

13. Pierard GE. EEMCO guidance for the assessment of skin color. *J Eur Acad Dermatol Venereol* 1998;10:1–11.

14. Weatherall IL, and Coombs BD. Skin color measurements in terms of CIELAB color space values. *J Invest Dermatol* 1992;99:468–73.

Chapter 18

INVASIVE TESTS

Hemant Kumar Kar and Gunjan Verma

CONTENTS

INTRODUCTION

Vitiligo may be associated with other autoimmune diseases, especially thyroid disease and diabetes mellitus. Other associated autoimmune diseases include pernicious anemia, Addison disease, and alopecia areata. Patients should be made aware of signs and symptoms that suggest the onset of hypothyroidism, diabetes, or other autoimmune diseases and if any signs or symptoms occur, appropriate tests should be performed.

A CBC count with indices helps rule out anemia. To rule out thyroid dysfunction, thyrotropin testing is the most cost-effective screening test. Clinicians should also consider investigating for serum antithyroglobulin and antithyroid peroxidase antibodies, particularly, as antithyroid peroxidase antibodies are regarded as a sensitive and specific marker of autoimmune thyroid disease. Screening for diabetes can be accomplished with fasting blood glucose or glycosylated hemoglobin testing. Antinuclear antibody screening is also helpful.

HISTOPATHOLOGICAL EXAMINATION OF SKIN BIOPSY

The histopathological changes in vitiligo in sections stained with hematoxylin and eosin (H&E) are often very subtle and may be inconclusive. Special staining procedures like Fontana-Masson staining is helpful in reaching a definitive diagnosis. The DOPA reaction which demonstrates viable and functional melanocytes may also be used but is technically difficult to perform [1].

Microscopic examination of involved skin shows a complete absence of melanocytes in association with a total loss of epidermal pigmentation. Superficial perivascular and perifollicular lymphocytic infiltrates may be observed at the margins of vitiliginous lesions, consistent with a cell-mediated process destroying melanocytes. Degenerative changes have been documented in keratinocytes and melanocytes in both border lesions and adjacent skin. Other documented changes include increased numbers of Langerhans cells, epidermal vacuolization, and thickening of the basement membrane.

Loss of pigment and melanocytes in the epidermis is highlighted by Fontana-Masson staining and immunohistochemistry testing.

In a recent study it was found that histologically, lesions of vitiligo showed more basal hypopigmentation and dermal inflammation than perilesional normal skin. With Fontana-Masson staining, 16% of cases of vitiligo showed the presence of melanin. In NKI/beteb staining, 12% of vitiligo showed the presence of melanocytes, and their average number was 7.68 per square millimeter [2].

Skin biopsy samples can also be examined by Melan-A (A103 clone)+ for melanocyte expression by immunohistochemical analysis and for melanin by histochemical studies with section staining by Fontana-Masson method. Melan-A+ cells and melanin granules were detected in depigmented skin as indication that the residual melanocytes are preserved in vitiligo lesions. More than threefold decrease of Melan-A+ melanocytes amount was revealed in perilesional normally pigmented skin of vitiligo patients [3].

Invasive tests are needed to study the vitiligo at a microscopic level. Because defects in adhesion impairment seem to be involved in the etiopathogenesis of vitiligo, various studies compared the immunohistochemical expression of several adhesion molecules in the epidermis of vitiligo and non-lesional skin, which showed that impairment in adhesion exists in vitiligo skin, which is supported by the diminished immunohistochemical expression of laminin, β1 integrin, ICAM-1, and VCAM-1.[4].

MINIMALLY INVASIVE TECHNIQUES

BIOMARKERS FROM BLISTER FLUID

In a published study, authors investigated the potential biomarkers of disease activity directly in the skin of vitiligo subjects and healthy subjects. Patient skin was sampled via a modified suction-blister technique, allowing for minimally invasive, objective assessment of cytokines and T-cell infiltrates in the interstitial skin fluid. Measuring CXCL9 directly in the skin can be used for diagnosis and as an early marker of treatment response [5].

HOMOCYSTEINE LEVEL MEASUREMENT FROM BLISTER FLUID

In another study, the increase in homocysteine levels was found to be statistically significant in the patients' lesional induced bulla compared to the healthy controls. There was no significant difference in homocysteine levels between males and females and between patients with negative or positive family histories of vitiligo. The presence of a high homocysteine level in active vitiligo lesions points to a local event occurring in the lesion, which is not reflected as an increase in the patient's serum level [5].

LABORATORY TESTS INDICATED IN PATIENTS WITH VITILIGO

1. Antithyroid peroxidase antibody and antiparietal gastric cell antibody could be useful laboratory markers in a subpopulation of vitiligo patients. However, testing antinuclear antibody, antithyroglobulin antibody, folic acid, and vitamin B_{12} seems to have limited clinical implications and diagnostic relevance in clinical practice. Both the aforementioned tests could be useful for the characterization of specific subpopulations of vitiligo patients in terms of severity and comorbidity. Their determination could have a prognostic value [6].

2. A study indicated lipid disturbances in vitiligo-affected children. Lipid disturbances in vitiligo may result from disturbed metabolic processes in the adipose tissue as well as from oxidative stress [7].

CYTOKINE ESTIMATION

INTERLEUKIN LEVELS IN VITILIGO

There is a possible systemic role of IL-33 in the pathogenesis of vitiligo. A positive correlation of IL-33 serum levels has been noticed with extension of vitiligo and disease activity. This also suggests that inhibiting IL-33 activity might be a novel therapeutic strategy in the treatment of autoimmune inflammatory disease, like vitiligo [8]. However, it does not have any diagnostic significance.

MELATONIN LEVELS IN VITILIGO

In patients with nonsegmental vitiligo, the level of melatonin has been found below the normal level (12.5 pg/mL) [9]. The level of melatonin in the blood plasma is determined by ELISA; the results are expressed in units of pg/mL.

SERUM ANTIMELANOCYTE ANTIBODIES BY IMMUNOFLUORESCENCE

Serum antimelanocyte autoantibodies are found against melanocytes in serum samples of patients with vitiligo. High titers of anti-tyrosine-related protein 1 (TRP-1) antibody are also detected [10].

REFERENCES

1. Kumar S, Singh A, and Prasad RR. Role of histopathology in vitiligo. *J Indian Med Assoc* 2011 Sep;109(9):657–8, 665.

2. Kim YC, Kim YJ, Kang HY, Sohn S, and Lee ES. Histopathologic features in vitiligo. *Am J Dermatopathol* 2008 Apr;30(2):112–6.

3. Kubanov A, Proshutinskaia D, Volnukhin V, Katunin O, and Abramova T. Immunohistochemical analysis of melanocyte content in different zones of vitiligo lesions using the Melan-A marker. *Acta Dermatovenerol Alp Pannonica Adriat* 2016;25(1):5–9.

4. Reichert Faria A, Jung JE, Silva de Castro CC, and de Noronha L. Reduced immunohistochemical expression of adhesion molecules in vitiligo skin biopsies. *Pathol Res Pract* 2017 Mar;213(3):199–204.

5. Anbar T, Zuel-Fakkar NM, Matta MF, and Arbab MM. Elevated homocysteine levels in suction-induced blister fluid of active vitiligo lesions. *Eur J Dermatol* 2016 Jan-Feb;26(1):64–7.

6. Rodríguez-Martín M, Sáez M, Merino de Paz N, Ferrer PC, Eliche MP, Rodríguez-Martín B, and Cabrera AN. When are laboratory tests indicated in patients with vitiligo? *Dermatoendocrinol* 2012 Jan 1;4(1):53–7.

7. Pietrzak A, Bartosińska J, Dybiec E, Chodorowska G, Krasowska D, Hercogova J, and Lotti T. Hepato-splenic and lipid profile abnormalities--do they exist in children affected with vitiligo? *Acta Dermatovenerol Croat* 2014;22(1):19–25.

8. Vaccaro M, Cicero F, Mannucci C, Calapai G, Spatari G, Barbuzza O, Cannavò SP, and Gangemi S. IL-33 circulating serum levels are increased in patients with non-segmental generalized vitiligo. *Arch Dermatol Res* 2016 Sep;308(7):527–30.

9. Tsiskarishvili NI, Katsitadze A, Tsiskarishvili NV, Tsiskarishvil TS, and Chitanava L. Melatonin concentration in the blood of vitiligo patients with stress in anamnesis. *Georgian Med News* 2016 May;(254):47–53.

10. Zhu MC, Liu CG, Wang DX, and Zhan Z. Detection of serum anti-melanocyte antibodies and identification of related antigens in patients with vitiligo. *Genet Mol Res* 2015 Dec 7;14(4):16060–73.

Chapter 19

ASSESSMENT OF VITILIGO

Sneha Ghunawat

CONTENTS

INTRODUCTION

There is a lack of consensus on methods of assessment of disease severity in vitiligo, making it difficult to carry out meta-analysis and compare the findings from different studies for the same treatment options. Also, the course of the disease is varied and includes flareups, remissions, and spontaneous repigmentation. Therefore documentation of the current extent of the disease and also the repigmentation on treatment is extremely important. Various scoring systems are available to assess extent, stability, and repigmentation in vitiligo. In routine practice, the common methods used include visual and photographic analysis. However, these methods are subjective and thus cannot be used in clinical studies.

AREAS OF INVOLVEMENT

The severity of the disease can be assessed in terms of extent of involvement. Point counting, digital planimetry, and digital photography with computerized planimetry and computer-aided design software are some of the methods used to assess the area of involvement in vitiligo. Other methods include colorimetry-based image analysis, spectrophotometry, and more modern methods like reflectance confocal microscopy [1,2].

The Wallace rule of nine is a common measure used to measure the extent of involvement in vitiligo [3]. A similar technique is the Lund-Browder chart. However, assessment of vitiligo severity based on the area of involvement alone is an incomplete measure. The severity of a lesion is much greater when it is located on the face or sexually important sites, such as the genitalia and the breast.

The Vitiligo Area Severity Index (VASI) is a tool for assessment of the disease proposed by Hamzavi and coworkers [4] to assess the response to narrowband UVB in vitiligo. This tool has also been widely used to assess the disease response with other modes of treatment. On comparison with physician global assessment in 22 patients, VASI was found to be a valid clinical tool for vitiligo assessment. For its calculation, the body is divided into five segments. The hands, upper extremities (including axilla), trunk, lower extremities (including buttocks), and feet. For assessment of the area of involvement, the hand unit is used. Each hand unit, i.e., palm and volar aspect of hand, is approximately 1% of body surface area. The area of involvement is calculated in each segment using the hand unit. The residual depigmentation is calculated by a percentage as follows: 100% depigmentation, no pigmentation is present; 90%, specks of pigmentation present; 75%, depigmented area exceeds the pigmented area; 50%, depigmented area equals the pigmented area; 25%, the pigmented area exceeds the depigmented area; 10%, only specks of depigmentation are seen. The total score is calculated as follows:

$$\text{VASI} = \sum \left(\text{Hand unit}\right) \times \left(\text{Residual depigmentation}\right)$$

Another assessment method is the Vitiligo European Task Force assessment (VETFa) [5]. This is a more complex system, developed by the European group. It takes into account the extent, stage, and progression of the disease. For assessment, the body is divided into five units: the head and neck, arms, trunk, legs, and hands and feet. The extent is calculated by the rule of nine as used in atopic dermatitis. For calculation of extent, the hands and feet are included with arms and legs, respectively. Staging is assessed by cutaneous and hair depigmentation in the largest macule from 0–4. The hands and feet are treated as separate sites for staging of the disease. The staging is done as follows: stage 0: normal pigmentation (no depigmentation); stage 1: incomplete depigmentation (spotty depigmentation, trichrome pigmentation, and lighter homogenous pigmentation); stage 2: complete depigmentation (including hair whitening in <30%); stage 3: complete depigmentation (hair whitening in >30%). The progression/spreading of the lesions is assessed using a simple scale (+1 progressive, 0 = stable, −1: regressive). The limits of the macule are assessed using normal light followed by Woods lamp examination. The extent, staging, and spreading are evaluated in each site. The largest macule is assessed in each site.

Both the VASI and VETFa are semi-objective tools that have been shown to reliably assess the extent of disease in vitiligo cases. They are easy to use, can be used in widespread vitiligo, and have been used in clinical studies to assess the response to treatment.

DISEASE STABILITY

Vitiligo is a disease that runs a variable and unpredictable course. No definite criteria exist to define the stability of the disease. Different workers have used various criteria in their studies to assess disease stability. Presence of punctate depigmentation, differing shades of hypopigmentation, sharpness of the lesional margins, and Woods lamp examination are some of the criteria used to determine disease stability. The cessation of appearance of new lesions is also taken as criteria for disease stability. Recommendation for vitiligo surgery after 1 year of inactivity is based on this premise. However, there is a paucity of data on factors that influence disease stability.

The Vitiligo Disease Activity Score (VIDA) score has been used to evaluate the activity of the disease in vitiligo [6]. It was first used in 1999 by Njoo et al. It is a 6-point scale based on disease activity and time period. The scoring is as follows: score 4+ activity lasting 6 weeks or less; score 3+ activity lasting 6 weeks to 3 months; score 2 activity lasting 3–6 months; score 1 activity lasting 6–12 months; score 0 stable for 1 year or more; score −1 stable with repigmentation for 1 year or more. The lower the score, the lesser is the disease activity.

REPIGMENTATION INDICES

One assessment tool used is potential repigmentation index (PRI). It was developed by Benzekri and coworkers [7] for prediction of repigmentation potential in nonsegmental vitiligo. In their study, they showed that patients with higher PRI were more likely to obtain pigmentation following narrowband UVB treatment. Each lesion exceeding 10 cm^2 is classified based on the clinical type of vitiligo and the melanocyte reservoir (follicular and epidermal) into four types (A, B, C, and D). PRI is calculated as a ratio of number of lesions with good clinical response and number of refractory lesions, i.e., PRI = (Type A + B)/(Type C + D).

QUALITY-OF-LIFE INDICES

Vitiligo has significant impact on the quality of life of the patient. The assessment measures remain incomplete without the inclusion of this component, as vitiligo has a great impact on the psychosocial aspect of the patient. This impact has not been found to correlate with the extent of the disease. Health-related quality-of-life (HRQL) measures and dermatologically specific HRQL indices such as Skindex and Dermatology Life Quality Index have been used to assess the psychological impact of the disease [8,9].

DISFIGUREMENT INDICES

Vitiligo is a disease that greatly affects the psyche of the patient. The disfigurement index measures the alteration in appearance of the patient as perceived by others. It involves scoring the photographs of the patient on scales such as the visual analog scale based on the disfigurement as perceived by the observer (medical professionals, patients, and laymen). This measure has also been used for other diseases such as port wine stain and head and neck cancer surgery.

CONCLUSION

There is clearly lack of a composite scale to measure the involvement in vitiligo. The use of individual scales for different parameters is cumbersome in the clinical practice. However, in vitiligo, the emphasis should not only be on measuring the extent of depigmentation; other factors such as quality of life and repigmentation potential also should be considered to gauge a comprehensive picture of the disease.

REFERENCES

1. Taïeb A, and Picardo M; VETF Members. The definition and assessment of vitiligo: A consensus report of the Vitiligo European Task Force. *Pigment Cell Res* 2007;20:27–35.

2. Kanthraj GR, Srinivas CR, Shenoi SD, Deshmukh RP, and Suresh B. Comparison of computer-aided design and rule of nines methods in the evaluation of the extent of body involvement in cutaneous lesions. *Arch Dermatol* 1997;133:922–3.

3. Hettiaratchy, S., and Papini, R. Initial management of a major burn: II–assessment and resuscitation. *BMJ* 2004;329:101–3.

4. Hamzavi I, Jain H, McLean D, and Shapiro J. Parametric modelling of narrowband UV-B phototherapy for vitiligo using a novel quantitative tool, the vitiligo area scoring index. *Arch Dermatol* 2004;140:677–83.

5. Komen L, da Graca V, Wolkerstorfer A et al. The VASI and the VETF assessment: Reliable and responsive instruments to measure the degree of depigmentation in vitiligo. *Br J Dermatol* 2015;172(2):437–43.

6. Menchini G, and Commacchio C. Vitiligo activity index, a new activity evaluation index for bilateral vitiligo vulgaris. *J Plast Dermatol* 2007;3:35–9.

7. Benzekri L, Ezzedine K, and Gauthier Y. Vitiligo Potential Repigmentation Index: A simple clinical score that might predict the ability of vitiligo lesions to repigment under therapy. *Br J Dermatol* 2013;168:1143–6.

8. van Geel N, Ongenae K, Vander Haeghen Y, and Naeyaert JM. Autologous transplantation techniques for vitiligo: How to evaluate treatment outcome? *Eur J Dermatol* 2004b;14:46–51.

9. Choi S, Kim DY, Whang SH, Lee JH, Hann SK, and Shin YJ. Quality of life and psychological adaptation of Korean adolescents with vitiligo. *J Eur Acad Dermatol Venereol* 2010;24:524–9.

Chapter 20

QUALITY-OF-LIFE MEASURES AND PSYCHOLOGICAL ASPECTS IN VITILIGO (COUNSELING AND SUPPORT GROUPS)

Rashmi Sarkar and Shilpa Garg

CONTENTS

INTRODUCTION

Vitiligo affects about 1%–4% of the world's population and presents as milky-white macules involving the skin and/or mucosa. It does not cause much physical impairment but causes impairment in mental health and quality of life (QoL) due to its disfiguring appearance, causing discrimination and segregation in certain cultures. Quality of life is defined by the World Health Organization as an individual's perception of their position in life in context of the culture and value systems in which they live and in relation to their goals, expectations, standards, and concerns [1]. Quality-of-life measures evaluate the extent of disability due to a disease in a standardized and quantitative manner. In India, patients with vitiligo face social problems due to its association with social beliefs (i.e., people with vitiligo are considered to have done "Guru Droh" (sin) in their previous life) and stigmatization due to its resemblance to leprosy (referred as "Sweta Kustha," meaning "white leprosy"). Those affected may be unable to find employment, get married, or even get divorced if they develop the disease after marriage. Quality of life is measured in three domains: physical functioning, which includes functional difficulties and symptoms; psychological state, which includes emotional and cognitive functions; and social interaction, which includes public relations, daily activities, and work. Vitiligo affects physical, social, psychological, and occupational aspects of QoL [2]. Dermatology-specific questionnaires are available for measuring the QoL in vitiligo patients, such as the Dermatology Life Quality Index (DLQI), and recently a vitiligo-specific scale was introduced by Senol et al. [3] (Table 20.1).

EMOTIONAL IMPACT OF VITILIGO

The psychosocial impact of vitiligo is the most important factor that affects the QoL in vitiligo patients and is derived from depression, anger, anxiety, self-consciousness, and embarrassment [2]. Due to disgust and fear of infection, these patients are often glared at and avoided. In a review of 21 studies of the DLQI score in vitiligo, 10 studies showed that women with vitiligo had significantly higher impairment in their QoL as compared to men with vitiligo ($p = 0.019$), while the remaining 11 studies showed no relation between gender and DLQI [4]. Dolatshahi et al. reported a statistically significant difference ($p = 0.033$) in the mean DLQI score in married individuals (mean DLQI 9.22) as compared to singles (mean DLQI 6.91) [5]. There was no significant difference in the DLQI between married men and single men; however, married women had a statistically higher DLQI score as compared to single women. Several other studies found no relationship between the DLQI score and marital status of the patient. Most studies have found no statistically significant relationship between the DLQI score and age range, except one by Parsad et al. [10] Some studies have reported longer duration of vitiligo as a predictor of impaired QoL, while some found no significant correlation between the two [4]. Vitiligo located on the face, hands, and feet is particularly embarrassing. Vitiligo present on exposed areas adversely effects the patient's chances of getting a job, and vitiligo on the chest and genitalia is significantly associated with sexual dysfunction. Patients with vitiligo located on visible areas had higher DLQI score as compared to those whose lesions were present on covered sites [4]. Ongenae et al. [6] reported that patients with involvement of head, face, or neck were particularly bothered by the disease, whereas Schmid-Ott et al. [7] reported no relationship between location of vitiligo lesion and stigmatization experienced by the patient. Homan et al. [8] reported that vitiligo on the chest was significantly associated with emotion and functioning scales and the sum score of the Skindex-29 score, whereas vitiligo on the face and hands had no negative impact on health-related quality of life (HRQL). The majority of the studies have found a positive correlation between the body surface area affected by vitiligo and poor QoL, except for few studies by Kent and al-Abadie who found only a weak correlation, and Mishra et al., who found no correlation [9]. The majority of the studies on HRQL in vitiligo have used DLQI, which shows a negative impact on the psychosocial functioning of the patient, with the scores

Table 20.1 Vitiligo Life Quality Index (VLQI)

Please answer the questions in light of the past week
1. Have you had pain, irritation, or itching due to vitiligo?
2. Have you felt embarrassed or insecure about the appearance of your vitiligo?
3. Have you felt uneasy about others staring at you because of vitiligo?
4. Have you used makeup to conceal vitiligo?
5. Have you picked out clothing specifically to cover up vitiligo?
6. Has vitiligo reduced your self-esteem?
7. Have you not wanted others to see your body due to vitiligo?
8. Have you had concerns about vitiligo spreading to other parts of your body?
9. Have you had concerns about getting skin cancer because of vitiligo?
10. Have you had anxiety over vitiligo being permanent?
11. Have you worried that your children might inherit vitiligo from you?
12. Have you felt uncomfortable looking in the mirror due to vitiligo?
13. Have you stayed away from crowded areas (public transportation, shopping centers, etc.) due to vitiligo?
14. Have you had difficulty with sun exposure or protection due to vitiligo?
15. Has vitiligo affected your vacation plans?
16. Has vitiligo had an impact on what you do on your free time, your activities, and hobbies?
17. Have you had any challenges at school or work due to vitiligo?
18. Have you felt uncomfortable with questions asked about your vitiligo and the explanations you had to make?
19. Have you felt isolated or been made fun of due to vitiligo?
20. Have you had issues with your partner due to vitiligo?
21. Have you avoided physical contact with others (shake hands, give hugs or kisses, etc.) because of vitiligo?
22. Have you had family issues due to vitiligo?
23. Have you felt uneasy about sharing personal items with the household due to vitiligo?
24. Have you had difficulty keeping up with vitiligo therapy (spending too much time or money, applying medicine, etc.)?
25. Have you had problems in your sexual relations because of vitiligo?

ranging from 4.94 to 15 in various studies [6,10]. In one study, 35% of patients scored above the threshold on the general health questionnaire (GHQ), indicating psychological distress [11]. The mean DLQI score was 4.82, which was related to the perceived stigma, GHQ, race, and self-esteem, suggesting that interventions made to target these variables may have a potential benefit on the level of disability [12]. Sampogna et al. [13] reported that worry of worsening of the disease (60%), anger (37%), embarrassment (34%), depression (31%), affect on social life (28%), and shame (28%) were problems experienced by vitiligo patients. Women, patients older than 40 years, and patients with vitiligo located on the feet, legs, and arms were at greater risk for impairment in QoL. Patients with a family history of vitiligo were significantly less worried by their disease in comparison to those with no family history. Low HRQL was seen in the emotional and functioning scales in 20 vitiligo patients in another study [14].

Porter et al. [15] reported that two-thirds of the patients were embarrassed by vitiligo, one-third reported interference in their sex life, and over 50% felt ill at ease, anxious, concerned, and worried about vitiligo. Friends and family members were perceived as supportive by 80% of the patients, while meeting strangers was uncomfortable as they felt that strangers were less understanding. Patients felt stigmatized by vitiligo, as they often felt stared at, discriminated against, and subjected to rude remarks. They experienced psychological problems such as depression, shame, and anxiety which led to social isolation and low self-esteem. Patients younger than 40 years and those belonging to the working class felt more embarrassed, self-conscious, and discriminated against.

Porter et al. [16] reported negative impact on sexual relationship in <23% of patients mostly due to embarrassment, and this was seen predominantly in men, singles, and those with low self-esteem and to whom appearance was more important. However, another study reported that women felt more embarrassed and more self-conscious of their disease, which impaired their social life, sexual activity, personal relationships, and choice of clothing [17].

IMPACT ON OCCUPATION

Majority of the studies observed that although vitiligo caused significant reduction in work and study, these were some of the least effected items as compared to other items of DLQI [4]. Vitiligo patients may suffer financial losses, as they often have to take leave from their jobs due to their appointments for treatment, such as psoralen-ultraviolet-A (PUVA) therapy. These patients face restricted career choices, as lesions present on the exposed body sites adversely affect their chances in job interviews. Parents of children with vitiligo have to take leave from work to accompany the child to various appointments [18].

PSYCHIATRIC MORBIDITY

In India, vitiligo patients face more social problems as compared to other countries [18]. Picardi et al. [19] reported increased psychiatric morbidity in women with vitiligo on visible body parts. Sampogna et al. [13] reported psychiatric morbidity to be strongly associated with poorer HRQL in the emotions and functioning scales. Vitiligo patients had higher prevalence of anxiety or depression (39%) and alexithymia (24%) than the general population. Mood disturbances like irritability and depression were seen especially in teenagers. Children with vitiligo avoided or restricted their sport activities and lost vital days at school. Vitiligo beginning in childhood caused significantly greater psychological trauma with lasting impact on self-esteem [18]. The manner in which children dealt with their disease depended on the attitudes of their sibling(s), parents, friends, teachers, babysitters, etc. [20].

The prevalence of psychiatric comorbidities in patients with vitiligo in the UK [11] and Italy [21] was 35% and 25%, respectively. Indian studies [22–24] showed adjustment disorders in 56%–75% of GHQ-positive patients. Psychiatric diagnosis and symptoms seen in patients with vitiligo were dysthymia (7%–9%), depression (10%), depressive episode (18%–22%), sleep disturbance (20%), suicidal thoughts (10%), anxiety (3.3%), and suicide attempts (3.3%). Psychiatric comorbidity in vitiligo patients correlated significantly with psychological dysfunction and change in the social behavior, and did not correlate with the extent or severity of the disease [23,25]. Severe depression was found to lead to suicide attempts [25]. The psychiatric morbidity was predicted better by the impact of the disease on the QOL than by the physician's assessment of clinical severity [21]. Owing to high prevalence of psychiatric morbidity, psychiatric evaluation is suggested for chronic and stigmatizing diseases like vitiligo. Patients with psychological distress and formal psychiatric disorders may need referral. It is important to screen and identify patients with psychiatric disorders to reduce psychological distress, improve QoL, enhance the adherence to treatment, and increase patient satisfaction.

PSYCHOLOGICAL INFLUENCE AND VITILIGO

There is no clear evidence of role of stress in vitiligo. Papadopoulos et al. [26] suggested the role of psychological distress in the onset of vitiligo and reported that patients with vitiligo encountered a significantly higher number of stressful situations as compared to patients with skin disease not thought to be associated with stress. In contrast to this study, stress events were not found to have a role in vitiligo by Picardi et al. [27].

The potential of therapeutic implication of psychosocial intervention and counseling in vitiligo is not very well established. Papadopoulos et al. [28] reported that counseling may have a positive effect on the course of vitiligo. Parsad et al. [10] reported that a less favorable response to treatment in vitiligo in patients with higher DLQI scores suggested the need for recognizing and dealing with the psychological problems, which would help in improving the treatment outcome in these patients.

COMPARISON OF QOL BETWEEN VITILIGO AND OTHER DISEASES

Finlay and Khann reported that vitiligo had a lower impact on the QoL as compared to atopic dermatitis, psoriasis, and generalized pruritus [29]. Ghajarzadeh et al. reported that QoL in vitiligo patients was more impaired than in patients with alopecia areata but better than in patients with psoriasis [30]. Ongenae et al. [6], Karelson et al. [31], and Radtke et al. [32] found that the DLQI score in patients with vitiligo was significantly lower than patients with psoriasis. Beikert et al. [33] reported that patients with vitiligo had higher QoL than patients with rosacea and lower QoL than patients with atopic dermatitis. Emotional problems in vitiligo patients are comparable to patients with acne, psoriasis, eczema, and chronic hand dermatitis. The mean DLQI score in women with vitiligo was comparable to patients with psoriasis in a study by Ongenae et al. [6]. However, Porter et al. [34] reported less impairment in vitiligo patients as compared to patients with psoriasis in terms of choice of clothes, job discrimination, social relations, and embarrassment. Radtke et al. [35] reported mean DLQI and EuroQol (EQ-5D) in

vitiligo patients as 7.0 and 83.6, respectively, as compared to 8.6 and 75.3 in psoriasis patients. The QoL was severely reduced in 24.6% patients with vitiligo as compared to 34.1% patients with psoriasis, and 32.9% of vitiligo patients were willing to pay greater than 5000 Euro for achieving complete remission. Willingness to pay in vitiligo patients correlated significantly with DLQI scores, duration of the disease, and affected body surface area.

Being associated with the feeling of embarrassment, vitiligo interferes with the patient's choice of clothing. A study on children showed that DLQI score in children with vitiligo was 11.68, which was higher than children with atopic dermatitis (7.74). The low QoL in children with vitiligo was found to be critical in the psychosocial development.

Psychiatric comorbidities in vitiligo patients from India were present in 16%−34% patients as compared to 24%−53% in patients with psoriasis. In a study by Sharma et al. [36] found statistically significant difference ($p = 0.0028$) in psychiatric morbidity seen in 16.7% of vitiligo patients as compared to 53.3% patients with psoriasis. Depression was seen in 23.3% of patients with psoriasis and 10% of patients with vitiligo, with anxiety being present in 3.3% in each group. Sleep disturbance was present in 56.6% patients with psoriasis and 20% in patients with vitiligo, and was the most common complaint in both the groups. Suicidal ideation and suicidal attempt were present in 23.3% and 3.3%, respectively in patients with psoriasis and 13.3% and 6.7%, respectively in patients with vitiligo. There was no statistically significant difference between interpersonal conflicts and somatic complaints between patients of vitiligo and psoriasis. No correlation was present between the extent of the skin disfigurement and psychiatric morbidity in patients with vitiligo and psoriasis, suggesting that the extent of skin involvement was not important as a single factor. In another Indian study by Mattoo et al. [24], psychiatric morbidity was present in 33.63% patients with vitiligo and 24.7% patients with psoriasis. Adjustment disorders (56% vs 62%), depressive episodes (22% vs 29%), and dysthymia (9% vs 4%) were seen in patients with vitiligo and psoriasis, respectively. Depression, anxiety, and total psychopathology levels were found to be similar in patients with vitiligo and psoriasis in the study by Mattoo et al. [24].

COMPARISON OF DERMATOLOGY LIFE QUALITY SCORES BETWEEN DIFFERENT NATIONS

Vitiligo is especially disfiguring for people with dark skin due to the strong contrast. The highest scores in DLQI was found in a Turkish study (DLQI 15.00), followed by Saudi Arabia (DLQI 11.86). The mean DLQI in 10 Indian studies was 9.51. The lowest DLQI score was found in Italy with a mean DLQI score of 1.82 [37]. The impact of vitiligo on QoL in India is the same as leprosy, where the affected individuals are considered "not clean." However, a study on Malaysian people reported significantly higher DLQI scores as compared to Indians who are of darker skin type [37]. Portel and Beuf found no significant difference in the degree of disturbance caused by vitiligo amongst the white and black patients [38]. Houman et al. [39] reported negative impact on HRQL in patients with generalized vitiligo in dark-skinned individuals with Fitzpatrick skin type IV−VI. In vitiligo patients of African descent, QoL was found to be moderately impaired, with a mean DLQI score of 7.2 due to sharp contrast of vitiligo patches with the dark skin. In Indian patients [40] with greater than 10% body surface area involvement, the mean DLQI was 10.67, higher than that found in patients with African descent. In contrast to these studies, Porter and Beuf reported no significant association between the race and the overall self-esteem and degree of disturbance caused by vitiligo [38].

COPING STRATEGIES ADOPTED BY THE PATIENT

To cope with the chronic illness, patients develop strategies for regaining equilibrium. Porter et al. [41] reported that around 20% of patients adopted a strategy of "active mastery," where patients learned to accept vitiligo with less embarrassment by learning about it. About 40% of patients had "passive acceptance" of vitiligo. These patients were not overly embarrassed by vitiligo, ignored it, and made no special efforts to hide it. The remaining 40% of patients showed "poor adjustment" to their disease. They made extra efforts to hide their lesions, were chronically embarrassed, depressed, and withdrew from social interactions. The ability to cope with vitiligo is related to self-esteem, as individuals with positive self-image cope better.

Lowered self-esteem in patients with psoriasis and vitiligo was comparable to those without skin disease, but vitiligo patients were better adjusted to their disease as compared to psoriasis patients, probably due to greater physical discomfort and negative social response in patients with psoriasis. In an attempt to hide their disease, many patients adapted their clothing and used large quantities of cosmetics. Negative response by others led to greater embarrassment for vitiligo patients, leading to poorer adjustment to their disease. Poor adjustment in vitiligo patients was related to discrimination by others and was significantly affected by the perceived stigmatization. Age, race, gender, severity, and visibility had no significant direct effect but had an indirect effect on the adjustment to the disease by its effect on stigmatization and perceived discrimination.

EFFECTIVENESS OF THERAPEUTIC INTERVENTIONS ON QOL IN VITILIGO PATIENTS

In a study where narrowband ultraviolet B (NB-UVB) was given to children with generalized vitiligo, a significant improvement in QoL paralleled the degree of repigmentation. Camouflage improves the "feeling of embarrassment and self-consciousness" and "choice of clothing" in patients with vitiligo, and studies have shown its beneficial effect on DLQI. Studies on either lifestyle-altering (psychological therapy using cognitive group therapy and camouflage) or disease-altering interventions (pharmacological therapy) showed improvement in QoL in vitiligo patients regardless of their effect on repigmentation. This should instill confidence in dermatologists to recommend treatment for vitiligo, as it improves the QoL even if complete repigmentation is not achieved.

APPROACH TO A PATIENT WITH VITILIGO

Vitiligo patients need reassurance and information as they experience anxiety due to the spreading lesions and are worried because they appear different from others. Mishra et al. [9] reported that higher education in vitiligo patients decreases the burden of the disease on QoL of those effected and leads to rational thinking about vitiligo in these patients. However, Dolatshahi et al. found that DLQI score and level of education were unrelated [5]. Studies have reported shortcomings in the interaction of patients with physicians, as 45%

of patients felt that their queries were inadequately answered by the doctor and around 50% felt they were inadequately informed about the cause, course, and treatment of vitiligo. The patients perceived their physicians to be unconcerned and insensitive. The patients who were embarrassed by vitiligo received limited emotional support from their physicians and wished they were assured of the physician's interest, suggesting the significance of supportive physician-patient interaction. Dermatologists in the Netherlands considered "giving information and reassurance regarding the nature of the disease" as the most important aim in the treatment of vitiligo. Providing supportive measures and counseling the patients regarding the cause and the natural course of the disease form essential components of good treatment. Counseling improves body image, QoL, and self-esteem of vitiligo patients and influences their ability to cope and live with the disease and its consequences. The benefit of counseling was found to be sustained at 5 months of follow-up. Psychosocial and psychiatric comorbidity seen in vitiligo patients can be treated with psychotropic agents and psychotherapeutic interventions which target the perceived stigma or self-esteem on the level of disability caused by vitiligo. Parsad et al. [42] found an inverse correlation between the DLQI scores and response to treatment, suggesting the role of an additional psychological approach.

Significance of treatment in vitiligo is underestimated. In studies, around 60%–80% of patients had never been treated for vitiligo, 72% of patients were not currently on any treatment at the time of survey, and many were told that there was no treatment [43]. Dermatologists in the Netherlands and Belgium were reluctant to treat vitiligo due to the poor treatment outcome, whereas around 60% of patients treated for vitiligo found the treatment to be partially effective and worthwhile. The new emerging therapies and evidence-based guidelines should help to change the outlook of the physicians toward the disease. Even incomplete response to treatment can help to reduce the psychological burden of the disease. Vitiligo patients should be treated promptly irrespective of the localization and size of lesion(s).

MEASURES TO IMPROVE THE QOL IN VITILIGO PATIENTS

In addition to dermatological evaluation, management should include psychological (psychiatric comorbidity and psychological aspects) and social (occupational and social effects) evaluation. Psychosocial evaluation is a good predictor of the psychiatric comorbidity and can be done by a standardized questionnaire or by asking the patient how vitiligo is affecting their daily life. Evaluation of psychosocial aspects should include the attitudes of the patient's intimates, social support network, and work. The location of vitiligo lesions is important, as even mild disease located on emotionally charged body sites such as the face, head, and neck areas may be debilitating. Online groups and support communities for vitiligo can improve the QoL by providing support, educational resources, and advice.

CONCLUSION

Vitiligo has a definite effect on the QoL of the affected patient. This varies according to site affected, Fitzpatrick skin types, and sex of the patient. Psychological counseling as well as proper information about the nature and course of disease will play an important role in improving the QoL of the patient along with medical and surgical treatment.

REFERENCES

1. WHOQOL Group. *Measuring Quality of Life: The Development of the World Health Organization Quality of Life Instrument (WHOQOL).* Geneva: WHO, 1993.

2. Mitrevska NT, Eleftheriadou V, and Guarneri F. Quality of life in vitiligo patients. *Dermatol Ther* 2012;25:S28–31.

3. Senol A, Yucelten AD, and Ay P. Development of a quality of life scale for vitiligo. *Dermatology* 2013;226:185–90.

4. Amer AA, and Gao XH. Quality of life in patients with vitiligo: An analysis of the dermatology life quality index outcome over the past two decades. *Int J Dermatol* 2016;55(6):608–14.

5. Dolatshahi M, Ghazi P, Feizy V, and Hemami MR. Life quality assessment among patients with vitiligo: Comparison of married and single patients in Iran. *Indian J Dermatol Venereol Leprol* 2008;74:700.

6. Ongenae K, van Geel N, De Schepper S, and Naeyaert JM. Effect of vitiligo on self-reported health-related quality of life. *Br J Dermatol* 2005;152:1165–72.

7. Schmid-Ott G, Kunsebeck HW, Jecht E et al. Stigmatization experience, coping and sense of coherence in vitiligo patients. *J Eur Acad Dermatol Venereol* 2007;21:456–61.

8. Homan MWL, Spuls PI, Korte J, Bos JD, Sprangers MA, and Veen W. The burden of vitiligo: Patient characteristics associated with quality of life. *J Am Acad Dermatol* 2009;61:411–20.

9. Mishra N, Rastogi MK, Gahalaut P, and Agrawal S. Dermatology specific quality of life in vitiligo patients and its relation with various variables: A hospital based cross-sectional study. *J Clin Diagn Res* 2014;8(6):YC01–3.

10. Parsad D, Pandhi R, Dogra S, Kanwar AJ, and Kumar B. Dermatology life quality index score in vitiligo and its impact on the treatment outcome. *Br J Dermatol* 2003;148:363–84.

11. Kent G, and Al'Abadie M. Psychologic effects of vitiligo: A critical incident analysis. *J Am Acad Dermatol* 1996;35:895–8.

12. Kent G, and Al'Abadie M. Factors affecting responses on dermatology life quality index items among vitiligo sufferers. *Clin Exp Dermatol* 1996;21:330–3.

13. Sampogna F, Raskovic D, Guerra L, Pedicelli C, Tabolli S, Leoni L, Alessandroni L, and Abeni D. Identification of categories at risk for high quality of life impairment in patients with vitiligo. *Br J Dermatol* 2008;159:351–9.

14. Zghal A, Zeglaoui F, Kallel L et al. Quality of life in dermatology: Tunisian version of the Skindex-29 [French]. *Tunis Med* 2003;81:34–7.

15. Porter JR, Beuf AH, Lerner AB, and Nordlund JJ. Response to cosmetic disfigurement: Patients with vitiligo. *Cutis* 1987;39:493–4.

16. Porter JR, Beuf AH, Lerner AB, and Nordlund JJ. The effect of vitiligo on sexual relationships. *J Am Acad Dermatol* 1990;22:221–2.

17. Al Robaee AA. Assessment of quality of life in Saudi patients with vitiligo in a medical school in Qassim province, Saudi Arabia. *Saudi Med J* 2007;28:1414–7.

18. Parsad D, Dogra S, and Kanwar AJ. Quality of life in patients with vitiligo. *Health Qual Life Outcomes* 2003;1:58–60.

19. Picardi A, Abeni D, Renzi C, Braga M, Puddu P, and Pasquini P. Increased psychiatric morbidity in female outpatients with skin lesions on visible parts of the body. *Acta Derm Venereol* 2001;81:410–4.

20. Hill-Beuf A, and Porter JDR. Children coping with impaired appearance. Social and psychologic influences. *Gen Hosp Psychiatry* 1984;6:294–300.

21. Picardi A, Abeni D, Melchi CF, Puddu P, and Pasquini P. Psychiatric morbidity in dermatological outpatients: An issue to be recognized. *Br J Dermatol* 2000;143:983–91.

22. Sharma N, Koranne RV, and Singh RK. Psychiatric morbidity in psoriasis and vitiligo: A comparative study. *J Dermatol* 2001;28:419–23.

23. Mattoo SK, Handa S, Kaur I, Gupta N, and Malhotra R. Psychiatric morbidity in vitiligo: Prevalence and correlates in India. *J Eur Acad Dermatol Venereol* 2002;16:573–8.

24. Mattoo SK, Handa S, Kaur I, Gupta N, and Malhotra R. Psychiatric morbidity in vitiligo and psoriasis: A comparative study from India. *J Dermatol* 2001;28:424–32.

25. Cotterill JA, and Cunliffe WJ. Suicide in dermatological patients. *Br J Dermatol* 1997;137:246–50.

26. Papadopoulos L, Bor L, Legg C, and Hawk JLM. Impact of life events on the onset of vitiligo in adults: A preliminary evidence for a psychological dimension in aetiology. *Clin Exp Dermatol* 1998;23:243–8.

27. Picardi A, Pasquini P, Cattaruzza MS et al. Stressful life events, social support, attachment security and alexithymia in vitiligo. A case-control study. *Psychother Psychosom* 2003;72:150–8.

28. Papadopoulos L, Bor R, and Legg C. Coping with the disfiguring effects of vitiligo: A preliminary investigation into the effects of cognitive-behaviour therapy. *Br J Med Psychol* 1999;72:385–96.

29. Finlay AY, and Khan GK. Dermatology Life Quality Index (DLQI): A simple practical measure for routine clinical use. *Clin Exp Dermatol* 1994;19:210–6.

30. Ghajarzadeh M, Ghiasi M, and Kheirkhah S. Associations between skin diseases and quality of life: A comparison of psoriasis, vitiligo, and alopecia areata. *Acta Med Iran* 2012;50:511–5.

31. Karelson M, Silm H, and Kingo K. Quality of life and emotional state in vitiligo in an Estonian sample: Comparison with psoriasis and healthy controls. *Acta Derm Venereol* 2013;93(4):446–50.

32. Radtke A, Sachafer I, and Gagur E. Willingness-to-pay and life quality in patients with vitiligo. *Br J Dermatol* 2009; 161:134–9.

33. Beikert FC, Langenbruch AK, Radtke MA et al. Willingness to pay and quality of life in patients with atopic dermatitis. *Arch Dermatol Res* 2014;306:279–86.

34. Porter JR, Beuf AH, Lerner A, and Nordlund J. Psychosocial effect of vitiligo: A comparison of vitiligo patients with "normal" control subjects, with psoriasis patients, and with patients with other pigmentary disorders. *J Am Acad Dermatol* 1986;15(2 Pt 1):220–4.

35. Radtke A, Sachafer I, and Gagur E. Willingness-to-pay and life quality in patients with vitiligo. *Br J Dermatol* 2009; 161:134–9.

36. Sharma N, Koranne RV, and Singh RK. Psychiatric morbidity in psoriasis and vitiligo: A comparative study. *J Dermatol* 2001;28:419–23.

37. Chen D, Tuan H, Zhou EY et al. Quality of life of adult vitiligo patients using camouflage: A survey in a Chinese vitiligo community. *PLOS ONE* 2019;14(1):e0210581.

38. Porter JR, and Beuf AH. Racial variation in reaction to physical stigma: A study of degree of disturbance by vitiligo among black and white patients. *J Health Soc Behav* 1991;32(2):192–204.

39. Homan MWL, Spuls PI, Korte J, Bos JD, Sprangers MA, and Veen W. The burden of vitiligo: Patient characteristics associated with quality of life. *J Am Acad Dermatol* 2009;61:411–20.

40. Jayaprakasam A, Darvay A, Osborne G, and McGibbon D. Comparison of assessments of severity and quality of life in cutaneous disease. *Clin Exp Dermatol* 2002;27:306–8.

41. Porter J, Beuf AH, Nordlund JJ, and Lerner AB. Psychological reaction to chronic skin disorders: A study of patients with vitiligo. *Gen Hosp Psychiatry* 1979 Apr;1(1):73–7.

42. Parsad D, Dogra S, and Kanwar AJ. Quality of life in patients with vitiligo. *Health Qual Life Outcomes* 2003;1:58–60.

43. Njoo MD, Bossuyt PM, and Westerhof W. Management of vitiligo. Results of a questionnaire among dermatologists in The Netherlands. *Int J Dermatol* 1999 Nov;38(11):866–72.

TOPICAL TREATMENT FOR VITILIGO

Chapter 21

TOPICAL CORTICOSTEROIDS

Deepika Pandhi and Vandana Kataria

CONTENTS

INTRODUCTION

Vitiligo is an acquired skin disease reported to affect approximately 1% of the population worldwide. It has a variable age of onset, but the peak prevalence is observed in the second and third decade of life [1]. Besides skin, mucosal as well as hair involvement corresponding to substantial loss of melanocytes in the epithelium and hair is observed. Although vitiligo is asymptomatic, treatment is important because the visible cosmetic disfigurement has a devastating effect on patients' psychosocial well-being, with significant impairment in quality of life. Current treatment modalities are directed toward stopping the progression of vitiligo and achieving repigmentation by regaining functional deficiencies in the depigmented skin areas.

Topical corticosteroids are one of the most commonly used topical medicines in dermatology and have been in use for more than 60 years. Early attempts to use corticosteroids failed, as the corticosteroid with a ketone group at the C11 position (cortisone) had to be reduced to the 11-hydroxyl analog (hydrocortisone) to be active, and this process could not occur effectively in the skin. Therefore, it was only in 1952 that Sulzberger and Witten reported success in use of topical corticosteroids (TCS) in dermatology. Subsequently, TCS have been indicated and used for the last four decades for treatment of limited areas of vitiligo [2].

Treatment of vitiligo is chiefly directed at achieving repigmentation, whereas in progressive or unstable vitiligo, arresting the spread of areas of depigmentation is the main target. Therefore, treatment strategies for vitiligo are decided by multiple factors including type of vitiligo, generalized or localized, stable or progressive, as well as the total body surface area involved [3]. To prescribe any TCS it is necessary to consider the etiology and extent of the disease to be treated as well as steroid potency, delivery vehicle, frequency of administration, duration of treatment, and side effects. Broadly, TCS are effective for dermatoses that are characterized by hyperproliferation, inflammation, and immunologic involvement. Vitiligo being an autoimmune disorder, TCS are a logical therapeutic option [3].

VITILIGO ETIOPATHOGENESIS

Among the many etiological hypotheses that have been put forward to explain vitiligo, the most longstanding and popular is that it is an autoimmune disease with an interplay of genetic and immunologic factors that results in autoimmune melanocyte destruction. Sporadic generalized vitiligo is also associated with other autoimmune diseases like pernicious anemia, Addison disease, and systemic lupus erythematosus. Familial generalized vitiligo is also characterized by a broad spectrum of autoimmune diseases, such as thyroiditis, rheumatoid arthritis, psoriasis, adult-onset dependent diabetes mellitus, pernicious anemia, and Addison disease [4]. Recent evidence has emerged for a role for T cell-mediated infiltrate with activated CD4 and CD8 T cells in the margins of inflammatory vitiligo. The presence of several circulating antibodies in the sera of vitiligo patients suggests a role of humoral immunity. Antibody-dependent immunity against melanosome membrane protein-1 (TYRP-1) of melanocytes leads to autoimmune hypopigmentation. Recently, new hypotheses such as disorder of melanocyte survival, melanocyte growth factor deficiency, post-viral infections, and melanocyte-defective adhesion have also been proposed to play some role [4].

MODE OF ACTION AND RATIONALE FOR USE IN VITILIGO

Topical corticosteroids seem to affect all cells involved in inflammation including the epidermal Langerhans cells. The antigen-presenting cells responsible for initiation of nonspecific and acquired immune responses are reduced in numbers and demonstrate decreased cellular receptors. Lymphocytes demonstrate decreased antibody-dependent cellular cytotoxicity and decreased natural killer cell activity. Topical corticosteroids induce lipocortins, which inhibit phospholipase A_2 and subsequent cell surface liberation of platelet-activating factor (PAF) and arachidonic acid as well as associated potent inflammatory mediators [5]. The negative regulation of transcription factors by glucocorticoid receptor has become the paradigm for the inflammatory

Table 21.1   Classification of topical corticosteroids

Class (potency)	Topical corticosteroid
Class I Superpotency	Clobetasol propionate 0.05%, halobetasol propionate 0.05%, desoximetasone 0.25%
Class II High potency	Betamethasone dipropionate 0.05% cream, halcinonide 0.1%
Class III Medium high potency	Fluticasone propionate 0.005% ointment
Class IV Medium potency	Mometasonefuroate 0.1% cream
Class V Medium potency	Betamethasone valerate 0.1% cream, fluocinolone acetonide 0.025% cream
Class VI low potency	Desonide 0.05% cream, fluocinolone acetonide 0.01% cream
Class VII low potency	Hydrocortisone acetate, dexamethasone acetate 0.1%

and immunosuppressive effect of glucocorticoids. This is achieved by reduction in the number of epidermal antigen-presenting Langerhans cells and of lymphocytes, leading to decrease in antibody-dependent cellular toxicity. Further, TCS reduce the synthesis and secretion of IL-1, IL-2, IFN-γ, and TNF, thereby suppressing vitiligo activity. Interestingly, studies have revealed that patients with a positive Koebner phenomenon indicative of active vitiligo respond significantly better to TCS. The anti-inflammatory effects of TCS may be beneficial in the inflammatory phase and is well evidenced at the margin of vitiligo lesions. Conversely, TCS are used in the treatment of hypermelanosis in combination with tretinoin and hydrocortisone. They suppress the biosynthetic and secretory functions of melanocytes and thereby reduce melanin production. If used alone, they may also act as depigmenting agents, and the loss of pigment or delay in pigmentation induced may help the migration of cells from the follicular compartment during repigmentation [6].

Steroid vehicles: Potency of steroids may differ based on the vehicle in which they are formulated. Some vehicles should be used only on certain parts of the body. Ointments should be avoided over hairy areas and intertriginous areas as they may cause maceration and folliculitis. Further, the greasy nature may result in poor patient satisfaction and compliance, while creams with good lubricating qualities and ability to vanish into the skin are cosmetically appealing. However, creams are less potent than ointments of the same medication and often contain preservatives that can cause irritation, stinging, and allergic reactions.

Potency: Vasoconstrictor assay that classifies steroids based on their ability to cause cutaneous vasoconstriction ("blanching effect") in normal, healthy people is the most preferred way of determining topical steroid potency. However, anti-inflammatory potency may vary depending on the frequency of administration, duration of treatment, and site of application [7,8].

Intraepidermal de-esterification is one of the principal mechanisms of metabolism of topical corticosteroids. Biotransformation of topical corticosteroids in the skin, for instance by halogenation, imparts resistance to de-esterification, thereby prolonging the active state of the compound (e.g., clobetasol propionate). As per the currently used potency-based classification system, topical corticosteroids can be divided into seven classes (Table 21.1) [9].

THERAPEUTIC GUIDELINES

Several treatment options are available for vitiligo, but none is universally effective and there is a high potential for relapse. However, as the disease results in visible cosmetic disfigurement and may produce profound adverse psychological effects due to low self-esteem, early treatment is warranted. Among the therapeutic options, TCS are most effective on small, newly depigmented lesions. Moderately potent topical corticosteroids can be used on the face, while ultrapotent and potent steroids are usually reserved for the body lesions. The topical steroid can be applied daily for a period of months and

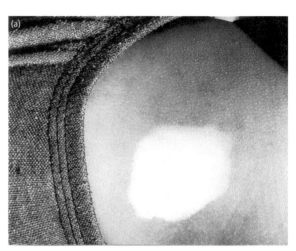

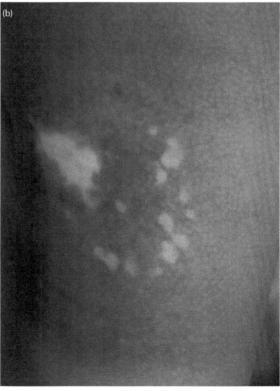

Figure 21.1   (a) Single depigmented macule over the left thigh of an 8-year-old girl. (b) More than 80% repigmentation with betamethasone dipropionate 0.05% cream at 3 months in the lesion in (a).

then tapered depending on the response. They have been shown to be effective in only 57% of adult patients and 64% of childhood vitiligo patients (Figures 21.1 and 21.2) [10]. A meta-analysis by Njoo et al. concluded that potent and superpotent TCS are effective treatment for localized vitiligo [11]. Optimum administration of TCS involves choosing a TCS preparation, estimating the necessary amount,

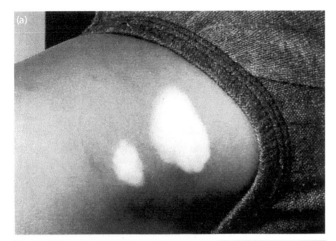

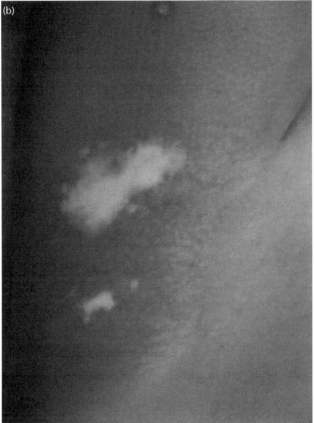

Figure 21.2 (a) Two localized depigmented macules over the right thigh of an 8-year-old girl. (b) More than 50% repigmentation with beta-methasone dipropionate 0.05% cream at 3 months in the lesion in (a).

and then supervising the therapy [5]. The decision to choose a TCS depends on (i) TCS potency, (ii) vehicle choice, (ii) brand name versus generic products, (iv) price and cost effectiveness considerations, and (v) proper amount to dispense. Desired potency is decided based on the patient's age, type, severity, extent, location, and duration of the vitiligo. Steroid-induced repigmentation occurs within 1–4 months of treatment in a perifollicular pattern or from the margins of the lesions [4]. The most important factors in selecting an appropriate vehicle for the steroid are the required site of application, the potential for irritation, and past allergic reaction to any of constituent vehicle. Unfortunately, there is no comparative potency labeling to ensure efficacy between generic and brand name products. Usually, increasing concentration of TCS in a product correlates with increasing cost, but may not necessarily result in increased efficacy [5]. If a prolonged treatment duration is required, TCS should

be gradually tapered to avoid rebound, and treatment should be resumed after ensuring a minimum of a 1-week steroid-free period.

A study conducted by Singh et al. [3]. observed reservoir effect of topical steroids in vitiliginous skin and showed that a significant amount of a reservoir of clobetasol propionate and fluticasone propionate persisted for at least 5 days in vitiliginous skin after a single application. The reservoir effect may be present for up to 7 days in case of clobetasol propionate, and for up to 6 days for fluticasone propionate on the basis of wheal suppression maintained for up to 7 and 6 days, respectively. The presence of a cutaneous reservoir of topical corticosteroids is an important factor that influences dosing frequency. As a result of the reservoir effect, it may be possible to reduce the frequency of application without compromising the efficacy and thus minimizing the local and systemic side effects, cost of treatment, and improving patient compliance.

STUDIES (LEVEL OF EVIDENCE)

Vitiligo is a steroid-responsive autoimmune disorder with a chronic course and usually requires long-term application of steroids [3]. Complete repigmentation of all the patches of vitiligo is seldom achieved, and approximately 15%–30% of patients have a failure to any form of treatment. Therefore most studies consider repigmentation of more than 75% as marked improvement [12]. However, comparison of different modalities in the treatment of vitiligo is hampered by the lack of standardized scoring system for vitiligo, and the Vitiligo Area Scoring Index (VASI) was not employed in most of the earlier trials. Another confounding factor could be the occurrence of spontaneous repigmentation in 10%–20% of patients with vitiligo. This repigmentation is usually partial and is most evident in children over the photo-exposed areas

In 1977, Bleehen conducted a placebo-controlled study of 20 patients with vitiligo, treated with either 0.1% betamethasone valerate or with 0.05% clobetasol propionate creams and similar control areas with placebo preparations and concluded that both topical corticosteroids can induce repigmentation of the skin and could be used for the treatment of selected patients with vitiligo [13].

Meta-analyses have shown medium potency TCS to have a success rate of approximately 55% in vitiligo [5]. Marked repigmentation can be achieved with potent TCS; however, TCS of low potency have not shown any tangible therapeutic effects. In a meta-analysis of non-surgical modalities of treatment in vitiligo, data from three randomized control trials (RCT) [13–15] on potent and two RCT on very potent corticosteroids [13,16] demonstrated 75% repigmentation in one-third of the patients treated with potent corticosteroids, while surprisingly no significant difference was found between very potent corticosteroids and placebo.

In 2008, Sassi et al. compared topical hydrocortisone 17-butyrate in combination with laser versus laser used as a monotherapy. A statistically significant difference in favor of the combination treatment was observed. Participants on combination therapy were more than twice as likely to achieve 75% repigmentation than those receiving laser treatment alone [17]. Combination treatment of hydrocortisone 17-butyrate with 308 excimer laser has also been documented to be synergistic in the same study.

In a study in patients with segmental vitiligo, the effect of 0.05% fluticasone propionate cream 0.1% once daily with 0.1% tacrolimus ointment twice daily for 6 months was evaluated; only one participant in the fluticasone group achieved greater than 75% repigmentation compared to none in the tacrolimus group. This suboptimal response to both therapies is not surprising given the usual lack of response to medical therapy in segmental vitiligo [18]. In a controlled randomized trial by Kandil [15], 0.1% betamethasone valerate in 50% isopropyl alcohol was compared to the alcohol base alone in 19 patients with vitiligo. A higher percentage of lesions had complete repigmentation when treated with the active product as compared to placebo. A randomized parallel group study [19] reported excellent response with combination treatment of topical 0.05% clobetasol propionate (or 0.1% triamcinolone acetonide for flexures) with oral zinc sulfate. An equivocal to slightly higher rates of repigmentation with topical corticosteroids has been observed in comparative studies between TCS and topical calcineurin inhibitor (TCI), thereby making TCS as a better choice of treatment compared to TCI [20]. Sanclemente et al. [21]. compared the effect of topical 0.05% betamethasone valerate to catalase/dismutase superoxide (C/DSO) in a randomized, matched-paired, double-blind trial with 25 patients and concluded that vitiligo repigmentation with topical C/DSO at 10 months is similar to repigmentation with topical 0.05% betamethasone valerate. A single-blinded pilot study compared the efficacy and safety of 0.1% tacrolimus ointment with 0.1% mometasone furoate cream in adult patients with symmetrical, non-acral vitiligo, and the patients on each side were randomized to receive either 0.1% tacrolimus ointment or 0.1% mometasone furoate cream, applied twice daily for 6 months. Repigmentation outcome at 6 months was compared with baseline. Of 18 cases, 22% and 33% in tacrolimus and mometasone groups, respectively, displayed more than 50% repigmentation. Telangiectasias were noticed in one-third of cases on the mometasone-treated side. Both treatments were effective in vitiligo; however, 0.1% tacrolimus ointment had fewer adverse effects.

In children, the use of the high potency steroid clobetasol dipropionate for 6 months was found to induce better repigmentation than PUVAsol alone, with more than 50% repigmentation evident in 68% as compared to 12% for PUVAsol [22]. In another trial, the efficacy of topical fluticasone propionate alone or in combination with UVA was evaluated in 135 adults over 9 months. It was demonstrated that fluticasone alone induced mean repigmentation of only 9% as compared to UVA alone in 8%. Remarkably, the fluticasone–UVA combination resulted in mean repigmentation of 31% [23]. A study by Lepe et al. compared (left-right) 0.05% clobetasol propionate with 0.1% tacrolimus for the treatment of vitiligo in children and showed a repigmentation rate of 49.3% for clobetasol and 41.3% for tacrolimus [21]. A synergistic effect of TCS with UVB and calcipotriol has been observed clinically but not proven through randomized trials [24]. However, combination therapy of TCS and calcipotriol could produce a significantly more rapid and stable repigmentation associated with minimization of side effects.

The repigmentation in vitiligo occurs in the following patterns: marginal, perifollicular, diffuse, and combinations of these. A study evaluating the repigmentation patterns in 352 vitiligo lesions reported that perifollicular repigmentation was the most prevalent, and marginal pattern the most stable pattern (93.3%), followed by perifollicular (91.7%) and combination type (84.4%), whereas the diffuse pattern of repigmentation was the least stable (78.5%). PUVA predominantly achieved a perifollicular or a marginal pattern. TCS demonstrated a diffuse type and also showed a faster repigmentation speed. Therefore, corticosteroids may induce faster but less stable repigmentation in comparison with PUVA. It was also suggested that combination therapies may be more effective than monotherapy, as they achieve a variety of repigmentation patterns [25]. The evidence available in favor of using TCS in vitiligo is tabulated in Table 21.2.

GENERAL GUIDELINES FOR APPLICATION OF TOPICAL CORTICOSTEROIDS

The efficacy of topical steroids in achieving repigmentation of vitiliginous skin is not uniform, and often the treatment period is prolonged by the time repigmentation occurs. Patients have to be counseled that more frequent application of TCS does not provide better results [26]. Usually once- or twice-daily application is recommended for most preparations. Interestingly, usage of intermittent topical clobetasol propionate resulted in 90%–100% repigmentation in more than 80% of patients with vitiligo over the face and in more than 40% with lesions elsewhere over the body. It should be remembered that chronic application of topical steroids can induce tolerance and tachyphylaxis. Therefore, ultra-high-potency steroids should not be applied for more than 3 weeks continuously [26]. In cases where a longer duration of treatment is needed, gradual tapering is required to avoid rebound symptoms, with a steroid-free period of at least 1 week before resuming the treatment. The standardized technique devised by Long and Finley [27] that uses the "fingertip unit" (FTU) has been recommended to measure the amount of ointment necessary for a specific anatomic area. An FTU is defined as the amount that can be squeezed from the fingertip to the first crease of the finger with a 5 mm diameter nozzle. Using a standard nozzle tube, one FTU equals 0.5 g cream/ointment [28].

Optimal duration of TCS for vitiligo, as well as the use of continuous versus discontinuous regimens, are not established [29]. However, if no repigmentation is evident after 3 months of treatment, the therapy should be discontinued [4]. The amount of TCS should be monitored, with accounting for number of tubes utilized per month being considered as the most practical method for quantification akin to atopic dermatitis [6]. The recommendation would be to start the treatment with potent TCS at first, and if no results are observed after 3 months of treatment, switch to super-potent TCS if no adverse effects have been noted, or stop the medication.

ADVERSE EFFECTS

As discussed earlier, vitiligo requires prolonged use of these agents, often much longer than the usual recommended periods of use for inflammatory dermatoses. This leads to an increased incidence of local and systemic adverse effects. Further occlusion that increases penetration of topical corticosteroids and leads to higher frequency of side effects should be avoided.

- *Local:* Topical corticosteroids are widely misused by patients due to their ease of application. Localized side effects include dermal atrophy, striae, telangiectasias, purpura, acneiform eruptions, hypertrichosis, hypopigmentation, localized infections, and tachyphylaxis.
- *Systemic:* Prolonged application of steroids causes systemic absorption significant enough to cause systemic side effects. Although rare, hypothalamic-pituitary-adrenal suppression, glaucoma, hyperglycemia, hypertension, and other systemic side effects have been reported [30].

Moderate- to high-potency topical corticosteroids are efficacious in children with vitiligo but may be associated with systemic absorption. Abnormal cortisol levels and steroid-induced adrenal suppression have been reported, especially in children treated with medium- to high-potency topical steroids with head- and/or

Table 21.2 Studies evaluating topical steroids in vitiligo

Name and year of study	Type of study	Drugs used	Comment
Kandil 1974 [15]	Randomized control trial	0.1% betamethasone valerate in 50% isopropyl alcohol vs alcohol base	More lesions showed complete repigmentation with active product
Clayton 1977 [16]	Randomized control trial	0.05% clobetasol proprionate in a cream base vs cream base alone	Active product was significantly better than base alone
Khalid et al. 1995 [22]	Randomized parallel group study	PUVAsol vs clobetasol propionate (0.05%) b.d.	Clobetasol showed favorable response
Westerhof et al. 1999 [23]	Randomized, parallel group, left/right comparison study	Fluticasone propionate 0.5% alone on one side of body and FP + UVA on other vs UVA alone on one side and FP+UVA on the other side	Combination treatment with fluticasone propionate and UV-A is much more effective
Lepe et al. 2003 [21]	Randomized control trial	0.1% tacrolimus versus 0.05% clobetasol	Tacrolimus and clobetasol propionate, both were equally effective
Agarwal et al. 2005 [35]	Randomized, placebo-controlled, double-blind, parallel study	Levamisole (150 mg adults and 100 mg children) on 2 consecutive days in a week plus mometasone 0.1% o.d. vs oral placebo plus mometasone o.d.	Levamisole was not much effective. Cessation of spread of disease was similar in both groups
Kumaran et al. 2006 [24]	Randomized trial	Betamethasone dipropionate (0.05%) vs calcipotriol (0.005%) b.d. vs betamethasone dipropionate (0.05%) morning and calcipotriol (0.005%) evening	Combined therapy showed faster and stable repigmentation with fewer side effects
Sanclemente et al. 2008 [36]	Randomized, matched-paired, double-blind trial	0.05% betamethasone vs topical catalase/ dismutase superoxide	Both showed good results
Sassi et al. 2008 [17]	Randomized, matched-paired, double-blind trial	308 nm laser phototherapy twice weekly plus hydrocortisone 17-butyrate cream b.d. vs 308 nm laser phototherapy twice weekly alone	Recalcitrant vitiligo of face and neck showed good results with combination of excimer laser phototherapy with topical HC 17-butyrate
Wazir et al. 2010 [37]	Randomized parallel group study	Mometasone 0.01% vs tacrolimus 0.03% mometasone 0.01%	Combination therapy showed good results
Köse et al. 2010 [38]	Randomized parallel group study	0.1% mometasone o.d. vs 1% pimecrolimus b.d.	Mometasone was found to be effective in vitiligo on any part of the body but pimecrolimus was effective on face only
Yaghoobi et al. 2011 [19]	Randomized parallel group study	0.05% Clobetasol propionate for body and 0.1% triamcinolone acetonide for the face and flexures, used twice daily for both groups Oral zinc was added for one group	Combination therapy showed excellent results in vitiligo
Xing and Xu 2012 [39]	Open, uncontrolled trial	Calcipotriol 0.005% vs betamethasone dipropionate 0.05% b.d.	Both were effective
Kathuria et al. 2012 [18]	Randomized parallel group study	0.1% Tacrolimus b.d. vs 0.05% fluticasone propionate o.d.	Both produced variable results in segmental vitiligo
Akdeniz et al. 2014 [40]	Randomized parallel group study	Calcipotriol, NB-UVB, and betamethasone vs NB-UVB and calcipotriol vs NB-UVB	Group receiving calcipotriol, NB-UVB, and betamethasone showed excellent results

neck-affected areas compared with children with other body areas affected [31]. According to the existing literature, over the past 35 years more than 40 cases of iatrogenic Cushing syndrome have been documented; the majority were in children and few were in adults. Infancy was the most commonly affected age group (86%), and the major primary dermatoses were diaper dermatitis followed by psoriasis, burn, non-bullous ichthyosiform erythroderma, and skin xerosis. The median duration of application was 2.75 months in children and 18 months in adults, and the mean recovery period of HPA axis suppression recorded was 3.49 ± 2.92 months and 3.84 ± 2.51 months in children and adults, respectively [2].

Most of the adverse reactions may be reversible to some extent upon discontinuation, with the exception of persistent atrophic striae [30]. The risk of adverse events is high when topical corticosteroids are applied on areas with high absorption potential such as genitals, eyelids, skin folds, armpits, and vulva. Also, there is lack of evidence regarding the safety profile of newer lipophilic TCS (mometasone furoate, fluticasone propionate, and methylprednisolone aceponate) with a good therapeutic index [32].

The usage of novel delivery systems may increase the efficacy and improve the safety profile of TCS. To illustrate this, improvement in skin penetration ability of hydrocortisone and dexamethasone was demonstrated by the suspension of these molecules in elastic vesicles-transferosomes. The latter ensures delivery of the drug into the skin with high efficacy. Increased biological potency, prolonged effect, and reduced therapeutic dosage were obtained [33].

SAFETY CONCERNS

PEDIATRIC POPULATION

Childhood vitiligo has a higher incidence of segmental vitiligo and is less frequently associated with systemic autoimmune and endocrine disorders. However, in this age group a marked psychosocial impact on the quality of life of the affected child and the parents may occur. Therefore, adequate and timely treatment is imperative, and usually medical therapy is preferred in this age group. Topical therapy is the first choice if the body surface area involvement is less than 20% and the disease is not spreading rapidly. Low to high potency TCS are the first line of treatment because of the ease of usage, the documented efficacy, and the excellent patient compliance. As in adults, moderate success of between 45%–60% has been reported, the best results being obtained in localized, recent-onset vitiligo. Morelli, in a meta-analysis, concluded that potent TCS had the highest odds for success compared to placebo [12].

Long-term steroid usage and potency of steroids used in children is associated with epidermal atrophy, striae, telangiectasia, systemic absorption, glaucoma, tachyphylaxis, and hypothalamus pituitary (HPA) axis suppression. Cushing syndrome and growth retardation are the most worrisome side effects in children and infants.

Topical corticosteroids should be used with caution in children as well as elderly individuals due to a larger surface area-to-body weight ratio and poor skin barrier function in the former and skin fragility in the latter [34]. In children, especially with head and neck lesions of vitiligo, systemic absorption with relevant effects should be considered, and TCIs are preferred at this location [6].

PREGNANCY

When large amounts of TCS are used, birth defects have been reported in animals, but this effect has not been reported so far in humans. They are therefore categorized as Pregnancy Category C and recommended only if the potential benefit justifies the potential risk to the fetus [30]. During lactation, they are to be used with caution.

CONCLUSION

There are many different therapeutic options with varying degrees of nonpermanent repigmentation in vitiligo. Topical treatment with corticosteroids shows only moderate efficacy. Local as well as systemic adverse effects have led investigators to search for newer therapeutic agents such as immunomodulators and vitamin D analogs. However, TCS are still first-line therapy for new-onset localized vitiligo in children and adults, and are often employed as adjunctive treatment with other topical and systemic therapies. A search for TCS molecule or vehicle with a better safety profile will greatly improve the therapeutic index of TCS in vitiligo.

REFERENCES

1. Whitton ME, Ashcroft DM, Barrett CW, and Gonzalez U. Interventions for vitiligo. *Cochrane Database Syst Rev* 2006 Jan 25;(1):CD003263.

2. Dhar S, Seth J, and Parikh D. Systemic side-effects of topical corticosteroids. *Indian J Dermatol* 2014 Sep;59:460–4.

3. Singh S, Nasir F. The reservoir effect of topical steroids in vitiliginous skin: A cross-sectional study. *Indian J Dermatology, Venereol Leprol* 2015;81:370–5.

4. Coleman WP. Pathogenesis of vitiligo. In: Gupta S, Olsson MJ, Kanwar AJ, and Ortonne J-P. (eds), *Surgical Management of Vitiligo*, pp. 3–13. UK: Blackwel publications limited.

5. Wolverton SE. *Comprehensive Dermatology Drug Therapy*, 3rd ed. Elsevier Saunders.

6. Picardo M, and Taieb A. *Vitiligo*. Springer Berlin Heidelberg; 2010.

7. Goa KL. Clinical pharmacology and pharmacokinetic properties of topically applied corticosteroids. A review. *Drugs* [Internet]. 1988 [cited 2017 Jun 17];36 Suppl 5:51–61. Available from: http://www.ncbi.nlm.nih.gov/pubmed/3076132

8. McKenzie AW. Comparison of steroids by vasoconstriction. *Br J Dermatol* [Internet]. 1966 Mar 1 [cited 2017 Jun 17];78(3):182–3. Available from: http://doi.wiley.com/10.1111/j.1365-2133.1966.tb12200.x

9. Ference JD, and Last AR. Choosing topical corticosteroids. *Am Fam Physician*. 2009;79(2):135–40.

10. Cho S, Kang HC, and Hahm JH. Characteristics of vitiligo in Korean Children. *Pediatr Dermatol*. 2000;17(3);189–93.

11. Njoo MD, and Spuls PI BJ. Non surgical repigmentation therapies in vitiligo. Meta-analysis of literature. *Arch Dermatol*. 1998;134:1186–91.

12. Morelli JG. Vitiligo: Is there a treatment that works? *Pediatr Dermatol* [Internet]. 2000 Jan [cited 2017 Jul 6];17(1):75–83. Available from: http://www.ncbi.nlm.nih.gov/pubmed/10721021

13. Bleehen S. The treatment of vitiligo with topical corticosteroids. Light and electron microscopic studies [Internet]. *Br J Dermatol* 1976;94 suppl 1:43–50. Available from: http://onlinelibrary.wiley.com/o/cochrane/clcentral/articles/554/CN-00701554/frame.html

14. Koopmans-van Dorp B, Goedhart-van Dijk B, Neering H, and van Dijk E. Treatment of vitiligo by local application of betamethasone valerate in dimethyl sulfoxide cream base. *Dermatologica* 1973;146:310–4.

15. Kandil E. Treatment of viltiligo with 0.1% betamethasone 17-valerate in isopropyl alcohol—a double blind trial. *Br J Dermatol* 1974;91:457–60.

16. Clayton R. A double blind trial of 0.05% clobetasol propionate in the treatment of vitiligo. *Br J Dermatol.* 1977;96:71–3.

17. Sassi F, Cazzaniga S, Tessari G et al. Randomized controlled trial comparing the effectiveness of 308-nm excimer laser alone or in combination with topical hydrocortisone 17-butyrate cream in the treatment of vitiligo of the face and neck. *Br J Dermatol* [Internet]. 2008 Aug [cited 2017 Jun 11];159(5):1186–91. Available from: http://www.ncbi.nlm.nih.gov/pubmed/18717675

18. Kathuria S, Khaitan BK, Ramam M, and Sharma VK. Segmental vitiligo: A randomized controlled trial to evaluate efficacy and safety of 0.1% tacrolimus ointment vs 0.05% fluticasone propionate cream. *Indian J Dermatol Venereol Leprol* [Internet]. 2012 [cited 2017 Jun 11];78(1):68–73. Available from: http://www.ncbi.nlm.nih.gov/pubmed/22199063

19. Yaghoobi R, Omidian M, and Bagherani N. Comparison of therapeutic efficacy of topical corticosteroid and oral zinc sulfate-topical corticosteroid combination in the treatment of vitiligo patients: A clinical trial. *BMC Dermatol* [Internet]. 2011 Dec 31 [cited 2017 Jun 11];11(1):7. Available from: http://www.ncbi.nlm.nih.gov/pubmed/21453467

20. Allam M, and Riad H. Concise review of recent studies in vitiligo. *Quatar Med J* [Internet]. 2013 [cited 2017 Jun 11];13. Available from: https://www.ncbi.nlm.nih.gov/pmc/articles/PMC4080492/pdf/qmj-2013-010.pdf

21. Lepe V, Moncada B, Castanedo-Cazares JP, Torres-Alvarez MB, Ortiz CA, and Torres-Rubalcava AB. A double-blind randomized trial of 0.1% tacrolimus vs 0.05% clobetasol for the treatment of childhood vitiligo. *Arch Dermatol* [Internet]. 2003 May 1 [cited 2017 Jun 20];139(5):581–5. Available from: http://www.ncbi.nlm.nih.gov/pubmed/12756094

22. Khalid M, Mujtaba G, and Haroon T. Comparison of 0.05% clobetasol propionate cream and topical PUVAsol in childhood vitiligo. *Int J Dermatol.* 1995;34:203–5.

23. Westerhof W, Nieuweboer-Krobotova L, Mulder PG, and Glazenburg EJ. Left-right comparison study of the combination of fluticasone propionate and UV-A vs. either fluticasone propionate or UV-A alone for the long-term treatment of vitiligo. *Arch Dermatol* [Internet]. 1999 Sep [cited 2017 Jun 20];135(9):1061–6. Available from: http://www.ncbi.nlm.nih.gov/pubmed/10490110

24. Kumaran MS, Kaur I, and Kumar B. Effect of topical calcipotriol, betamethasone dipropionate and their combination in the treatment of localized vitiligo. *J Eur Acad Dermatology Venereol.* 2006;20(3):269–73.

25. Parsad D, Pandhi R, Dogra S, and Kumar B. Clinical study of repigmentation patterns with different treatment modalities and their correlation with speed and stability of repigmentation in 352 vitiliginous patches. *J Am Acad Dermatol* [Internet]. 2004 Jan [cited 2017 Jul 6];50(1):63–7. Available from: http://www.ncbi.nlm.nih.gov/pubmed/14699367

26. Drake LA, Dinehart SM, Farmer ER et al. Guidelines of care for the use of topical glucocorticosteroids. American Academy of Dermatology. *J Am Acad Dermatol* [Internet]. 1996 Oct [cited 2017 Jun 17];35(4):615–9. Available from: http://www.ncbi.nlm.nih.gov/pubmed/8859293

27. Long CC, and Finlay AY. The finger-tip unit--a new practical measure. *Clin Exp Dermatol* [Internet]. 1991 Nov [cited 2017 Jun 19];16(6):444–7. Available from: http://www.ncbi.nlm.nih.gov/pubmed/1806320

28. Tadicherla S, Ross K, Shenefelt PD, and Fenske NA. Topical corticosteroids in dermatology. *J Drugs Dermatol [Internet].* 2009 Dec [cited 2017 Jun 19];8(12):1093–105. Available from: http://www.ncbi.nlm.nih.gov/pubmed/20027937

29. Gawkrodger DJ, Ormerod A D, Shaw L et al. Guideline for the diagnosis and management of vitiligo. *Br J Dermatol* 2008;159(5):1051–76.

30. Rathi SK, and D'Souza P. Rational and ethical use of topical corticosteroids based on safety and efficacy. *Indian J Dermatol* [Internet]. 2012 Jul [cited 2017 Jun 18];57(4):251–9. Available from: http://www.ncbi.nlm.nih.gov/pubmed/22837556

31. Kwinter J, Pelletier J, Khambalia A et al. High-potency steroid use in children with vitiligo: A retrospective study. *J Am Acad Dermatol* [Internet]. 2007 Feb [cited 2017 May 13];56(2):236–41. Available from: http://linkinghub.elsevier.com/retrieve/pii/S0190962206022584

32. Das A, and Panda S. Use of topical corticosteroids in dermatology: An evidence-based approach. *Indian J Dermatol* [Internet]. 2017 [cited 2017 Jun 20];62(3):237. Available from: http://www.e-ijd.org/article.asp

33. Cevc G, and Blume G. Hydrocortisone and dexamethasone in very deformable drug carriers have increased biological potency, prolonged effect, and reduced therapeutic dosage. *Biochim Biophys Acta Biomembr* [Internet]. 2004 May 27 [cited 2017 Jul 6];1663(1–2):61–73. Available from: http://www.ncbi.nlm.nih.gov/pubmed/15157608

34. Saraswat A. Topical corticosteroid use in children: Adverse effects and how to minimize them. *Indian J Dermatol Venereol Leprol* [Internet]. 2010 [cited 2017 Jun 19];76(3):225–8. Available from: http://www.ncbi.nlm.nih.gov/pubmed/20445290

35. Agarwal S, Ramam M, Sharma VK, Khandpur S, Pal H, and Pandey RM. A randomized placebo-controlled double-blind study of levamisole in the treatment of limited and slowly spreading vitiligo. *Br J Dermatol* [Internet]. 2005 Jul [cited 2017 Jun 20];153(1):163–6. Available from: http://www.ncbi.nlm.nih.gov/pubmed/16029343

36. Sanclemente G, Garcia J, Zuleta J, Diehl C, Correa C, and Falabella R. A double-blind, randomized trial of 0.05% betamethasone vs. topical catalase/dismutase superoxide in vitiligo. *J Eur Acad Dermatology Venereol* [Internet]. 2008 Nov [cited 2017 Jun 20];22(11):1359–64. Available from: http://www.ncbi.nlm.nih.gov/pubmed/18624857

37. Wazir SM, Muhammad Wazir S, Paracha MM, and Khan SU. Efficacy and safety of topical mometasone furoate 0.01% vs. tacrolimus 0.03% and mometasone furoate 0.01%in vitiligo. *J Pakistan Assoc Dermatologists* [Internet]. 2010 [cited 2017 Jun 20];20:89–92. Available from: http://www.jpad.com.pk/index.php/jpad/article/viewFile/427/402

38. Kose O, and Arca E KZ. Mometasone cream versus pimecrolimus cream for the treatment of childhood localized vitiligo. *J Dermatolog Treat* [Internet]. 2010 [cited 2017 Jun 11];21(3):133–9. Available from: https://www.researchgate.net/profile/Osman_Koese/publication/43159034_Mometasone_cream_versus_pimecrolimus_cream_for_the_treatment_of_childhood_vitiligo/links/542a5ae40cf277d58e8716a3/Mometasone-cream-versus-pimecrolimus-cream-for-the-treatment-of-childho

39. Chenjing Xing and Aie Xu; Department of Dermatology AHCCAMUHC. The effect of combined calcipotriol and betamethasone dipropionate ointment in the treatment of vitiligo: An open, uncontrolled trial. *J Drugs Dermatol* [Internet]. 1348 [cited 2017 Jun 20];11(10):e52. Available from: http://jddonline.com/articles/dermatology/S1545961612E0052X

40. Akdeniz N, Yavuz IH, Gunes Bilgili S, Ozaydin Yavuz G, and Calka O. Comparison of efficacy of narrow band UVB therapies with UVB alone, in combination with calcipotriol, and with betamethasone and calcipotriol in vitiligo. *J Dermatolog Treat* [Internet]. 2014 Jun 6 [cited 2017 Jun 20];25(3):196–9. Available from: http://www.ncbi.nlm.nih.gov/pubmed/23441902

Chapter 22

TOPICAL CALCINEURIN INHIBITORS

Iffat Hassan and Safia Bashir

CONTENTS

INTRODUCTION

Vitiligo is a common pigmentary disorder affecting 0.5%–2% of the world population [1]. Despite several treatment options available, the treatment of vitiligo is usually unsatisfactory, and most of the treatments used are long and cumbersome with unpredictable results.

Immune alterations appear to play an important role in the etiopathogenesis of this disease, so immunosuppressants and immunomodulators have increasingly been investigated for the treatment of vitiligo [2]. Calcineurin inhibitors are immunosuppressive drugs that were developed primarily for use in transplantation medicine. Though systemic calcineurin inhibitors have not been used in vitiligo, topical calcineurin inhibitors have shown promise in the treatment of vitiligo because of their immunomodulatory effects without the side effect profile of corticosteroids.

TACROLIMUS

Tacrolimus is a macrolide produced by a soil fungus, *Streptomyces tsukubaensis*. The efficacy of tacrolimus in the treatment of vitiligo was first demonstrated by Grimes et al. in 2002 who used topical tacrolimus in six patients of generalized vitiligo, and five of the patients achieved moderate to excellent results (>50% repigmentation of skin lesions) by the end of the study period [3]. Since then, several studies have demonstrated the efficacy of topical tacrolimus in vitiligo [4–7].

MECHANISM OF ACTION

Tacrolimus exerts its therapeutic effects by inhibition of calcineurin in the skin. Tacrolimus binds to the cytosolic 12 Kd macrophilin FK506 binding protein (FK-BP) forming a complex (tacrolimus/FK-BP complex) which in turn inhibits the calcineurin-mediated phosphorylation of the transcription factor, nuclear factor of activated T-cells (NFAT). This in turn downregulates the proinflammatory cytokines like IL-2, IL-3, IL-4, IL-6, IFN-γ, TNF-α, and granulocyte-stimulating factors.

Tacrolimus may also enhance melanocyte growth by direct stimulation of tyrosinase activity and may also increase cell migration. In addition, tacrolimus provides a favorable environment to foster the proliferation of melanocytes by direct interaction with keratinocytes [8]. Also, TNF-α has been shown to have an inhibitory effect on melanogenesis. It inhibits melanocyte proliferation and also upregulates the expression of intercellular adhesion molecule-1 (ICAM-1) on melanocytes, leading to lymphocyte–melanocyte attachment and destruction of melanocytes. Tacrolimus, by inhibiting TNF-α and other cytokines, promotes melanogenesis [9,10].

It is important to note that the most beneficial effects of tacrolimus are seen in the head and neck region. The ability of topical calcineurin inhibitors to induce repigmentation in photoprotected areas is controversial, as minimal improvement was observed in these areas in most of the studies. The better response on the head and neck regions may be explained by the stimulatory effect of sun exposure on melanogenesis, better penetration of the drug on the face and neck, or due to the greater melanocyte reservoir provided by greater density of hair follicles in these areas.

Although topical corticosteroids may be equally or even more effective than topical calcineurin inhibitors in the treatment of vitiligo, the adverse effects associated with long-time corticosteroid use like skin atrophy, telangiectasia, hypertrichosis, and acne cannot be ignored. Several studies comparing tacrolimus with clobetasol propionate 0.05% in adults as well as children with vitiligo have shown both treatments to be equally effective [3,11,12]. However, the pigmentation induced by tacrolimus is mainly perifollicular, in contrast to topical corticosteroids which result in a diffuse pattern of repigmentation [13]. This points toward the effect of tacrolimus on proliferation of melanoblasts leading to formation of perifollicular pigment islands [14]. Topical tacrolimus may serve as an effective alternative to topical corticosteroids in childhood vitiligo where the apprehension of topical corticosteroid induced adverse effects is more. In a survey of 25 Asian children affected by vitiligo, topical tacrolimus was found to be an effective and well tolerated treatment [15].

Tacrolimus may also be effective in the treatment of segmental vitiligo. In a study involving 30 vitiligo patients, 66.7% of patients with segmental vitiligo responded to topical tacrolimus therapy. The response was even better in patients with segmental vitiligo involving the face, where 80% of the patients responded to the treatment [16].

A twice-daily application of tacrolimus ointment has been found to be superior to once-daily application in the treatment of vitiligo [17,18]. In a randomized controlled study comparing once- with twice-daily application of tacrolimus, a significantly better treatment outcome was observed in patients treated with twice-daily tacrolimus compared to controls, but when compared with once-daily application the difference remained just below the level of statistical significance [17]. No minimal or ideal treatment period has been described, and treatment for several months may be required to produce satisfactory results [17].

A placebo-controlled, prospective study showed that additional occlusion may significantly enhance the therapeutic effect of tacrolimus and shorten the time required for initiation of repigmentation, especially in the extremities and non-photo-exposed areas. Side effects noted were minimal and also there was no significant elevation in tacrolimus blood levels, probably due to use of tacrolimus in limited body parts [19].

Topical tacrolimus may also be effective in preventing relapses in previously treated vitiligo lesions. A twice-weekly application of tacrolimus to previously repigmented lesions may inhibit the low-grade immune reaction against melanocytes thus preventing recurrences. Cavalie et al. in their study showed that the maintenance therapy using 0.1% tacrolimus is effective in preventing the depigmentation of vitiligo patches that have been previously successfully repigmented irrespective of the initial treatment modality used [20].

The synergistic use of topical calcineurin inhibitors with other therapeutic modalities has shown a reasonable increase in efficacy of these drugs [6,21–23]. The therapies usually combined with tacrolimus include narrowband UVB, microphototherapy, helium-neon laser, or narrowband excimer laser. Exposure to UVB radiation induces keratinocytes to secrete endothelin, which is a prodifferentiation factor for melanoblasts. Thus combination of tacrolimus with UVB leads to optimal melanoblast differentiation, leading to better treatment response [24].

Studies combining topical tacrolimus with 308-nm excimer laser have shown even more promising results. In a study combining twice-daily topical tacrolimus with twice-weekly 308-nm xenon chloride excimer laser for the treatment of vitiligo lesions, a synergistic activity of the combination was demonstrated. The combination treatment shows a statistically significant efficacy compared to controls in achieving a repigmentation rate of at least 75%. It was also seen that the combination was superior to laser monotherapy in treating resistant areas [6]. Combination of excimer laser rather than narrowband UVB with tacrolimus offers the advantage of more efficient photobiological effects due to induction of lymphocyte apoptosis and that of selectively targeting vitiliginous lesions with sparing of healthy skin.

PIMECROLIMUS

Pimecrolimus is a macrolide with structure similar to that of tacrolimus. The lipophilicity of pimecrolimus is, however, greater than that of tacrolimus and it binds to macrophilin-12 with high affinity [25]. While tacrolimus is available as an ointment, pimecrolimus has a cream base and thus may be cosmetically more acceptable.

Pimecrolimus acts by a similar mechanism as that of tacrolimus but is less potent due to its lesser protein binding capacity and lesser permeability through skin.

The efficacy of pimecrolimus in the treatment of vitiligo was first reported in 2003 in a female patient with facial vitiliginous lesions who showed >90% repigmentation with the use of 1% pimecrolimus for a period of 5 months [26]. Later, a trial including 10 patients with bilaterally symmetrical vitiliginous lesions showed comparable rate of pigmentation with 1% pimecrolimus and 0.05% clobetasol

propionate. Side effects like atrophy and telangiectasia were seen in the clobetasol group, whereas the side effects in pimecrolimus included only mild burning sensation in two patients [27]. Several studies since then have proved the efficacy of pimecrolimus in the treatment of vitiligo [28–30]. In a study by Seirafi et al., 30 patients with 135 vitiligo lesions involving <20% of the body surface area were treated with 1% pimecrolimus cream for 12 weeks. Among these, 28 patients developed repigmentation in at least one of their vitiligo lesions at the end of 12 weeks [30].

Pimecrolimus, like tacrolimus, has also been used in combination therapies. In a randomized controlled study, pimecrolimus combined with narrowband UVB therapy showed significantly better improvement in facial vitiligo lesions compared to narrowband UVB alone. However, the repigmentation rate of other body parts was not different in the two groups [31]. In another study, microdermabrasion was combined with 1% pimecrolimus cream in the treatment of nonsegmental vitiligo in children. Of lesions treated with the combination, 60.4% showed a positive clinical response and 43.4% of lesions showed complete repigmentation. In patients treated with pimecrolimus alone, 32.1% of lesions showed repigmentation, whereas only 1.7% of lesions responded in the placebo group [32]. The better efficacy of this combination in the treatment of vitiligo may be due to modulation of immune response and autoinoculation of melanocytes as well as improved absorption of pimecrolimus through the erosions and inflammation of skin caused by microdermabrasion.

ADVERSE EFFECTS

Transient local reactions such as burning, irritation, and pruritis are commonly seen. Folliculitis and acneiform eruptions have also been reported with the use of tacrolimus in vitiligo patches [12,33]. There is also a theoretical risk of local skin carcinogenesis (including non-melanoma skin cancers and lymphomas) with the use of topical calcineurin inhibitors, although epidemiological analyses and clinical data have failed to demonstrate any relationship between the use of topical calcineurin inhibitors and development of malignancy [34]. The risk of carcinogenesis may be especially relevant in cases of combination treatments using topical calcineurin inhibitors and phototherapy.

SAFETY

Topical calcineurin inhibitors are safe for short-term or intermittent long-term use. Patients should be encouraged to use sun protective measures, including the use of high SPF broad spectrum sunscreens to the exposed sites while using topical calcineurin inhibitors. The Food and Drug Administration (FDA) recommends the use of 0.1% tacrolimus above the age of 16 years, while 0.03% tacrolimus can be used in children aged 2–15. Pimecrolimus 1% cream can be used in patients 2 years or older. Both topical tacrolimus and pimecrolimus are Pregnancy Category C drugs and thus should be used with caution and only if benefits outweigh the risks.

CONCLUSION

Given the lack of local side effects and a comparable efficacy to topical corticosteroids, topical calcineurin inhibitors may be effective treatment alternatives for both adults and children with vitiligo. Face and neck lesions show the best responses, while the efficacy of treatment in other areas may be improved by occlusion or by combination with other treatment modalities like phototherapy, excimer laser, and microdermabrasion.

REFERENCES

1. Passeron T, and Ortonne JP. Physiopathology and genetics of vitiligo. *J Autoimmun* 2005;25(Suppl.):63–8.

2. Laddha NC, Dwivedi M, Mansuri MS et al. Role of oxidative stress and autoimmunity in onset and progression of vitiligo. *Exp Dermatol* 2014:23: 352–3.

3. Grimes PE, Soriano T, and Dytoc MT. Topical tacrolimus for repigmentation of vitiligo. *J Am Acad Dermatol* 2002 Nov;47(5):789–91.

4. Lepe V, Moncada B, Castanedo-Cazares JP, Torres-Alvarez MB, Ortiz CA, and Torres Rubalcava AB. A double-blind randomized trial of 0.1% tacrolimus vs 0.05% clobetasol for the treatment of childhood vitiligo. *Arch Dermatol* 2003;139:581–5.

5. Kawalek AZ, Spencer JM, and Phelps RG. Combined excimer laser and topical tacrolimus for the treatment of vitiligo: A pilot study. *Dermatol Surg* 2004;30:130–5.

6. Mehrabi D, and Pandya AG. A randomized, placebo-controlled, double-blind trial comparing narrowband UV-B plus 0.1% tacrolimus ointment with narrowband UV-B plus placebo in the treatment of generalized vitiligo. *Arch Dermatol* 2006;142:927–9.

7. Passeron T, Ostovari N, Zakaria W et al. Topical tacrolimus and the 308-nm excimer laser: A Synergistic combination for the treatment of vitiligo. *Arch Dermatol* 2004;140(9):1065–9

8. Lan CC, Chen GS, Chiou MH, Wu CS, Chang CH, and Yu HS. FK506 promotes melanocyte and melanoblast growth and creates a favourable milieu for cell migration via keratinocytes: Possible mechanisms of how tacrolimus ointment induces repigmentation in patients with vitiligo. *Br J Dermatol* 2005;153:498–505

9. Swope VB, Abdel-Malek Z, Kassem LM, and Nordlund JJ. Interleukins 1a and 6 and tumor necrosis factor-a are paracrine inhibitors of human melanocyte proliferation and melanogenesis. *J Invest Dermatol* 1991;96:180–5.

10. Yohn JJ, Critelli M, Lyons MB, and Norris DA. Modulation of melanocyte intercellular adhesion molecule-1 by immune cytokines. *J Invest Dermatol* 1990;90:233–7.

11. Vijayalakshmi P, Rao N, and Priseela T. A comparative study of clobetasol propionate (0.05%) cream and tacrolimus (0.1%) ointment in the management of vitiligo. *J Evid Based Healthc* 2015;2:724–8

12. Ho N, Pope E, Weinstein M, Greenberg S, Webster C, and Krafchik BR. A double-blind, randomized, placebo controlled trial of topical tacrolimus 0·1% vs. clobetasol propionate 0·05% in childhood vitiligo. *Br J Dermatol* 2011;165:626–32.

13. Imokawa G, Miyagishi M, and Yada Y. Endothelin-1 as a new melanogen: Coordinated expression of its gene and the tyrosinase gene in UVB-exposed human epidermis. *J Invest Dermatol* 1995;105:32–7.

14. Kang HY, and Choi YM. FK506 increases pigmentation and migration of human melanocytes. *Br J Dermatol* 2006;155(5):1037–40.

15. Kanwar AJ, Dogra S, and Parsad D. Topical tacrolimus for treatment of childhood vitiligo in Asians. *Clin Exp Dermatol* 2004;29:589–92.

16. Xu AE, Zhang DM, Wei XD, Huang B, and Lu LJ. Efficacy and safety of tacrolimus cream 0.1% in the treatment of vitiligo. *Int J Dermatol* 2009;48:86–90

17. Radakovic S, Breier-Maly J, Konschitzky R et al. Response of vitiligo to once- vs. twice-daily topical tacrolimus:a controlled prospective, randomized, observer-blinded trial. *J Eur Acad Dermatol Venereol* 2009:23:951–953

18. Stinco G, Piccirillo F, Forcione M, Valent F, and Patrone P. An open randomized study to compare narrow band UVB, topical pimecrolimus and topical tacrolimus in the treatment of vitiligo. *Eur J Dermatol* 2009;19:588–593

19. Hartmann A, Bröcker EB, and Hamm H. Occlusive treatment enhances efficacy of tacrolimus 0.1% ointment in adult patients with vitiligo: Results of a placebo controlled 12-month prospective study. *Acta Derm Venereol* 2008;88:474–79.

20. Cavalie M, Ezzedine K, Fontas E et al. Maintenance therapy of adult vitiligo with 0.1% tacrolimus ointment: A randomized, double blind, placebo-controlled study. *J Invest Dermatol* 2015;135:970–4.

21. Lotti T, Buggiani G, Troiano M et al. Targeted and combination treatments for vitiligo. Comparative evaluation of different current modalities in 458 subjects. *Dermatol Ther* 2008;21 (Suppl 1):S20–6.

22. Fai D, Cassano N, and Vena GA. Narrow-band UVB phototherapy combined with tacrolimus ointment in vitiligo: Review of 110 patients. *J Eur Acad Dermatol Venereol* 2007;21(7):916–20.

23. Majid, I. Does topical tacrolimus ointment enhance the efficacy of narrowband ultraviolet B therapy in vitiligo? A left–right comparison study. *Photodermatol Photoimmunol Photomed.* 2010; 26: 230–4.

24. Imokawa G, Miyagishi M, and Yada Y. Endothelin-1 as a new melanogen: Coordinated expression of its gene and the tyrosinase gene in UVB-exposed human epidermis. *J Invest Dermatol* 1995;105:32–7.

25. Billich A, Aschauer H, Aszódi A, and Stuetz A. Percutaneous absorption of drugs used in atopic eczema: Pimecrolimus permeates less through skin than corticosteroids and tacrolimus. *Int J Pharm* 2004;269:29–35.

26. Mayoral FA, Gonzalez C, Shah NS, and Arciniegas C. Repigmentation of vitiligo with pimecrolimus cream: A case report. *Dermatology* 2003;207(3):322–3.

27. Coskun B, Saral Y, and Turgut D. Topical 0.05% clobetosol propionate versus 1% pimecrolimus ointment in vitiligo. *Eur J Dermatol* 2005;15(2):88–91.

28. Mayoral FA, Vega JM, Stavisky H, McCormick CL, and Parneix-Spake A. Retrospective analysis of pimecrolimus cream 1% for treatment of facial vitiligo. *J Drugs Dermatol* 2007;6(5):517–21.

29. Boone B, Ongenae K, Van Geel N, Vernijns S, Keyser S, and Naeyaert JM. Topical pimecrolimus in the treatment of vitiligo. *Eur J Dermatol* 2006;17(1):1–7.

30. Seirafi H, Farnaghi F, Firooz A, Farahani AV, Alirezaie NS, and Dowlati Y. Pimecrolimus cream in repigmentation of vitiligo. *Dermatology* 2007;214:253–9.

31. Esfandiarpour I, Ekhlasi A, Farajzadeh S, and Shamsadini S. The efficacy of pimecrolimus 1% cream plus narrow-band ultraviolet B in the treatment of vitiligo: A double-blind,

placebo-controlled clinical trial. *J Dermatolog Treat* 2009;20(1):14–18.

32. Farajzadeh S, Daraei Z, Esfandiarpour I, and Hosseini SH. The efficacy of pimecrolimus 1% cream combined with microdermabrasion in the treatment of nonsegmental childhood vitiligo: A randomized placebo-controlled study. *Pediatr Dermatol* 2009;26(3):286–91.

33. Baldo A, Lodi G, Di Caterino P, and Monfrecola G. Vitiligo, NB-UVB and tacrolimus: Our experience in Naples. *G Ital Dermatol Venereol* 2014;149:123–30.

34. Siegfried EC, Jaworski JC, and Hebert AA. Topical calcineurin inhibitors and lymphoma risk: Evidence update with implications for daily practice. *Am J Clin Dermatol* 2013;14:163–178.

Chapter 23

TOPICAL VITAMIN D ANALOGS

Mualla Polat and Özge Uzun

CONTENTS

INTRODUCTION

Vitiligo is a commonly acquired idiopathic, depigmenting disease characterized by the loss of normal melanin pigments in the skin. The etiology of this disorder is unknown; however, vitiligo is frequently associated with autoimmune diseases, and patients also have an increased incidence of various autoantibodies in sera, including antibodies reacting to melanocytes in the skin [1].

Today we know that the human epidermis is a natural source of vitamin D and is the main regulator of skin physiology. Vitamin D is a fat-soluble vitamin that is produced endogenously via skin exposure to ultraviolet (UV) light and exogenously through dietary intake. Two forms of dietary vitamin D are available: vitamin D_2 (ergocalciferol) and vitamin D_3 (cholecalciferol) [2]. Humans can synthesize vitamin D_3 when 7-dehydrocholesterol that is present in epidermal keratinocytes interacts with UV light. 7-Dehydrocholesterol absorbs light at wavelengths in the range of 270–300 nm; however, optimal vitamin D_3 synthesis occurs at wavelengths of 295–300 nm [3]. In addition, if whole-body exposure to UVB radiation occurs for 15–20 minutes (~1 minimal erythemal dose) it can produce up to 10,000 IU (250 μg) of vitamin D. Vitamin D-binding protein binds vitamin D molecules and transports them from skin to circulation. In the liver, vitamin D is metabolized into calcifediol, and then in the kidney into calcitriol, and it can be stored in the body as fat to later be released into circulation [4]. The molecular mechanism of vitamin D is dependent on receptor activation. This receptor is a 427-amino acid peptide that belongs to the superfamily of steroid/thyroid nuclear receptor. Vitamin D and its synthetic analogs coordinate the function of various cells mainly by acting at their transcriptional machinery. The machinery consists of genomic and non-genomic controls in the target cells [5]. Vitamin D is a very important tool for dermatologists because of the synthesis in the skin and its role in skin disease. In addition, it is understood that vitamin D insufficiency or receptor deficiency can lead to dermatological or autoimmune diseases such as psoriasis, atopic dermatitis, acne, rosacea, skin cancers, and vitiligo. Therefore, clinical application of vitamin D and its analogs is useful in dermatological diseases.

Recent data show that there is a relationship between vitamin D and vitiligo pathogenesis. The presence of cytotoxic T cells, which target melanocyte antigens and create an imbalance in the cytokine network, are described as the characteristics of the disease. Vitamin D ligands are designed to target the local immune response in vitiligo, therefore acting on specific T cell activation, mainly by inhibiting the transition of T cells from early to late G1 phase [5]. Moreover, it is known that the proinflammatory and proapoptotic cytokines such as IL-6, IL-8, TNF-α, and TNF-γ are inhibited by vitamin D analogs [2,6]. In addition, vitamin D_3 is known to affect melanocyte maturation, differentiation, and also to upregulate melanogenesis through pathways that are activated by specific ligand receptors, such as endothelin receptor and c-kit [5]. Another interesting finding is that the Apa-I polymorphism of the vitamin D receptor (VDR) gene is associated with vitiligo [7]. All this emphasizes the important role of vitamin D and its receptor in the etiopathogenesis of skin pigmentation. Moreover, several studies have shown that vitamin D levels were found to be insufficient in most patients who had vitiligo [8,9].

Generally, steroids are the first line of therapy for vitiligo. However, apart from topical treatment with steroids, in most cases a combination of psoralen-UVA therapy (PUVA) and a vitamin D analog is used and is highly effective [10]. Finally, calcitriol and tacalcitol have been used as topical therapeutic agents in vitiligo, which is an autoimmune pigmentary disorder characterized by aberrant loss of functional melanocytes from the affected epidermis [5].

HISTORICAL BACKGROUND

The first clinical observation of topical vitamin D analogs affecting the human skin were noticed in patients who had psoriasis and were receiving calcitriol treatment [11]. Physicians subsequently began investigation of the topical effect of vitamin D analogs in vitiligo. The two low-calcemic synthetic analogs (calcitriol and tacalcitol) were the main focus in the treatment of vitiligo as a monotherapy.

THE ACTION MECHANISMS OF VITAMIN D ANALOGS IN VITILIGO TREATMENT

At the molecular level, vitamin D and its synthetic analogs via VDR have both genomic and non-genomic effects. It can either regulate expression of the vitamin D-responsive gene positively or negatively by binding to the vitamin D-responsive elements (VDREs) [5]. However, vitamin D may inhibit the expression of some genes such as nuclear factor of activated T cells (NF-AT) and nuclear factor kappa B (NF-κB). Those genes are the ones whose expression is induced by VDR, and they have important roles in inflammation, proliferation, differentiation, and adhesion function in the skin. Thus vitamin D acts as a coordinator of the skin cell functions that target keratinocyte, melanocyte, fibroblast, and macrophage and T cells [5]. On the other hand, vitamin D exerts a non-genomic effect due to activating several signal transduction pathways via binding to a second class of receptor residing in the plasma membrane or its caveolae component [12].

CALCIUM HOMEOSTASIS

Defective calcium (Ca^{2+}) transport has been shown in vitiliginous keratinocytes and melanocytes [13]. Furthermore, a decrease in intracellular Ca^{2+} inhibits tyrosine activity and results in the lowering of melanin synthesis and of melanocyte-expressing VDRs which take part in the regulation of melanin synthesis [6]. It is likely that calcitriol helps to regulate Ca^{2+} by 1,25-dihydroxyvitamin D_3 receptors in melanocytes and/or by regulating the defective Ca^{2+} homeostasis [14].

MELANOGENESIS

Vitamin D protects the epidermal melanin unit and restores melanocyte integrity via two main mechanisms: first by controlling the activation, proliferation, and migration of melanocytes and pigmentation pathway, and also by modulating T-cell activation, which apparently correlates with melanocyte disappearance in vitiligo. The coordination in T cell activation is exerted mainly by the ability of vitamin D to inhibit the T cell transition from the early to the late G1 phase, and by inhibiting several cytokine genes, such as those encoding TNF-α and IFN-γ [5]. Vitamin D is also believed to be involved in melanocyte physiology, since it can coordinate melanogenic cytokines and the activity of the SCF/c-Kit system, which is one of the most important regulators in melanocyte viability and maturation [5].

IMMUNOLOGICAL RESPONSE

The skin includes all the elements of the intrinsic immune system, and vitamin D mediates the immunological response in the immune cell type. A significantly high level of proinflammatory cytokines such as IL-6 and IL-2 has been found in the serum and TNFα in the lesioned vitiligo skin [15]. As mentioned earlier, vitamin D might inhibit the expressions of these cytokines and also have a modulatory effect on the dendritic cell maturation, differentiation, and activation in both human and murine culture systems [16]. Furthermore, vitamin D compounds are shown to induce the inhibition of antigen presentation.

ANTIAPOPTOTIC EFFECTS

It has been suggested that apoptosis is an important mechanism in the vitiligo pathogenesis. A variety of factors, including immune cytokines, some environmental chemicals, and/or other molecular mechanisms induce apoptosis. Because of that, it can be assumed that anti-apoptotic therapy might be able to prevent or to stop the progression of the disease [6]. As a medical therapy, vitamin D is a good alternative because it reduces the apoptotic activity induced by UVB in keratinocytes and melanocytes [17,18].

ANTIOXIDANT PROPERTIES

The onset of vitiligo can be initiated by various factors such as sunburn and exposure to various chemicals. These chemicals can induce oxidative stress. The presence of an imbalance in the oxidant—antioxidant system might play a role in melanocyte degeneration in generalized vitiligo. Therefore, it has been proposed that vitamin D should be used in the protection of vitiliginous skin due to its antioxidant properties and the regulatory function it carries out toward the reactive oxygen species that can produce vitiligo epidermis. Moreover, evidence has shown that calcitriol decreased the level of MDA (malondialdehyde) and increased the activity of superoxide dismutase (SOD) in melanocyte [19]. In addition, observation by transmission electron microscopy suggested that calcitriol might help to reduce the injury of mitochondria in melanocytes under oxidative stress [19].

SIDE EFFECTS OF VITAMIN D ANALOGS

Topical calcipotriol causes skin irritation and in rare instances hypercalcemia after excessive or prolonged application by patients with concomitant renal impairment. It is not recommended in patients with atopic dermatitis, neurodermatitis, or nummular eczema. A relatively high pH is required for stability and it should therefore not be mixed with other agents [20].

Tacalcitol side effects are similar to calcitriol. Local skin reactions such as itching, burning, or redness may be experienced. On rare occasions, mild contact dermatitis or worsening of the skin condition may occur. These are usually mild effects and do not last very long. Calcium levels in the blood may increase due to tacalcitol but this cannot currently be substantiated based on the available data, and its frequency is not known [21].

STUDIES OF VITAMIN D ANALOGS IN THE TREATMENT OF VITILIGO

The first study of a vitamin D analog being used in vitiligo treatment was presented by Parsad et al. in 1998 [22]. The purpose of this study was to determine the efficacy of combining PUVAsol with topical calcitriol in the treatment of vitiligo. The experiment was a randomized, double-blind, and right/left comparative study, which evaluated 19 patients for a duration of 18 months. The test also gave the patients 8-methoxypsoralen before they were exposed to sun, and the patients were advised to apply calcitriol (50 microgram/g) twice daily on one side of the body and placebo ointment on the lesions on the other side. At the end of treatment, 76% of patients showed a marked improvement in calcitriol-treated lesions whereas 53% patients showed moderate to marked improvement in placebo-treated lesions. In addition, it was reported that the repigmentation of hands and feet was much better with the combination of PUVAsol and calcitriol. Therefore, Parsad et al. suggested that the combination of PUVA and calcitriol is highly effective and works faster, and may be used for short-term therapy along with PUVA in the treatment of vitiligo [22]. Parsad et al. used calcipotriol in pediatric vitiligo patients who had serious side effects to PUVA and/or topical steroids, and in 1999 they published their second study [23]. In this study the children were advised to apply calcitriol 50 μg/g in the evening and expose themselves to sunlight the next day for 10–15 minutes. Repigmentation occurred in the majority of children after 6–12 weeks of treatment. Complete repigmentation was seen in 10 of the 18 patients. As a result of this study, calcitriol became a new and potentially efficacious treatment agent for pigmentation disorder in children [23]. After the initial studies, vitamin D analogs were further evaluated in vitiligo treatment in a number of studies [24–36]. In most of these studies, topical vitamin D analogs are compared to commonly used treatment methods in vitiligo [26–39].

The effect of monotherapy with topical calcipotriol was evaluated by Chiaverini et al. in 2002 [24]. In this study, which was a right/left comparative, open study, they found that the calcipotriol in monotherapy was not effective in treatment of vitiligo [24].

In a randomized, double-blind, vehicle-controlled study, Rodriguez-Martin et al. investigated the efficacy and safety of tacalcitol ointment along with sunlight exposure in the treatment of nonsegmental vitiligo [25]. At the end of the study there was no significant difference in the repigmentation response at the 16-week time point between the vehicle + sunlight exposure and the tacalcitol + sunlight exposure groups. Their study clearly shows that topical tacalcitol and sunlight exposure does not induce better effects in repigmentation than solar exposure alone [25].

COMPARISON OF VITAMIN D ANALOGS WITH OTHER TREATMENT METHODS IN VITILIGO

TOPICAL VITAMIN D ANALOGS AND PHOTOTHERAPY

Phototherapy has been used as the main treatment in patients with vitiligo. Different forms of phototherapy for vitiligo include broadband UVB (BB-UVB), narrowband UVB (NB-UVB), excimer light and excimer laser, and PUVA. One of these treatments, PUVA, is an effective treatment, but it carries potential risk of leading to various skin cancers such as squamous cell carcinoma and malignant melanoma. An alternative to PUVA therapy is NB-UVB phototherapy which uses lamps that have a maximum emission of 311–312 nm. In addition, NB-UVB treatment does not require photosensitizers, which is a benefit. As with many other treatments, PUVA and NB-UVB therapies generally result in good repigmentation of the face, but not as good in the hands and feet [26].

PUVA

PUVA is the oldest phototherapy method for vitiligo treatment, but there are not many studies available regarding the use of a topical vitamin D analog and PUVA together. Ameen et al. conducted an open study to determine the efficacy and tolerability of calcipotriol cream as monotherapy in conjunction with PUVA in the treatment of vitiligo [10]. They found that topical calcipotriol appears to be an effective and well-tolerated treatment for vitiligo and can be safely used in conjunction with PUVA [10]. The first placebo-controlled double-blind study in the use of topical calcipotriol and PUVA in the treatment of vitiligo was reported by Ermis et al. [14]. They investigated whether the effectiveness of PUVA treatment could be enhanced by combining it with topical calcipotriol in the treatment of vitiligo. Results of the study showed that the use of topical calcipotriol before the exposure to PUVA increased the efficacy in treatment of vitiligo, and that this combination achieves earlier pigmentation with a lower total UVA dosage [14].

NB-UVB

Because of the side effects of PUVA, the studies are mostly done with UVB. Arca et al. investigated the safety and efficacy of NB-UVB as monotherapy in combination with topical calcipotriol in the treatment of generalized vitiligo [1]. However, addition of topical calcipotriol to NB-UVB did not show any positive results. Khullar et al. wanted to compare the efficacy and safety of topical calcipotriol (0.005%) in combination with NB-UVB versus NB-UVB alone in 27 generalized vitiligo patients [27]. Their results show that addition of calcipotriol to NB-UVB does not enhance the efficacy of treatment in terms of the extent of repigmentation and time to initial

repigmentation. The combination of tacalcitol and NB-UVB is more effective than when used alone. Sahu et al. conducted a study to define the clinical efficacy and safety of NB-UVB when combined with topical tacalcitol versus NB-UVB alone in vitiligo. The results of this study reported that topical tacalcitol increased the efficacy of NB-UVB as it enhances the extent of pigmentation, decreased time to repigmentation, and lowered the cumulative doses of NB-UVB required, thereby leading to greater patient satisfaction and improved compliance [28]. According to a meta-analysis, adding either topical calcineurin inhibitors or topical vitamin D_3 analogs to NB-UVB can yield significantly superior outcomes than simple NB-UVB monotherapy for the treatment of vitiligo [29]. The authors think that NB-UVB monotherapy is a good therapeutic option, but the possible increased risk of skin cancers needs to be taken into consideration [29].

EXCIMER LASER 308 NM

The first study that used 308-nm excimer laser and topical calcipotriol was reported by Goldinger et al. [30]. It was a pilot study whose purpose was to determine if the addition of topical calcipotriol increased the efficacy of the 308-nm xenon chloride excimer laser in the treatment of vitiligo. Ten patients received 308-nm XeCl excimer laser therapy three times weekly. Calcipotriol ointment was applied to lesions on one side of the body twice daily. After 8 weeks, evidence of faster repigmentation did not occur, as there was no significant difference between the side treated with calcipotriol and excimer laser and the side treated with excimer laser alone [30]. The first clinical study to investigate whether adding high-concentration tacalcitol ointment to excimer laser treatment would enhance repigmentation in nonsegmental vitiligo was reported by Oh et al. [31]. In this open-label, prospective, randomized, single-blinded, paired comparative study, it was found that patient satisfaction scores in the combination treatment were slightly better. The authors concluded that the use of high-concentration tacalcitol had a limited effect as either monotherapy or as combination therapy with excimer laser for the treatment of vitiligo [31].

Finally, a study reported by Abdel Latif et al. aimed to compare the efficacy of excimer light (308 nm) versus topical combination therapy of vitamin D_3 analog along with steroid in the treatment of nonsegmental vitiligo [32]. Forty-four patients participated in the study and were divided into two groups; group A was treated with a daily topical combination of calcipotriol and betamethasone, and group B was treated with biweekly sessions of monochromatic excimer light for 3 months. Efficacy based on repigmentation percentages was blindly evaluated. The results showed that there was significant improvement in both groups but without any significant differences in the two groups. They proposed that both treatment modalities offered encouraging results, and both are promising lines for the treatment of vitiligo, and excimer light may be more effective in obtaining rapid regimentation than topical combination of vitamin D_3 analog and steroids [32].

TOPICAL VITAMIN D ANALOGS AND TOPICAL STEROIDS

Topical corticosteroids are generally the first line of therapy in both children and adults for treatment of vitiligo. However, prolonged use of topical steroids can lead to many side effects, such as cutaneous atrophy, telangiectasia, and perioral dermatitis. Calcipotriol has been studied as a treatment both by itself and/or in combination with topical steroids to reduce these side effects. Kumaran et al. evaluated the effect of topical calcipotriol ointment and betamethasone dipropionate cream, when given alone or in combination, in treatment of localized vitiligo. They found that combined therapy appeared to provide a significantly faster onset of repigmentation along with better stability of the achieved pigmentation and with fewer side effects [33]. Another study with betamethasone dipropionate was reported by Xing and Xu [34]. They evaluated the efficacy and safety of calcipotriol when used along with betamethasone dipropionate ointment in the treatment of vitiligo. The result of this study was that calcipotriene 0.005%/betamethasone dipropionate 0.05% ointment is effective and well tolerated in the treatment of patients with vitiligo [34]. Travis et al. conducted a study to define the effects and the side effects of calcipotriene and corticosteroid combination [35]. Their results show that topical calcipotriene in combination with corticosteroids can repigment vitiligo, even in those patients where topical corticosteroids failed when used alone, and the side effect profile of both agents improved if lower concentrations and amounts of both agents were used in dual therapy. This study suggests that the combination of these two agents may be more efficacious than topical corticosteroids alone [35].

TOPICAL VITAMIN D ANALOGS AND PIMECROLIMUS

Topical calcineurin inhibitors such as tacrolimus and pimecrolimus are immunomodulatory agents and are recommended as the first-line treatments in vitiligo. There is only one case report in the English written literature. In this case report, Bilaç et al. observed significant improvement with topical application of pimecrolimus and calcipotriol creams on facial vitiligo lesions [36].

CHILDHOOD VITILIGO AND VITAMIN D ANALOGS

Childhood vitiligo differs from that in adults in that there is a higher incidence in females, and segmental vitiligo is more common and less frequently associated with other systemic autoimmune and endocrine disorders. Treatment of childhood vitiligo is indeed a tougher challenge for dermatologists. Therapy for vitiligo in a child is chosen based on the location of the lesions, lesion age, and extent of lesions in the context of the child's age and developmental status [37]. Although multiple therapeutic modalities are available in the treatment of vitiligo, not all can be used in children.

The data regarding use of vitamin D analogs in childhood vitiligo is limited. The first report was presented by Parsad et al. in 1999 as a prospective uncontrolled study. In this study, calcipotriol was used as once-daily application with sunlight for 10–15 min on all lesions for varying periods. Repigmentation was reported in 55.6% of 18 treated children [23]. The second report was presented by Gargoom et al. in 2004. Topical calcipotriol was used alone on all lesions. Repigmentation of 80%–100% of lesions was reported in 21.4% of 14 treated patients [38]. A study with topical calcipotriol and sunlight was presented by Samar et al. in 2014 [6], where the mean percentage of repigmentation was 41.5%. The adverse effects due to calcipotriol were mild burning and irritation of the skin [39]. There are two case reports for the use of vitamin D analog tacalcitol in childhood vitiligo. The first was presented by Amano et al. in a 11-year-old girl who had an 8-month history of vitiligo on her post-cervical, periocular, and periauricular regions [40]. The authors suggested that the use of a combination therapy with tacalcitol ointment and sunlight exposure instead of UV irradiation should be carried out as an alternative therapy for vitiligo vulgaris because the treatment is safer and increases compliance in children [40]. The second was presented by Oiso and Kawada in a boy with left eyelid vitiligo [41]. They reported that after using the topical tacalcitol to treat the vitiligo lesion on and around the left eyelid, moderate repigmentation and worsening of freckles occurred. The reason for this could be that the topical tacalcitol might have induced and worsened the freckles, because the change in freckles occurred during the treatment. The authors suggested that dermatologists should be aware that applying topical application of tacalcitol to the cheeks can cause freckling and

worsen existing freckles in predisposed children, as described here [41]. However, there is no information about using vitamin D analogs in segmental vitiligo, which is common occurrence in children.

CONCLUSION

The role of vitamin D is a very interesting subject in the autoimmune disease pathogenesis for researchers, since vitamin D analogs are a new therapy candidate for treating vitiligo as an autoimmune disease. Laboratory research has demonstrated their effect in mechanisms of melanogenesis. Furthermore, recent studies of vitamin D analogs and their role in the vitiligo treatment in humans have been done [26–28,31,32,34]. These studies suggested that vitamin D analogs are not sufficiently effective if used as a monotherapy. However, good effectiveness of vitamin D analogs when used in a combination therapy along with other treatments such as PUVA, NB-UVB, topical corticosteroids, sunlight, and pimecrolimus has been shown. Therefore, we need more controlled studies to decide whether vitamin D analogs are an effective cure in the treatment of vitiligo.

PRACTICAL TIPS

1. Topical calcipotriol as monotherapy is not effective in the treatment of vitiligo.

2. Topical calcipotriol provides earlier pigmentation with a lower total UVA dosage when it is used before exposure to PUVA in the treatment of vitiligo.

3. Topical tacalcitol increases the efficacy of NB-UVB.

4. Therapy results show that vitamin D analogs with topical steroids cause significantly faster onset of repigmentation with fewer side effects.

5. A few case reports declare that topical application of pimecrolimus and calcipotriol creams achieve significant improvement in facial vitiligo lesions.

REFERENCES

1. Arca E, Taştan HB, Erbil AH, Sezer E, Koç E, and Kurumlu Z. Narrow-band ultraviolet B as monotherapy and in combination with topical calcipotriol in the treatment of vitiligo. *J Dermatol* 2006;33:338–43.

2. Shahriari M, Kerr PE, Slade K, and Grant-Kels JE. Vitamin D and the skin. *Clin Dermatol* 2010;28:663–8.

3. Holick MF, Chen TC, Lu Z, and Sauter E. Vitamin D and skin physiology: A D-lightful story. *J Bone Miner Res* 2007;22 Suppl 2:V28–33.

4. Juzeniene A, Grigalavicius M, Juraleviciute M, and Grant WB. Phototherapy and vitamin D. *Clin Dermatol* 2016;34:548–55.

5. Birlea SA, Costin GE, and Norris DA. Cellular and molecular mechanisms involved in the action of vitamin D analogs targeting vitiligo depigmentation. *Curr Drug Targets* 2008;9:345–59.

6. AlGhamdi K, Kumar A, and Moussa N. The role of vitamin D in melanogenesis with an emphasis on vitiligo. *Indian J Dermatol Venereol Leprol* 2013;79:750–8.

7. Birlea S, Birlea M, Cimponeriu D et al. Autoimmune diseases and vitamin D receptor Apa-I polymorphism are associated with vitiligo in a small inbred Romanian community. *Acta Derm Venereol* 2006;86:209–14.

8. Beheshti A, Ghadami H, Barikani A, and Haj Manouchehri F. Assessment of vitamin D plasma levels in patients with vitiligo vulgaris. *Acta Med Iran* 2014;52:601.

9. Upala S, and Sanguankeo A. Low 25-hydroxyvitamin D levels are associated with vitiligo: A systematic review and meta-analysis. *Photodermatol Photoimmunol Photomed* 2016;32:181–90.

10. Ameen M, Exarchou V, and Chu AC. Topical calcipotriol as monotherapy and in combination with psoralen plus ultraviolet A in the treatment of vitiligo. *Br J Dermatol* 2001;145:476–9.

11. Gläser R, Röwert J, and Mrowietz U. Hyperpigmentation due to topical calcipotriol and photochemotherapy in two psoriatic patients. *Br J Dermatol* 1998;139:148–51.

12. Brown AJ. Mechanisms for the selective actions of vitamin D analogues. *Curr Pharm Des* 2000;6:701–16.

13. Schallreuter-Wood KU, Pittelkow MR, and Swanson NN. Defective calcium transport in vitiliginous melanocytes. *Arch Dermatol Res* 1996;288:11.

14. Ermis O, Alpsoy E, Cetin L, and Yılmaz E. Is the efficacy of psoralen plus ultraviolet A therapy for vitiligo enhanced by concurrent topical calcipotriol? A placebo-controlled double-blind study. *Br J Dermatol* 2001;145:472–5.

15. Singh S, Singh U, and Pandey SS. Serum concentration of IL-6, IL-2, TNF-α, and IFNγ in vitiligo patients. *Indian J Dermatol* 2012;57:12–4.

16. Penna G, and Adorini L. 1 Alpha, 25-dihydroxyvitamin D3 inhibits differentiation, maturation, activation, and survival of dendritic cells leading to impaired alloreactive T cell activation. *J Immunol* 2000;164:2405–11.

17. De Haes P, Garmyn M, Degreef H, Vantieghem K, Bouillon R, and Seqaert S. 1,25-Dihydroxyvitamin D3 inhibits ultraviolet B-induced apoptosis, Jun kinase activation, and interleukin-6 production in primary human keratinocytes. *J Cell Biochem* 2003;89:663–73.

18. Sauer B, Ruwisch L, and Kleuser B. Antiapoptotic action of 1alpha, 25-dihydroxyvitamin D3 in primary human melanocytes. *Melanoma Res* 2003;13:339–47.

19. Gong Q, Li X, Sun J, Ding G, Zhou M, Zhao W, and Lu Y. The effects of calcipotriol on the dendritic morphology of human melanocytes under oxidative stress and a possible mechanism: Is it a mitochondrial protector? *J Dermatol Sci* 2015;77:117–24.

20. Khandpur S, Sharma VK, and Sumanth K. Topical immunomodulators in dermatology topical immunomodulators in dermatology. *J Postgrad Med* 2004;50:131–9.

21. *Curatoderm® 4 micrograms/G ointment; Talcacitol [package insert]. Reinbek, Germany; Almirall Hermal GmbH*. 2019. Available at: https://www.medicines.org.uk/emc/PIL.23578.latest.pdf

22. Parsad D, Saini R, and Verma N. Combination of PUVAsol and topical calcipotriol in vitiligo. *Dermatology* 1998;197:167–70.

23. Parsad D, Saini R, and Nagpal R. Calcipotriol in vitiligo: A preliminary study. *Pediatr Dermatol* 1999;16:317–20.

24. Chiavérini C, Passeron T, and Ortonne JP. Treatment of vitiligo by topical calcipotriol. *J Eur Acad Dermatol Venereol* 2002;16:137–8.

25. Rodríguez-Martín M, García Bustínduy M, Sáez Rodríguez M, and Noda Cabrera A. Randomized, double-blind clinical trial to evaluate the efficacy of topical tacalcitol and sunlight exposure in the treatment of adult nonsegmental vitiligo. *Br J Dermatol* 2009;160:409–14.

26. Leone G, Pacifico A, Iacovelli P, Paro Vidolin A, and Picardo M. Tacalcitol and narrow-band phototherapy in patients with vitiligo. *Clin Exp Dermatol* 2006;31:200–5.

27. Khullar G, Kanwar AJ, Singh S, and Parsad D. Comparison of efficacy and safety profile of topical calcipotriol ointment in combination with NB-UVB vs. NB-UVB alone in the treatment of vitiligo: A 24 week prospective right-left comparative clinical trials. *J Eur Acad Dermatol Venereol* 2015;29:925–32.

28. Sahu P, Jain VK, Aggarwal K, Kaur S, and Dayal S. Tacalcitol: A useful adjunct to narrow-band ultraviolet-B phototherapy in vitiligo. *Photodermatol Photoimmunol Photomed* 2016;32:262–8.

29. Li R, Qiao M, Wang X, Zhao X, and Sun Q. Effect of narrow band ultraviolet B phototherapy as monotherapy or combination therapy for vitiligo: A meta-analysis. *Photodermatol Photoimmunol Photomed* 2017;33:22–31.

30. Goldinger SM, Dummer R, Schmid P, Burg G, Seifert B, and Läuchli S. Combination of 308–nm xenon chloride excimer laser and topical calcipotriol in vitiligo. *J Eur Acad Dermatol Venereol* 2007;21:504–8.

31. Oh SH, Kim T, Jee H, Do JE, and Lee JH. Combination treatment of nonsegmental vitiligo with a 308-nm xenon chloride excimer laser and topical high concentration tacalcitol: A prospective, single-blinded, paired, comparative study. *J Am Acad Dermatol* 2011;65:428–30.

32. Abdel Latif AA, and Ibrahim SM. Monochromatic excimer light versus combination of topical steroid with vitamin D3 analogue in the treatment of nonsegmental vitiligo: A randomized blinded comparative study. *Dermatol Ther* 2015;28:383–9.

33. Kumaran MS, Kaur I, and Kumar B. Effect of topical calcipotriol, betamethasone dipropionate and their combination in the treatment of localized vitiligo. *J Eur Acad Dermatol Venereol* 2006;20:269–73.

34. Xing C, and Xu A. The effect of combined calcipotriol and betamethasone dipropionate ointment in the treatment of vitiligo: An open, uncontrolled trial. *J Drugs Dermatol* 2012;11:e52–54.

35. Travis LB, and Silverberg NB. Calcipotriene and corticosteroid combination therapy for vitiligo. *Pediatr Dermatol* 2004;21:495–8.

36. Bilaç DB, Ermertcan AT, Sahin MT, and Oztürkcan S. Two therapeutic challenges: Facial vitiligo successfully treated with 1% pimecrolimus cream and 0.005% calcipotriol cream. *J Eur Acad Dermatol Venereol* 2009;23:72–3.

37. Van Driessche F, and Silverberg N. Current management of pediatric vitiligo. *Paediatr Drugs* 2015;17:303–13.

38. Gargoom AM, Duweb GA, Elzorghany AH, Benghazil M, and Bugrein OO. Calcipotriol in the treatment of childhood vitiligo. *Int J Clin Pharmacol Res* 2004;24:11–4.

39. Sarma N, and Singh AK. Topical calcipotriol in childhood vitiligo: An Indian experience. *Int J Dermatol* 2004;43:856–9.

40. Amano H, Abe M, and Ishikawa O. First case report of topical tacalcitol for vitiligo repigmentation. *Pediatr Dermatol* 2008;25:262–4.

41. Oiso N, and Kawada A. Freckling promoted by topical tacalcitol in a Japanese boy with left eyelid vitiligo. *Pediatr Dermatol* 2012;29:671–2.

Chapter 24

NEWER AGENTS FOR TOPICAL TREATMENT

Devinder Mohan Thappa and Malathi Munisamy

CONTENTS

INTRODUCTION

The exact cause of vitiligo has not been identified despite ongoing research in this field. The most prevalent hypotheses that form the basis for the existing therapeutic options include autoimmune, genetic, neural, self-destruction, growth factor deficiency, viral, and convergence theories. However, recent genetic profiling and research on the pathogenesis of vitiligo have identified immune-mediated mechanisms and oxidative stress to be the key pathogenetic mechanisms involved in melanocyte destruction. Genome-wide association studies have demonstrated an interplay between immunoregulatory genes and melanocyte-specific genes [1].

Oxidative stress has been reported to be the primary event initiating the immune dysfunction in genetically susceptible individuals resulting in melanocyte destruction mediated by activated cytotoxic CD8 + T lymphocytes and interferon gamma–induced chemokine CXCL10. In addition, the differentiation of melanocyte stem cells is also affected due to impaired Wnt signaling pathway as demonstrated in recent transcriptomic analysis [1,2]. These pathways are now the primary targets for the newer therapeutic options currently being developed for vitiligo.

The therapy of vitiligo aims at achieving three outcomes: [2]

- To arrest the disease progression—immune dysfunction and oxidative stress needs to be targeted
- To induce repigmentation—differentiation and migration of melanocytes needs to be targeted
- To prevent relapse

Hence it is quite obvious that to achieve a complete cure for vitiligo, different therapeutic approaches need to be used to achieve each outcome, which points to the fact that the best therapeutic responses are possible only with combination therapy [3].

Topical therapy with or without phototherapy has been the mainstay of treatment for vitiligo, with topical corticosteroids and topical calcineurin inhibitors targeting the immune dysfunction and narrowband ultraviolet B (NV-UVB) therapy inducing repigmentation being the first-line treatment for vitiligo. Other topical agents commonly used include vitamin D analogs, pseudocatalase, and depigmenting agents [3–5].

Though these current treatments are effective, not all patients and not all sites respond well to the available therapies, thus posing a therapeutic challenge and the need for newer therapeutic options.

NEWER TOPICAL AGENTS IN VITILIGO

The newer topical agents that have been investigated in vitiligo include capsaicin, curcumin, *Cucumis melo* extracts, piperine, prostaglandin E2 (PGE2) analogs, prostaglandin F2 alpha (PGF2α) analogs, basic fibroblast growth factor (bFGF), afamelanotide, L-carnosine, photocil, topical phenytoin gel, topical histamine, topical mycophenolate mofetil (MMF), and ruxolitinib [3,6].

TOPICAL ANTIOXIDANTS

i. *Capsaicin and curcumin*: Capsaicin (8-methyl-N-vanillyl-6-none-namide) obtained from chili pepper and curcumin (diferuloylmethane) obtained from turmeric are known to possess potent anti-inflammatory, antioxidant, and anti-apoptotic properties. Pretreatment of perilesional skin of patients with vitiligo with capsaicin and curcumin demonstrated a beneficial effect by protecting the keratinocytes from perilesional vitiligo skin from mitochondrial damage and apoptosis by restoring mitochondrial permeability and mitochondrial membrane potential, and inhibiting the intrinsic apoptotic pathway, respectively. Both curcumin and capsaicin inhibited apoptosis by inhibiting caspase 8 and 9, p38 and NF-kB activation, and increasing ERK phosphorylation. Curcumin was more effective than capsaicin in protecting from mitochondrial damage. Since both these natural antioxidants were found to increase the total antioxidant capacity, repress the intracellular reactive oxygen species generation and lipid peroxidation, and improve the mitochondrial activity, they have been suggested as alternative approaches to protect against progression of vitiligo [7]. Synergistic therapeutic effects have been demonstrated with slightly improved repigmentation on combining targeted NB-UVB with tetrahydrocurcuminoid cream when compared to phototherapy alone in a preliminary randomized controlled trial on patients with focal and generalized vitiligo [8]. However, an in vivo study on Asian patients with acute vitiligo who consumed turmeric daily demonstrated dietary curcumin to contribute to oxidative stress in acute vitiligo and prevent repigmentation [9].

ii. *Cucumis melo extracts*: The vegetable extracts obtained from muskmelon (*C. melo*) were found to have superoxide dismutase and catalase activities, and were formulated into microsphere gel for topical application in vitiligo and marketed as Vitix gel [10]. However, this preparation failed to demonstrate reduction in hydrogen peroxide in both in vitro and in vivo studies [10]. Though there are reports of this preparation being effective in vitiligo [11] when combined with phototherapy, recent studies [12,13] report no beneficial effect on vitiligo repigmentation when used alone or when combined with phototherapy.

Though these topical antioxidants are often prescribed, the consensus guidelines do not recommend the use of topical antioxidants as their efficacy has been observed in only limited number of trials [5].

TOPICAL AGENTS AFFECTING MELANOCYTE PROLIFERATION, DIFFERENTIATION, AND MELANOGENESIS

i. *Piperine and its synthetic analogs*: Piperine (1-piperoylpiperidine), an alkaloid obtained from black pepper fruit extract, was found to have a stimulatory effect on the growth of cultured melanocytes and induced melanocyte proliferation and dendrite formation in mouse models. However, synthesis of melanin occurred only in the presence of UV radiation. Hence piperine and its analogs, when used for treatment of vitiligo, should be used with concomitant UVA exposure. However, the application of piperine and phototherapy needs to be staggered to avoid photoisomerization [3,6].

ii. *Prostaglandin E2 (PGE2) analogs*: Prostaglandins are effective in vitiligo due to their role in immunomodulation, melanogenesis, proliferation, and maturation of melanocytes. The therapeutic efficacy of ultraviolet radiation (UVR) to cause repigmentation in vitiligo is attributed to increased production of PGE2. UVR induces cyclooxygenase 2 enzyme, which is a mitogenic and inflammatory stimuli that causes PGE2 production by keratinocytes. Animal studies demonstrated increased melanocyte density on topical application of PGE2 gel, and studies on vitiligo patients have demonstrated significant repigmentation with the minor side effect of transient burning sensation when applied twice daily for 6 months [6,14].

iii. *Prostaglandin F2 alpha (PGF2α) analogs*: PGF2α analogs have been reported to be promising therapeutic options in vitiligo in both human and animal studies, with increased efficacy when combined with phototherapy or topical steroids. The therapeutic efficacy is mediated indirectly through induction of COX-2 and PGE2 and not due to direct effect on melanogenesis. Latanoprost (0.005%), Bimatoprost (0.03%), and Travoprost (0.004%) ophthalmic solutions are the PGF2α analogs that are being investigated in various studies [15–17].

iv. *Basic fibroblast growth factor (bFGF)*: bFGF exerts effects on melanocyte migration and proliferation, and the lesional and perilesional skin of vitiligo patients has demonstrated reduced expression of bFGF. UVR-induced pigmentation has been attributed to the increase in residual cutaneous melanocytes in vitiligo skin stimulated by melanocyte growth factors like bFGF and endothelin-1. However, its role in vitiligo is still controversial, as its levels were found to be both higher and lower in different subpopulations of vitiligo patients [3,6].

v. *Alpha-melanocyte–stimulating hormone agonistic analog*: Afamelanotide, a potent and longer lasting synthetic α-MSH analog, is a potentially effective treatment for vitiligo which is available as a monthly 16-mg subcutaneous implant. It targets the key pathway of melanogenesis by binding to melanocortin-1 receptor (MC1R) and stimulates pigmentation and increases proliferation of melanocytes. Since MC1R is not expressed by melanocyte stem cells, afamelanotide has no effect on the differentiation of melanocyte stem cells. Hence afamelanotide needs to be combined with phototherapy for increased

efficacy, as phototherapy induces melanoblast differentiation, proliferation, and eumelanogenesis and thus combination therapy would increase the speed and extent of repigmentation. Afamelanotide causes potent tanning, causing a major concern in fair-skinned individuals, as it results in sharp color contrast. Hence the best results were obtained in dark-skinned individuals [3,6,18].

vi. *Histamine*: The role of topical histamine on skin pigmentation in vitiligo was studied based on the observation that histamine stimulates melanogenesis, and melanocyte proliferation in vitro and vitiligo skin had reduced expression of histamine receptor 2 (H2r). It was observed that topically applied histamine (1% histamine in distilled water applied twice daily for 5 weeks) stimulated repigmentation in a receptor-dependent mechanism mediated by H2r. Histamine also accelerated the permeability barrier recovery in vitiligo by upregulating the expression of cornified envelope proteins, thereby improving permeability barrier homeostasis. Apart from direct effect on melanocytes, histamine can also indirectly stimulate melanocyte proliferation and differentiation by stimulating keratinocytes to secrete granulocyte-macrophage colony-stimulating factor. Based on these observations, H2r agonists and topical histamine can be considered as alternative approaches for vitiligo, especially in those with longer duration of disease, as the efficacy of histamine was not affected by disease duration [19].

vii. *Phenytoin*: Two percent phenytoin gel for 3 months has been recently reported to have beneficial effects in vitiligo owing to its immunomodulatory activity and stimulatory effect on melanocytes without any observed side effects during the study period. Phenytoin has been reported to suppress mitogen-induced activation of lymphocytes and cytotoxic T lymphocyte activity, decrease suppressor T cells, and increase the helper/suppressor ratio, thereby shifting to a TH2 immune response. In addition, the hydantoin moiety of phenytoin directly stimulates the melanocytes and stabilizes the melanosome membrane. Though three types of phenytoin topical preparations are available as gel, hydrophilic cream, and ointment, the gel preparation has been reported to give the highest release of phenytoin. Whether combination therapy of phenytoin with steroids and phototherapy would potentiate their therapeutic effects needs to be studied in the future, although no additional benefit was observed when phenytoin was combined with PUVA therapy [20].

TOPICAL IMMUNOSUPPRESSANTS

i. *Mycophenolate mofetil*: Fifteen percent MMF topical preparation (obtained by dissolving the MMF tablets in Eucerin) when applied twice daily over vitiligo patches for 3 months was reported to cause repigmentation and hence can be considered an alternative and safe topical drug therapy for vitiligo in a recent pilot study. The therapeutic efficacy of MMF could be improved by the use of permeation enhancers like eucalyptol and N-methyl-2-pyrrolidone. MMF targets the immune dysregulation in vitiligo as it induces apoptosis of activated lymphocytes, decreases the recruitment of CD4 and CD8 lymphocytes and monocytes at sites of inflammation, and inhibits the production of antibodies by B cells. Though found to be effective, MMF may not be indicated in steroid-resistant cases and can be used in cases where topical steroids are contraindicated [21].

ii. *5-fluorouracil*: Five percent 5-fluorouracil (5-FU) has been used in the topical treatment of vitiligo as early as 1983 [22]; currently, it is regaining popularity for its efficacy when used as combination therapy with dermabrasion or laser ablation and phototherapy wherein it reduces the treatment duration of phototherapy. 5-FU is used for its immunomodulatory property, which helps in stabilizing the depigmentation process. In addition, 5-FU on dermabraded or ablated epidermis, by distorting the epidermis, results in stable migration of melanocytes and spread of pigments by stimulating the amelanotic melanocytes of the infundibulum for melanin synthesis and migration to epidermis and also by stimulating the melanocyte division that leads to melanocyte colonization in the epidermis. 5-FU also exerts a detrimental effect on the inhibitor cells or factors in dermis or epidermis that are harmful for melanocytes [23,24].

TARGETED IMMUNOTHERAPY

i. *Ruxolitinib*: Ruxolitinib, a JAK1/JAK2 (Janus kinase) inhibitor approved for treating myelofibrosis and polycythemia vera is currently undergoing trials for its role as a topical therapeutic agent for vitiligo based on two case reports reporting complete repigmentation with oral JAK inhibitors tofacitinib citrate and ruxolitinib. In a recent phase 2, investigator-initiated open label, proof of concept trial, twice-daily application of ruxolitinib 1.5% cream for 20 weeks has been proven to be safe and effective in inducing repigmentation in facial vitiligo with minor adverse events like erythema, hyperpigmentation, and transient acne. Ruxolitinib targets the IFN-γ/JAK/CXCL10 pathway, the key pathogenetic mechanism underlying the depigmentation process of vitiligo, and hence is a promising new therapeutic option that needs to be explored in detail. Well-conducted large-scale randomized controlled trials should be conducted in the future to provide a better understanding of the long-term safety and efficacy of these newer agents [5,25].

OTHERS

i. Photocil is an innovative topical agent composed of diethylamino hydroxybenzoil hexyl benzoate and alpha-glucosyl hesperidin (glucosylated derivative of a natural plant flavonoid) developed to selectively deliver NB-UVB by filtering out harmful radiation to improve patient compliance with phototherapy [26].

ii. Another novel agent with a combination of phenylalanine, *C. melo* extract, and acetylcysteine in a gel formulation has been found to be effective in inducing repigmentation either as monotherapy or in combination with NB microphototherapy [27].

iii. Elastic cationic niosomes (liposomes) to deliver tyrosinase plasmid (pMEL34) to increase tyrosinase gene expression to increase tyrosinase have been developed which have a potential role in gene therapy for vitiligo [28].

iv. L-carnosine (Beta-alanyl-l-histidine), a dipeptide with high antioxidant properties, has been proposed as a promising agent, as it protects the cell membranes from oxidative damage and reduces age-related mitochondrial dysfunction which is responsible for keratinocyte damage in vitiligo skin [3,6].

v. Psoralen and resveratrol (a sirtuin activator and a potential antioxidant) co-loaded ultradeformable liposomes have been developed as a promising therapeutic option for combined PUVA and antioxidant therapy in a special formulation to improve percutaneous permeability of psoralen and improve solubility of resveratrol for effective topical administration [29].

FUTURE PERSPECTIVES

Recent translational research has identified the IFN-γ-CXCL 10 chemokine axis as a potential target for targeted immunotherapies for vitiligo, of which ruxolitinib is already under trials. Other agents targeting various downstream signals should be developed and investigated. Consistent elevation of cytokines (IL-17, IL-2, IL-22, IL-23, and IL-33) has been reported in vitiligo, and these cytokines are also potential therapeutic targets [1]. Sirtuins that function as histone deacetylase and/or adenosine diphosphate ribosyltransferase are involved in cellular pathways related to skin structure and function. SIRT1-positive modulation has been recently reported as a potential preventive therapy to reduce keratinocyte oxidative stress and promote activation of antiapoptotic pathways. Resveratrol, a natural SIRT1 activator, has already been investigated and has shown promising results in vitiligo. However, future studies are needed to elucidate the protective role of SIRT1 activators in the protection of perilesional skin keratinocytes in vitiligo [30]. Another interesting therapeutic target would be the Wnt/b catenin signaling, which regulates melanocyte stem cell differentiation and Kit signaling which induces the migration of differentiated melanoblasts in UVB-irradiated skin. Since the Wnt pathway is deregulated in vitiligo skin, Wnt agonists can be considered as potential therapeutic options [1,2]. Another area that needs to be explored is the development of efficient and skin-friendly topical drug delivery systems with improved drug penetration, with drug deposition at the desired site(s) of action for prolonged periods without allowing systemic absorption, and shielding the drug from the local metabolic milieu of the skin [31].

CONCLUSION

New information as a result of ongoing research on the pathogenesis of vitiligo has opened avenues to a variety of exciting therapeutic options that need to be explored in detail. Many of the newer agents like ruxolitinib, afamelanotide, and resveratrol have shown promising results in various studies. However, their long-term safety and efficacy in terms of sustained effects needs to be explored further in large-scale, well-designed controlled trials. With recent establishment of the core outcome measures for vitiligo, new measurement instruments, biomarkers, and key pathogenetic targets, a new generation of targeted treatments needs to be developed and investigated. Owing to its complex pathogenesis, vitiligo might benefit most from combination treatments targeting the various aspects of the pathogenesis, which is essential to achieve all three therapeutic outcomes; namely, to stop progression, achieve repigmentation, and prevent relapse.

REFERENCES

1. Speeckaert R, and van Geel N. Vitiligo: An update on pathophysiology and treatment options. *Am J Clin Dermatol* 2017;18(6):733–44.

2. Passeron T. Medical and maintenance treatments for vitiligo. *Dermatol Clin* 2017;35:163–70.

3. Malathi M, and Thappa DM. Topical therapy in vitiligo: What is new? *Pigment Int* 2016;3:1–4.

4. Whitton M, Pinart M, Batchelor JM et al. Evidence-based management of vitiligo: Summary of a Cochrane systematic review. *Br J Dermatol* 2016;174:962–9.

5. Rodrigues M, Ezzedine K, Hamzavi I, Pandya AG, Harris JE; Vitiligo Working Group. Current and emerging treatments for vitiligo. *J Am Acad Dermatol* 2017;77:17–29.

6. Lotti TM, Hercogová J, Schwartz RA et al. Treatments of vitiligo: What's new at the horizon. *Dermatol Ther* 2012;25 Suppl 1:S32–40.

7. Becatti M, Prignano F, Fiorillo C, Pescitelli L, Nassi P, Lotti T, and Taddei N. The involvement of Smac/DIABLO, p53, NF-kB, and MAPK pathways in apoptosis of keratinocytes from perilesional vitiligo skin: Protective effects of curcumin and capsaicin. *Antioxid Redox Signal* 2010;13:1309–21.

8. Schallreuter KU, and Rokos H. Turmeric (curcumin): A widely used curry ingredient, can contribute to oxidative stress in Asian patients with acute vitiligo. *Indian J Dermatol Venereol Leprol* 2006;72:57–9.

9. Asawanonda P, and Klahan SO. Tetrahydrocurcuminoid cream plus targeted narrowband UVB phototherapy for vitiligo: A preliminary randomized controlled study. *Photomed Laser Surg* 2010;28:679–84.

10. Schallreuter KU, Panske A, and Chiuchiarelli G. Ineffective topical treatment of vitiligo with Cucumis melo extracts. *Int J Dermatol* 2011;50:374–5.

11. Kostović K, Pastar Z, Pasić A, and Ceović R. Treatment of vitiligo with narrow-band UVB and topical gel containing catalase and superoxide dismutase. *Acta Dermatovenerol Croat* 2007;15:10–4.

12. Yuksel EP, Aydin F, Senturk N, Canturk T, and Turanli AY. Comparison of the efficacy of narrow band ultraviolet B and narrow band ultraviolet B plus topical catalase-superoxide dismutase treatment in vitiligo patients. *Eur J Dermatol* 2009;19:341–4.

13. Naini FF, Shooshtari AV, Ebrahimi B, and Molaei R. The effect of pseudocatalase/superoxide dismutase in the treatment of vitiligo: A pilot study. *J Res Pharm Pract* 2012;1:77–80.

14. Kapoor R, Phiske MM, and Jerajani HR. Evaluation of safety and efficacy of topical prostaglandin E2 in treatment of vitiligo. *Br J Dermatol* 2009;160:861–3.

15. Anbar TS, El-Ammawi TS, Barakat M, and Fawzy A. Skin pigmentation after NB-UVB and three analogues of prostaglandin F(2alpha) in guinea pigs: A comparative study. *J Eur Acad Dermatol Venereol* 2010;24:28–31.

16. Anbar TS, El-Ammawi TS, Abdel-Rahman AT, and Hanna MR. The effect of latanoprost on vitiligo: A preliminary comparative study. *Int J Dermatol* 2015;54:587–93.

17. Bagherani N, and Smoller BR. Efficacy of bimatoprost in the treatment of non-facial vitiligo. *Dermatol Ther* 2017;30(2).

18. Lim HW, Grimes PE, Agbai O et al. Afamelanotide and narrowband UV-B phototherapy for the treatment of vitiligo: A randomized multicenter trial. *JAMA Dermatol* 2015;151:42–50.

19. Liu J, Xu Y, Lin TK, Lv C, Elias PM, and Man MQ. Topical histamine stimulates repigmentation of nonsegmental vitiligo by a receptor-dependent mechanism. *Skin Pharmacol Physiol* 2017;30:139–45.

20. Abdou AG, Abdelwahed Gaber M, Elnaidany NF, and Elnagar A. Evaluation of the effect and mechanism of action of local phenytoin in treatment of vitiligo. *J Immunoassay Immunochem* 2017; 22:1–15.

21. Handjani F, Aghaei S, Moezzi I, and Saki N. Topical mycophenolate mofetil in the treatment of vitiligo: A pilot study. *Dermatol Pract Concept* 2017;7:31–3.

22. Tsuji T, and Hamada T. Topically administered fluorouracil in vitiligo. *Arch Dermatol* 1983;119:722–7.

23. Anbar TS, Westerhof W, Abdel-Rahman AT, Ewis AA, and El-Khayyat MA. Effect of one session of ER: YAG laser ablation plus topical 5fluorouracil on the outcome of short-term NB-UVB phototherapy in the treatment of non-segmental vitiligo: A left-right comparative study. *Photodermatol Photoimmunol Photomed* 2008;24:322–9.

24. Mohamed HA, Mohammed GF, Gomaa AH, and Eyada MM. Carbon dioxide laser plus topical 5-fluorouracil: A new combination therapeutic modality for acral vitiligo. *J Cosmet Laser Ther* 2015;17:216–23.

25. Rothstein B, Joshipura D, Saraiya A et al. Treatment of vitiligo with the topical Janus kinase inhibitor ruxolitinib. *J Am Acad Dermatol* 2017;76:1054–60.

26. Wang X, McCoy J, Lotti T, and Goren A. Topical cream delivers NB-UVB from sunlight for the treatment of vitiligo. *Expert Opin Pharmacother* 2014;15:2623-7.

27. Buggiani G, Tsampau D, Hercogovà J, Rossi R, Brazzini B, and Lotti T. Clinical efficacy of a novel topical formulation for vitiligo: Compared evaluation of different treatment modalities in 149 patients. *Dermatol Ther* 2012;25:472–6.

28. Gude D. Vitiligo: Newer insights in pathophysiology and treatment. *Indian J Paediatr Dermatol* 2012;13:27–33.

29. Doppalapudi S, Mahira S, and Khan W. Development and in vitro assessment of psoralen and resveratrol co-loaded ultradeformable liposomes for the treatment of vitiligo. *J Photochem Photobiol B* 2017;174:44–57.

30. Gianfaldoni S, Zanardelli M, and Lotti T. Vitiligo repigmentation: What's new? *J Dermatolog Clin Res* 2014; 2:1023.

31. Garg BJ, Saraswat A, Bhatia A, and Katare OP. Topical treatment in vitiligo and the potential uses of new drug delivery systems. *Indian J Dermatol Venereol Leprol* 2010;76:231–8.

Chapter 25

COSMETIC CAMOUFLAGE IN VITILIGO

Feroze Kaliyadan, Karalikkattil T. Ashique, and Ambika Kumar

CONTENTS

INTRODUCTION

Skin camouflage refers to special products or techniques that can be used to disguise skin disfigurement [1]. Camouflage can be used for providing customized, immediate appearance normalization for a variety of skin conditions [2]. One of the most common conditions in which camouflage is used, in the context of dermatological disorders, is vitiligo.

HISTORICAL BACKGROUND

The concept of skin camouflage has been described since ancient Roman times. It is said that slaves applied camouflage to mask the mark made on the forehead with a hot iron, which was used to brand them. During the same period, camouflage was used to mask freckles [1]. Skin camouflage creams were first developed during the Second World War, when plastic surgeons associated with the British Royal Air Force (RAF) began searching for durable skin-colored preparations to help conceal severely disfiguring scars of war victims [3]. Max Factor (originally Maksymilian Faktorowicz) is credited with coining the term "makeup," and he worked with plastic surgeons to create makeups to camouflage scars of movie actors injured in war [2]. Lydia O'Leary developed Covermark™ in 1928, which helped skin camouflage gain importance in Great Britain. Sir Archibald McIndoe, a plastic surgery consultant to the RAF, established a patient support group called the " Guinea Pig Club," members of which were to try camouflage creams prepared by Thomas Blake, a chemist from the Veil company. Meanwhile in the United States, Elizabeth Arden created "scar cream" during World War II, and she toured hospitals to promote its use. In the 1950s, Joyce Allsworth trained members of the British Red Cross in techniques of skin camouflage and helped in the founding of British Association of Skin Camouflage (BASC) in 1985. BASC offers courses in skin camouflage and has set up clinics in hospitals throughout Great Britain [2,3].

IMPORTANCE OF CAMOUFLAGE IN VITILIGO

Even though vitiligo affects only the skin, as many as 30% of patients suffer from psychological problems that affect their quality of life [4]. Indian studies have shown that vitiligo has significant psychosocial impact, including features like anxiety, depression, and sleep disturbances [5,6]. Increased prevalence of avoidance behavior has been noted [7]. One of the primary concerns of patients with vitiligo is the presence of lesions on visible areas like the face. While there are currently quite a few treatment options available for vitiligo, they are limited by fact that most of them take time to produce results. Camouflage can be very useful in addressing the psychosocial aspects in such cases. It is especially useful in areas like the face and difficult-to-treat areas like the hands and feet [1].

Camouflage can also be used to cover lesions when treatments fail to obtain adequate results or when lesions occur on exposed areas and the patients are not motivated to treat their disease [8]. Many studies have suggested that appropriate camouflage can improve the quality of life for patients with vitiligo [8–11]. Cosmetic camouflage can help the patient to achieve a better self-image [1].

CLASSIFICATION OF CAMOUFLAGE

Broadly, skin camouflage products are classified as temporary or permanent [3,12]. Temporary camouflage consists of liquid dyes, indigenous products, foundation-based cosmetic camouflages, and self-tanning products, and permanent camouflage consists of micropigmentation.

TEMPORARY CAMOUFLAGE
LIQUID DYES
Some of the commonly used liquid dyes include potassium permanganate, indigo carmine, Bismarck brown, and henna paste. The disadvantages are that they are washed away easily, and it is difficult to make an appropriate color match.

INDIGENOUS PRODUCTS

Iron filings (Loha Bhasma) and Suvarna Karini (clay mixed with henna and oils) are some traditional Indian preparations used for vitiligo camouflage [13]. A disadvantage is an inappropriate color match.

FOUNDATION-BASED COSMETIC CAMOUFLAGE

These are the most common type of camouflage products used for vitiligo. Cosmetic camouflage preparations contain up to 25% more pigment compared to normal makeup foundations. The texture is denser, and they may contain up to 50% mineral oils/waxes. These are waterproof and last up to 24 hours.

There are four basic foundation formulations [3,12,14]:

- *Oil-based*: These are water-in-oil emulsions with the pigment held within the oil. They are best suited for dry skin and for skin that requires considerable coverage. The water evaporates from the foundation after application, leaving the pigment in the oily base.
- *Water-based*: These are oil-in-water preparations and are suitable for dry to normal skin. They are less stable compared to oil-based preparations but tend to be more popular.
- *Oil-free*: These replace the oil with non-comedogenic ingredients like dimethicone or cyclomethicone; they provide a "dry feel" to oily skin.
- *Water-free*: Comprised of oils, alcohols, and artificial esters and are waterproof; they contain combinations of titanium dioxide with iron oxide, sometimes combined with ultramarine blue. These are suited for patients requiring intensive facial camouflage [15].

The most popular foundation cosmetic camouflage is the liquid oil-in-water emulsion type that contains a small amount of oil in which the pigment is emulsified with a relatively large quantity of water. Foundations are available in a variety of finishes like matte, semi-matte, moist semi-matte, and shiny. Foundations are also manufactured in various forms: liquid, mousse, water-containing cream, soufflé, anhydrous cream, stick, cake, and shake lotion [3,14].

CRITERIA FOR IDEAL COSMETIC CAMOUFLAGE [1,3,14,15]

- Color—must match all skin tones, must blend easily with the surrounding normal skin
- Opacity—must conceal all types of skin discoloration
- Waterproof
- Sweat resistant—should not smudge as a result of sweating
- Holding power—must adhere to the skin without sliding off
- Longer wear—must last for a long duration
- Ease of application—must be easy to apply
- Non-allergic/non-comedogenic/non-photosensitizing
- Sun-screening capacity—must have a good, homogenous sun protection capacity
- Ease of removal—must be easy to remove with non-alcohol/non-acetone—based makeup removers
- Cost effective—should be easily affordable

Some of the popular and well established brands available in the market are Dermablend™ (Division of L'Oreal USA, New York, NY), CoverBlend™ (Neostrata, Princeton, NJ), Cover FX™ (Cover FX Skin Care Inc, Toronto, Ontario, Canada), Covermark (Covermark, Northvale, NJ), Dermacolor™ (Dermacolor, London, UK), Keromask™ (Christy, London, UK), Veil Cover™ (Durham, UK) and PerfectCover™ (Tokyo, Japan).

PRACTICAL TIPS

Before advising cosmetic camouflage, the physician needs to keep in mind the patient's medical history, concomitant topical and systemic medications, allergies, patient expectations, and the patient's social and occupational activities [14].

For applying foundation-based products, first the area needs to be cleaned to remove any previous makeup. Patients must be advised regarding proper makeup removal techniques (especially keeping in mind the need to avoid Koebnerization). The color palette can be held next to the patient's skin to get a rough idea of the best matching shades. Encourage the patient to experiment with the color palettes until they get the best match; it is best to try to achieve a match with no more than two shades. Mixing more than two shades might become costly and cumbersome (although some camouflage products do require a greater number of shades to get the correct color match). Apply the product with the ball of the middle finger. Feather out the edges with a brush. Apply the fixing powder with a small cotton pad to stabilize the foundation and make it waterproof and smudge-proof. The powder should remain for 8 to 10 minutes on the skin to absorb the excess oil (especially if the patient has oily skin). Fixing sprays contain silicone and polymers to produce an elastic film, which gives coverage that is more durable. Removal of the camouflage requires a water-in-oil—based cleansing solution, followed by soap and water cleansing (Figures 25.1 through 25.4). For the lips, camouflage foundation creams in the form of lipsticks can be used [1,3,14].

SELF-TANNING PRODUCTS

Self-tanning products are available in different preparations—gels, creams, lotions, and sprays. The active ingredient in most self-tanning preparations is dihydroxyacetone (DHA); the most common strength is 5%. DHA is a sugar that combines with the keratin in the cornified layer, producing a tan that resembles a normal suntan. The chemical reaction is considered to be a variant of the Maillardreaction (golden brown crusting of bread in an oven).

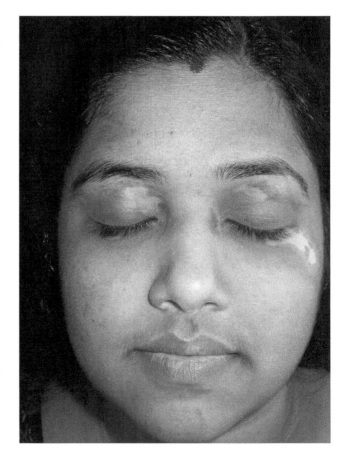

Figure 25.1 Vitiligo over face.

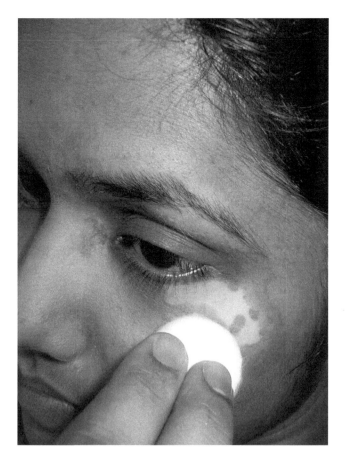

Figure 25.2   Application of camouflage cream.

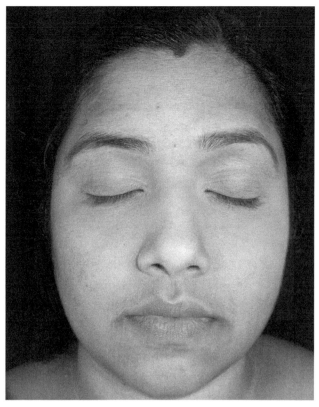

Figure 25.4   Appearance after application of foundation-based camouflage.

The advantages of DHA are that the tan is waterproof (although seawater can cause it to fade faster) and does not stain clothing. The tanning develops within a day of application and lasts for about 3–5 days

Practical Tips for Application of Self-Tanning Products

● Gently brush the skin with a soft brush prior to application to remove dead cells. This helps to ensure a uniform color. The rubbing should not be rough, to avoid Koebnerization.

● Some products such as alpha hydroxyl acids, zinc, and titanium can inactivate the DHA, so it is important to avoid topical preparations containing these chemicals prior to application of DHA.

● Excessive sweating can result in uneven pigmentation, so it should not be applied when it is very hot. The product is to be used on completely dry skin, and washing should be avoided for up to 3 hours after application.

● DHA does not have any sun protective action, so additional sunscreens need to be prescribed.

● Self-tanning products are effective mainly in people with lighter skin types, so this should be kept in mind when advising patients [1,16–18].

PERMANENT CAMOUFLAGE

Micropigmentation/cosmetic tattooing is a technique used for permanent camouflage in vitiligo, especially over the lips and the nipple area. The results of color matching are better in dark complexions and on mucous membranes [19]. Different techniques for the procedure have been described using either manual or motorized devices [20]. The advantage of cosmetic tattooing is that it is simple and cost-effective [21]; however with the advent of more effective surgical techniques for the treatment of stable vitiligo, the utility of this procedure has decreased. Although labeled as "permanent," most cases show significant fading of the pigmentation after a few years.

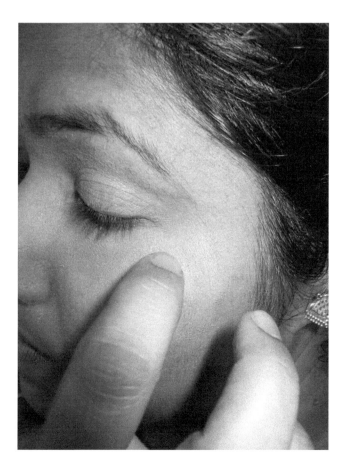

Figure 25.3   Application of camouflage cream.

In addition, the dropping down of the pigment to the dermis some-times gives the skin a bluish hue due to the Tyndall effect, which is cosmetically unpleasing. Tattooing itself has been associated with vitiligoid achromia. The possibility of Koebnerization after tattooing should also be kept in mind [22–25].

Micropigmentation requires a dermatosurgeon with good exper-tise and experience, and the patient needs to be counseled carefully regarding the expected results, both in the short and long term [1,3].

LEUKOTRICHIA

The simplest way to camouflage white hair over the patches of vit-iligo is to use normal hair dyes. Special hair colors are available for use in sensitive areas like the eyebrows and eyelashes [1].

THE ROLE OF THE DERMATOLOGIST

Dermatologists should be aware of all the camouflage products available for vitiligo. The dermatologist must be well-versed with the techniques of application and the relative advantages/disadvan-tages of different products. It is also important to know the actual chemical composition of these products, especially in the context of patients having previous allergic reactions to various cosmetics. Ideally, specialized consultations should be available for patients to educate them on camouflage techniques. Dermatology clinics should have a "camouflage therapist," a specialist who educates and helps the patient choose an appropriate color and teaches them how to apply the color to normalize their appearance [3]. Ideally, these consultations should involve a multidisciplinary team includ-ing trained nurses, camouflage specialists, and the dermatologist. Studies have shown that attendance at specialized camouflage clin-ics can improve the quality of life in vitiligo patients [10,26]. One of the primary aims must to be to train patients to effectively choose and apply the cosmetic camouflage by themselves. For children, the guardians should be trained in the process [1,14].

WHAT IS NEW?

An innovative method to prevent smudging of camouflage cream using the Cavilon™ 3M No-Sting Barrier Film (3M, St. Paul, MN) has been described. This is essentially used to protect delicate skin around stoma sites but has also been found to increase the durability of makeup by making it less water soluble. This prevented rub-off in high-friction areas such as the neckline and cuffs. It is available as a spray, containing a siliconized material, and is especially useful to swimmers due to its waterproof nature [27].

Tanioka and Miyachi have also described a technique to camouflage large areas of vitiligo by simply blurring the border of the lesion. The principle is that vitiligo is more conspicuous due to contrast with the normal skin, and blurring of this border makes the lesions less evident. It reduces the time and amount of camouflage product required. However, this is obviously more effective only in patients with a lighter skin type [28].

One of the new breakthroughs in cosmetic camouflage industry is Microskin (Microskin, Brisbane, Queensland, Australia); it is an oil- and alcohol-based cosmetic agent. It acts in two steps; first

the evaporation of the alcohol component leaves a water-resistant pigment-containing film on the skin, and second, the oil component enters the stratum corneum and helps to bind the overlying film more strongly. It lasts for a longer duration of about 1–2 days on the face and several days on the body. Color match is obtained using a computer color-matching program. It can be applied using an air-brush (for large areas) or with sponge applicators [15].

CONCLUSION

Effective camouflage can help improve the quality of life in patients with vitiligo. Foundation-based camouflage creams are the most effective preparations that can be used in vitiligo. The dermatolo-gist must be aware of the various products available for camouflage as well as the practical and technical aspects of their use.

PRACTICAL TIPS

- Cosmetic camouflage for vitiligo is something that needs proper patient guidance to be effective. During the first session it is important that the dermatologist/camouflage specialist works with the patient to choose the most suitable product and to clarify any questions the patient might have.
- Foundation-based products are the most effective camouflage products. The patient's specific needs related to occupation/life-style should be kept in mind when choosing a product.
- Always keep a complete palette of the common camouflage products in your office to help the patient choose the best color match.
- Always ask for allergies before choosing a product.
- Explain properly the procedure for removal of the products.
- For extensive areas of involvement, simply blurring the borders with the camouflage product can reduce the visual impact of the lesion and is more cost effective.
- Self-tanning products do not work well for darker skin types. Sweating during or immediately after application can lead to lesser efficacy of self-tanning products.
- For any cosmetic camouflage, avoid vigorous rubbing during application or removal to avoid Koebnerization.
- Micropigmentation is most effective on areas like the lips and areolae, but here too the patient must be counseled regarding fading/leaching of pigment with time.

REFERENCES

1. Jouary T, and DePase A. Camouflage. In: Taïeb A, and Picardo M, eds. *Vitiligo*. Berlin: Springer-Verlag; 2010, pp. 423–9.

2. Steinman DA, and Steinman HK. Skin camouflage. In: Kaminer MS, Arndt KA, and Dover JS, eds. *Atlas of Cosmetic Surgery*. Philadelphia: Saunders-Elseiver; 2009, pp. 107–16.

3. Kaliyadan F, and Kumar A. Camouflage for patients with vit-iligo. *Indian J Dermatol Venereol Leprol* 2012;78:8–15.

4. Porter J, Beuf AH, Nordlund JJ, and Lerner AB. Psychological reaction to chronic skin disorders: A study of patients with vitiligo. *Gen Hosp Psychiatry* 1979;1(1):73–7.

5. Sharma N, Koranne RV, and Singh RK. Psychiatric morbidity in psoriasis and vitiligo: A comparative study. *J Dermatol* 2001;28:419–23.

6. Pahwa P, Mehta M, Khaitan BK et al. The psychosocial impact of vitiligo in Indian patients. *Indian J Dermatol Venereol Leprol* 2013;79:679–85.

7. Picardi A, Pasquini P, Cattaruzza MS et al. Stressful life events, social support, attachment security and alexithymia in vitiligo: A case control study. *Psychother Psychosom* 2003;72:150–8.

8. Tanioka M, Yamamoto Y, Kato M, and Miyachi Y. Camouflage for patients with vitiligo vulgaris improved their quality of life. *J Cosmet Dermatol* 2010;9:72–5.

9. Levy LL, and Emer JJ. Emotional benefit of cosmetic camouflage in the treatment of facial skin conditions: Personal experience and review. *Clin Cosmet Investig Dermatol* 2012;5:173–82.

10. Holme SA, Beattie PE, and Fleming CJ. Cosmetic camouflage advice improves quality of life. *Br J Dermatol* 2002;147:946–49.

11. Ongenae K, Dierckxsens L, Brochez L et al. Quality of life and stigmatization profile in a cohort of vitiligo patients and effect of the use of camouflage. *Dermatology* 2005;210:279–85.

12. Sarveswari KN. Cosmetic camouflage in vitiligo. *Indian J Dermatol* 2010;55:211–4.

13. Sugathan P, and Najeeba R. A new camouflage for vitiligo. *Indian J Dermatol Venereol Leprol* 1991;57:45–6.

14. Antoniou C, and Stefanaki C. Cosmetic camouflage. *J Cosmet Dermatol* 2006;5:297–301.

15. Hossain C, Porto DA, Hamzavi I, and Lin HW. Camouflaging agents for vitiligo patients. *J Drugs Dermatol* 2016;15:384–7.

16. Fesq H, Brockow K, Strom K et al. Dihydroxyacetone in a new formulation—A powerful therapeutic option in vitiligo. *Dermatology.* 2001;203:241–3.

17. Rajatanavin N, Suwanachote S, and Kulkollakarn S. Dihydroxyacetone: A safe camouflaging option in vitiligo. *Int J Dermatol* 2008;47:402–6.

18. Hsu S. Camouflaging vitiligo with dihydroxyacetone. *Dermatol Online J* 2008;14:23.

19. Mahajan BB, Garg G, and Gupta RR. Evaluation of cosmetic tattooing in localised stable vitiligo. *J Dermatol* 2002;29:726–30.

20. Singal A, Thami GP, and Bhalla M. Watchmaker's pinvise for manual tattooing of vitiligo. *Dermatol Surg* 2004;30:203–4.

21. Singh AK, and Karki D. Micropigmentation: Tattooing for the treatment of lip vitiligo. *J Plast Reconstr Aesthet Surg* 2010;63:988–91.

22. Korsaga-Somé N, Barro-Traoré F, Andonaba JB et al. Vitilgoid achromia after temporary tattooing. *Int J Dermatol* 2012;51 Suppl 1:54–6, 60-2.

23. Pan H, Song W, and Xu A. A case of vitiligo induced by tattooing eyebrow. *Int J Dermatol* 2011;50:607–8.

24. Garg G, and Thami GP. Micropigmentation: Tattooing for medical purposes. *Dermatol Surg* 2005;31:928–31.

25. De Cuyper C. Permanent makeup: Indications and complications. *Clin Dermatol* 2008;26:30–4.

26. Padilla-España L, del Boz J, Ramírez-López MB, and Fernández-Sánchez ME. Camouflage therapy workshop for pediatric dermatology patients: A review of 6 cases. *Actas Dermosifiliogr* 2014;105:510–4.

27. Tanioka M, and Miyachi Y. Waterproof camouflage age for vitiligo of the face using Cavilon 3M as a spray. *Eur J Dermatol* 2008;18:93–4.

28. Tanioka M, and Miyachi Y. Camouflage for vitiligo. *Dermatol Ther* 2009;22:90–3.

SYSTEMIC TREATMENT FOR VITILIGO

Chapter 26

ORAL CORTICOSTEROIDS

Sanjeev Handa and Manju Daroach

CONTENTS

INTRODUCTION

Vitiligo is a common, idiopathic, acquired disorder of pigmentation of skin, hair, and mucosa in which there is loss of normal melanin-producing cells from the epidermis and follicular reservoirs leading to depigmented patches of skin. The etiology of vitiligo is largely unknown. Many pathogenic mechanisms have been linked to melanocyte destruction; these include autoimmune hypothesis, neural hypothesis, intrinsic defect of melanocyte adhesion, biochemical hypothesis, defective-free radical defense, deficiency of unidentified melanocyte growth factors, and some genetic factors. No single mechanism can fully explain the pathogenesis of vitiligo. The integrated convergence theories have been formulated in which environmental, biochemical, and immunological mechanisms combine in a background of genetic defect [1]. The natural course of vitiligo is its slow progression, but it may exacerbate rapidly, regress, or stabilize.

Two main goals of vitiligo treatment are, first, to halt the process of depigmentation and then to induce repigmentation. Treatments for vitiligo include topical, physical, and systemic therapies. Oral corticosteroids have been found to be the most effective method for controlling disease activity in rapidly progressive vitiligo. However, appropriate dose and duration of systemic corticosteroids must be used, as many patients have reactivation of the disease after corticosteroid withdrawal, and long-term use often leads to undesirable side effects. This chapter summarizes the current status of use of systemic corticosteroids in vitiligo.

CORTICOSTEROIDS IN VITILIGO

There is no proven curative treatment of vitiligo. As a conventional therapy, topical corticosteroids are widely used in treatment of vitiligo. Better efficacy is seen when these are combined with other therapies like topical calcipotriol, topical tacrolimus, and phototherapy. Systemic corticosteroids are currently not used as conventional therapy. However, this remains the most important medical therapy to halt the disease progression through their immunosuppressive role. Combining corticosteroids with other topical or physical modalities like phototherapy improves the efficacy rates.

MECHANISM OF ACTION OF CORTICOSTEROIDS

Glucocorticosteroids exert their effect through four mechanisms [2]

1. Classic genomic mechanism
2. Nongenomic mechanism through cytosolic glucocorticoid receptors
3. Nongenomic mechanism through membranous glucocorticoid receptors
4. Nonspecific nongenomic effect exerted by interaction with cell membranes

According to the classic genomic theory of action, glucocorticoids bind to the cytosolic glucocorticoid receptor, after which glucocorticosteroid receptor complex is formed. This complex transactivates the nucleus to produce anti-inflammatory proteins, and it also decreases the production of proinflammatory molecules by preventing the translocation of other transcription factors into the nucleus [3]. Along with the delayed genomic actions, corticosteroids also have rapid nongenomic effects [3]. These effects are exerted through second-messenger cascades, which include phospholipase C and protein kinase C [3].

Lipocortins (annexins) inhibit the activity of phospholipase A2. Phospholipase A2 releases arachidonic acid from phospholipids for production of prostanoids and leukotrienes, which produces an inflammatory response. Corticosteroids act as anti-inflammatories by stimulating the production of lipocortins. Corticosteroids also inhibit formation of interleukin-1 by inhibiting mRNA. By altering arachidonic acid metabolism and reducing interleukin-1 formation, corticosteroids produce immunosuppressive, anti-inflammatory, and anti-mitogenic effects [4,5].

Various proposed mechanisms for corticosteroids in vitiligo are as follows.

1. *Reduction of antigen-presenting cells.* In vitiligo lesions, there is increase in number of Langerhans cells. Langerhans cells have a role in antigen presentation to the immune system and provoke an immune response [6]. Corticosteroids reduce the number of these epidermal Langerhans cells. Corticosteroids also decrease Langerhans cell receptors, thereby decreasing their function of antigen presentation [5].

2. *Reduction of number of lymphocytes.* Corticosteroids decrease the lymphocytes and their antibody-dependent cell cytotoxicity [5].

There is an imbalance of cytotoxic and helper T lymphocytes in active lesions of vitiligo [7]. Also, the increased levels of soluble IL-2 receptor, Il-6, and IL-8 in vitiligo lesions indicate the role of T cells in its pathogenesis [8]. Corticosteroids decrease the number and function of lymphocytes and thus help in treating vitiligo.

3. *Reduction of synthesis of proinflammatory cytokines.* Corticosteroids are known to reduce the synthesis of proinflammatory cytokines IL-1, IL-2, IFN-γ, and TNF [5]. In vitiligo, the expression of these cytokines is greater, indicating their role in disease causation [8]. Corticosteroids, by decreasing these cytokines, suppress the vitiligo activity.

4. *Suppression of abnormal immune response.* It is hypothesized that vitiligo occurs due to abnormal immune response of body against own melanocytes. Corticosteroids due to its immunosuppressive properties help in treating and stabilizing active vitiligo.

5. *Reduction of antibody-mediated cytotoxicity.* Systemic corticosteroids suppress anti-melanocyte antibodies, thereby reducing antibody-mediated melanocyte cell toxicity [9,10].

6. *Role of bFGF and ICAM-1.* Basic fibroblast growth factor (bFGF) is a well-known melanocyte mitogen [11]. bFGF deficiency could be one of the etiological factors in the pathogenesis of vitiligo [12]. Intracellular adhesion molecule-1 (ICAM-1) is a cell surface glycoprotein which is increased in patients with active vitiligo and those with early age of onset [13]. Corticosteroids are known to decrease transcription of ICAM-1 through inhibition of NF-kβ [5].

7. *Upregulation of zinc α-2 glycoprotein.* In a study by Bagherani, it has been shown that there is decrease in level of zinc α-2 glycoprotein in lesions of vitiligo [14]. Corticosteroids are known to increase zinc α-2 glycoprotein expression and are thus effective in treating vitiligo.

INDICATIONS OF SYSTEMIC CORTICOSTEROIDS IN VITILIGO

- Systemic steroids are not indicated as first-line treatment for vitiligo. However, they are beneficial to arrest the disease progression in rapidly progressing vitiligo and also have some effect in repigmentation of lesions.
- Systemic corticosteroids are used in combination with phototherapy in unstable vitiligo.
- Systemic corticosteroids are used in patients not responding to other topical and physical therapies.

MODES OF ADMINISTERING SYSTEMIC CORTICOSTEROIDS

DAILY SYSTEMIC CORTICOSTEROIDS

Oral low-dose corticosteroids are used in vitiligo and are found to be effective in controlling disease activity in more than 80% of patients. However, daily systemic corticosteroids are less popular because of side effect profile and more risk of HPA suppression than oral minipulse (OMP) corticosteroids [15].

ORAL PULSE SYSTEMIC CORTICOSTEROIDS

Pulse therapy is defined as the administration of higher (suprapharmacologic) doses of drugs in an intermittent manner so that the therapeutic effects are enhanced and the side effects are reduced.

In vitiligo, OMP therapy is widely used [16,17]. OMP is usually given at doses of 2.5–7.5 mg per day dexamethasone or betamethasone, or 0.5–0.8 mg per kg body weight methylprednisolone on two consecutive days per week in patients with progressive disease until control of disease activity or maximum 6 months. OMP corticosteroids have been shown to stop the disease progression in rapidly progressing vitiligo but are less effective in inducing repigmentation. Side effects seen are also fewer as compared to conventional daily regimen. In a study in which 2.5 mg per day was given on two consecutive days per week, 91.8% of patients had control of disease progression achieved at mean duration of 13.1 weeks, and mean disease-free interval until relapse was 55 weeks [18]. In another study, oral dexamethasone minipulse with 10 mg per week on two consecutive days showed arrest of disease activity in 88% of patients, moderate to marked repigmentation in 16% of patients, and side effects in 69% of patients [19]. In another study, 5 mg betamethasone per day used for two consecutive days in a week, for a duration of 16 weeks, showed arrest of disease progression in 90% of patients and repigmentation of more than 10% of area in 65% of patients, while side effects occurred in 42% of patients [20].

PARENTERAL PULSE CORTICOSTEROIDS

Intravenous methylprednisolone pulse therapy has also been tried in vitiligo patients. It has been shown that this therapy halts the progression in 85% of patients and induces repigmentation in 71% of patients with progressive disease, but has a great deal less repigmentation in those with stable disease, and the side effects seen are also greater with intravenous therapy. It is contraindicated in high-risk patients and is not commonly used [21].

COMBINATION THERAPY

Studies have shown that response to treatment is better when combination therapy is used in vitiligo along with systemic steroids. In one such study, patients were divided into three groups. One group was given OMP corticosteroid alone, another group received OMP along with narrowband UVB (NB-UVB), and third group received NV-UVB alone. The combination group showed statistically significant improvement as compared to the monotherapy groups, with a decrease in markers of disease activity like ICAM-1, and increased bFGF levels [22]. In combination therapy with physical modalities, PUVA and NB-UVB both have similar efficacy when combined with OMP and have better results than OMP alone [23,24]. Combination of OMP has also been tried along with surgery for vitiligo and has shown good results [25].

ADVERSE EFFECTS RELATED TO CORTICOSTEROIDS

One of the most important limiting factors for corticosteroids is the adverse effects seen with them. Long-term use of corticosteroids can lead to osteoporosis, osteonecrosis, growth retardation, various metabolic complications like diabetes, hypertriglyceridemia, iatrogenic Cushing disease, peptic ulcer disease, menstrual irregularities, psychosis, cataract, and glaucoma.

With pulse therapy corticosteroids, side effects are less common. In a study with OMP, side effects have been seen in around 69% of patients in form of weight gain, agitation, insomnia, menstrual disturbance, acne, and hypertrichosis [19]. The most common side effect of OMP corticosteroids is weight gain. Other side effects are headache, generalized weakness, and a metallic taste in the mouth. However, HPA suppression does not occur significantly with OMP. Decreased cortisol and corticotrophin levels are seen after 48 hours of intake of drug but return to normal before next corticosteroid pulse [19].

SPECIAL SITUATIONS
PREGNANCY
Corticosteroids are considered Pregnancy Category C. Management of vitiligo in pregnancy does not differ from that in other patients.

CHILDREN

In children, immunosuppressants and psoralens are not widely used because of side effects seen with these drugs. Steroids are used in children in both topical and oral routes and have shown good results. However, in children, oral steroids can lead to serious and irreversible side effects like Cushing syndrome and premature closure of the epiphysis, which leads to stunted growth. Therefore, low-dose OMP is preferred to minimize the side effects. In children, various doses used in OMP are 0.1 mg per kg body weight for dexamethasone or 0.5–0.8 mg per kg body weight for methylprednisolone. Response rates for disease control are more than 90% [26].

MONITORING OF PATIENTS ON CORTICOSTEROIDS

Patients should be monitored closely for side effects if given treatment for more than 2 months, and there is an indication to stop corticosteroids if despite 2 months of therapy there are no signs of improvement [27].

PATTERN OF REPIGMENTATION AND LONG-TERM PROGNOSIS WITH SYSTEMIC CORTICOSTEROIDS

The pattern of repigmentation with corticosteroids is diffuse as compared to PUVA, in which the pattern of repigmentation is usually perifollicular. In vitiligo patches, it has been shown that some melanocytes still remain in the epidermis, and reactivation of these DOPA-negative melanocytes may be the cause for the diffuse type of repigmentation. When repigmentation occurs in a diffuse pattern it occurs faster, but the perifollicular type of repigmentation lasts longer, as perifollicular repigmentation occurs due to activation of stem cells in the reservoir in hair follicles [28]. The diffuse pattern has been shown to be the least stable repigmentation, so the chances of relapse are greater on stopping corticosteroids.

Long-term prognosis of vitiligo depends on many factors such as age, sex, duration of disease, ethnicity, location on the body, and extent of disease.

A better response to therapy is seen in patients with the following characteristics [15]:

- Male sex
- Children
- Disease on exposed areas, face, and thorax
- Disease of shorter duration
- Dark-skinned individuals

CONCLUSION

Systemic corticosteroids play a better role in arresting rapidly progressive vitiligo than in inducing repigmentation. OMP has advantages over other modes of administration in terms of patient compliance and side effect profile. The risk-benefit ratio should be considered in patients planned for systemic corticosteroids to avoid undesirable side effects.

REFERENCES

1. Taïeb A. Vitiligo as an inflammatory skin disorder: A therapeutic perspective. *Pigment Cell Melanoma Res* 2012;25:9–13.

2. Spies CM, Strehl C, van der Goes MC, Bijlsma JWJ, and Buttgereit F. Glucocorticoids. *Best Pract Res Clin Rheumatol* 2011;25:891–900.

3. Falkenstein E, Tillmann HC, Christ M, Feuring M, and Wehling M. Multiple actions of steroid hormones--a focus on rapid, nongenomic effects. *Pharmacol Rev* 2000;52:513–56.

4. Kragballe K. Topical corticosteroids: Mechanisms of action. *Acta Derm Venereol Suppl (Stockh)* 1989;151:7–10; discussion 47–52.

5. Wolverton SE. *Comprehensive Dermatologic Drug Therapy.* 3rd ed. Elsevier Saunders; 2013.

6. Kao CH, Yu HS. Depletion and repopulation of Langerhans cells in nonsegmental type vitiligo. *J Dermatol* 1990;17:287–96.

7. Pichler R, Sfetsos K, Badics B, Gutenbrunner S, Berg J, and Auböck J. Lymphocyte imbalance in vitiligo patients indicated by elevated CD4+/CD8+ T-cell ratio. *Wien Med Wochenschr* 2009;159:337–41.

8. Mandelcorn-Monson RL, Shear NH, Yau E et al. Cytotoxic T lymphocyte reactivity to gp100, MelanA/MART-1, and tyrosinase, in HLA-A2-positive vitiligo patients. *J Invest Dermatol* 2003;121:550–6.

9. Hann SK, Kim H Il, Im S, Park YK, Cui J, and Bystryn JC. The change of melanocyte cytotoxicity after systemic steroid treatment in vitiligo patients. *J Dermatol Sci* 1993;6:201–5.

10. Hann S-K, Chen D, and Bystryn J-C. Systemic steroids suppress antimelanocyte antibodies in vitiligo. *J Cutan Med Surg* 1997;1.

11. Wu CS, Yu CL, Wu CS, Lan CCE, and Yu HS. Narrow-band ultraviolet-B stimulates proliferation and migration of cultured melanocytes. *Exp Dermatol* 2004;13:755–63.

12. Seif El Nasr H, Shaker OG, Fawzi MMT, and El-Hanafi G. Basic fibroblast growth factor and tumour necrosis factor alpha in vitiligo and other hypopigmented disorders: Suggestive possible therapeutic targets. *Eur Acad Dermatol Venereol J* 2013;27:103–8.

13. Laddha NC, Dwivedi M, Gani AR, Mansuri MS, and Begum R. Tumor necrosis factor B (TNFB) genetic variants and its increased expression are associated with vitiligo susceptibility. *PLOS ONE* 2013;8.

14. Bagherani N. The newest hypothesis about vitiligo: Most of the suggested pathogeneses of vitiligo can be attributed to lack of one factor, zinc-α2–glycoprotein. *ISRN Dermatol* 2012;2012:405268.

15. Kim SM, Lee HS, and Hann SK. The efficacy of low-dose oral corticosteroids in the treatment of vitiligo patients. *Int J Dermatol* 1999;38:546–50.

16. Pasricha JS, and Srivastava G. Cure in pemphigus a possibility. *Indian J Dermatol Venereol Leprol* 1986;52:185–6.

17. Pasricha JS, and Khaitan BK. Oral mini pulse therapy with betamethasone in vitiligo patients having extensive or fast spreading disease. *Int J Dermatol* 1993;32:753–7.

18. Kanwar AJ, Mahajan R, and Parsad D. Low-dose oral minipulse dexamethasone therapy in progressive unstable vitiligo. *J Cutan Med Surg* 2013;17:259–68.

19. Radakovic-Fijan S, Fürnsinn-Friedl AM, Hönigsmann H, and Tanew A. Oral dexamethasone pulse treatment for vitiligo. *J Am Acad Dermatol* 2001;44:814–7.

20. Goldsmith LA, Katz SI, Gilchrest BA, Paller AS, Leffell DJ, and Wolff K. *Fitzpatrick's Dermatology in General Medicine.* 8th ed. McGraw Hill; 2012; 150:22.

21. Seiter S, Ugurel S, Tilgen W, and Reinhold U. Use of high-dose methylprednisolone pulse therapy in patients with progressive and stable vitiligo. *Int J Dermatol* 2000;39(8):624–7.

22. El Mofty M, Essmat S, Youssef R et al. The role of systemic steroids and phototherapy in the treatment of stable vitiligo: A randomized controlled trial. *Dermatol Ther* 2016;29:406–12.

23. Agarwal A, Nath J, and Barua KN. Twice weekly 5 mg beta-methasone oral pulse therapy in the treatment of alopecia areata. *J Eur Acad Dermatol Venereol* 2006;20:1375–6.

24. Lee J, Chu H, Lee H, Kim M, Kim DS, and Oh SH. A ret-rospective study of methylprednisolone mini-pulse therapy combined with narrow-band UVB in non-segmental vitiligo. *Dermatology* 2016;232:224–9.

25. Mulekar SV. Stable vitiligo treated by a combination of low-dose oral pulse betamethasone and autologous, noncultured melanocyte-keratinocyte cell transplantation. *Dermatologic Surg* 2006;32:536–41.

26. Majid I, Masood Q, Hassan I, Khan D, and Chisti M. Childhood vitiligo: Response to methylprednisolone oral minipulse therapy and topical fluticasone combination. *Indian J Dermatol* 2009;54:124–7.

27. Mahmoud BH, Hexsel CL, and Hamzavi IH. An update on new and emerging options for the treatment of vitiligo. *Skin Therapy Lett* 2008;13:1–6.

28. Parsad D, Pandhi R, Dogra S, and Kumar B. Clinical study of repigmentation patterns with different treatment modalities and their correlation with speed and stability of repigmentation in 352 vitiliginous patches. *J Am Acad Dermatol* 2004;50:63–7.

Chapter 27

OTHER IMMUNOSUPPRESSIVE AGENTS IN VITILIGO

Sanjeev Handa and Manju Daroach

CONTENTS

INTRODUCTION

Vitiligo is a chronic autoimmune skin disease leading to depigmentation in otherwise normal skin. It is often associated with other autoimmune disorders and has an unpredictable course. The average age of presentation is 20 years, although it may develop in children also [1]. The disease is familial in about 18% of cases [2]. Vitiligo has a great psychological impact on patients' quality of life. They suffer the social and emotional consequences of low self-esteem, anxiety, depression, and stigmatization [3].

Treatment of vitiligo includes topical, systemic, physical, and surgical modalities [4]. The modalities may focus on any or all of the following: stopping the progression of disease, repigmentation of lesions, and prevention of relapse [5].

No single treatment is proven to completely cure the disease. Medical treatments alone or in combination with phototherapy are key approaches in treatment of vitiligo. Topical corticosteroids are common first-line and adjunctive therapies [6]. Medical therapies for halting the disease progression include systemic corticosteroids, methotrexate, minocycline, and antioxidants, while topical agents like steroids, calcineurin inhibitors, and vitamin D analogs are beneficial in repigmentation of lesions. Phototherapy is effective in halting progression of the disease and repigmentation of lesions as well [5,7].

TREATMENT ALGORITHMS PROPOSED FOR VITILIGO

Segmental vitiligo: A medical approach, including topical steroids and topical calcineurin inhibitors, is the first-line therapy. Surgical treatment can be planned as first-line therapy in stable disease or after trying medical therapy [5].

Nonsegmental vitiligo: If active ongoing depigmentation exists, phototherapy and/or systemic corticosteroids should be considered. In inactive localized disease, topical steroids and/or calcineurin inhibitors are preferred. In inactive widespread disease, phototherapy alone or in combination should be considered. In widespread disease, depigmentation of left-out pigment specks can be considered.

This chapter summarizes the use of systemic immunosuppressants other than corticosteroids in vitiligo. Data available for these therapies are very limited. No randomized controlled trials are available with these agents in vitiligo. Data are present in the form of limited case reports or studies only. When systemic corticosteroids are contraindicated, use of these therapies can be considered in active disease.

Various immunosuppressive therapies discussed in this chapter include:

1. Methotrexate
2. Azathioprine
3. Cyclosporine
4. Janus kinase inhibitors
5. Biologics

METHOTREXATE

Methotrexate is an antimetabolite, antifolate immunosuppressant drug which acts by inhibiting conversion of dihydrofolate to tetrahydrofolate by binding to dihydrofolate reductase enzyme. Methotrexate possibly suppresses tumor necrosis factor-alpha (TNF-α) production by suppressing T cells. It has been used in autoimmune disorders, cancers, psoriasis, and psoriatic arthritis, in addition to other dermatologic conditions such as vasculitis, mycosis fungoides, and immunobullous and proliferative disorders. There are a few conflicting reports of its use in vitiligo.

An initial documentation of the use of methotrexate comes from a case report in a 54-year-old female with rheumatoid arthritis and rapidly progressive vitiligo. She was given a 7.5-mg/week dose of methotrexate for her arthritis. After 3 months of methotrexate, not only did her new lesions of vitiligo stop, but she also had repigmentation of her lesions [8].

In a case study including six vitiligo patients with body surface area involvement of more than 6%, methotrexate was given at a dose of 25 mg/week for 6 months. No repigmentation was seen in the patients at the end of 6 months of treatment, showing lack of its efficacy in the treatment vitiligo [9].

In another larger study of 50 vitiligo patients, methotrexate was compared with oral minipulse steroids. Twenty-five patients received methotrexate at a dose of 10 mg/week and the rest received oral minipulse steroids. At the end of 6 months, disease stabilization was seen in 76% of patients in the methotrexate group and in 72% in the oral minipulse steroid group. Repigmentation was seen in both groups. The pattern of repigmentation was diffuse in 64% of patients, perifollicular in 20%, and combined in 8% of patients. No serious side effects were seen in any of the patients [10].

AZATHIOPRINE

Azathioprine is an immunosuppressive agent which is widely used in autoimmune disorders. It has a good safety profile and is also more cost effective. Its use in vitiligo is limited. It has been tried as combination therapy with oral PUVA and compared with oral PUVA therapy alone. Azathioprine was given at a dose of 0.6–0.75 mg/kg (max dose 50 mg per dose). After a follow-up for 4 months, 58.4% body surface repigmentation was seen in the azathioprine and PUVA therapy combination group, while only 28.4% repigmentation was seen in the PUVA therapy only group. Repigmentation of the acral areas was better in the azathioprine only group while perifollicular repigmentation was earlier in the azathioprine and PUVA combination group. Two patients developed gastric upset while on azathioprine. This was the only side effect seen [11].

CYCLOSPORINE

Cyclosporine (CsA) is a calcineurin inhibitor that acts selectively on T cells and has been routinely used in preventing organ transplant rejection. It has been used in preventing perilesional halo and achieving uniform repigmentation in vitiligo post-surgery. In a recent study involving 50 patients of stable vitiligo who underwent autologous melanocyte–keratinocyte cell transplant surgery, 25 patients were given CsA at a dose of 3 mg/kg for 3 weeks post-surgery followed by 1.5 mg/kg for the next 6 weeks. Another group of 25 patients were not given any oral or topical treatment. In the CsA group, all the patients achieved more than 75% repigmentation, while in the other group only 28% of patients achieved more than 75% repigmentation. The mechanism behind perilesional halo involves destruction of autologous melanocytes by CD8+ T cells. CsA inhibits these perilesional CD8+ T cells and thus has a role in bringing about uniform pigmentation post-surgery. Side effects seen in this study were minor, including nausea, vomiting, transient rise in blood pressure, and headache [12].

JANUS KINASE INHIBITORS

Janus kinase (JAK) inhibitors (JAK1/3 inhibitor tofacitinib and JAK 1/2 inhibitor ruxolitinib) act as immunosuppressants. Their use in vitiligo is limited to case reports.

Tofacitinib is US Food and Drug Administration (FDA)-approved for rheumatoid arthritis and is used off-label for alopecia areata and plaque psoriasis. In vitiligo, it was given to a female who was refractory to other topical and physical therapies at a dose of 5 mg every other day for 2 months and then increased to 5 mg per day. At 2 months, repigmentation started on the face and upper limb, and it was complete at 5 months, while partial repigmentation was seen at other sites. No side effects were observed in this patient [13]. Recent advances in the understanding of the pathogenesis of vitiligo support the use of JAK inhibitors for this condition. It has been proposed that because interferon-gamma (IFN-g) signal transduction occurs through the JAK pathway, the use of the JAK 1/3 inhibitor tofacitinib effectively blocks IFN-g signaling and downstream CXCL10 expression, thus giving rise to repigmentation in vitiligo [13].

Ruxolitinib is a potent small-molecule JAK inhibitor approved by the FDA for the treatment of intermediate or high-risk myelofibrosis and polycythemia vera. It was used in a patient with coexistent alopecia areata and vitiligo at a dose of 20 mg/day. At week 12 the patient started having repigmentation of the skin, which increased at 20 weeks along with hair regrowth [14]. Ruxolitinib interferes with IFN-g signaling. CXCL10 is an IFN-g-induced chemokine and is critical for auto reactive T-cell recruitment to the skin during the progression and maintenance of vitiligo, and the authors hypothesized that targeting the IFN-g CXCL10 cytokine axis might be an effective treatment by reducing the production of CXCL10 [14].

CYCLOPHOSPHAMIDE

Cyclophosphamide is a cytotoxic drug which acts by alkylation and DNA cross-linking, and also suppresses the suppressor T cells. In an early single study, twice-daily oral cyclophosphamide (50 mg) was given to patients. Twenty-nine patients demonstrated repigmentation, with good results in the difficult-to-treat areas like acral sites. Significant side effects were reported in this study [15].

BIOLOGICS

RITUXIMAB
Rituximab has been used in five patients with active and generalized vitiligo. They were given 1 g single IV infusion of rituximab and followed up for 6 months. Of them, three patients showed an overt clinical and histological improvement of disease [16]. Rituximab is proposed to act via suppressing B-cell antibody response.

ANTI-TNF-α INHIBITORS
TNF-α is proposed to be involved in the pathogenesis of vitiligo [17]. TNF-α potentially plays both a harmful and a protective role in vitiligo, by activating the cytotoxic T cells that are detrimental to melanocytes and stimulating T regs, respectively [18]. On this basis, etanercept, which is a TNF-α inhibitor, was used in two patients. At 6 months follow-up there was complete response [17]. In another study including six patients with progressive vitiligo, infliximab, etanercept, or adalimumab were tried. The patient receiving infliximab reported worsening of the disease while other patients reported improvement and no relapse even after 6 months of cessation of treatment [19]. Of four men treated with etanercept in another study, improvement was seen at 16 weeks of treatment [18]. There are as of today no recommendations for the use of biologics in vitiligo since the evidence is very limited.

REFERENCES

1. Nordlund JJ, and Majumder PP. Recent investigations on vitiligo vulgaris. *Dermatol Clin* 1997;15:69–78.

2. Mason CP, and Gawkrodger DJ. Vitiligo presentation in adults. *Clin Exp Dermatol* 2005;30:344–5.

3. Papadopoulos L, Bor R, and Legg C. Coping with the disfiguring effects of vitiligo: A preliminary investigation into the effects of cognitive-behavioural therapy. *Br J Med Psychol* 1999;72:385–96.

4. Rodrigues M, Ezzedine K, Hamzavi I, Pandya AG, and Harris JE. Current and emerging treatments for vitiligo. *J Am Acad Dermatol* 2017;77:17–29.

5. Passeron T. Medical and maintenance treatments for vitiligo. *Dermatol Clin* 2017;35:163–70.

6. Alikhan A, Felsten LM, Daly M, and Petronic-Rosic V. Vitiligo: A comprehensive overview. *J Am Acad Dermatol* 2011;65:473–91.

7. Gawkrodger DJ, Ormerod AD, Shaw L et al. Guideline for the diagnosis and management of vitiligo. *Br J Dermatol* 2008;159:1051–76.

8. Sandra A, Pai S, and Shenoi SD. Unstable vitiligo responding to methotrexate. *Indian J Dermatol* 1998;64:309.

9. AlGhamdi K, and Huma K. Methotrexate for the treatment of generalized vitiligo. *Saudi Pharm J* 2013;21:423–4.

10. Singh H, Kumaran MS, Bains A, and Parsad D. A randomized comparative study of oral corticosteroid minipulse and low-dose oral methotrexate in the treatment of unstable vitiligo. *Dermatology* 2015;231:286–90.

11. Radmanesh M, and Saedi K. The efficacy of combined PUVA and low-dose azathioprine for early and enhanced repigmentation in vitiligo patients. *J Dermatolog Treat* 2006;17:151–3.

12. Mutalik S, Shah S, Sidwadkar V, and Khoja M. Efficacy of cyclosporine after autologous noncultured melanocyte transplantation in localized stable vitiligo—A pilot, open label, comparative study. *Dermatol Surg* 2017;43.

13. Craiglow BG, and King BA. Tofacitinib citrate for the treatment of vitiligo: A pathogenesis-directed therapy. *JAMA Dermatol* 2015;151:11–3.

14. Mackay-Wiggan J, Jabbari A, Nguyen N et al. Oral ruxolitinib induces hair regrowth in patients with moderate-to-severe alopecia areata. *JCI Insight* 2016;1:e89790.

15. Gokhale BB. Cyclophosphamide and vitiligo. *Int J Dermatol* 1979;18:92.

16. Ruiz-Argüelles A, García-Carrasco M, Jimenez-Brito G et al. Treatment of vitiligo with a chimeric monoclonal antibody to CD20: A pilot study. *Clin Exp Immunol* 2013;174:229–36.

17. Kim NH, Torchia D, Rouhani P, Roberts B, and Romanelli P. Tumor necrosis factor-α in vitiligo: Direct correlation between tissue levels and clinical parameters. *Cutan Ocul Toxicol* 2011;30:225–7.

18. Webb KC, Tung R, Winterfield LS et al. Tumour necrosis factor-α inhibition can stabilize disease in progressive vitiligo. *Br J Dermatol* 2015;173:641–50.

19. Alghamdi KM, Khurrum H, Taieb A, Ezzedine K. Treatment of generalized vitiligo with anti-TNF-α agents. *J Drugs Dermatol* 2012;11:534–9.

Chapter 28

ROLE OF ANTIOXIDANTS IN VITILIGO

Mehmet Yildirim, Selma Korkmaz, and İjlal Erturan

CONTENTS

INTRODUCTION

Vitiligo is an acquired depigmenting disorder which is characterized by loss of epidermal melanocytes because of multifactorial and overlapping pathogenetic mechanisms. It affects approximately 1% of the world population. Although it is usually asymptomatic, the psychosocial effect of vitiligo can be severe [1].

The etiology of vitiligo is still not clear, although many mechanisms have been implicated. The generally accepted idea is that the loss of melanocytes results in the development of depigmentation of the skin. It is considered that intrinsic factors such as autoimmunity, genetic mutations, self-destruction of melanocytes, disorders involved in the migration and proliferation of melanocytes, and oxidative stress and extrinsic factors including toxic compounds, infectious agents, and Koebnerization have roles in the onset and progression of the disease [2].

It has been suggested that one of the most important factors that play a role in the pathogenesis of vitiligo is impairment of the balance between oxidative stress and the oxidant antioxidant system [3–5]. During the production of melanin from melanocytes, reactive oxygen species (ROS) are formed as toxic intermediates. Overproduction of ROS causes damage to melanocytes and the antioxidant system that protects melanocytes. Studies have shown that oxidative stress is increased in vitiligo and there are negative effects on the antioxidant defense system [2,6,7].

OXIDANT AND ANTIOXIDANT SYSTEMS

Reactive oxygen species are atoms or molecules that contain unpaired electrons in natural metabolic processes. These molecules are short lived and have the ability to chemically induce cellular damage. In addition to being formed due to exogenous factors such as UV and chemicals, ROS are also produced under certain pathogenic conditions including cancer, inflammation, and stress. However, ROS produced by regular activities of the body are removed by the antioxidant defense systems. The impairment of this balance leads to increased ROS and cell damage, a process called oxidative stress, which damages nucleic acids, lipids, and proteins in the body, leading to cell death or mutations. Damage caused by ROS in the body can be reversed by antioxidant mechanisms. To prevent oxidative damage during natural metabolic processes in the body, oxidant and antioxidant systems need to be maintained in balance. Effective antioxidant should be sufficient in tissues and body fluids and it should be eliminate the negative effects of ROS [4,8].

Antioxidant mechanisms involved in organisms are composed of enzymatic and non-enzymatic micro- and macromolecules (Table 28.1). Enzymes such as superoxide dismutase (SOD), catalase (CAT), and glutathione peroxidase (GPx) are examples of enzymatic antioxidants. It is known that non-enzymatic molecules such as vitamins, polyphenols, carotenoids, transferrin, ferritin, bilirubin, thiol-containing compounds, and coenzyme Q also have antioxidant properties and are synthesized and released at an increased level during oxidative stress [9,10].

VITILIGO AND OXIDATIVE STRESS

The skin is the largest organ of the body and is in constant interaction with the external environment. Melanocytes are adversely affected by the overproduction of ROS due to their specific tasks such as melanin synthesis [4,11]. Tyrosinase, a rate-limiting enzyme converting tyrosine to DOPA, that results in the formation of Dopaquinone which is intermediate product in melanin synthesis. The activity of tyrosinase decreases with increased levels of ROS. Excessive accumulation of ROS caused by chemical or physical stimuli in the epidermis of vitiligo patients results in lipid, protein, and DNA damage and increases apoptosis in melanocytes, followed by the destruction of melanocytes [11].

Studies have shown that oxidative stress markers such as malondialdehyde (MDA) and the total oxidant status (TOS) are elevated in tissue

Table 28.1 Enzymatic and non-enzymatic antioxidants

Enzymatic antioxidants	Non-enzymatic antioxidants
SOD	Vitamins (vitamins A, E, and C)
Catalase	Polyphenols
Glutathione peroxidase	Carotenoids (β-carotene, α-carotene, lycopene) Transferrin Ferritin Bilirubin Uric acid Selenium Glutathione Koenzim Q Thiol-containing compounds (N-acetyl cysteine)

and blood samples of vitiligo patients. Studies conducted in recent years have reported that ROS accumulate in the skin of vitiligo patients as a result of oxidative stress. In particular, hydrogen peroxide (H_2O_2) has been found to play a major role in the onset and progression of vitiligo. It is also considered that low concentrations of H_2O_2 play a role in the regulation of human pigmentation by increasing melanin synthesis and transferring melanosomes to keratinocytes. However, it has been suggested that high concentrations of H_2O_2 suppress these mechanisms and affect melanocytes, leading to the development of vitiligo [1,12].

These findings support the theory that melanocytes and even antioxidant defense systems in vitiligo may have oxidative damage [11]. However, the molecular roles of oxidant and antioxidant systems in the etiopathogenesis of vitiligo are still under investigation [8,13,14]. Many studies in the literature have examined oxidative stress and antioxidant parameters in vitiligo by measuring the serum or tissue levels of CAT, SOD, glutathione, and GPx. These studies have been conducted on clinical subtypes such as generalized and localized forms of the disease, and some have also evaluated the activation of the disease.

When studies conducted with generalized vitiligo patients are examined, it is observed that in these patients the oxidative stress parameters are increased while the antioxidant system parameters are decreased. Yildirim et al. examined the levels of MDA, SOD, and GPx in vitiligo tissues and found them to be significantly higher compared to healthy controls [7]. In another study, serum GPx levels were reported to be significantly lower in generalized vitiligo patients than in the control group [15]. Furthermore, in patients with active localized vitiligo, the plasma MDA and SOD levels were significantly higher and CAT activities were significantly lower compared to the healthy controls [16]. In other studies that evaluated the localized and generalized vitiligo cases together, the serum MDA, TOS, and oxidative stress index (OSI) levels were reported to be significantly higher, and the levels of SOD, GPx, vitamin C, and vitamin E were significantly lower [2,16]. Also, in a study evaluating the association of antioxidants with disease activity, the SOD, GPx, and MDA levels were found to be significantly higher, and the CAT levels were significantly lower in patients with active vitiligo [6]. These results suggest that changes in oxidant and antioxidant parameters may play a role in the activation of the disease rather than vitiligo types.

THE ROLE OF ANTIOXIDANTS IN THE TREATMENT OF VITILIGO

The increased oxidative stress markers and the reduction of antioxidant mechanisms reported in many studies conducted with vitiligo patients have led researchers to consider the possibility of supplementing vitiligo treatment with antioxidants to reduce oxidative stress. Review of the literature shows that various antioxidants have been administered either alone or in combination with other conventional treatments (Table 28.2).

Table 28.2 Clinical trials involving antioxidant treatments in vitiligo

Study/year	Study design	Treatment	Number of subjects	Clinical characteristics of vitiligo	Comments
Soliman et al. [21] 2016	Prospective, comparative, randomized	Excimer light 2 × week 24 sessions, ± antioxidant hydrogel	30	Localized	Topical antioxidant and excimer light effective therapy for localized vitiligo
Dell'Anna et al. [18] 2007	Randomized, placebo-controlled	NB-UVB, 2 × week, ±2 tablets of oral antioxidants (containing α-lipoic acid, vitamin C, vitamin E, polyunsaturated fatty acids)	35	Generalized	Oral supplementation with antioxidants during NB-UVB significantly improves the clinical effectiveness of NB-UVB
Elgoeini et al. [19] 2009	Randomized, placebo-controlled	NB-UVB, 3 × week ±400 IU/day of vitamin E one a day	20	Stable disease	Oral vitamin E may represent a valuable adjuvant therapy, increasing the effectiveness of NB-UVB
Parsad et al. [26] 2003	Randomized, double blind, controlled	Ginkgo biloba 40 mg 3 × day	47	Localized and acrofacial	Gingko biloba extract seems to be a safe and fairly effective therapy for vitiligo
Szczurko et al. [25] 2011	Prospective, open-label, non-randomized, uncontrolled	60 mg Ginkgo biloba 2 × day	12	Progressive disease ($n=7$) Non progressive disease ($n=5$)	Gingko biloba seems to be effective for vitiligo treatment
Middelkamp-Hup et al. [29] 2004	Randomized, placebo-controlled	NB-UVB 2 × week ±3 tablets daily of oral *Polypodium leucotomos* for 26 wk	50		*P. leucotomos* showed a trend toward more repigmentation in all four body areas, most prominent in head and neck
Bakis-Petsoglou et al. [28] 2010	Randomize, double blind	NB-UVB 3 × week × 24 wk + pseudocatalase cream or placebo	32	Active disease	No statistical significance was found between combination pseudocatalase dismutase and NB-UVB vs NB-UVB and placebo

The most commonly used systemic antioxidants in vitiligo treatment are vitamins A, C, and E and minerals such as selenium and zinc. In the study by Colucci et al., phototherapy and topical treatments of nonsegmental vitiligo patients were supplemented with 10 mg/day vitamin E and 4.7 mg carotenoids three times a day for 6 months. The authors reported significantly increased repigmentation in the antioxidant group compared to the control group, whereas erythema and inflammation were higher, and the disease progressed rapidly in the control group [17]. In another study in nonsegmental vitiligo cases, one group received narrowband UVB (NB-UVB) phototherapy (placebo group) while the phototherapy of the other group was supplemented with oral tablets containing α-lipoic acid, vitamin C, and vitamin E twice a day for 8 weeks. In the oral antioxidant group, the increase in repigmentation was clinically significant compared to the placebo group. Furthermore, in the oral antioxidant group, after 2 months of treatment, the CAT activity significantly increased and H_2O_2, an oxidative stress marker, significantly decreased compared to the placebo controls [18]. Similarly, Elgoweini et al. treated one group of vitiligo patients with only NB-UVB while supplementing the other group with vitamin E in addition to UVB. The authors reported a significant increase in the level of repigmentation and a significant decrease in the MDA level in the antioxidant group [19]. In contrast, Jayanth et al. evaluated the combined use of vitamin C, vitamin E, beta carotene, selenium, zinc, copper, and manganese with photochemotherapy and did not observe a significant difference between the control group and the combined treatment group [20]. In another study, a group of vitiligo patients received 308-nm excimer light alone, and the other group was treated with topical hydrogel containing antioxidant enzyme and minerals along with the excimer light treatment. Higher repigmentation was reported in antioxidant group compared to the control group [21].

Jalel et al. reported that minerals such as zinc and selenium provided high repigmentation (70%) in mouse models with vitiligo similar to antioxidant vitamins [22]. In a similar study, topical corticosteroids were supplemented with 440 mg/day systemic zinc and the clinical responses were found to be higher in the combined treatment group compared to the control patients, although the difference between the two groups was statistically insignificant [23].

Topical preparations containing CAT/SOD and ginkgo biloba are among vitiligo treatment options due to their immunomodulator, anti-inflammatory, and antioxidant effects [12,24]. For example, Szczurko et al. administered 120 mg/day ginkgo biloba to vitiligo patients for 12 weeks and found that their post-treatment vitiligo area scoring index (VASI) was significantly reduced and the total area of vitiligo lesions decreased [25]. Similarly, Parsad et al. reported successful outcomes in localized/acrofacial vitiligo cases following 120 mg/day gingko biloba treatment [26]. However, there are contradicting reports about the therapeutic effects of pseudo-catalase on vitiligo, another group of antioxidant enzymes. In their study to evaluate patients with bilateral vitiligo lesions, Naini et al. treated one group of patients with a pseudocatalase/SOD gel and the other group with a placebo gel for 6 months. The authors reported no significant differences between the two groups in terms of their perifollicular pigmentation scores evaluated at 2-month intervals [27]. Similarly, in another randomized placebo-controlled study, it was reported that there was no significant difference in terms of repigmentation in the active vitiligo group using cream to the face twice a day with three sessions/week of NB-UVB therapy for 24 weeks compared to placebo [28].

Polypodium leucotomos extract with antioxidant, immunomodulatory properties and polyphenol content has also been shown to have clinical benefits for vitiligo treatment. Middelkamp-Hup et al. applied NB-UVB and oral *P. leucotomos* in one group and NB-UVB

and a 250-mg placebo capsule three times a day for the other group. They reported statistically significantly higher percentages of repigmentation in the *P. leucotomos* group, particularly in the head and neck areas [29].

CONCLUSION

Although there are some discrepancies between the results of the studies mentioned previously, it has demonstrated that oxidative stress is generally increased, and the antioxidant system does not function properly in vitiligo. This imbalance between the oxidant and antioxidant systems may play a role in the pathogenesis of vitiligo. It has also been observed that supplementing vitiligo treatment with antioxidants results in increased treatment efficacy. Since oxidants and antioxidants are effective in physiological and pathological processes, the balance between these two systems is important. However, despite the availability of findings regarding the role of oxidants, antioxidants, and cytokines in the pathogenesis of vitiligo, the biomolecular mechanisms of these processes are still not fully understood. Therefore, there is a need for future work to further elucidate this mechanism.

REFERENCES

1. Glassman SJ. Vitiligo, reactive oxygen species and T-cells. *Clin Sci (Lond)* 2011;120(3):99–120.

2. Akoglu G, Emre S, Metin A et al. Evaluation of total oxidant and antioxidant status in localized and generalized vitiligo. *Clin Exp Dermatol* 2013;38(7):701–6.

3. Dell'anna ML, and Picardo M. A review and a new hypothesis for non-immunological pathogenetic mechanisms in vitiligo. *Pigment Cell Res* 2006;19:406–11.

4. Qiao Z, Wang X, Xiang L, and Zhang C. Dysfunction of autophagy: A possible mechanism involved in the pathogenesis of vitiligo by breaking the redox balance of melanocytes. *Oxid Med Cell Longev* 2016;2016:3401570.

5. Shajil EM, and Begum R. Antioxidant status of segmental and non-segmental vitiligo. *Pigment Cell Res* 2006;19(2):179–80.

6. Dammak I, Boudaya S, Ben Abdallah F et al. Antioxidant enzymes and lipid peroxidation at the tissue level in patients with stable and active vitiligo. *Int J Dermatol* 2009;48(5):476–80.

7. Yildirim M, Baysal V, Inaloz HS, and Can M. The role of oxidants and antioxidants in generalized vitiligo at tissue level. *J ur Acad Dermatol Venereol* 2004;18(6):683–6.

8. Xie H, Zhou F, Liu L, Zhu G, Li Q, Li C, and Gao T. Vitiligo: How do oxidative stress-induced autoantigens trigger autoimmunity? *J Dermatol Sci* 2016;81(1):3–9.

9. Lü JM, Lin PH, Yao Q, and Chen C. Chemical and molecular mechanisms of antioxidants: Experimental approaches and model systems. *J Cell Mol Med* 2010;14(4);840–60.

10. Rahal A, Kumar A, Singh V, Yadav B, Tiwari R, Chakraborty S, and Dhama K. Oxidative stress, prooxidants, and antioxidants: The interplay. *Biomed Res Int* 2014;2014:761264.

11. Denat L, Kadekaro AL, Marrot L, Leachman SA, and Abdel-Malek ZA. Melanocytes as instigators and victims of oxidative stress. *J Invest Dermatol* 2014;134:(6)1512–8.

12. Khan R, Satyam A, Gupta S, Sharma VK, and Sharma A. Circulatory levels of antioxidants and lipid peroxidation in Indian patients with generalized and localized vitiligo. *Arch Dermatol Res* 2009;301(10):731–7.

13. Zhang Y, Liu L, Jin L, Yi X, Dang E, Yang Y, Li C, and Gao T. Oxidative stress-induced calreticulin expression and translocation: New insights into the destruction of melanocytes. *J Invest Dermatol* 2014;134(1):183–91.

14. Laddha NC, Dwivedi M, Mansuri MS, Gani AR, Ansarullah M, Ramachandran AV, Dalai S, and Begum R. Vitiligo: Interplay between oxidative stress and immune system. *Exp Dermatol* 2013;22(4):245–50.

15. Beazley WD, Gaze D, Panske A, Panzig E, and Schallreuter KU. Serum selenium levels and blood glutathione peroxidase activities in vitiligo. *Br J Dermatol* 1999;141(1):301–3.

16. Arian O, and Kurutas EB. Oxidative stress in the blood of patients with active localized vitiligo. *Acta Dermatovenerol Alp Pannonica Adriat* 2008;17(1):12–6.

17. Colucci R, Dragoni F, Conti R, Pisaneschi L, Lazzeri L, and Moretti S. Evaluation of an oral supplement containing Phyllanthus emblica fruit extracts, vitamin E, and carotenoids in vitiligo treatment. *Dermatol Ther* 2015;28(1):17–21.

18. Dell'Anna ML, Mastrofrancesco A, Sala R et al. Antioxidants and narrow band-UVB in the treatment of vitiligo: A double-blind placebo controlled trial. *Clin Exp Dermatol* 2007;32(6):631–6.

19. Elgoweini M, Nour El, and Din N. Response of vitiligo to narrowband ultraviolet B and oral antioxidants. *J Clin Pharmacol* 2009;49(7):852–5.

20. Jayanth DP, Pai BS, Shenoi SD, and Balachandran C. Efficacy of antioxidants as an adjunct to photochemotherapy in vitiligo: A case study of 30 patients. *Indian J Dermatol Venereol Leprol* 2002;68(4):202–5.

21. Soliman M, Samy NA, Abo Eittah M, and Hegazy M. Comparative study between excimer light and topical antioxidant versus excimer light alone for treatment of vitiligo. *J Cosmet Laser Ther* 2016;18(1):7–11.

22. Jalel A, Soumaya GS, and Hamdaoui MH. Vitiligo treatment with vitamins, minerals and polyphenol supplementation. *Indian J Dermatol* 2009;54(4):357–60.

23. Yaghoobi R, Omidian M, and Bagherani N. Comparison of therapeutic efficacy of topical corticosteroid and oral zinc sulfate-topical corticosteroid combination in the treatment of vitiligo patients: A clinical trial. *BMC Dermatol* 2011;11:7.

24. Colucci R, Lotti T, and Moretti S. Vitiligo: An update on current pharmacotherapy and future directions. *Expert Opin Pharmacother* 2012;13(3):1885–99.

25. Szczurko O, Shear N, Taddio A, and Boon H. Ginkgo biloba for the treatment of vitiligo vulgaris: An open label pilot clinical trial. *BMC Complement Altern Med* 2011;11:21.

26. Parsad D, Pandhi R, and Juneja A. Effectiveness of oral Ginkgo biloba in treating limited, slowly spreading vitiligo. *Clin Exp Dermatol* 2003;28(3):285–7.

27. Naini FF, Shooshtari AV, Ebrahimi B, and Molaei R. The effect of pseudocatalase/superoxide dismutase in the treatment of vitiligo: A pilot study. *J Res Pharm Pract* 2012;1(2):77–80.

28. Bakis-Petsoglou S, Le Guay JL, and Wittal R. A randomized, double-blinded, placebo-controlled trial of pseudocatalase cream and narrowband ultraviolet B in the treatment of vitiligo. *Br J Dermatol* 2009;161(4):910–7.

29. Middelkamp-Hup MA, Bos JD, Rius-Diaz F, Gonzalez S, and Westerhof W. Treatment of vitiligo vulgaris with narrow-band UVB and oral Polypodium leucotomos extract: A randomized double-blind placebo-controlled study. *J Eur Acad Dermatol Venereol* 2007;21(7):942–50.

Chapter 29

NEWER AGENTS IN SYSTEMIC TREATMENT

Rachita Dhurat and Shilpi Agarwal

CONTENTS

INTRODUCTION

Vitiligo is a chronic pigmentary condition with varying etiology. Genetics, familial inheritance, stress, infections, toxic productions, neurologic factors, autoimmunity, melanocytorrhagy, apoptosis, and oxidative stress are many of the postulated etiological factors for vitiligo [1]. As vitiligo causes significant psychological distress for patients, it is imperative for us as dermatologists to treat it. Treatment options available are multiple due to the many etiological factors. Hence, there is a need for further research and advent of newer molecules to treat vitiligo. In this chapter, we summarize the systemic options for vitiligo available in our armamentarium.

CORTICOSTEROID THERAPY

As vitiligo is considered an auto-inflammatory process, corticosteroids are the mainstay of treatment. Various ways in which steroids are used in vitiligo include topical, intralesional, daily low-dose prednisolone, oral minipulse (OMP), and high-dose intravenous pulse therapy. Corticosteroids may be combined with immunomodulators for additional benefit [2].

IMMUNOMODULATORS

Cyclophosphamide has been used in vitiligo for its immunosuppressive effect with or without systemic corticosteroids. In a study by Gokhale, cyclophosphamide in a dose of 50 mg twice daily was used in 33 vitiligo patients, of which 29 showed repigmentation following therapy [3]. It has also shown good result in another study by Pasricha along with OMP therapy. It is a useful adjunct in fast spreading vitiligo that cannot be controlled by OMP alone [4].

Cyclosporine in a dose of 50 mg twice daily, azathioprine 50 mg twice daily, methotrexate 7.5 mg per week, and levamisole 150 mg on two consecutive days every week have also been used in conjunction with corticosteroids or alone in treatment of unstable vitiligo [4,5].

ANAPSOS

Anapsos is an extract of a fern called *Polypodium leucotomos* and has immunomodulator properties. It was used by Pathak in an oral dose of 120–360 mg per day followed by exposure to UV-A on 12 patients having vitiligo vulgaris. In 3–9 month, three patients developed 25%–30% repigmentation and three other patients developed minimal repigmentation. Its role in vitiligo has also been shown in

Pacifico and colleagues enrolled 57 patients with generalized vitiligo to receive NBUVB phototherapy twice daily with or without 480 mg of P. leucotomos daily. At 6 months, 47.8% of patients responded to treatment in the P. leucotomos and NBUVB group versus 22% with NBUVB alone [6].

CLOFAZIMINE

Clofazimine is an iminophenazine dye used as part of multidrug therapy treatment of leprosy. Hyperpigmentation is a noted side effect in the majority of patients. In the study by Shah, repigmentation was seen in patients treated with clofazimine, which was reversible on stopping treatment [7]. In other study done by Guha et al., there was no evidence of repigmentation of the affected areas in any of the patients treated [8].

QUINOLONE COMPOUNDS

Chloroquine in a dose of 250 mg per day and hydroxychloroquine 400 mg/day can be given with or without PUVA therapy. Christiansen treated a 49-year-old patient with extensive vitiligo of 37 years of duration, using chloroquine in a dose of 500 mg per day for the first month and then reducing the dose to 250 mg per day [9]. He observed repigmentation to an extent of 50% on the body and 90% on the face in a span of 4 months [9].

PLACENTAL EXTRACTS

Placental extract can be used topically, intralesionally, and intramuscularly. It is thought to contain tyrosine, which is a precursor of melanin. It also contains copper, vitamins, and trace elements, all playing a role in treatment of vitiligo. Pantothenic acid and folic acid in placental extracts help in the copper-tyrosinase linkage during synthesis of melanin. Placental extracts also enhance body immunity to combat vitiligo. It has also been shown that placenta is a rich source of fibroblast growth factor promoting proliferation of melanocytes.

The dosage is intramuscular injection of placental extract 2 cc on alternate days or intralesional injection of the extract in small isolated patches [10–12].

AFAMELANOTIDE

Afamelanotide (melanotan I, CUV1647; brand name Scenesse) [13] is a potent synthetic peptide and analog of the naturally occurring α-melanocyte stimulating hormone (α-MSH).

Afamelanotide was initially developed as a sunless tanning agent and is now being used in Europe to prevent phototoxicity in adults with erythropoietic protoporphyria and solar urticaria. The photoprotective mechanism is by inducing melanin to act as a photoprotective filter [14,15]. It has been approved for marketing authorization under exceptional circumstances by the European Medicines Agency for the prevention of phototoxicity in adults with erythropoietic protoporphyria.

Its role in vitiligo is now being evaluated. Let us first understand the molecular basics of afamelanotide in melanin synthesis.

The cutaneous melanocortin system comprises the following bioactive peptides: α-MSH, β-endorphin, corticotropin, and various other peptides that are obtained from the precursor proopiomelanocortin [16–22]. The peptide α-MSH has a pivotal role in melanogenesis and stimulating melanocyte proliferation [16–22]. It acts via melanocortin-1 receptor present on the melanoblasts and increases melanin synthesis via production of eumelanin [16–22]. When combined with NB-UVB phototherapy, it increases differentiation of melanoblasts and upregulates melanocortin-1 receptor [22].

A multicenter randomized controlled trial has been carried out to study the safety and efficacy of afamelanotide with phototherapy versus NB-UVB phototherapy alone [22]. Patients were randomized in equal numbers to one of two treatment groups (combination therapy and NB-UVB monotherapy). Both groups received NB-UVB phototherapy 2–3 times weekly for 6 months, for a maximum of 72 treatments. The combination therapy group received 4 monthly subcutaneous afamelanotide implants (on days 28, 56, 84, and 112). During the 6-month active treatment phase, participants underwent weekly evaluation for onset of repigmentation [22].

The afamelanotide implant is a sterile biodegradable and biocompatible poly (D,L-lactide-co-glycolide) polymer implant core (Sigma-Aldrich Corp.) containing 16 mg of the drug. It is about the size of a grain of rice. Implants were placed subcutaneously above the supra-iliac crest, using sterile technique with a 14-gauge catheter after injection of 1% lidocaine hydrochloride anesthesia [22].

This study found a statistically significant superior response in the combination therapy group, with repigmentation (represented by a relative reduction in the VASI) of 48.64% (95% CI, 39.49%−57.80%) at day 168 versus 33.26% (95% CI, 24.18%−42.33%) in the NB-UVB monotherapy group.

Adverse effects of afamelanotide included erythema, pruritis, nausea, and abdominal pain. No serious adverse effects were noted.

This study could serve as a gateway to understanding and exploring the role of afamelanotide for treatment of vitiligo.

APREMILAST

Apremilast is an oral small-molecule phosphodiesterase-4 (PDE4) inhibitor that regulates inflammatory mediators. It elevates levels of cyclic adenosine monophosphate, which is a modulator of inflammatory responses [23,24], thus decreasing proinflammatory mediators, like tumor necrosis factor (TNF)-α, interleukin (IL)-23, and interferon gamma, and increased production of IL-10, an anti-inflammatory cytokine [25]. Apremilast is shown to modulate the inflammatory cycle in many studies. Other mechanisms for decreased proinflammatory cytokine production include toll-like receptor 4 agonism in peripheral blood mononuclear cells, T-cell receptor agonism, cytokine and immunoglobulin receptor agonism on natural killer cells, and ultraviolet light exposure of keratinocytes. All these mechanisms have proven their role in psoriasis and psoriatic arthritis [26]. In March 2014, the Food and Drug Administration (FDA) approved apremilast for adults with active psoriatic arthritis [27].

The hypothesis for use of apremilast in vitiligo is that it will shut down the inflammatory insult in vitiligo, and NB-UVB phototherapy will then be able to regenerate melanocytes and their activity. It is been postulated that UV radiation in vitiligo produces an increased number and activity of melanocytes, increased melanin density, and elongation and branching of dendrites, with increased transfer of more heavily melanized melanosomes to keratinocytes [28].

A randomized placebo control study done by Khemis et al. for apremilast in combination therapy with narrowband (NB)-UVB versus NB-UVB in 40 patients each with vitiligo. Authors have reported no statistical difference in vitiligo Area Scoring Index score between the two groups [28]. A single case report of a 52-year-old female with chronic, tenacious vitiligo who responded to apremilast 30 mg BD after 6 months of treatment has been reported [29].

JANUS KINASE INHIBITORS

These molecules have long been evaluated for their role in alopecia areata and vitiligo. Both oral and topical forms are available.

WHAT ARE JANUS KINASE ENZYMES?

The JAK family of enzymes is linked with cytokine receptors on the cell surface. They play a role in the signal transducer and activation of transcription pathway which is involved in inflammatory and immune responses [30].

JANUS KINASE-SIGNAL TRANSDUCER AND ACTIVATION OF TRANSCRIPTION SIGNALING

Cytokines including interleukins, interferons, and colony-stimulating factors play a critical role in cell proliferation and differentiation, hematopoiesis, apoptosis, and immunoregulation [31]. Cytokines function by binding to specific receptors on cell membranes.

There are two subgroups of cytokine-receptor interactions that cause signal transduction via the Janus kinase-signal transducer and activation of transcription (JAK-STAT) pathway [32]. This pathway is a crucial intracellular conduit by which many cytokines interact with their receptors (see Figure 29.1).

Type I receptors bind several interleukins, colony stimulating factors, and hormones such as erythropoietin and prolactin. Type II receptors bind interferons and interleukin-10 related cytokines [33].

JANUS KINASE INHIBITION

Currently, four important members of the JAK family are known. Janus kinase 1 and Janus kinase 2 are involved in host defense, hematopoiesis, neural development, and growth. Janus kinase 3 and tyrosine kinase 2 have a role in the immune response [32].

Inhibiting JAK will interrupt the JAK-STAT pathway. In myelofibrosis there is a significant reduction in splenomegaly with overall improvement in associated symptoms due to this inhibition [34].

JAK inhibition has been widely studied in rheumatoid arthritis, as there is overproduction of interleukin-6, interleukin-12, interleukin-15, interleukin-23, granulocyte-macrophage colony stimulating factor, and interferons [35]. Inhibition of Janus kinase 1 and 3 will inhibit signaling and therefore suppress immune responses.

Due to the critical role of JAK in host defense, autoimmunity, and hematological cancers, they have become an attractive target for therapeutics for a variety of disorders [30].

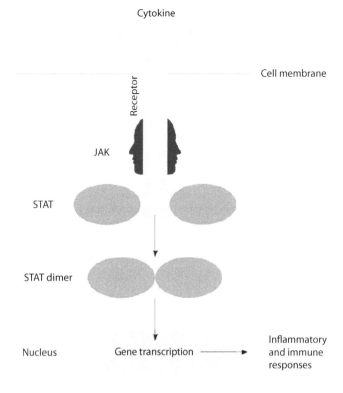

Figure 29.1   Signaling through the JAK-STAT pathway.

TOFACITINIB

Tofacitinib is principally an inhibitor of Janus kinase 1 and 3. It also inhibits Janus kinase 2 to some extent but has very little effect on tyrosine kinase 2.

RUXOLITINIB

This is a Janus kinase 1 and 2 inhibitor that selectively targets myeloproliferative disorders involving the gain-of-function mutation in Janus kinase 2 (V617F mutation). It reduces splenomegaly and systemic symptoms and improves overall survival in myelofibrosis. It is also being studied in rheumatoid arthritis and skin psoriasis [36].

ROLE OF TOFACITINIB IN VITILIGO

Tofacitinib was approved by the FDA in 2012 for the treatment of moderate to severe rheumatoid arthritis. Its oral form has been established in treating plaque psoriasis and alopecia universalis [37–43].

Alopecia areata and vitiligo have common genetic risk factors and possibly pathogenesis [44]. Recent advances in the understanding of vitiligo support the use of JAK inhibitors for this condition (Table 29.1). Interferon-gamma–induced expression of C-X-C motif

Table 29.1 Depicts the various JAK-STAT inhibitors available [27]

Drug	Janus kinase inhibition		
	Janus kinase		
	1	2	3
Ruxolitinib	Yes	Yes	No
Baricitinib	Yes	Yes	No
Tofacitinib	Yes	Yes	Yes
Pacritinib	No	Yes	No
Momelotinib	Yes	Yes	No

chemokine10 (CXCL10) in keratinocytes is a mediator of depigmentation in vitiligo [39]. Antibody neutralization of interferon gamma or CXCL10 will reverse depigmentation [44]. Thus, the use of the JAK1/3 inhibitor tofacitinib will lead to blockade of interferon gamma pathway and downstream CXCL10 expression, thus inducing repigmentation in vitiligo [37].

A 50-year-old female with generalized vitiligo vulgaris was treated by Craiglow et al. with oral tofacitinib citrate (Xeljanz). Treatment was initiated at a dosage of 5 mg alternate day. After 3 weeks, the dosage was increased to 5 mg/day. After 2 months of treatment, partial repigmentation of the face and upper extremities was seen. After 5 months, repigmentation of the forehead and hands was nearly complete, and the remaining involved areas demonstrated partial repigmentation. Approximately 5% of the total body surface area remained depigmented. The patient tolerated the drug well with no adverse effects [37].

Thus, JAK inhibitors need to be studied more in detail to evaluate their role in skin diseases including vitiligo.

SIMVASTATIN AND ATORVASTATIN

The 3-hydroxy-3-methylglutaryl-coenzyme (HMG-CoA) reductase inhibitors, also known as statins, are the most effective class of drugs for lowering serum low-density lipoprotein cholesterol concentrations [45]. After its ingestion, the inactive lactone is hydrolyzed in β-hydroxyl acid and inhibits the hydroxy-3 methyl-3 glutaryl coenzyme A (HMG-CoA) reductase [46]. The role of the regulatory enzyme HMG-CoA essentially limits the mevalonate pathway through which cells synthesize cholesterol. Some examples of statins include atorvastatin, simvastatin, rosuvastatin, etc.

ROLE OF STATINS IN VITILIGO

There is presence of circulating antibodies and T lymphocytes reacting against melanocyte antigens in sera of patient with vitiligo [47]. A higher proportion of activated peripheral T cells as determined by expression of HLA-DR is also seen in vitiligo patients [48,49]. Lesional T cells rather than circulatory anti-melanocytic antibody may also be responsible for the autoimmune patchy destruction on cutaneous melanocytes in vitiligo [49]. It has been seen that normal melanocytes present antigenic peptide fragment to well-defined proliferative cytotoxic T cells in a MHC class II−restricted manner [50]. This may contribute to abnormal immune responses seen in vitiligo.

Interestingly, the use of lipid lowering agents, specifically HMG-CoA reductase inhibitors, has been reported to have immunosuppressive effects in a study of heart transplant recipients [51]. The immunosuppressive effect is due to blockade of interleukin-2 synthesis in activated T lymphocytes [52]. Kwak et al. [53] showed that statins act as direct inhibitors of the induction of MHC-II expression by

interferon gamma (IFN-γ) and thus as repressor of MHC-II mediated T-lymphocyte activation in human endothelial cells.

A report has been published of a patient with pre-myocardial infarction and vitiligo whose vitiligo lesions improved on taking 80 mg Simvastatin at bedtime and worsened on stopping it [54]. Clinical trials are currently underway for establishing a role of statins in vitiligo.

CONCLUSION

Abatacept is known to decrease T cell activity in rheumatoid arthritis and hence its role is being deciphered in psoriasis and vitiligo. It acts via CTLA4 pathway and is self-administered weekly 125 mg subcutaneously [55]. Few studies are underway for treatment of vitiligo via TNF-α inhibitors like infliximab, etanercept, and adalimumab [56]. Vitiligo patients have a defective WNT signaling pathway and hence WNT activation could play a role in treatment of vitiligo. Further large-scale studies and trials are needed to bring all these newer systemic agents in clinical practice.

REFERENCES

1. Njoo MD, and Westerhof W. Vitiligo. Pathogenesis and treatment. *Am J Clin Dermatol.* 2001;2(3):167–81.

2. Hann SK, and Nordlund JJ, editors. *Vitiligo: A Monograph on the Basic and Clinical Science*, 1st ed. Oxford, London: Blackwell Science Ltd; 2000; pp. 1–386.

3. Gokhale BB. Cyclophosphamide and vitiligo. *Int J Dermatol* 1979;18:92.

4. Pasricha JS, and Khaitan BK. *Drugs for Vitiligo.* New Delhi: New Age International (P) Limited; 1996.

5. Pasricha JS, and Khera V. Effect of prolonged treatment with levamisole on vitiligo with limited and slow spreading disease. *Internat J Dermatol* 1984;33:584–7.

6. Pacifico A, Vidolin AP, Leone G, and Iacovelli P. Combined treatment of narrowband ultraviolet B light (NBUVB) phototherapy and oral Polypodium leucotomos extract versus NB UVB phototherapy alone in the treatment of patients with vitiligo. *J Am Acad Dermatol.* 2009;3(Suppl 1):AB154.

7. Shah KC. Clinical evaluation of clofazimine in vitiligo. *Indian J Dermatol Venereol Leprol.* 1981;47(1):40–1.

8. Guha PK, Pandey SS, and Singh G. Clofazimine in vitiligo. *Indian J Dermatol Venereol Leprol.* 1980;46(1):35–7.

9. Christiansen J. Vitiligo treated with chloroquine; a preliminary report. *Acta Derm Venereol.* 1955;35(6):453–56.

10. Punshi SK, and Aggrawal A. Placental extract therapy. *Asian Clin Dermatol* 1994;1(1):53–7.

11. Punshi SK et al. Vitiligo. *Probe.* 1969;1:18.

12. Punshi SK. *A Handbook of Vitiligo and Colour Atlas*, 1st ed. Jaypee; 2003.

13. Minder El. Afamelanotide, antagonistic analog of α-melanocyte-stimulating hormone, in dermal phototoxicity of erythropoietic protoporphyria. *Expert Opin Investig Drugs* 2010;19(12):1591–602.

14. Harms J, Lautenschlager S, Minder CE, and Minder EI. An α-melanocyte-stimulating hormone analogue in erythropoietic protoporphyria. *N Engl J Med* 2009;360(3):306–7.

15. Haylett AK, Nie Z, Brownrigg M, Taylor R, and Rhodes LE. Systemic photoprotection in solar urticarial with α-melanocyte-stimulating hormone analogue [Nle4-D-Phe7]-α-MSH. *Br J Dermatol* 2011;164(2):407–14.

16. Abdel-Malek Z, Swope VB, Suzuki I et al. Mitogenic and melanogenic stimulation of normal human melanocytes by melanotropic peptides. *Proc Natl Acad Sci U S A* 1995;92(5):1789–93.

17. Abdel-Malek Z, Scott MC, Suzuki I et al. The melanocortin-1 receptor is a key regulator of human cutaneous pigmentation. *Pigment Cell Res* 2000;13(suppl 8):156–62.

18. Luger TA, Scholzen TE, Brzoska T, and Böhm M. New insights into the functions ofα-MSH and related peptides in the immune system. *Ann N Y Acad Sci* 2003;994:133–40.

19. Böhm M, Luger TA, Tobin DJ, and García-Borrón JC. Melanocortin receptor ligands: New horizons for skin biology and clinical dermatology. *J Invest Dermatol* 2006;126(9):1966–75.

20. Scott MC, Suzuki I, and Abdel-Malek ZA. Regulation of the human melanocortin 1 receptor expression in epidermal melanocytes by paracrine and endocrine factors and by ultraviolet radiation. *Pigment Cell Res* 2002;15(6):433–9.

21. Brzoska T, Luger TA, Maaser C, Abels C, and Böhm M. α-Melanocyte-stimulating hormone and related tripeptides: Biochemistry, anti-inflammatory and protective effects invitro and in vivo, and future perspectives for the treatment of immune-mediated inflammatory diseases. *Endocr Rev* 2008;29(5):581–602.

22. Lim HW, Grimes PE, Agbai O et al. Afamelanotide and narrowband UV-B phototherapy for the treatment of vitiligo: A randomized multicenter trial. *JAMA Dermatol* 2015;15:42–50.

23. Serezani CH, Ballinger MN, Aronoff DM, and Peters-Golden M. Cyclic AMP: Master regulator of innate immune cell function. *Am J Respir Cell Mol Biol* 2008;39:127–32.

24. Tasken K, and Aandahl EM. Localized effects of cAMP mediated by distinct routes of protein kinase A. *Physiol Rev* 2004;84:137–67.

25. Schafer P. Apremilast mechanism of action and application to psoriasis and psoriatic arthritis. *Biochem Pharmacol* 2012;83:1583–90.

26. Schafer PH, Parton A, Gandhi AK et al. Apremilast, a cAMP phosphodiesterase-4 inhibitor, demonstrates anti-inflammatory activity *in vitro* and in a model of psoriasis. *Br J Pharmacol* 2010;159:842–55.

27. Food and Drug Administration. FDA news release: FDA approves Otezla to treat psoriatic arthritis. Mar 21, 2014. Available at: http://www.fda.gov/newsevents/newsroom/pressannouncements/ucm390091.htm.

28. Khemis A, Fontas E, Moulin S, Montaudié H, Lacour JP, and Passeron T. Apremilast in combination with narrowband UVB in the treatment of vitiligo: A 52-week monocentric prospective randomized placebo-controlled study. *J Invest Dermatol.* 2020;S0022-202X(20)30067-1. doi:10.1016/j.jid.2019.11.031.

29. Huff SB, and Gottwald LD. Repigmentation of tenacious vitiligo on apremilast. *Case Rep Dermatol Med* 2017;2017:3–6.

30. Kubler P. Janus kinase inhibitors: Mechanisms of action. *Aust Prescr* 2014;37:154–71.

31. O'Shea JJ, Holland SM, and Staudt LM. JAKs and STATs in immunity, immunodeficiency, and cancer. *N Engl J Med* 2013;368:161–70.

32. Leonard WJ, and O'Shea JJ. JAKs and STATS: Biological implications. *Annu Rev Immunol* 1998;16:293–322.

33. O'Shea JJ, Kontzias A, Yamaoka K, Tanaka Y, and Laurence A. Janus kinase inhibitors in autoimmune diseases. *Ann Rheum Dis* 2013;72(Suppl 2):ii111–5.

34. Laurence A, Pesu M, Silvennoinen O, and O'Shea J. JAK kinases in health and disease: An update. *Open Rheumatol J* 2012;6:232–44.

35. McInnes IB, and Schett G. The pathogenesis of rheumatoid arthritis. *N Engl J Med* 2011;365:2205–19.

36. Kwatra SG, Dabade TS, Gustafson CJ, and Feldman SR. JAK inhibitors in psoriasis: A promising new treatment modality. *J Drugs Dermatol* 2012;11:913–8.

37. Craiglow BG, and King BA. Tofacitinib citrate for the treatment of vitiligo. A pathogenesis-directed therapy. *JAMA Dermatol* 2015;151(10):1110–2.

38. Boy MG, Wang C, Wilkinson BE et al. Double-blind, placebo-controlled, dose-escalation study to evaluate the pharmacologic effect of CP-690,550 in patients with psoriasis. *J Invest Dermatol* 2009;129(9):2299–302.

39. Papp KA, Menter A, Strober B et al. Efficacy and safety of tofacitinib, an oral Janus kinase inhibitor, in the treatment of psoriasis: A phase 2b randomized placebo-controlled dose-ranging study. *Br J Dermatol* 2012;167(3):668–77.

40. Ports WC, Khan S, Lan S et al. A randomized phase 2a efficacy and safety trial of the topical Janus kinase inhibitor tofacitinib in the treatment of chronic plaque psoriasis. *Br J Dermatol* 2013;169(1):137–45.

41. Strober B, Buonanno M, Clark JD et al. Effect of tofacitinib, a Janus kinase inhibitor, on haematological parameters during 12 weeks of psoriasis treatment. *Br J Dermatol* 2013;169(5):992–9.

42. Mamolo C, Harness J, Tan H, and Menter A. Tofacitinib (CP-690,550), an oral Janus kinase inhibitor, improves patient-reported outcomes in a phase 2b, randomized, double-blind, placebo-controlled study in patients with moderate-to-severe psoriasis. *J Eur Acad Dermatol Venereol* 2014;28(2):192–203.

43. Craiglow BG, and King BA. Killing two birds with one stone: Oral tofacitinib reverses alopecia universalis in a patient with plaque psoriasis. *J Invest Dermatol* 2014;134(12):2988–90.

44. Harris JE. Vitiligo and alopecia areata: Apples and oranges? *Exp Dermatol* 2013;22(12):785–9.

45. Smith MEB, Lee NJ, Haney E, and Carson S. Drug Class Review: HMG-CoA reductase inhibitors (statins) and fixed-dose combination products containing a statin, final report update 5. *Drug Class Reviews* 2009.

46. Palinski W, and Tsimikas S. Immunomodulatory effects of statins: Mechanisms and potential impact on arteriosclerosis. *J Am Soc Nephrol* 2002;13:1673–81

47. al-Fouzan A, al-Arbash M, Fouad F, Kaaba SA, Mousa MA, and al-Harbi SA. Study of HLA class I/IL and T lymphocyte subsets in Kuwaiti vitiligo patients. *Eur J Immunogenet* 1995;22:209–13.

48. Abdel-Naser MB, Ludwig WD, Gollnick H, and Orfanos CE. Nonsegmental vitiligo: Decrease of the CD45RA+ T-cell subset and evidence for peripheral T-cell activation. *Int J Dermatol* 1992;31:321–6.

49. Badri AM, Todd PM, Garioch JJ, Gudgeon JE, Stewart DG, and Goudie RB. An immunohistological study of cutaneous lymphocytes in vitiligo. *J Pathol* 1993;170:149–55.

50. Le Poole IC, Mutis T, van den Wijngaard RM, Westerhof W, Ottenhoff T, de Vries RR, and Das PK. A novel, antigen-presenting function of melanocytes and its possible relationship to hypopigmentary disorders. *J Immunol* 1993;151:7284–92.

51. Kobashigawa JA. Statins as immunosuppressive agents. *Liver Transpl* 2001;7:559–61.

52. Wenke K, Meiser B, Thiery J, Nagel D, von Scheidt W, Steinbeck G, Seidel D, and Reichart B. Simvastatin reduces graft vessel disease and mortality after heart transplantation: A four-year randomized trial. *Circulation* 1997;96:1398–402.

53. Kwak B, Mulhaupt F, Myit S, and Mach F. Statins as a newly recognized type of immunomodulator. *Nat Med* 2000;6:1399–402.

54. Noël M, Gagné C, Bergeron J, Jobin J, and Poirier P. Positive pleiotropic effects of HMG-CoA reductase inhibitor on vitiligo. *Lipids Health Dis* 2004;3:7.

55. ClinicalTrials.gov Brigham and Women's Hospital. *2014 Nov 3. Identifier: NCT02281058, Open-Label pilot study of Abetacept for the treatment of vitiligo*;2017 Aug 9; Available at: https://clinicaltrials.gov/ct2/show/NCT02281058.

56. Lv Y, Li Q, Wang L, and Gao T. Use of anti-tumor necrosis factor agents: A possible therapy for vitiligo. *Med Hypotheses* 2009;72(5):546–7.

PHOTOTHERAPY AND LASERS

Chapter 30

UVA THERAPY IN VITILIGO

Surabhi Dayal and Priyadarshini Sahu

CONTENTS

INTRODUCTION

Phototherapy is one of the most significant treatment modalities available for the management of vitiligo. It is also known as "light therapy," in particular, ultraviolet (UV) light. This UV-based therapy includes photochemotherapy (psoralens with UVA [PUVA]), phototherapy (narrowband UVB [NB-UVB]), and targeted phototherapy (excimer laser and excimer lamp). It is essential for the dermatologist to understand UV-based therapy to take full advantage in terms of patient treatment and its consequent adverse effects. Numerous studies have shown the beneficial effect of UV radiation for the treatment of various dermatological conditions, one of which is vitiligo, which can be distressing and is a potentially disfiguring condition, especially in darker skin phototypes. PUVA and PUVAsol therapy are usually preferred in the treatment of widespread vitiligo in adults. However, currently it is being surpassed by ultraviolet B (UVB), which is equally or slightly more efficacious, with a better side effect profile [1]. This chapter is reviews UVA therapy in vitiligo based on the current evidence.

HISTORICAL BACKGROUND

More than 3500 years ago, ancient Indians and Egyptians were using the pigment-stimulating properties of psoralen-containing plants such as the Babchi plant (*Psoralea corylifolia*) and Ammi majus, respectively in addition to sunlight for treating "leukoderma," which was mistakenly thought to be a part of leprosy. In 1895, Niels Ryberg Finsen, the father of modern UV therapy, demonstrated the effect of UV therapy in treatment of lupus vulgaris, for which he was awarded the Nobel Prize in medicine.

Photochemotherapy use was resumed in 1947, when the active ingredients of Ammi majus, 8-methoxypsoralen (8-MOP) and 5-methoxypsoralen (5-MOP), were isolated. The first trials with 8-MOP and sun exposure were performed in vitiligo patients by El-Mofty in Egypt in 1947. Various publications by Parrish, Fitzpatrick, Tanenbaum, and Pathak reported the beneficial effect of this new type of UVA tube in combination with oral 8-MOP in the treatment of psoriasis. The use of psoralen baths and subsequent UVA exposure (bath PUVA) originated in Scandinavia and is still in use, as it avoids 8-MOP side effects such as nausea and dizziness. However, topical and bath PUVA did not gain as much popularity as the oral form. Hence, photochemotherapy revolutionized dermatological management and in fact was the driving force for a whole new series of discoveries during the next two decades, such as narrowband UVB (NB-UVB), and later UVA1 (340–400 nm) [2].

In 1992, UVA1 (340–400 nm) was first introduced for the treatment of atopic dermatitis. Few studies with small numbers of patients showed efficacy in some other dermatoses such as vitiligo, morphea, urticaria pigmentosa, and mycosis fungoides. However, the published evidence on UVA1 has still remained limited and of variable quality [3].

SPECTRUM OF ULTRAVIOLET RADIATION

The solar electromagnetic spectrum is made up of x-rays, UV radiation (UVR), and visible light. Further, UVR consists of UVA (320–400 nm), UVB (280–320 nm), and UVC (<280 nm). UVA is further subdivided into UVA1 (340–400 nm) and UVA2 (320–340 nm).

UVC has the shortest wavelength and is filtered out by the ozone layer before it reaches the Earth's surface. Both UVA and UVB reach the Earth's surface. With respect to production of erythema, cellular effects, and DNA damage, UVB is 100–1000 times more effective as compared to UVA. Although UVA is less energetic, it penetrates deeper into the skin, resulting in chronic photobiologic events [4].

PHOTOCHEMOTHERAPY

Photochemotherapy is a photochemical reaction between exogenous photosensitizer (i.e., psoralen) and UVA radiation, which has beneficial effects in various dermatological diseases. It is mainly of two types: PUVA and PUVAsol. In PUVA, UVA radiation is produced by an artificial light source which is equipped with a fluorescent bulb. In centers where artificial chambers are not available, sunlight is used as the source of UVA irradiation and is known as PUVAsol.

Pharmacology of Psoralens: Psoralens are derived from naturally occurring tricyclic furocoumarins. 8-MOP, (methoxsalen) is the most widely used derivative in PUVA; it is principally of plant origin but it is also available as a synthetic drug. 4,5,8-trimethyl psoralen (TMP; trioxsalen) is a synthetic drug and is primarily used for the treatment of vitiligo. It is less phototoxic after oral administration as compared to 8-MOP. 5-MOP (bergapten) which has a lower potential for phototoxicity, is also sometimes used.

On oral administration, 8-MOP is absorbed from the gastrointestinal tract, and after 1 hour photosensitivity develops, reaches a peak at about 2 hours, and disappears after about 8 hours [1]. The rate of absorption of psoralens depends upon the physical characteristics of the preparation (i.e., hard gelatin capsules or soft gelatin capsules), concomitant food intake, and individual factors. Soft gelatin capsules are better absorbed than hard gelatin capsules as they yield peak serum levels in relatively reproducible time in all patients. Concomitant diet intake, especially food rich in fat content, retards and decreases the absorption. Drugs inducing cytochrome P-450 enzymes enhance and accelerate the metabolism of methoxalen, so they reduce the biological effect. Inter-patient variability in response to PUVA is based on biochemical markers such as glutathione S-transferase genotype [5].

When 8-MOP is applied locally, it rapidly penetrates the skin and can be detected in the urine after 4 hours [6]. The plasma levels of 8-MOP in patients receiving total body topical 8-MOP are comparable to those found during oral 8-MOP ingestion [7].

MECHANISM OF ACTION OF PSORALENS

The rationale for photochemotherapy is to maintain an adequate level of psoralen in the target organ (skin) only at the time of exposure to UV radiation. It is a unique form of therapy where the drug psoralen has no therapeutic effect by itself but produces an effect when the patient is exposed to UVA radiation. Thus, an unintentional exposure may be harmful if psoralen is present in skin before and after the exposure. The erythema induced by PUVA therapy usually appears after 36–48 hours of exposure to UVA radiation and peaks after 48–96 hours or up to 120 hours [8].

The exact mechanism of pigment induction by PUVA in vitiligo is still speculative. In vitiligo, PUVA therapy acts primarily via stimulation of melanocytes and by manipulating the abnormal immune response. The photo-conjugation of psoralens to the melanocyte DNA is followed by mitosis, replication and proliferation of melanocytes, and increased number of melanosomes and their further transfer to keratinocytes. Furthermore, PUVA therapy increases the number and activity of epidermal melanocytes and decreases the degenerative changes in both melanocytes and keratinocytes in both

the vitiliginous areas and normal skin. The reversal of degeneration in both leucodermic and apparently normal skin after PUVA points toward the role of this modality in both repigmentation and protection against further depigmentation [9].

PUVA also affects immunological processes and may induce a suppressor T cell population and release IL-10, which is important for differentiation and activation of T-regulatory cells that may suppress the autoimmune stimulus responsible for melanocyte destruction [10]. PUVA also induces basic fibroblast growth factor (bFGF) and hepatocyte growth factor, which may aid in regrowth and migration of follicular melanocytes to the basal layer of skin [11].

SOURCES OF UVA RADIATION

Currently most UVA treatment units are equipped with fluorescent lamps or high-pressure metal halide lamps. The action spectrum ranges from 320–380 nm. The typical fluorescent PUVA lamp has an emission peak at 352 nm and emits approximately 0.5% in UVB range also. UVA doses are expressed in J/cm^2, measured using a photometer with a maximum sensitivity at 350–360 nm [1].

TREATMENT METHODOLOGY IN VITILIGO

PUVA THERAPY

Initially, methoxsalen is administrated orally; that is 8-MOP in a dose of 0.4–0.6 mg/kg and 5-MOP in a dose of 0.5 mg/kg followed by UVA radiation after 1–2 hours. There are three protocols for the administration of UVA radiation [1]:

- *U.S. protocol*: Initial treatment exposure is based on skin type and patients are given UVA radiation twice or thrice a week. Depending on erythema production and therapeutic response, the dose is increased by 0.5–1.5 J/cm^2 for each subsequent visit.

- *European protocol*: In this protocol, the initial dose is administered after determination of the patient's minimum phototoxic dose (MPD). It is defined as the minimal dose of UVA that produces barely perceptible well-defined erythema when a small test area is exposed to increasing doses of UVA ranging from 0.5 to 1.5 J/cm^2 in a patient who has ingested the requisite dose of psoralen before exposure. For MPD, the erythema reading is taken 48–72 hours after giving the test dose, when the phototoxicity has reached a peak.

- *Indian protocol*: The Indian association of Dermatology, Venereology, and Leprology (IADVL) therapeutic guidelines recommend a modified US regimen that suits Indian patients. Initially the dose is started at 2–3 J/cm^2 and is increased by 0.5 J/cm^2 subsequently until the patient has not developed erythema or burning sensation over apparently normal skin.

Indications of oral PUVA include vitiligo involving more than 10% body surface area and localized lesions not responding to topical PUVA or other treatment modalities [1]. Lesions of the lower limbs tend to respond more slowly so additional doses may be needed. Ideally, 8-MOP should be taken on an empty stomach, but in practice it is taken after breakfast in order to prevent nausea. Generally, UV radiation is given two to three times a week with at least 48-hour intervals between treatments. If mild erythema develops, the dose may either be reduced or kept constant, but if moderate to severe erythema develops, treatment is deferred. Therapy is continued until repigmentation is achieved, which may last for months to years.

PUVASOL

The name stands for psoralen and UVA obtained by solar light. Sunlight is a rich source of UVA, so it can be used instead of UVA units. However, a major disadvantage of solar irradiation is the difficultly in quantifying UV light. It is usually recommended for those patients who cannot visit the hospital for phototherapy. The total amount of UVA reaching the skin depends on the season, time of the day, latitude, and atmospheric conditions. Other disadvantages are lack of privacy and difficulty in monitoring the dose of UV rays in addition to UVA, UVB, infrared rays, and visible light, which are not needed for PUVA therapy, leading to undesirable effects. The best time of day for PUVAsol is between 9:15–11:15 am and 2:30–3:30 pm [12]. There is minimal unwanted exposure to UVB and infrared light at these times. Treatment should be given twice to thrice weekly, with a minimum gap of 1 day between treatments.

PUVAsol can also be given after oral 8-MOP or after topical methoxsalen. Oral 8-MOP is given in the dose of 0.6 mg/kg. Nearly after 1.5–2 hours after intake of 8-MOP, sun exposure is advised for 10 mins. The time of exposure is increased by 5 mins every week until there is mild erythema of the involved area, after which the exposure time can be kept constant. It should be discontinued if there is no improvement after 30–40 sittings. Oral TMP is preferred over 8-MOP due to its weaker phototoxic effects.

Sunglasses should be recommended for all the patients on oral PUVA for 12–24 hours after the treatment to prevent eye toxicity. To avoid inadvertent excessive exposure to sunlight, sunscreen can be used to cover the vitiligo lesions that are exposed to PUVA. Oral PUVA is contraindicated in children and in pregnancy. However, bath PUVA may be used in children as it provides a wider margin of safety. Male genital areas should be shielded during PUVA treatments as they have increased susceptibility to skin cancers [1].

TOPICAL PUVASOL

Topical PUVAsol uses 8-MOP in patients with smaller lesions involving less than 5% of body surface area. Application of 0.01%–0.1% 8-MOP in a cream or lotion base to the affected area is done followed by irradiation after 30 min, starting with 0.5–1 min. Treatment is done 2–3 times/week and duration of sun exposure should be slowly increased by 0.5–1 min every week until slight erythema appears, after which the time is kept constant. Sunscreen should be applied to the surrounding uninvolved skin, so as to prevent undue tanning. Topically, TMP and 5-MOP are more phototoxic. Commercially available 8-MOP lotion can be diluted with nine parts of eau-de-cologne or propylene glycol [1].

MODIFICATIONS OF PUVA

Bath PUVA, bathing suit PUVA, and soak PUVA are various modifications of PUVA. These are mainly used for alopecia areata and psoriasis. However, a single study by Mai et al. [13] used bath PUVA successfully for the treatment of childhood vitiligo.

ULTRAVIOLET A1 PHOTOTHERAPY

The UVA1 phototherapy is available as long-wave UVA1 (340–400 nm) therapy with low dose (10–30 J/cm^2), medium dose (40–70 J/cm^2), and high dose (up to 130 J/cm^2). The biological effect of UVA1 phototherapy overlaps with NB-UVB and is relatively free of side effects such as phototoxicity and possible carcinogenesis as associated with other phototherapy regimens [14]. According to a recent study by El-Zawahry et al. [14], NB-UVB was found to be statistically significantly better than UVA1. This may be due to the fact that UVA therapy without psoralen shows a delayed onset of response compared to UVA therapy preceded by psoralen intake. Therefore, UVA1 can have an effect on vitiligo, but seems to be of limited use as monotherapy in treatment of vitiligo.

CONTRAINDICATIONS FOR PUVA THERAPY

- Age limit: Very young age, especially children less than 10 years of age (although in exceptional cases, young age groups may be considered for treatment provided regular ophthalmologic evaluation is done to rule out ocular toxicity)
- History of photosensitivity disorder
- Pregnancy and lactation
- Severe cardiac, liver, or renal disease
- History of skin cancer or chronic photodamage
- History or family history of melanoma [15]

PROGNOSTIC FACTORS DETERMINING RESPONSE TO UVA THERAPY IN VITILIGO

- Darker-skinned patients respond better than those who are fair skinned
- Head and neck lesions and lesions on hairy parts of the body are the most responsive sites; certain areas such as lips, dorsa of hands, acral parts, bony prominences, palms, soles, and nipples are resistant to treatment
- Usually, duration of disease does not affect the response rate to PUVA
- Patients having 30%–40% affected body surface area have a poor response to PUVA therapy [1]

MONITORING GUIDELINES FOR PUVA THERAPY

- Baseline liver function test and renal function test
- If there is any history of photosensitivity or other evidence of autoimmune connective tissue disease, then lupus laboratory panel (or ANA alone) is suggested
- Baseline ocular examination and repeated yearly or more often if there are abnormal ocular findings
- Cutaneous examination for skin cancer and actinic damage [1]

EFFICACY OF PUVA IN VITILIGO

According to various studies, the results of PUVA therapy vary considerably from one patient to another, and seldom achieve complete repigmentation [16,17]. According to a retrospective study of 10 years by Kwok et al. [18], PUVA therapy is only moderately effective in widespread vitiligo and needs careful patient counseling before therapy, as it seldom achieves extensive repigmentation that is cosmetically acceptable, and there is a high relapse rate after therapy. Repigmentation with PUVA, as with other modes of treatment, is usually observed around the hair follicles and/or from the periphery of the lesions. For optimal and maximum pigment induction, prolonged duration of phototherapy should be encouraged, with as many as 100–200 exposures given 2–3 times a week. If response occurs and patient discontinues treatment, the newly acquired repigmentation may be lost. Completely repigmented areas may remain stable for as long as 10 years.

A study by Singh et al. [19] found that PUVA is more efficacious as compared to PUVAsol and also provides greater psychological benefit in treatment of generalized vitiligo, although it is associated with more phototoxic adverse effects. However, according to various studies, it was found that NB-UVB is more effective in terms of efficacy, stability, and color match achieved in comparison to PUVA therapy in a comparable time period [20,21].

COMBINATION OF PUVA WITH OTHER MODALITIES

- Combination of calcipotriol with PUVA: Various studies have shown quicker response to this combination therapy with more intense repigmentation as compared to PUVA monotherapy, although acral vitiligo does not respond well. This combination therapy may shorten the duration of exposure to UVA, thus reducing the PUVA-induced side effects [22,23]. However, there is an isolated study which does not demonstrate any beneficial effect of combined treatment over PUVA [24].
- Combination of topical phenytoin with PUVA: Topical phenytoin suppresses type 1 immunoresponse, inhibits the production of free radicals and norepinephrine, and has direct melanocyte-stimulating effects. Therefore, topical phenytoin had also been tried in conjunction with PUVA therapy in treatment of vitiligo but showed that it cannot enhance the therapeutic response of PUVA [25].
- Low dose of azathioprine (0.6–0.75 mg/kg) has also been tried with oral PUVA therapy and found to potentiate the repigmentary efficacy of PUVA in vitiligo patients [26].

ADVERSE EFFECTS OF PUVA

SHORT-TERM SIDE EFFECTS
- *Nausea and vomiting*: This is the most common adverse effect. It can be relieved by taking the drug with food, preferably of high fat content, or milk. If nausea persists, the dose can be reduced or antiemetics can be given.
- *Erythema, pruritus, and xerosis*: This is the most common phototoxic reaction and can be managed by supportive measures, such as emollients, antihistamines, and other antipruritic agents.
- Reactivation of herpes simplex.
- Hypertrichosis, photo-onycholysis, melanonychia, friction blisters, and ankle edema.
- *Pigmentation*: Excessive darkening can occur of vitiliginous skin with repeated treatments, especially in dark-skinned patients. Treatment can also stimulate pigmentation of normal skin, which can accentuate the difference between normal and lesional skin.
- *Others*: Central nervous system side effects such as headache, insomnia, hyperactivity, and mild depression may be seen. Bronchoconstriction, hepatic toxicity, drug fever, and exanthems can be seen [1].

LONG-TERM SIDE EFFECTS
- *Photoaging*: This occurs in all patients with Fitzpatrick skin types I–IV after long-term PUVA therapy. Photoaging includes hyper- or hypopigmentation, telangiectasia, wrinkles, lentigines, solar elastosis, and actinic keratosis.
- *Cutaneous malignancies*: This is a major concern for non-melanoma skin cancer (especially squamous cell carcinoma [SCC]) and is associated with high cumulative UVA dose (more than 160 treatments or a cumulative UVA dose of 1000 J/cm^2). Most

of the SCC associated after long-term PUVA therapy has been reported in psoriatic patients, but there are few case reports of SCC in vitiligo patients [27,28]. Men exposed to PUVA have an increased risk of genital skin cancer [29].
- Concerns such as cataracts and immunosuppression are also raised with long-term PUVA therapy. However, the data in the literature do not support their occurrence.

CONCLUSION

PUVA is a well-known treatment modality in the management of generalized vitiligo. There are abundant case control studies of PUVA therapy in vitiligo, but there is no concrete multicentric randomized control trial suggesting its efficacy and safety. Most of these studies and case reports have a level of evidence that is B and C. Further improved understanding of its adverse effects, such as cutaneous malignancy, is also required. There remains the need for long-term prospective studies to gain a better understanding of its clinical efficacy, recurrence rate following PUVA therapy, and adverse effects associated with PUVA.

PRACTICAL TIPS

1. PUVA therapy is only moderately effective in widespread vitiligo, as it leads to moderate repigmentation in generalized vitiligo with a color match not cosmetically acceptable to the patient, and a high relapse rate after therapy.
2. PUVA therapy is contraindicated in pregnancy, lactation, and for children.
3. A high cumulative dose of oral PUVA therapy is associated with a dose-related increase in risk of nonmelanoma skin cancer, especially squamous cell carcinoma.
4. Sunscreens should be used to cover the vitiligo lesions exposed to PUVA therapy, to avoid the inadvertent effect of UVA radiation present in sunlight.
5. To prevent ocular toxicity, sunglasses are recommended for all patients on oral PUVA for 12–24 hours after PUVA therapy.

REFERENCES

1. Prabhu S, and Shenoi SD. Photochemotherapy (PUVA) in psoriasis and vitiligo. *Indian J Dermatol Venereol Leprol* 2014;80:497–504.
2. Hönigsmann H. History of phototherapy in dermatology. *Photochem Photobiol Sci* 2013;12:16–21.
3. Dawe RS. Ultraviolet A1 phototherapy. *Br J Dermatol* 2003;148(4):626–37.
4. Griffiths CEM, Barker J, Bleiker T, Chalmers R, and Creamer D. *Rook's Textbook of Dermatology*. Chichester. West Sussex (UK): Wiley Blackwell; 2016.
5. Ibbotson SH, Dawe RS, Dinkova-Kostova AT, Weidlich S, Farr PM, Ferguson J, Wolf CR, and Smith G. Glutathione S-transferase genotype is associated with sensitivity to

psoralen-ultraviolet a photochemotherapy. *Br J Dermatol* 2012;166:380–8.

6. Srinivas CR, and Rai R. Phototherapy: An Indian perspective. *Indian J Dermatol* 2007;52:169–75.

7. Neild VS, and Scott LV. Plasma levels of 8-methoxypsoralen in psoriatic patients receiving topical 8-methoxypsoralen. *Br J Dermatol* 1982;106:199–203.

8. Ibbotson SH, and Farr PM. The time-course of psoralen ultraviolet A (PUVA) erythema. *J Investig Dermatol* 1999;113:346–9.

9. Anbar TS, El-Sawy AE, Attia SK, Barakat MT, Moftah NH, El-Ammawy TS, Abdel-Rahman AT, and El-Tonsy MH. Effect of PUVA therapy on melanocytes and keratinocytes in non-segmental vitiligo: Histopathological, immuno-histochemical and ultrastructural study. *Photodermatol Photoimmunol Photomed* 2011;28:17–25.

10. Falabella R, and Barona MI. Update on skin repigmentation therapies in vitiligo. *Pigment Cell Melanoma Res* 2009;22:42–65.

11. Wu C-S, Lan C-CE, Wang L-F, Chen G-S, Wu C-S, and Yu H-S. Effects of psoralen plus ultraviolet A irradiation on cultured epidermal cells in vitro and patients with vitiligo in vivo. *Br J Dermatol* 2007;156:122–9.

12. Balasaraswathy P, Kumar U Srinivas CR, and Nair S. UVA and UVB in sunlight: Optimal utilization of UV rays in sunlight for phototherapy. *Indian J Dermatol* 2002;68:198–201.

13. Mai DW, Omohundro C, Dijkstra JW, and Bailin PL. Childhood vitiligo successfully treated with bath PUVA. *Pediatr Dermatol* 1998;15:53–5.

14. El-Zawahry BM, Bassiouny DA, Sobhi RM, Abdel-Aziz E, Zaki NS, Habib DF, and Shahin DM. A comparative study on efficacy of UVA1 vs. narrow-band UVB phototherapy in the treatment of vitiligo. *Photodermatol Photoimmunol Photomed* 2012;28:84–90.

15. Wolverton SE. *Comprehensive Dermatologic Drug Therapy*. Elsevier; 2013.

16. Tallab T, Joharji H, Bahamdan K, Karkashan E, Mourad M, and Ibrahim K. Response of vitiligo to PUVA therapy in Saudi patients. *Int J Dermatol* 2005;44:556–8.

17. Westerhof W. Treatment of vitiligo with UV-B radiation vs topical psoralen plus UV-A. *Arch Dermatol* 1997;133:1525–8.

18. Kwok YKC, Anstey AV, and Hawk JLM. Psoralen photochemotherapy (PUVA) is only moderately effective in widespread vitiligo: A 10-year retrospective study. *Clin Exp Dermatol* 2002;27:104–10.

19. Singh S, Khandpur S, Sharma VK, and Ramam M. Comparison of efficacy and side-effect profile of oral PUVA vs. oral PUVA sol in the treatment of vitiligo: A 36-week prospective study. *J Eur Acad Dermatol Venereol* 2012;27:1344–51.

20. Parsad D, Kanwar AJ, and Kumar B. Psoralen-ultraviolet A vs. narrow-band ultraviolet B phototherapy for the treatment of vitiligo. *J Eur Acad Dermatol Venereol* 2006;20:175–7.

21. Bhatnagar A, Kanwar AJ, Parsad D, and De D. Psoralen and ultraviolet A and narrow-band ultraviolet B in inducing stability in vitiligo, assessed by vitiligo disease activity score: An open prospective comparative study. *J Eur Acad Dermatol Venereol* 2007;21:1381–5.

22. Parsad D, Saini R, and Verma N. Combination of PUVAsol and topical calcipotriol in vitiligo. *Dermatology* 1998;197:167–70.

23. Ameen M, Exarchou V, and Chu AC. Topical calcipotriol as monotherapy and in combination with psoralen plus ultraviolet A in the treatment of vitiligo. *Br J Dermatol* 2001;145:476–9.

24. Baysal V, Yildirim M, Erel A, and Kesici D. Is the combination of calcipotriol and PUVA effective in vitiligo? *J Eur Acad Dermatol Venereol* 2003;17:299–302.

25. Bahmani M, Fallahzadeh MK, Jowkar F, Khalesi M, Bahri-Najafi R, and Namazi MR. Can topical phenytoin augment the therapeutic efficacy of PUVA against vitiligo? A double-blind, randomized, bilateral-comparison, placebo-controlled study. *J Dermatolog Treat* 2010;22:106–8.

26. Radmanesh M, and Saedi K. The efficacy of combined PUVA and low-dose azathioprine for early and enhanced repigmentation in vitiligo patients. *J Dermatolog Treat* 2006;17:151–3.

27. Buckley DA, and Rogers S. Multiple keratoses and squamous carcinoma after PUVA treatment of vitiligo. *Clin Exp Dermatol* 1996;21:43–5.

28. Takeda H, Mitsuhashi Y, and Kondo S. Multiple squamous cell carcinomas in situ in vitiligo lesions after long-term PUVA therapy. *J Am Acad Dermatol* 1998;38:268–70.

29. Park HS, Lee YS, and Chun DK. Squamous cell carcinoma in vitiligo lesion after long-term PUVA therapy. *J Eur Acad Dermatol Venereol* 2003;17:578–80.

Chapter 31

UVB THERAPY IN VITILIGO

Surabhi Dayal and Priyadarshini Sahu

CONTENTS

INTRODUCTION

Ultraviolet (UV)-based therapy has been the mainstay of treatment for vitiligo for long time [1]. The earliest form is photochemotherapy (psoralen and ultraviolet A [PUVA]), which was the mainstay of treatment of vitiligo for a long period until the discovery of UVB phototherapy. Narrowband UVB (NB-UVB) has revolutionized the management of vitiligo with better efficacy, tolerability, and a lower adverse effect profile [2]. NB-UVB is found to be effective alone and in combination with other topical and systemic adjuncts with encouraging results. Newer phototherapeutic modalities such as excimer light and laser are being introduced into the dermatological armamentarium. In this chapter, the authors review the course of UVB therapy in vitiligo, various adjunctive therapies, and recommendation based on the current evidence and authors' experience with NB-UVB.

HISTORICAL BACKGROUND

The history of ancient phototherapy and photochemotherapy was been discussed in the previous Chapter 30. The development of PUVA led to the discovery of NB-UVB (311–313 nm) irradiation. Consequently, in 1976, Parish and Jaenicke explained the action spectrum for the clearance of psoriasis with a peak at 313 nm. This research paved the way for development of NB-UVB. In 1978, broadband UVB was introduced for the treatment of psoriasis but was unable to gain popularity due to lower efficacy and increased side effects. In 1984, Van Weelden et al. demonstrated the clinical efficacy of NB-UVB. Westerhof and Nieweboer-Krobotova, in 1997, introduced NB-UVB in the treatment of vitiligo [3].

MECHANISM OF ACTION OF NB-UVB IN VITILIGO

There are two main steps by which NB-UVB exerts its effects in treatment of vitiligo. The first is stabilization of the depigmenting process, and the second, stimulation of residual follicular melanocytes. Both steps may occur simultaneously or individually [4].

IMMUNOMODULATION

Immunomodulation is the most important effect of UV radiation. Nuclear DNA is the major molecular target of UVB. When UVB radiation is absorbed by nucleotides of nuclear DNA, it leads to induction of various DNA photoproducts, especially pyrimidine dimers, leading to its destruction, thereby stabilizing the depigmentation process. NB-UVB also induces the immunosuppressive effect by inducing interleukin-10, lowering the peripheral natural killer cell activity, and lymphocyte proliferation. NB-UVB irradiation also stimulates the release of basic fibroblast growth factor (bFGF) and endothelin-1 (ET-1) from keratinocytes, which induces melanocyte proliferation [4].

MIGRATION OF MELANOCYTES FROM THE OUTER HAIR ROOT SHEATH

NB-UVB also stimulates the dopa-negative, amelanotic melanocytes in the outer hair root sheaths. These melanocytes get activated to proliferate and migrate outward to adjacent depigmented skin, resulting in perifollicular repigmentation, and later these melanocytes migrate downward to the hair matrices to produce melanin [5].

ROLE OF VITAMIN D

The role of calcium imbalance and low levels of circulating 25(OH) vitamin D has been implicated in the etiopathogenesis of vitiligo. Studies have shown that vitamin D modulates melanogenesis at the cellular level by inducing tyrosinase enzyme and immature melanocytes to produce melanin. NB-UVB exposures have shown an increase in the serum levels of vitamin D [6].

EQUIPMENT FOR THE DELIVERY OF PHOTOTHERAPY

A wide variety of NB-UVB units are available. The most common means of producing artificial UV radiation is by the passage of electric current through mercury vapor enclosed in a fluorescent tube [7]. These excited electrons of mercury are absorbed by phosphorus coated tubes, which results in emission of radiation of longer wavelengths by the process of fluorescence. By changing this phosphorus content, a variety of UV radiation of different spectra are produced. The tube commonly used for production of NB-UVB is TL-01, and for broadband UVB is TL-12. This fluorescent tube delivers UVB in the range of 310–315 nm with a peak of 312 nm.

Commercially, NB-UVB cabins either incorporate TL-01 alone or in combination with UVA tubes [7]. Commercially available NB-UVB cabins incorporating TL-01 alone are shown in Figures 31.1 and 31.2. Whole-body panels necessitate rotation of the patient to provide uniform irradiation. Recently, a home phototherapy unit, the SS-01UV phototherapy instrument, bearing two TL-9 W/01 lamps, has also been introduced [8]. Point source devices avoid unnecessary irradiation of unaffected skin, but care must be taken to avoid under- or overdosing at the overlap area.

DOSING SCHEDULE

Based on expert opinion, there is no clear consensus with regard to initial dosing and the dosing schedule. There are two dosing regimens that are most commonly used; one based on the calculation of

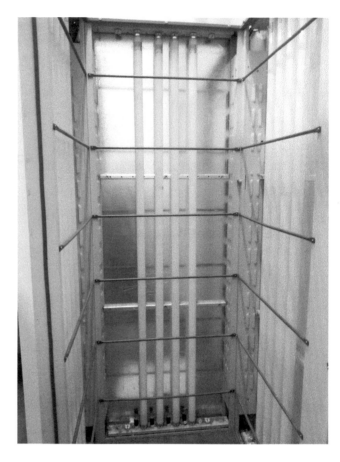

Figure 31.2   Commercially available NB-UVB unit, inner view.

minimal erythema dose (MED) and the other based on fixed dosing protocol. The ideal strategy for initial dosing is based on the patient's MED; however, determining MED for each individual is quite time consuming. According to the Vitiligo Working Group (VWG) phototherapy committee [9], a fixed dosing protocol initiated at 200 mJ/cm^2 regardless of skin type is convenient, with stepwise increase (usually 10%–20%) per treatment, depending on the patient's erythema response. The maximum acceptable dose for the face is 1500 mJ/cm^2, while for the body it is 3000 mJ/cm^2. Before assessing the treatment response, at least 18–36 exposures are required. Forty-eight NB-UVB sessions should be administered before discontinuing phototherapy due to lack of response. According to the VWG committee, some patients may be slow responders. Therefore, more than 72 exposures may be considered before stopping the treatment [9]. The following are the recent recommendations given by the VWG phototherapy committee: [9]

a. *Frequency of treatment*: Repigmentation depends on the total number of sessions, with earlier onset of pigmentation associated with a greater number of treatment sessions. However, there are no direct comparisons between twice- versus thrice-weekly regimens using NB-UVB. According to the VWG phototherapy committee, a twice-weekly regimen has better acceptability due to lower cost, and increases patient compliance, but a thrice-weekly regimen is optimal due to earlier repigmentation leading to decrease of patient's psychological distress.

b. *Dose adjustment based on degree of erythema*: The desirable response to phototherapy is "pink asymptomatic erythema" lasting for less than 24 hours. In the case of no erythema, the subsequent dose should be increased by 10%–20%. When the desirable erythema appears, the current dose should be held constant until erythema disappears, and then the dose can

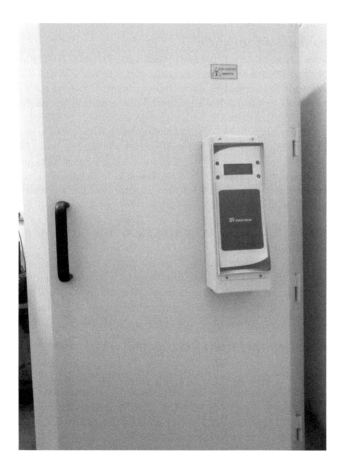

Figure 31.1   Commercially available NB-UVB unit, outer view.

be increased by 10%–20%. For bright red asymptomatic erythema, NB-UVB sessions should be withheld until the affected site becomes light pink, then treatment can be resumed at the previous dose. In the case of symptomatic erythema (including pain and blistering), phototherapy should be stopped until erythema fades to light pink, then the treatment can be resumed at the last tolerated dose. Up to one-third of vitiliginous patients are "non-photoadapters," meaning they are unable to tolerate increased doses of NB-UVB at subsequent exposures and have increased risk of developing burns. These patients should be identified as early as possible because they may benefit from alternative therapies.

c. *Recommendation for special sites*: If the face is not involved, it should be covered during the phototherapy sessions. If the face is involved but eyelids are spared, then patients must wear black goggles. Patients with eyelid lesions are recommended to keep their eyes closed without goggles during the treatment, as in vitro examination has shown negligible penetration of UVB through the eyelid [10]. Genitalia should be shielded because of the possible risk of genital malignancy. Sunscreen must be applied on female areola before exposure to avoid burns from phototherapy, especially in skin types I–III.

d. *Dose adjustment following missed dose*: The dose should be held constant if 4–7 days pass between treatments. The dose should be decreased by 25% if 8–14 days pass between treatments. Similarly, the dose should be decreased by 50% if there is lapse of 15–21 days of treatment. If more than 3 weeks have passed between treatments, then phototherapy should be resumed at the initial dose.

e. *Pre- and post-exposure recommendations*: Before phototherapy sessions, all topical products should be avoided, with exception of mineral oil, for ≥4 hours, as they may deactivate or interfere with the transmission of NB-UVB phototherapy. However, in the areas of dry and thickened skin, such as on elbows and knees, mineral oil can be used to enhance light penetration. Regardless of skin phototypes, all patients should be advised to avoid sun exposure and apply a broad-spectrum sunscreen with a skin protection factor (SPF) of greater than 30, with reapplication after every 2 hours according to American Academy of Dermatology sunscreen guidelines.

f. *Maintenance regimen for NB-UVB*: The dose of NB-UVB should be tapered once the maximum repigmentation has been achieved. During the first month, phototherapy should be continued twice weekly. The frequency should be decreased to weekly during the second month and then to every other week during the third and fourth month. If there is no disease recurrence, the phototherapy can be discontinued. However, there is no sufficient data in the literature for the stability of repigmentation with NB-UVB.

g. *Follow-up*: For patients with phototype I–III, yearly follow-up for cutaneous examination and to monitor for adverse effects of phototherapy, including cutaneous malignancy, is recommended. For skin phototypes IV–VI, yearly follow-up is not required, as no reports of malignancy exist with this group.

GOOD PROGNOSTIC FACTORS DETERMINING RESPONSE TO NB-UVB

- Stable vitiliginous lesions
- Darker skin phototypes (IV–VI)
- Lesions in non-acral areas, especially facial lesions (except for perioral lesions)

- Patients with nonsegmental vitiligo have a good outcome as compared to segmental vitiligo
- Patients having early response (e.g., by 1 month)
- Adherence to treatment (patient must be committed for twice to thrice-weekly treatment at least for 2 months in order to determine response)
- Shorter duration of disease

EFFICACY OF NB-UVB MONOTHERAPY IN VITILIGO

Westerhof and Nieuweboer-Krobotova [11] first reported the efficacy of twice-weekly NB-UVB phototherapy in vitiligo with 75% or greater improvement in 63% of patients at 12 months. A positive correlation between repigmentation and number of NB-UVB exposure has also been reported in other studies [12,13]. Figure 31.3 shows improvement in vitiligo with NB-UVB in one of our patients. NB-UVB phototherapy is also an effective and well-tolerated treatment modality in pediatric patients with vitiligo [14].

COMBINATION THERAPIES WITH NB-UVB

Recently, combination therapies of NB-UVB with topical calcineurin inhibitors ([TCIs] e.g., tacrolimus and pimecrolimus), topical vitamin D analogs ([VDAs] e.g., calcipotriol and tacalcitol), antioxidants, and other therapies have attracted the interest of various dermatologists. The rationale of these combination therapies is to:

a. Achieve a synergistic effect with NB-UVB, especially in causing repigmentation of vitiligo lesions

b. Decrease the total duration, number of sessions, and cumulative dosage of NB-UVB

c. Increase the compliance and satisfaction of patients

NB-UVB WITH TOPICAL CALCINEURIN INHIBITORS

Various authors have investigated TCIs such as tacrolimus and pimecrolimus in combination with NB-UVB. TCIs are presumed to act synergistically with UVB through activation of pathways influencing melanocyte mitogenesis, melanocyte migration, and melanogenesis [15].

According to various studies, the adjunctive use of tacrolimus ointment with NB-UVB increases the extent of repigmentation and decreases the duration of treatment on the combination side as compared to NB-UVB-treated side [16,17]. Dayal et al. have also reported combination of tacrolimus ointment with NB-UVB to be a safe and a more effective option than NB-UVB alone in pediatric vitiligo where treatment options are very limited [14]. Similarly, another TCI, i.e., pimecrolimus, when combined with NB-UVB, has been shown to result in faster and more extensive repigmentation in facial lesions as compared to NB-UVB monotherapy, although this effect was not apparent on other body areas [18].

Of note, there is a perceived risk of skin carcinogenesis with these combination therapies (i.e., tacrolimus or pimecrolimus with NB-UVB), but Tran et al. [19] and Park et al. [20] have separately shown that on a long-term basis the combination of TCIs and NB-UVB is safe and is not associated with increased risk of carcinogenesis. The drug information of these TCIs also recommends protection from the sunlight.

NB-UVB WITH VITAMIN D ANALOGS

Vitamin D analogs (VDAs) include both naturally occurring and synthetic analogs. The naturally occurring analogs include calcitriol

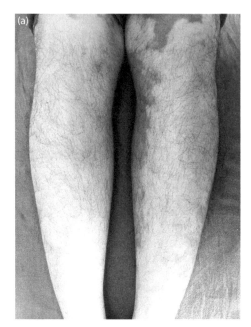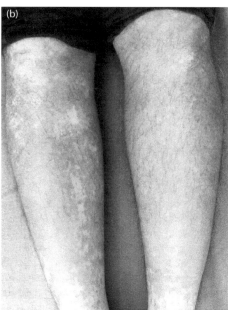

Figure 31.3 NB-UVB in vitiligo patient. (a) Pretreatment photograph; (b) post-treatment improvement photograph.

(1,25-dihydroxyvitamin D₃), and two synthetic analogs are calcipotriol (1,24-dihydroxy-22-ene-24-cyclopropylvitamin D₃) and tacalcitol (1α,24(R)-dihydroxyvitamin D₃). All have been shown to be effective when applied topically in vitiligo [21].

VDAs act by correcting decreased calcium levels in melanocytes in vitiliginous lesions and via immunomodulation [4]. Initially, a case report by Dogra and Parsad [22] showed that the combination of NB-UVB and calcipotriene is effective and well tolerated in vitiligo. Subsequently, calcipotriol has been examined in a number of small prospective studies. However, in these studies the combination showed an equivocal result or did not lead to significantly improved outcome [23,24]. Tacalcitol, another VDA, was also combined with NB-UVB in two clinical trials by Leone et al. [25] and Sahu et al. [26] and revealed that when tacalcitol is combined with NB-UVB, the combination side achieved statistically significant higher repigmentation as compared to NB-UVB alone; however, more studies are required to reach a definite conclusion regarding the potential benefits of these combinations.

NB-UVB WITH ORAL AND TOPICAL ANTIOXIDANTS

Recently, the role of increased oxidative stress has been elucidated in the pathogenesis of vitiligo, which has led to the use of topical and oral antioxidants in its management. Topical preparations, including pseudocatalase, superoxide dismutase, and oral polypodium leucotomas have been studied with NB-UVB in several case studies. Some showed beneficial results [27,28], while others showed no additional benefits [29,30]. NB-UVB, when combined with topical tetrahydrocurcuminoid [31] and placental extract [32], did not produce significant additive effects.

Oral vitamin E and C, alpha lipoic acid, polyunsaturated fatty acids, and cysteine monohydrate, when combined with NB-UVB, showed increased repigmentation [33]. Oral polypodium leucotomus extract, with its antioxidative and immunomodulating properties, when combined with NB-UVB also significantly increased repigmentation in the head and neck area [34].

NB-UVB WITH AFAMELANOTIDE

Afamelanotide, a potent long-lasting synthetic analog of naturally occurring α-MSH (melanocyte stimulating hormone) when combined with NB-UVB results in clinically apparent earlier and superior repigmentary response [35,36].

NB-UVB WITH 5-FLUOROURACIL

Two weekly intradermal injections of 5-fluorouracil (5-FU) in combination with NB-UVB, in localized nonsegmental vitiligo, resulted in significantly higher repigmentation in all body areas except acral areas [37]. With its immunomodulatory properties, 5-FU combination with NB-UVB may stimulate reservoir of follicular melanocytes or persistent dopa-negative melanocytes in depigmented epidermis

NB-UVB WITH LASER ADJUVANTS

Excimer laser, erbium-YAG laser-assisted dermabrasion, and fractional carbon dioxide (CO_2) laser have been examined as an adjunctive therapy with NB-UVB. In generalized vitiligo, treatment with a combination of NB-UVB and excimer laser promotes a synergistic effect through the high energy of the excimer laser and prevents occurrence of new lesions through the immunomodulating effect of NB-UVB to make up for the weakness of excimer laser alone [38].

NB-UVB with prior erbium-YAG laser dermabrasion has also proven to be effective for UV-resistant sites such as hands, feet, and bony prominences [39,40]. As fractional CO_2 laser is associated with better wound healing, it has also been combined with NB-UVB. This combination therapy also resulted in significantly better clinical outcomes as compared to NB-UVB therapy alone, and was well tolerated, with higher patient satisfaction scores [41]. Thus, NB-UVB combination with laser adjuvants is a newer breakthrough in treatment of vitiligo, although a costlier option, but results in improved clinical outcome with a shorter duration of therapy.

NB-UVB WITH SYSTEMIC TREATMENT

NB-UVB has been combined with oral minipulse by Rath et al. [42] indicating additional benefits. Lee et al. [43] have shown that oral methylprednisolone minipulse when combined with NB-UVB is effective in arresting vitiligo progression and rapidly induced repigmentation.

SAFETY AND TOLERABILITY

NB-UVB is a safe and well-tolerated therapeutic modality for vitiligo. It has remarkably very few side effects as compared to PUVA therapy.

SHORT-TERM ADVERSE EFFECTS
The most common short-term adverse effects of NB-UVB include xerosis, pruritus, erythema, and blistering. Among these adverse effects, erythema is the most common, with incidence varying from 10% to 94% [44]. Precautionary measures should be taken in those with a history of herpes simplex, as reactivation of herpes simplex virus can occur with UVB treatment. Exposure keratitis and conjunctivitis can also occur.

LONG-TERM ADVERSE EFFECTS
The long-term side effect of association with carcinogenic risk is well established with PUVA therapy in patients with chronic plaque psoriasis, although it has not been elucidated with NB-UVB either with vitiligo or psoriasis [45]. However, according to some recent studies in cultured lymphoblasts and melanocytes [46] and animal models [47], it has been found that NB-UVB is more carcinogenic than BB-UVB, but this finding is not consistent. While these findings are reassuring, additional follow-up data in vitiligo patients are needed to elucidate the relationship between NB-UVB phototherapy and carcinogenic risk.

CONCLUSION

Over the past two decades, NB-UVB has become the most widely used modality for generalized vitiligo due to its efficacy and favorable safety profile. NB-UVB is considered to be better than PUVA therapy due to its superior efficacy, lack of oral/topical photosensitizer agents, lower cumulative dose, and fewer adverse effects. The addition of systemic and topical adjuncts may provide additional benefits to NB-UVB alone, allowing for optimization of clinical outcome. However, further elaborate well-designed research is needed to determine other treatment modalities that can be safely combined with NB-UVB to increase its beneficial effect and to identify its long-term side effects so that dosing can be optimized.

PRACTICAL TIPS

1. To determine the responsiveness to NB-UVB phototherapy, at least 6 months of treatment duration is required.
2. To achieve a maximal treatment response, phototherapy requires at least 1 year, although the appropriate treatment duration cannot be assessed on the basis of various studies.
3. Certain shared host factors such as disease activity, autoimmune state, large involved body surface area, and presence of poliosis might hinder repigmentation.
4. The most effective response is anticipated on the face and neck, whereas hands and feet show minimal response.
5. NB-UVB is a safe and effective treatment modality in special circumstances such as generalized vitiligo in pregnancy and in childhood, where the treatment modalities are quite limited.
6. Various adjuvant treatments, including VDAs, TCIs, topical/oral antioxidants, and lasers can be used in addition to phototherapy to enhance the treatment response in practice.

REFERENCES

1. Hamzavi IH, Syed ZU, and Lim HW. Ultraviolet-based therapy for vitiligo: What's new? *Indian J Dermatol Venereol Leprol* 2012;78:42–8.
2. Sokolova A, Lee A, and Smith SD. The safety and efficacy of narrow band ultraviolet B treatment in dermatology: A review. *Am J Clin Dermatol* 2015;16:501–31.
3. Hönigsmann H. History of phototherapy in dermatology. *Photochem Photobiol Sci* 2013;12:16–21.
4. Dogra S, and Arora AK. Narrowband ultraviolet B and beyond: Evolving role of phototherapy in vitiligo. *Pigment Int* 2015;2:9.
5. Cui J, Shen L-Y, and Wang G-C. Role of hair follicles in the repigmentation of vitiligo. *J Investig Dermatol* 1991;97:410–6.
6. Schallreuter KU, Bahadoran P, Picardo M et al. Vitiligo pathogenesis: Autoimmune disease, genetic defect, excessive reactive oxygen species, calcium imbalance, or what else? *Exp Dermatol* 2008;17:139–40.
7. Griffiths CEM, Barker J, Bleiker T, Chalmers R, and Creamer D. *Rook's Textbook of Dermatology*. Chichester, West Sussex (UK): Wiley Blackwell; 2016.
8. Shan X, Wang C, Tian H, Yang B, and Zhang F. Narrow-band ultraviolet B home phototherapy in vitiligo. *Indian J Dermatol Venereol Leprol* 2014;80:336.
9. Mohammad TF, Al-Jamal M, Hamzavi IH, Harris JE, Leone G, Cabrera R, Lim HW, Pandya AG, and Esmat SM. The vitiligo working group recommendations for narrow band ultraviolet B light phototherapy treatment of vitiligo. *J Am Acad Dermatol* 2017;76:879–88.
10. Prystowsky JH, Keen MS, Rabinowitz AD, Stevens AW, and DeLeo VA. Present status of eyelid phototherapy. *J Am Acad Dermatol* 1992;26:607–13.
11. Westerhof W, and Nieuweboer-Krobotova L. Treatment of vitiligo with UV-B radiation vs topical psoralen plus UV-A. *Arch Dermatol* 1997;133:1525–8.
12. Kanwar AJ, Dogra S, Parsad D, and Kumar B. Narrow-band UVB for the treatment of vitiligo: An emerging effective and well-tolerated therapy. *Int J Dermatol* 2005;44:57–60.
13. Kishan Kumar YH, Rao GR, Gopal KV, Shanti G, and Rao KV. Evaluation of narrow-band UVB phototherapy in 150 patients with vitiligo. *Indian J Dermatol Venereol Leprol* 2009;75:162.
14. Dayal S, Sahu P, and Gupta N. Treatment of childhood vitiligo using tacrolimus ointment with narrowband ultraviolet B phototherapy. *Pediatr Dermatol* 2016;33:646–51.
15. Castanedo-Cazares JP, Lepe V, and Moncada B. Repigmentation of chronic vitiligo lesions by following tacrolimus plus ultraviolet-B-narrow-band. *Photodermatol Photoimmunol Photomed* 2003;19:35–6.
16. Nordal EJ, Guleng GE, and Rönnevig JR. Treatment of vitiligo with narrowband-UVB (TL01) combined with tacrolimus ointment (0.1%) vs. placebo ointment, a randomized right/left double-blind comparative study. *J Eur Acad Dermatol Venereol* 2011;25:1440–3.
17. Majid I. Does topical tacrolimus ointment enhance the efficacy of narrowband ultraviolet B therapy in vitiligo? A left-right comparison study. *Photodermatol Photoimmunol Photomed* 2010;26:230–4.

18. Esfandiarpour I, Ekhlasi A, Farajzadeh S, and Shamsadini S. The efficacy of pimecrolimus 1% cream plus narrow-band ultraviolet B in the treatment of vitiligo: A double-blind, placebo-controlled clinical trial. *J Dermatolog Treat* 2009;20:14–8.

19. Tran C, Lübbe J, Sorg O, Doelker L, Carraux P, Antille C, Grand D, Leemans E, Kaya G, and Saurat J-H. Topical calcineurin inhibitors decrease the production of UVB-induced thymine dimers from hairless mouse epidermis. *Dermatology* 2005;211:341–7.

20. Park KK, Murase JE, and Koo J. Long-term prognosis of vitiligo patients on narrowband UVB phototherapy. *J Am Acad Dermatol* 2012;66:326–7.

21. Wolverton SE. *Comprehensive Dermatologic Drug Therapy.* Elsevier; 2013.

22. Dogra S, and Prasad D. Combination of narrowband UV-B and topical calcipotriene in vitiligo. *Arch Dermatol* 2003;139:393.

23. Goktas EO, Aydin F, Senturk N, Canturk MT, and Turanli AY. Combination of narrow band UVB and topical calcipotriol for the treatment of vitiligo. *J Eur Acad Dermatol Venereol* 2006;20:553–7.

24. Hartmann A, Lurz C, Hamm H, Brocker E-B, and Hofmann UB. Narrow-band UVB311 nm vs. broad-band UVB therapy in combination with topical calcipotriol vs. placebo in vitiligo. *Int J Dermatol* 2005;44:736–42.

25. Leone G, Pacifico A, Iacovelli P, Paro Vidolin A, and Picardo M. Tacalcitol and narrow-band phototherapy in patients with vitiligo. *Clin Exp Dermatol* 2006;31:200–5.

26. Sahu P, Jain VK, Aggarwal K, Kaur S, and Dayal S. Tacalcitol: A useful adjunct to narrow-band ultraviolet-B phototherapy in vitiligo. *Photodermatol Photoimmunol Photomed* 2016;32:262–8.

27. Schallreuter KU, Krüger C, Würfel BA, Panske A, and Wood JM. From basic research to the bedside: Efficacy of topical treatment with pseudocatalase PC-KUS in 71 children with vitiligo. *Int J Dermatol* 2008;47:743–53.

28. Kostovic K, Pastar Z, Pasic A, and Ceovic R. Treatment of vitiligo with narrow-band UVB and topical gel containing catalase and superoxide dismutase. *Acta Dermatovenerologica Iugoslavica* 2007;15:10–4.

29. Bakis-Petsoglou S, Le Guay JL, and Wittal R. A randomized, double-blinded, placebo-controlled trial of pseudocatalase cream and narrowband ultraviolet B in the treatment of vitiligo. *Br J Dermatol* 2009;161:910–7.

30. Patel DC, Evans AV, and Hawk JLM. Topical pseudocatalase mousse and narrowband UVB phototherapy is not effective for vitiligo: An open, single-centre study. *Clin Exp Dermatol* 2002;27:641–4.

31. Asawanonda P, and Klahan S-O. Tetrahydrocurcuminoid cream plus targeted narrowband UVB phototherapy for vitiligo: A preliminary randomized controlled study. *Photomed Laser Surg* 2010;28:679–84.

32. Majid I. Topical placental extract: Does it increase the efficacy of narrowband UVB therapy in vitiligo? *Indian J Dermatol Venereol Leprol* 2010;76:254–8.

33. Dell'Anna, ML, Mastrofrancesco A, Sala R, Venturini M, Ottaviani M, Vidolin AP, Leone G, Calzavara PG, Westerhof W, and Picardo M. Antioxidants and narrow band-UVB in the treatment of vitiligo: A double-blind placebo controlled trial. *Clin Exp Dermatol* 2007;32:631–6.

34. Middelkamp-Hup MA, Bos JD, Rius-Diaz F, Gonzalez S, and Westerhof W. Treatment of vitiligo vulgaris with narrow-band UVB and oral polypodium leucotomos extract: A randomized double-blind placebo-controlled study. *J Eur Acad Dermatol Venereol* 2007;21:942–50.

35. Grimes PE, Hamzavi I, Lebwohl M, Ortonne JP, and Lim HW. The efficacy of afamelanotide and narrowband UV-B phototherapy for repigmentation of vitiligo. *JAMA Dermatol* 2013;149:68–73.

36. Lim HW, Grimes PE, Agbai O, Hamzavi I, Henderson M, Haddican M, Linkner RV, and Lebwohl M. Afamelanotide and narrowband UV-B phototherapy for the treatment of vitiligo. *JAMA Dermatol* 2015;151:42.

37. Abd El-Samad Z, and Shaaban D. Treatment of localized non-segmental vitiligo with intradermal 5-flurouracil injection combined with narrow-band ultraviolet B: A preliminary study. *J Dermatolog Treat* 2011;23:443–8.

38. Shin S, Hann SK, and Oh SH. Combination treatment with excimer laser and narrowband UVB light in vitiligo patients. *Photodermatol Photoimmunol Photomed* 2015;32:28–33.

39. Anbar TS, Westerhof W, Abdel-Rahman AT, Ewis AA, and El-Khayyat MA. Effect of one session of ER: YAG laser ablation plus topical 5 Fluorouracil on the outcome of short-term NB-UVB phototherapy in the treatment of non-segmental vitiligo: A left-right comparative study. *Photodermatol Photoimmunol Photomed* 2008;24:322–9.

40. Bayoumi W, Fontas E, Sillard L, Le Duff F, Ortonne J-P, Bahadoran P, Lacour J-P, and Passeron T. Effect of a preceding laser dermabrasion on the outcome of combined therapy with narrowband ultraviolet B and potent topical steroids for treating nonsegmental vitiligo in resistant localizations. *Br J Dermatol* 2011;166:208–11.

41. Shin J, Lee JS, Hann S-K, and Oh SH. Combination treatment by 10 600 Nm ablative fractional carbon dioxide laser and narrowband ultraviolet B in refractory nonsegmental vitiligo: A prospective, randomized half-body comparative study. *Br J Dermatol* 2012;166:658–61.

42. Rath N, Sabhnani S, and Kar HK. An open labeled, comparative clinical study on efficacy and tolerability of oral mini pulse of steroid (OMP) alone, OMP with PUVA and broad/narrow band UVB phototherapy in progressive vitiligo. *Indian J Dermatol Venereol Leprol* 2008;74:357–60.

43. Lee J, Chu H, Lee H, Kim M, Kim DS, and Oh SH. A retrospective study of methylprednisolone mini-pulse therapy combined with narrow-band UVB in non-segmental vitiligo. *Dermatology* 2015;232:224–9.

44. Ibbotson SH, Bilsland D, Cox NH et al. An update and guidance on narrow band ultraviolet B phototherapy: A British photodermatology group workshop report. *Br J Dermatol* 2004;151:283–97.

45. Archier E, Devaux S, Castela E et al. Carcinogenic risks of psoralen UV-a therapy and narrowband UV-B therapy in chronic plaque psoriasis: A systematic literature review. *J Eur Acad Dermatol Venereol* 2012;26:22–31.

46. Tzung T-Y, and Rünger TM. Assessment of DNA damage induced by broadband and narrowband UVB in cultured lymphoblasts and keratinocytes using the comet assay. *Photochem Photobiol* 1998;67:647–50.

47. Wulf HC, Hansen AB, and Bech-Thomsen N. Differences in narrowband ultraviolet B and broad-spectrum ultraviolet photocarcinogenesis in lightly pigmented hairless mice. *Photodermatol Photoimmunol Photomed* 1994;10:192–7.

Chapter 32

TARGETED PHOTOTHERAPY

Christopher Tzermias

CONTENTS

INTRODUCTION AND HISTORICAL BACKGROUND

Phototherapy entered the practitioner's armamentarium for the treatment of vitiligo long ago in the form of psoralen plus ultraviolet A (PUVA) therapy, a form of photochemotherapy, introduced in 1948, and widely used for a long time [1]. Phototherapy modalities have evolved since, as UVA was abandoned in favor of UVB, a wavelength range found to be more efficacious, especially at 311 nm, for the intended repigmentation of vitiliginous skin. This could be attributed to the higher levels of cis-urocanic acid produced, as well as to alterations caused in function and morphology of Langerhans cells [2]. The lesser efficacy, combined with PUVA's acute undesirable side effects, led to its being surpassed by the improved modality of narrowband ultraviolet B (NB-UVB) phototherapy, bearing fewer adverse effects and a better efficacy [3]. The NB-UVB not only includes the most efficacious wavelength for repigmentation (311 nm) but also excludes the spectral region of the most erythemogenic and carcinogenic wavelengths, unlike BB-UVB [4]. To date, NB-UVB remains a mainstay in vitiligo treatment, especially in the case of nonsegmental diffuse vitiligo [1].

However, at the dawn of the twenty-first century, new UVB-emitting devices started to emerge, intended for targeted phototherapy [1]. The concept of targeted phototherapy pertains to the restricted delivery of UV light selectively to the affected area, allowing also for higher fluencies while sparing the surrounding healthy skin. In contrast, during conventional phototherapy the whole skin is irradiated with lower UV fluencies by means of a whole-body unit and thus affected by the subsequent adverse effects, while the therapeutic effect is slower and dichromy can be retained between the lesional and perilesional skin [1,5]. Targeted phototherapy has been suggested as a therapeutic approach, mostly in cases of nonsegmental limited vitiligo, but can also be tried in the treatment of segmental vitiligo [1].

Herein, the different available targeted phototherapy modalities are presented, discussed with respect to their potential for vitiligo treatment, and compared with one another as well as with conventional phototherapy. It should be noted that for the sake of comprehensiveness, this chapter constitutes an overview of the current advances in targeted phototherapy rather than an extended critical review of all available research conducted on the matter over the years.

TARGETED PHOTOTHERAPY MODALITIES

MONOCHROMATIC EXCIMER LIGHT DEVICES: THE LASER AND THE LAMP

The 308-nm xenon-chloride (XeCl) excimer devices, used in dermatology, take advantage of the energy emitted as UV radiation during the decomposition of an XeCl excimer. A 308-nm XeCl excimer is an excited complex of xenon-chloride formed by the combination of a noble gas (xenon) and a reactive halogen (chlorine) that, upon decomposition, emits UV radiation at the 308-nm wavelength. The latter is designated as 308-nm monochromatic excimer light (MEL), while the emitting devices can be either a laser or a lamp, which, in turn, impacts on the light's properties [6].

XeCl EXCIMER LASER

The excimer laser device emits pulsing, monochromatic, and coherent light, and its application for the treatment of vitiligo has been approved by the U.S. Food and Drug Administration (FDA) [6]. Initially proved a more effective modality for the treatment of psoriasis compared with conventional NB-UVB, it was reported for the first time as a potential treatment for vitiligo in 2001, in a case report published by the same research group. In this report, a 24-year-old female, with a Fitzpatrick skin type III and enduring vitiliginous lesions on the elbows, achieved almost complete, and stable after at least 1 year, repigmentation after being treated with the laser for 6 months. The first signs of repigmentation were visible after the third month of treatment, while no adverse effects were observed [7]. Following this, one of the early studies, paving the way for further investigation of the therapeutic potential of the excimer laser in vitiligo, was a pilot study published in the *Journal of American Academy of Dermatology* in 2002 [8]. Employing 18 patients with a total of 29 enduring stable vitiligo patches to be treated with excimer laser thrice a week for a maximum of 4 weeks, the study showed the potential of this therapeutic modality to provide better results in terms of time efficiency compared with the types of phototherapy mainly used until then. In particular, 57% of lesions treated for at least 2 weeks showed some repigmentation by the end of the second week. Upon completion of all treatments (end of fourth week), 82% of the treated patches resulted in repigmentation. Such a degree of repigmentation, achieved that early in time, had no precedent with PUVA, broadband, or narrowband UVB, which may require up to a year to achieve a therapeutic effect. This is significant, since most patients who quit the therapeutic process state withdrawal results from an inability to comply with the frequency of treatment sessions over an extended period of time [8].

Since then, many studies assessing the excimer laser's efficacy and safety for the treatment of vitiligo have followed. A review of these studies indicates that excimer laser phototherapy is recommended as a first-line therapy for localized vitiligo and is considered suitable for application to children and all Fitzpatrick skin types (I–VI), although recipients with darker skin tend to respond better. Treatment sessions are usually performed two or three times per week for a variable period of 4–36 weeks, while more frequent sessions show better results [6,9]. Duration of treatment could also have an impact on efficacy [6]. The initial dose is usually determined as a function of minimal erythema dose (MED), while taking into account the area of treatment [9]. The best response is usually achieved from face, neck, axillae, and trunk, as opposed to hands, feet, and digits, which exhibit minimal results. Repigmentation seems to be persistent and even continue after the end of treatment [6]. Finally, a sole study investigating, for the first time, the impact of excimer laser treatment on vitiligo patients' quality of life and satisfaction suggests that there is an improvement in these, even if some of the treated lesions do not show significant repigmentation. This promotes the idea of patients being treated regardless of potentially poor results for some of the vitiligo patches [10].

XeCl EXCIMER LAMP

Soon after the advance of excimer laser, a second device emitting radiation at a similar wavelength was introduced and tested. The excimer lamp is a device emitting polychromatic or, expressed more precisely, quasi-monochromatic light, since it actually emits radiation at a range of 306–310 nm wavelength with a peak at 308 nm that constitutes the majority of light emitted. It is also incoherent and nondirectional. Thus there are in fact inherent differences between the two MEL devices, the excimer laser and lamp, which can differentiate the treatment offered, as will be discussed further down [6].

The first study to investigate the efficacy and safety of the excimer lamp in the treatment of vitiligo was conducted with the participation of 37 patients, both males and females, suffering from different types of the disease. The patients were treated with the lamp twice a week for 6 months and their overall repigmentation rates were assessed. Upon completion of the first 8 sessions, 36 patients showed some repigmentation, while by the completion of the treatment, 18 achieved an excellent and 16 a good repigmentation rate. Only one was a nonresponder and dropped out after the first 3 months. This study asserted that the potential for repigmentation using the excimer lamp can be evaluated early, based on responsiveness during the first treatment sessions. Moreover, although face and neck exhibit the best response, hands, which usually exhibit poor results, could also get repigmented. Both of these findings contradict what was known up to then for treatment with NB-UVB. Authors suggest that the laser lamp's operational mechanism could offer the advantage of higher fluencies, shorter treatment durations, and lower cumulative doses compared with conventional NB-UVB, rendering it worthy of further investigation [3]. More studies followed that confirmed the excimer lamp's utility in the treatment of vitiligo [6].

TARGETED NARROWBAND UVB PHOTOTHERAPY

Concurrently with the advent of excimer technology in the treatment of vitiligo, efforts were made to assess the efficacy of a targeted version of NB-UVB phototherapy and put it into practice. The most notable effort seems to be the use of the BIOSKIN® equipment to perform what the inventors originally called microphototherapy. It is a device capable of emitting both visible and UV light, which by use of a filter can be restricted to emitting at a spectrum ranging

from 300 to 320 nm, with a peak at 311 nm, allowing for targeted NB-UVB treatment of vitiligo patches. During a clinical study spanning 30 months, 734 patients between 6 and 78 years of age, with a skin type either II or III, were treated with the device and had their response levels assessed by comparison of their photos, by means of planimetry, as the treatment was progressing. Patients were treated only once every 2 weeks for 12 consecutive months. However, the authors eventually mention a mean of 40 treatment sessions for each patient. For most patients, repigmentation started after the second month of treatment, and by the end of the study period, 69.48% of all participants had achieved repigmentation on more than 75% of the treated lesions, while another 21.12% achieved repigmentation on 50%–75% of the patches. It is not mentioned whether the repigmentation persisted or not [2]. A more recent study, employing 40 patients with 97 lesions treated with a device emitting at a similar spectrum, the Levia® professional targeted UVB machine, yielded promising results. Repigmentation rates of 50% or higher were achieved by 77.5% of the patients, while 46.6% of the vitiliginous lesions achieved 90%–100% repigmentation. It should be noted, however, that no acral lesions were included in this study [5]. Acral lesions are known to be recalcitrant to treatment with the excimer technology [6] and thus their inclusion in or exclusion from a study could impact the overall repigmentation rate and should be taken into account during comparison with others. Although the author admits that a follow-up period of 3 months cannot establish the stability of repigmentation, he concludes the results are similar to those obtained with other targeted UVB devices, such as the BIOSKIN, but the early onset of repigmentation observed is similar to that achieved with MEL, probably due to the similarity of the treatment protocol used [5].

TARGETED BROADBAND UVB PHOTOTHERAPY

A targeted version of broadband UVB (BB-UVB) phototherapy has been also tested for the treatment of vitiligo. Proponents of testing the potential of this modality have warranted this investigation on the fact that although the excimer laser is effective, it is also expensive and difficult to maintain. Thus, Dua-Light™, a mercury lamp emitting either UVA or UVB with an average wavelength of 304 nm and peaks at 302 nm and 312 nm, was used as an irradiation source to treat 29 lesions from 6 patients during a pilot study. The treatment was delivered twice a week for 12 weeks. It was well tolerated, some repigmentation occurred in all patients, and in some cases it had an early onset. However, this is not conclusive for BB-UVB's efficacy as no significant repigmentation occurred on the face, as is usually the case in other studies, while the sample was very small and diverse [11]. However, during another study utilizing the same device, 53 lesions from 35 patients were treated twice per week for a maximum of 60 sessions, with an average of 44. In this case, 77.4% of the participants achieved a repigmentation rate equal to or higher than 75%. The best response was observed in the face and neck, while results were better for focal rather than segmental vitiligo [12]. A second, portable device, the BClear®, emitting incoherent light at a spectrum of 290–320 nm, was utilized to treat 47 vitiliginous patches in 12 patients. A total of 30 treatment sessions were applied, with a frequency of two per week. The first signs of repigmentation were visible after the 16th session for the face, which showed repigmentation >75%, and after the 20th for the trunk, neck, and genitalia, which showed a repigmentation rate of 26%–50%. Upper and lower extremities showed no repigmentation. Adverse effects, such as itching, pruritus, erythema, and desquamation were observed. One year later, repigmentation persisted in eight patients [13]. However, a retrospective study published during the same year showed that targeted BB-UVB phototherapy may be safe but not efficient to use in the treatment of vitiligo. In this study, a different device was used, namely the Daavlin T500ˣ High-Dose Targeted Phototherapy

System, emitting at 302–312 nm. A total of 32 patients were treated twice or thrice a week, undergoing a total of 20–60 sessions. Only 4 out of the 32 participants showed repigmentation, while mild adverse events were also present [14].

HELIUM-NEON LASER

The Helium-Neon (He-Ne) laser constitutes a different option for targeted phototherapy treatment of vitiligo. It is not a UV source but a device emitting monochromatic light within the visible spectrum, specifically at 632.8 nm [15,16]. It is considered a low-energy laser. That means that when applied, it does not confer a thermal effect but acts by exerting biostimulatory effects. It has been shown to promote repigmentation in vitiligo, possibly due to stimulation and proliferation of melanocytes, and has been suggested as a therapeutic option of equal efficacy to traditional phototherapy methods but also less costly, with no adverse effects and easier to apply [15]. More recent research has interestingly shown that He-Ne irradiation is capable of inducing differentiation of melanoblasts via interactions that cannot be elicited by UVB [16].

COMPARATIVE ASPECTS FOR TARGETED PHOTOTHERAPY TREATMENT CHOICE

Before proceeding to acknowledgment of the available comparative literature, it should be noted that comparison among studies treating vitiligo, by application either of the same modality or different modalities of phototherapy, involves major limitations, which could be accountable for potential variations in results. The author of this chapter suspects that, as investigators themselves have in part admitted, variability in the number [6,17,18], age [19], and skin types [20] of patients, the type and mean duration of vitiligo [6,18,19], the body areas where the vitiliginous lesions are located [6,17,18], the treatment scheme followed (namely the number [6,17]), frequency and length of treatment sessions [6,17–19] as well as the fluence used [6,17,19] and its pattern of alteration during the therapeutic period [17], the methodology for evaluating the efficacy of treatment [17–19], and the different devices employed [6] reduce the conclusiveness of the comparative deductions. Furthermore, taking into account that, as pointed out earlier, a sole study regarding the quality of life after treatment has been conducted [10], it seems there is a general disregard of this important aspect in the assessment of therapeutic modalities [17,19]. Finally, there is the inherent publication bias, which constitutes a tendency according to which results that do not confirm the hypothesis of interest are rejected and remain unpublished [18].

Studies comparing the effectiveness between targeted vs conventional phototherapy, mainly the excimer technology and conventional NB-UVB, have shown that a lower number of treatments is required for targeted phototherapy to achieve the same amount of repigmentation as conventional therapy does [21]. Furthermore, it has a rapid repigmentation potential, and consequently a faster therapeutic response [1,22] that, combined with the overall shorter treatment duration and frequency, could encourage patient compliance [6,22], while it also allows for a lower cumulative dose [19,21]. There has been a study that proposed, however, that there are no differences in repigmentation patterns [23], while two systematic reviews similarly agree for no differences in repigmentation efficacy according to the studies analyzed. However, both acknowledge some of the aforementioned limitations and indicate the necessity for further studies [19,24]. It should especially be noted that the previous reviews have included in their analyses studies employing either conventional or targeted NB-UVB in the same group indiscriminately when comparing with

the excimer technology (either laser or lamp) and also have classified studies, either with or without a combination of a treatment preceding phototherapy, in the same group too. Among other acknowledged targeted phototherapy advantages over the conventional method are the ease of therapeutic access to vitiliginous areas otherwise difficult to reach [1], the potential treatment of lesions conventional NB-UVB previously failed to treat [3], sparing of the healthy perilesional skin from UV exposure [1,19] as well as the subsequent potential for eliminating the location of the side effects [1] and reducing the risk of carcinogenicity [2,19], and last, the potential for delivering irradiation of higher intensity to the treating area in less time [1]. Furthermore, some of the targeted phototherapy devices are portable [13,19], and treatment sessions can even be conducted at home by the patients, as is the case for many of the author's patients. However, targeted phototherapy is more expensive than conventional and is regarded as unsuitable for vitiligo patients with more than 10% [19], 20% [1], or 30% [2] of the body surface area affected.

It is generally hypothesized that NB-UVB and MEL should have similar photobiological properties due to their similar wavelengths of 311 nm and 308 nm, respectively [9,18]. Their mechanism of action purportedly pertains to the enhancement of proliferation and migration of melanocytes to the depigmented area combined with effects on the immune response [18,19]. However, the different light (coherent or incoherent, polychromatic or monochromatic), the different emitting devices, and the way the irradiation is administered (targeted or not) can confer differing biological effects on the body [1,6]. During an early study on excimer lamp, Leone and colleagues noted an implication that higher fluences of NB-UVB could treat vitiliginous patches on hands similarly to what had been accomplished with MEL during their study [3]. Higher fluences can be achieved by targeted phototherapy. Although studies on targeted NB-UVB have been conducted, only one direct comparison study with the excimer lamp could be found. In this intrapatient study, targeted 311-nm NB-UVB appears to be more efficacious than 308-nm MEL. Investigators propose it as an effective alternative form of targeted phototherapy for localized vitiligo in view of its low cost and ease of accessibility [17].

Similarly, there is only one study directly comparing targeted BB-UVB with targeted NB-UVB. The efficacy of the two modalities was found to be similar for the treatment of localized nonsegmental vitiligo [25].

The correlation of efficacy and side effects between the excimer laser and excimer lamp seems to have sparked more interest in the scientific community. Both devices have been shown to share similar efficacy in direct comparison studies [18,26,27]. However, the lamp was found to produce more erythema than the laser [26], while it also demanded more time to deliver the same light dose, which could have an effect on the duration of treatment sessions. Despite this, its lower cost of acquisition, operation, and maintenance combined with its smaller dimensions that make it more easily accessible [6,26], and its potential for a larger irradiation field during treatment [6,27] could counterbalance its disadvantages and render the excimer lamp a more cost-effective and widely available option than the laser [6,26,27].

TARGETED PHOTOTHERAPY AS A COMBINATION TREATMENT

Targeted phototherapy modalities have not only been used as a monotherapy but also in combination with other vitiligo treatments, yielding significant results. Topical corticosteroids and calcineurin inhibitors, such as tacrolimus and pimecrolimus, increase the efficacy when combined with either the excimer lamp or laser [1,6,9]. Investigations on the potential of combination therapies in the treatment of vitiligo have also produced promising results in the case of targeted NB-UVB [28,29].

PRACTICAL EXPERIENCE

Experience at the author's dermatology practice, obtained by application of the excimer lamp to vitiligo patients, confirms many of the aforementioned observations. Therapeutic effects usually become visible after the 25th and before the 30th treatment session, while first and best repigmentation results are observed primarily on the face and also axillae, elbows, and genitalia, body areas in which repigmentation can reach 100% at the end of treatment. On the contrary, response is slower and complete repigmentation rare in the case of the feet and digits of the hands. Initial irradiation dose starts at 100 mJ/cm^2 and there is a stable increment of 50 mJ/cm^2 after the completion of each two successive sessions, unless erythema is presented. Frequency of sessions is either two or three times per week, and the duration of phototherapy treatment ranges from 3 to 9 months. More frequent treatment sessions usually correspond to faster results. Prospective patients are usually concerned with the overall duration of treatment and more importantly with safety and the level of expectable recovery. Therefore, they should be explicitly informed and advised about all aspects of this therapy to avoid misunderstanding. Finally, thorough examination of the body under a Woods lamp is recommended to allow for detection and prevention of future vitiligo patches before visible depigmentation occurs.

A similar protocol and results are observed in the case of a portable 311-nm NB-UVB device that some of our patients are provided with for domestic use. This device is convenient to carry from one place to another, eliminating even the need for mandatory presence at home. All vitiligo patches are initially recorded at the dermatology practice and patients undergo intensive training on how to perform the treatment and what they need to be cautious about. They also record the parameters of each treatment session they perform and need to give an oral report about their progress to the clinician, over the phone, once a month. An examination at the dermatology practice every 3 months is also required to evaluate the results and potentially adjust the protocol.

Combination of the aforementioned phototherapy modalities with the application of tacrolimus and Pigmerise™ ointments has been shown to improve results in our clinic. Both agents have an indication for long-term use and are applied once per day to the affected area as long as the treatment continues. Tacrolimus ointments exhibit fewer side effects compared to steroid creams but their application should be omitted the day before a phototherapy session. An ointment with reduced tacrolimus content is used for sensitive areas. Although Pigmerise has no contraindication for application the day before phototherapy, it is recommended that it not be used in sensitive areas that day since some patients may develop irritant dermatitis.

CONCLUDING REMARKS

Since its development in the early 2010s, targeted phototherapy has revolutionized our capabilities for selectively treating vitiligo with major efficiency but minor adverse effects. Notably, its immediate therapeutic response combined with the overall less demanded time and frequency of treatment sessions have strongly encouraged patients' commitment to therapy, which has been a major issue in the past. Taking the efficacy for granted, emphasizing the impact on patients' self-assessed quality of life and mental well-being is recommended for future investigators.

REFERENCES

1. Pacifico A, and Leone G. Photo(chemo)therapy for vitiligo. *Photodermatol Photoimmunol Photomed* Oct 2011;27(5): 261–77.

2. Menchini G, Tsoureli-Nikita E, and Hercogova J. Narrowband UV-B micro-phototherapy: A new treatment for vitiligo. *J Eur Acad Dermatol Venereol* Mar 2003;17(2):171–7.

3. Leone G, Iacovelli P, Paro Vidolin A, and Picardo M. Monochromatic excimer light 308 Nm in the treatment of vitiligo: A pilot study. *J Eur Acad Dermatol Venereol* Sep 2003;17(5):531–7.

4. Gambichler T, Breuckmann F, Boms S, Altmeyer P, and Kreuter A. Narrowband UVB phototherapy in skin conditions beyond psoriasis. *J Am Acad Dermatol* Apr 2005;52(4):660–70.

5. Majid I. Efficacy of targeted narrowband ultraviolet B therapy in vitiligo. *Indian J Dermatol* Sep 2014;59(5):485–9.

6. Park KK, Liao W, and Murase JE. A review of monochromatic excimer light in vitiligo. *Br J Dermatol* Sep 2012;167(3):468–78.

7. Baltás E, Nagy P, Bánis B, Novák Z, Ignácz F, Szabó G, Bor Z, Dobozy A, and Kemény L. Repigmentation of localized vitiligo with the xenon chloride laser. *Br J Dermatol* Jun 2001;144(6):1266–7.

8. Spencer JM, Nossa R, and Ajmeri J. Treatment of vitiligo with the 308-Nm excimer laser: A pilot study. *J Am Acad Dermatol* May 2002;46(5):727–31.

9. Alhowaish AK, Dietrich N, Onder M, and Fritz K. Effectiveness of a 308-nm excimer laser in treatment of vitiligo: A review. *Lasers Med Sci* May 2013;28(3):1035–41.

10. Al-Shobaili HA. Treatment of vitiligo patients by excimer laser improves patients' quality of life. *J Cutan Med Surg* 2015 Jan-Feb 2015;19(1):50–6.

11. Asawanonda P, Charoenlap M, and Korkij W. Treatment of localized vitiligo with targeted broadband UVB phototherapy: A pilot study. *Photodermatol Photoimmunol Photomed* Jun 2006;22(3):133–6.

12. Kim JE, Ahn HH, and Kye YC. Targeted broadband UVB phototherapy for the treatment of localized vitiligo. *Ann Dermatol* Sep 2008;20(3):107–12.

13. Welsh O, Herz-Ruelas ME, Gómez M, and Ocampo-Candiani J. Therapeutic evaluation of UVB-targeted phototherapy in vitiligo that affects less than 10% of the body surface area. *Int J Dermatol* May 2009;48(5):529–34.

14. Akar A, Tunca M, Koc E, and Kurumlu Z. Broadband targeted UVB phototherapy for localized vitiligo: A retrospective study. *Photodermatol Photoimmunol Photomed* Jun 2009;25(3):161–3.

15. Yu HS, Wu CS, Yu CL, Kao YH, and Chiou MH. Helium-neon laser irradiation stimulates migration and proliferation in melanocytes and induces repigmentation in segmental-type vitiligo. *J Invest Dermatol* Jan 2003;120(1):56–64.

16. Lan CC, Wu SB, Wu CS, Shen YC, Chiang TY, Wei YH, and Yu HS. Induction of primitive pigment cell differentiation by visible light (helium-neon laser): A photoacceptor-specific response not replicable by UVB irradiation. *J Mol Med (Berl)* Mar 2012;90(3):321–30.

17. Verhaeghe E, Lodewick E, van Geel N, and Lambert J. Intrapatient comparison of 308-nm monochromatic excimer light and localized narrow-band UVB phototherapy in the treatment of vitiligo: A randomized controlled trial. *Dermatology* 2011;223(4):343–8.

18. Sun Y, Wu Y, Xiao B, Li L, Chen HD, and Gao XH. Treatment of 308-nm excimer laser on vitiligo: A systemic review of randomized controlled trials. *J Dermatolog Treat* 2015;26(4):347–53.

19. Lopes C, Trevisani VF, and Melnik T. Efficacy and safety of 308-nm monochromatic excimer lamp versus other phototherapy devices for vitiligo: A systematic review with meta-analysis. *Am J Clin Dermatol* Feb 2016;17(1):23–32.

20. Chua S, Pitts M, and Li J. Phototherapy for vitiligo: Skin phototypes are important. *Pediatr Dermatol* 2015 Nov-Dec 2015;32(6):877.

21. Casacci M, Thomas P, Pacifico A, Bonnevalle A, Paro Vidolin A, and Leone G. Comparison between 308-nm monochromatic excimer light and narrowband UVB phototherapy (311–313 nm) in the treatment of vitiligo--a multicentre controlled study. *J Eur Acad Dermatol Venereol* Aug 2007;21(7):956–63.

22. Hong SB, Park HH, and Lee MH. Short-term effects of 308-nm xenon-chloride excimer laser and narrow-band ultraviolet B in the treatment of vitiligo: A comparative study. *J Korean Med Sci* Apr 2005;20(2):273–8.

23. Yang YS, Cho HR, Ryou JH, and Lee MH. Clinical study of repigmentation patterns with either narrow-band ultraviolet B (NBUVB) or 308 nm excimer laser treatment in Korean vitiligo patients. *Int J Dermatol* Mar 2010;49(3):317–23.

24. Xiao BH, Wu Y, Sun Y, Chen HD, and Gao XH. Treatment of vitiligo with NB-UVB: A systematic review. *J Dermatolog Treat* 2015;26(4):340–6.

25. Asawanonda P, Kijluakiat J, Korkij W, and Sindhupak W. Targeted broadband ultraviolet B phototherapy produces similar responses to targeted narrowband ultraviolet B phototherapy for vitiligo: A randomized, double-blind study. *Acta Derm Venereol* 2008;88(4):376–81.

26. Le Duff F, Fontas E, Giacchero D, Sillard L, Lacour JP, Ortonne JP, and Passeron T. 308-Nm excimer lamp vs. 308-nm excimer laser for treating vitiligo: A randomized study. *Br J Dermatol* Jul 2010;163(1):188–92.

27. Shi Q, Li K, Fu J, Wang Y, Ma C, Li Q, Li C, and Gao T. Comparison of the 308-nm excimer laser with the 308-nm excimer lamp in the treatment of vitiligo--a randomized bilateral comparison study. *Photodermatol Photoimmunol Photomed* Feb 2013;29(1):27–33.

28. Lotti T, Buggiani G, Troiano M, Assad GB, Delescluse J, De Giorgi V, and Hercogova J. Targeted and combination treatments for vitiligo. Comparative evaluation of different current modalities in 458 subjects. *Dermatol Ther* Jul 2008;21(Suppl 1):S20–6.

29. Klahan S, and Asawanonda P. Topical tacrolimus may enhance repigmentation with targeted narrowband ultraviolet B to treat vitiligo: A randomized, controlled study. *Clin Exp Dermatol* Dec 2009;34(8):e1029–30.

Chapter 33

LASERS IN VITILIGO

Manjunath Shenoy, Ganesh S. Pai, and Anusha H. Pai

CONTENTS

INTRODUCTION

Vitiligo therapy includes medical (both topical and systemic), surgical, and light-based treatments. The majority of new published studies involved use of light, either alone or in combination with other therapies. Among the light-based treatments, narrowband UVB (NB-UVB) is employed most commonly. Laser utility is becoming popular in vitiligo. It is designed primarily as a targeted therapy for resistant cases. Its efficacy and safety have been fairly well established, but large-scale studies should be undertaken. Response to treatment of vitiligo depends on many factors, including duration of disease and site of involvement. Laser therapies are not available to all patients in the world. They appear to have definite advantages over the conventional repigmentation therapies and hence should be used in a greater number of patients. This chapter reviews the efficacy, safety, and optimal utilization of the various laser devices and therapies in vitiligo.

PRINCIPLES OF LASER THERAPEUTICS

Melanogenesis is a complex process in which pigment melanin is produced and sequestered within melanosomes. Understanding the physiology of migration, distribution, differentiation, and function of melanocytes is crucial while managing vitiligo. This is true especially when light-based treatment in management is employed. Lasers can be used to promote pigment production, especially in treatment-resistant sites. These therapies can be combined with other modalities for enhanced results. Lasers can also be used to assist in surgical management, especially to create recipient sites for grafts. Finally, laser devices can be explored to achieve depigmentation of residual pigment in cases of universal vitiligo. The mechanisms underlying the commonly used laser- and light-based treatments are discussed here.

Monochromatic excimer laser or lights are the laser devices most frequently used in vitiligo treatment. The mechanism underlying their utility is similar to that of NB-UVB. It is believed that while the active melanocytes in the epidermis are destroyed, inactive melanocytes in the outer root sheaths of the hair follicles are not affected in vitiligo. Repigmentation following irradiation is initiated by activation, proliferation, and upward migration of these melanocytes. Perifollicular repigmentation in treated vitiligo lesions and poor repigmentation in the paucifollicular areas like fingers and mucosa are the evidence for these theories [1]. In addition, irradiation may also trigger T-lymphocyte depletion followed by suppression of autoimmunity.

Response to fractional CO_2 and erbium YAG lasers involves different mechanisms. These laser therapies can be grouped with the various "therapeutic wounding" procedures like dermabrasion, needling, and local application of phenol or trichloroacetic acid [2]. Wounding or fractional wounding therapies may increase the penetration and efficiency of UV radiation. They may also induce the activation, proliferation, and migration of melanoblasts from the border areas.

Helium-neon laser is a relatively newer option being explored in vitiligo. It stimulates the differentiation of melanocytes by enhanced $\alpha2$-$\beta1$ integrin expression. Studies indicate that primitive pigment cell proliferative effect is so pronounced that it cannot be replicable by UVB treatment even at high doses. It also stimulates mitochondrial DNA and the regulatory genes for mitochondrial biogenesis [3,4].

Lasers are also used to create recipient sites for the surgical therapies in vitiligo. Erbium YAG laser has been used to prepare the recipient site in both the punch grafting and suction blister grafting techniques. By these methods, survival of the grafts and the spread of the pigmentation has been accomplished [5,6]. Fractional CO_2 laser can also be employed for preparation of the recipient site [7].

Residual pigmentation can be unsightly in patients with universal vitiligo. Depigmentation therapy is the only option in such patients and can be achieved by monobenzyl ether of hydroquinone (MBEH), phenol peels, cryotherapy, and lasers. Q-switched ruby laser, Q-switched 755-nm alexandrite laser, and fractional CO_2 lasers can

Table 33.1   Lasers employed in vitiligo

Objective	Device	Description
Repigmentation	Excimer laser and light Fractional CO_2 laser Erbium YAG laser Helium-neon laser	Used alone or in combination with topical therapy, systemic therapy, or phototherapy
Recipient site preparation	Erbium YAG laser Fractional CO_2 laser	As an alternate to the conventional methods like dermabrasion or cryotherapy
Depigmentation	Q-switched ruby laser Q-switched alexandrite laser Fractional CO_2 lasers	An alternate to monobenzyl ether of hydroquinone in universal vitiligo

be employed to achieve depigmentation [8–10]. These laser irradiations cause selective photothermolytic and photoacoustic damage to melanosomes and melanocytes, leading to induced depigmentation.

DEVICES

Lasers are primarily used for achieving repigmentation in vitiligo. However, as discussed earlier, laser devices are also used for recipient site preparation and depigmentation. Various devices used in vitiligo are summarized in Table 33.1.

REPIGMENTATION DEVICES
- Excimer laser and light: Xenon chloride gas device that emits monochromatic 308 nm beam in the UVB region delivered through a fiber-optic cable. The excimer lamp is a noncoherent quasimonochromatic light source with a wavelength of 304–308 nm.
- Fractional CO_2 laser: Ablative fractional carbon dioxide laser emits radiation with a wavelength of 10,600 nm infrared region.
- Erbium YAG laser: Erbium-doped yttrium aluminum garnet typically emits light with a wavelength of 2940 nm infrared region.
- Helium-neon laser: A mixture of helium and neon excited by a DC electrical discharge emitting a wavelength of 632.8 nm in the red part of the visible spectrum.

RECIPIENT SITE PREPARATION DEVICES
- Erbium YAG laser
- Fractional CO_2 laser

DEPIGMENTATION DEVICES
- Q-switched ruby laser: A synthetic ruby crystal laser producing pulses of coherent visible light at a wavelength of 694.3 nm, which is a deep red color.
- Q-switched alexandrite laser: A weak laser similar to ruby laser that emits coherent far infrared light at a wavelength of 775 nm.
- Q-switched Nd-YAG laser: Delivers energy at two different wavelengths of 1064 nm and 532 nm, and later is commonly used for the epidermal depigmentation.
- Fractional CO_2 laser.

INDICATIONS

REPIGMENTATION
Achieving maximum repigmentation in the shortest period of time is the primary goal of vitiligo management. Topical, systemic, and

phototherapeutic modalities are effectively used to achieve this. Localized NB-UVB and excimer laser/lamp therapy are considered as the second line of treatment in limited segmental disease [11]. They can also be used as a first line in limited disease. Excimer devices are designed for targeted therapy. Devices like the fractional CO_2 laser have an adjustable spot size and can be used as a targeted therapy.

Indications for targeted laser therapy include the following:

1. *Localized segmental and nonsegmental vitiligo.* Segmental vitiligo and focal nonsegmental vitiligo (under 10% body surface) are ideal cases for targeted therapy using monochromatic laser devices. Larger areas are best treated using phototherapy chambers, usually NB-UVB. Smaller areas or lesions can be targeted with these devises with ease for optimal results. Excimer lamp can be used for the irradiation of relatively larger areas.
2. *Childhood vitiligo.* To avoid the risk of total body irradiation, targeted devices can be used. This can minimize the risk of melanoma, non-melanoma skin cancer, and photoaggravated diseases that prevail in childhood.
3. *Small lesions of recent onset.* These can be treated with targeted laser devices in order to obtain quick results.
4. *Difficult-to-treat regions.* Locations such as knees, elbows, and scalp are not easily accessible to irradiation in phototherapy. Lasers with maneuverable and pointing handpieces and with variable spot size allow free mobility and they can be directed to difficult-to-irradiate regions [12].
5. *Resistant anatomical sites.* Resistant sites like fingertips and bony prominences respond poorly to all forms of treatment including targeted therapies. However, combining them with other topical therapies may induce good response [13].

RECIPIENT SITE PREPARATION
Surgical therapy is indicated for all types of stable vitiligo including segmental, generalized, and acrofacial that do not respond to standard medical treatment. There is no universal consensus on stability, but 1 year of disease inactivity may be considered as stable vitiligo [14,15].

Recipient site preparation is crucial for grafts to take up. Various methods like use of liquid nitrogen, mechanical dermabrasion, suction blisters, PUVA, and lasers have been used for this purpose. Every method has its own advantages and disadvantages; operator preference, expertise, and availability of equipment are the main determinants for technique selection. Fractional CO_2 or erbium laser can be used for the preparation of the recipient site for noncultured cell suspension transplantation, punch grafting, and blister roof grafting.

DEPIGMENTATION
Vitiligo can progress with or without treatment to involve a majority of the body surface area, for which the term "universal vitiligo" is commonly used. In such patients, inducing depigmentation is impossible. Removal of residual pigmentation (depigmentation) can achieve a cosmetically acceptable outcome in such patients.

Depigmentation is indicated when vitiligo is widespread and involves over 50% of the body surface. The chance of cosmetically acceptable repigmentation in such cases is very low. Less extensive, progressive and treatment-resistant vitiligo has also been considered for the therapy. Vitiligo extensively involving the exposed parts of the body like the face and hands, where cosmetic coverage is difficult, may also be subjected to the therapy [16].

COMBINATION THERAPY WITH LASERS

Combination therapies are used to induce faster and more intense repigmentation, especially in cases of resistant lesions of vitiligo.

The principle behind the combination includes targeting the various aspects of pathogenesis such as immune suppression and repigmentation. Lasers, when used as repigmentation devices, can be supplemented with topical immune-suppressive therapies. Various combination treatments used with lasers are summarized in Table 33.2.

MONOCHROMATIC EXCIMER LASER AND LIGHT

Several topical and phototherapies are used in combination with monochromatic excimer laser and light therapies. Topical corticosteroids and tacrolimus are most frequently combined with this laser, and this is the ideal combination.

There are many published studies on the combination of laser with other modalities. A randomized controlled trial comparing 308-nm excimer laser alone or in combination with topical hydrocortisone 17-butyrate cream in the treatment of vitiligo of the face and neck showed that the combination was more efficacious [17]. A controlled study of the combination of tazorotene with excimer laser also showed a synergistic effect in achieving repigmentation. Combination therapy with 308-nm excimer laser, topical tazorotene, and short-term systemic corticosteroids for segmental vitiligo was also found effective [18]. A combined treatment of NB-UVB and excimer laser in vitiligo may also enhance the treatment response [19]. A combined treatment of NB-UVB and excimer laser in vitiligo may also enhance the treatment response [20].

A combination of twice-a-week 308-nm excimer laser therapy with 0.1% tacrolimus ointment applied twice daily seems to be the most effective combination for vitiligo lesions involving not only the UV-sensitive areas, but also in UV-resistant areas.

FRACTIONAL CO_2 LASER

Ablative fractional carbon dioxide laser and NB-UVB can be used in refractory nonsegmental vitiligo. Fractional CO_2 laser pretreatment in autologous hair transplantation along with phototherapy may improve perifollicular repigmentation in refractory vitiligo [21,22]. Triple-combination treatment with fractional CO_2 laser plus topical betamethasone solution and NB-UVB for refractory vitiligo has also yielded good therapeutic response [23].

Table 33.2   Combination or adjuvant therapies with lasers for repigmentation

Device	Therapies
Excimer laser	Narrowband UVB phototherapy, topical corticosteroids, topical calcineurin inhibitors, topical pseudocatalase, systemic corticosteroids, after vitiligo surgery
Fractional laser	Sunlight, phototherapy, topical corticosteroids, topical 5-fluorouracil, pretreatment to autologous hair transplantation in vitiligo

MONOCHROMATIC EXCIMER LASER AND LAMP FOR REPIGMENTATION

Vitiligo patches with 308-nm excimer laser are treated twice weekly with a starting dose of 50–100 mJ/cm^2, and dose increase of 50 mJ/cm^2 in each session until erythema appears [24]. Sensitive areas like eyelids and genitals can be started at a lower dose and other body parts at a higher dose. If the erythema persists beyond 48 hours, the dose must be reduced. Therapy should be discontinued if burns or blisters occur, and it can be restarted at a lower dose after recovery. There are no definite guidelines on the duration of therapy. Treatment is usually given twice or three times weekly and is continued as long as there is ongoing repigmentation. Doses varying from 5.5 to 100 mJ/cm^2 and increased by 10%–30% at each treatment have been used [25]. Therapy may be stopped if no repigmentation occurs within the 3 months or, in the case of unsatisfactory response (<25% repigmentation), after 6 months of treatment [11].

Excimer laser has also been compared with excimer lamp and found to give equivalent results. The excimer lamp treats a larger area since it is a light source, as opposed to a laser source, and therefore can be more efficient in supplying the required dose [26]. It can be used with topical steroid or tacrolimus for better results (Figures 33.1, 33.2).

FRACTIONAL CO_2 LASER FOR REPIGMENTATION

Fractional CO_2 laser has always been used as an adjunct to other forms of therapy like phototherapy or topical therapy. Authors are not aware of any standard guidelines, and treatments have been instituted weekly, monthly, and even once every 2 months by various authors using ablative fractional CO_2 lasers. Therapy protocol can also vary depending on the area treated and the operator's experience. Dermabrasion can also be performed using CO_2 or erbium lasers prior to the regular topical treatments for resistant lesions.

FRACTIONAL LASER FOR RECIPIENT SITE PREPARATION

Selective removal of the epidermis and superficial dermis without damaging the deeper tissue is the objective of laser treatment at the recipient surgical site of vitiligo. This is achieved by one to two passes of the laser at 1.0–3.0 W, with subsequent removal of tissue debris using saline-soaked cotton tips. Distance between the skin and the laser head can be increased in order to defocus and vaporize the tissue without cutting or coagulation (Figure 33.3). In order to prevent scarring from thermal necrosis by continuous CO_2 lasers, intermittent beams from pulsed or UltraPulse lasers can be used [8].

LASERS FOR DEPIGMENTATION

Lasers are the second-line options for depigmentation in universal vitiligo. Monobenzyl ether of hydroquinone (MBEH) is the most frequent and the only FDA-approved therapy for depigmentation. It

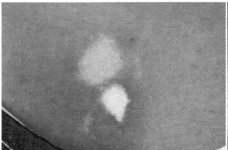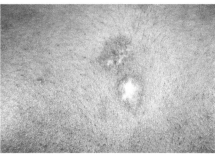

Figure 33.1   Response of focal vitiligo lesions on the trunk to excimer light. (Contributed by Dr. Shantiprasad Tippanawar.)

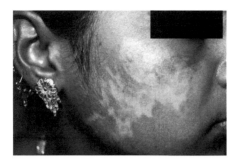
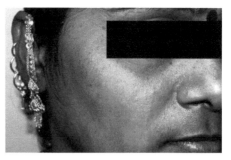

Figure 33.2   Response of segmental vitiligo lesions on the face to excimer light. (Contributed by Dr. Shantiprasad Tippanawar.)

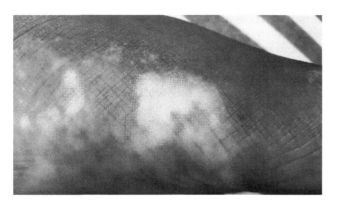

Figure 33.3   Fractional CO_2 laser treatment for resistant vitiligo lesions on the foot.

takes a long time for the induction of depigmentation, and it is often associated with local adverse effects. Lasers can be safely used for faster achievement of depigmentation.

It is preferable to do a test patch before doing the whole area. The Q-switched ruby laser can be used with energy intensity varying from $10-40$ J/cm^2 according to the skin type. The Q-switched alexandrite (QSA) laser has been used at an energy intensity of $3.4-6.0$ J/cm^2 [16]. For the frequency-doubled Q-switched Nd:YAG laser (532-nm), a range of $1-2$ J/cm^2 has been used [10]. Multiple sessions are

generally required. The author has used the fractional CO_2 laser and has obtained comparable results to the Nd:YAG laser (Figure 33.4). Fractional CO_2 may induce its benefit by exhibiting Koebnerization and epidermal exfoliation. Topical anesthesia can be used before doing the laser procedures for depigmentation.

ADVANTAGES AND DISADVANTAGES

Lasers are used in the comprehensive management of vitiligo that includes repigmentation, surgical management, and depigmentation.

ADVANTAGES
Using lasers has distinct advantages:

1. Repigmentation can be achieved rapidly as compared to phototherapy, especially in smaller lesions of recent onset. Studies indicate superiority of the excimer laser over the phototherapy.

2. The dose of irradiation is lower as compared to the phototherapy; hence, the total irradiation is less. This is an advantage, especially considering the carcinogenic risk of UV radiation, particularly in children.

3. Being a targeted therapy, irradiation of the unaffected skin can be avoided.

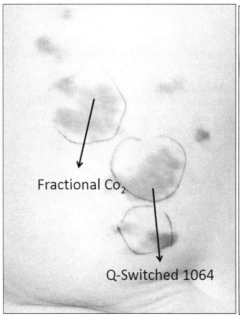
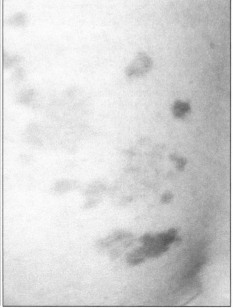

Fractional Co$_2$

Q-Switched 1064

Figure 33.4   Depigmentation induced by Q-switched laser and fractional CO_2 laser in universal vitiligo.

4. Excimer laser and the fractional CO_2 can be combined with phototherapy as well as topical therapies to optimize the therapeutic benefits.

5. Lasers are advantageous in recipient site preparation since the procedure can be done instantly as compared to other measures like cryotherapy.

6. Lasers have a definite advantage over MBEH in that depigmentation can be achieved early and there is no risk of sensitization.

DISADVANTAGES

1. Cost of therapy and availability of the devices are the major disadvantages of lasers.

2. Although considered safe, the risk of cancer cannot be ruled out in patients who have received long-term therapy, especially with the excimer laser.

CONCLUSION

Lasers are not curative in the treatment of vitiligo. They enhance the potential for repigmentation with excimer or CO_2 lasers, ablate stubborn pigmentary spots in an otherwise generalized vitiligo using Q-switched lasers, fractional CO_2, or erbium laser. A 4-mm spot size erbium laser can be used to punch holes preparatory to grafting.

Along with phototherapy, systemic use of psoralens and noncultured melanocyte grafting, many patients with vitiligo can achieve satisfactory though not complete repigmentation. Vitiligo often requires lifetime treatment, with chronic management of the active and stable phases. Administering the comprehensive medical, surgical, laser, and counseling therapies is the duty of dermatologists.

REFERENCES

1. Mouzakis JA, Liu S, and Cohen G. Rapid response of facial vitiligo to 308-nm excimer laser and topical calcipotriene. *J Clin Aesthet Dermatol* 2011;4(6):41–4.

2. Savant SS. Surgical therapy of vitiligo: Current status. *Indian J Dermatol Venereol Leprol* 2005;71:307–10.

3. Lan CC, Wu CS, Chiou MH, Chiang TY, and Yu HS. Low-energy helium-neon laser induces melanocyte proliferation via interaction with type IV collagen: Visible light as a therapeutic option for vitiligo. *Br J Dermatol* 2009;161(2):273–80.

4. Lan CC, Wu SB, Wu CS, Shen YC, Chiang TY, Wei YH, and Yu HS. Induction of primitive pigment cell differentiation by visible light (helium-neon laser): A photoacceptor-specific response not replicable by UVB irradiation. *J Mol Med (Berl)* 2012 Mar;90(3):321–30.

5. Pai GS, Vinod V, and Joshi A. Efficacy of erbium YAG laser-assisted autologous epidermal grafting in vitiligo. *J Eur Acad Dermatol Venereol* 2002 Nov;16(6):604–6.

6. Sachdev M, and Krupashankar DS. Suction blister grafting for stable vitiligo using pulsed erbium:YAG laser ablation for recipient site. *Int J Dermatol* 2000;39(6):471–3.

7. Komen L, Vrijman C, Wietze van der Veen JP, de Rie MA, and Wolkerstorfer A. Observations on CO_2 laser preparation of recipient site for noncultured cell suspension transplantation in vitiligo. *J Cutan Aesthet Surg* 2016;9(2):133–5.

8. Kim YJ, Chung BS, and Choi KC. Depigmentation therapy with Q-switched ruby laser after tanning in vitiligo universalis. *Dermatol Surg* 2001;27:969–70.

9. Rao J, and Fitzpatrick RE. Use of the Q-switched 755 nm alexandrite laser to treat recalcitrant pigment after depigmentation therapy for vitiligo. *Dermatol Surg* 2004;30:1043–5.

10. Majid I, and Imran S. Depigmentation therapy with Q-switched Nd:YAG laser in universal vitiligo. *J Cutan Aesthet Surg* 2013;6:93–6.

11. Taieb A, Alomar A, Böhm M et al. Guidelines for the management of vitiligo: The European Dermatology Forum consensus. *Br J Dermatol* 2013;168(1):5–19.

12. Mysore V, and Shashikumar BM. Targeted phototherapy. *Indian J Dermatol Venereol Leprol* 2016;82:1–6.

13. Nisticò S, Chiricozzi A, Saraceno R, Schipani C, and Chimenti S. Vitiligo treatment with monochromatic excimer light and tacrolimus: Results of an open randomized controlled study. *Photomed Laser Surg* 2012;30(1):26–30.

14. Al-Hadidi N, Griffith JL, Al-Jamal MS, and Hamzavi I. Role of recipient-site preparation techniques and post-operative wound dressing in the surgical management of vitiligo. *J Cutan Aesthet Surg* 2015;8:79–87.

15. Prasad D, and Gupta S. Standard guidelines of care for vitiligo surgery. *Indian J Dermatol Venereol Leprol* 2008;74:S37–45.

16. Gupta D, Kumari R, and Thappa DM. Depigmentation therapies in vitiligo. *Indian J Dermatol Venereol Leprol* 2012;78: 49–58.

17. Sassi F, Cazzaniga S, Tessari G et al. Randomized controlled trial comparing the effectiveness of 308-nm excimer laser alone or in combination with topical hydrocortisone 17-butyrate cream in the treatment of vitiligo of the face and neck. *Br J Dermatol* 2008;159(5):1186–91.

18. Lu-yan T, Wen-wen F, Lei-hong X, Yi J, and Zhi-zhong Z. Topical tacalcitol and 308-nm monochromatic excimer light: A synergistic combination for the treatment of vitiligo. *Photodermatol Photoimmunol Photomed* 2006;22(6):310–4.

19. Bae JM, Yoo HJ, Kim H, Lee JH, and Kim GM. Combination therapy with 308-nm excimer laser, topical tacrolimus, and short term systemic corticosteroids for segmental vitiligo: A retrospective study of 159 patients. *J Am Acad Dermatol* 2015;73(1):76–82.

20. Shin S, Hann SK, and Oh SH. Combination treatment with excimer laser and narrowband UVB light in vitiligo patients. *Photodermatol Photoimmunol Photomed* 2016;32(1):28–33.

21. Shin J, Lee JS, Hann SK, and Oh SH. Combination treatment by 10 600 nm ablative fractional carbon dioxide laser and narrowband ultraviolet B in refractory nonsegmental vitiligo: A prospective, randomized half-body comparative study. *Br J Dermatol* 2012;166(3):658–61.

22. Feily A, Seifi V, and Ramirez-Fort MK. Fractional CO_2 laser pretreatment to autologous hair transplantation and phototherapy improves perifollicular repigmentation in refractory vitiligo: A randomized, prospective, half-lesion, comparative study. *Dermatol Surg* 2016;42(9):1082–8.

23. Li L, Wu Y, Li L, Sun Y, Qiu L, Gao XH, and Chen HD. Triple combination treatment with fractional CO_2 laser plus topical

betamethasone solution and narrowband ultraviolet B for refractory vitiligo: A prospective, randomized half-body, comparative study. *Dermatol Ther* 2015;28(3):131–4.

24. Al-Otaibi SR, Zadeh VB, Al-Abdulrazzaq AH, Tarrab SM, Al-Owaidi HA, Mahrous R, Kadyan RS, and Najem NM. Using a 308-nm excimer laser to treat vitiligo in Asians. *Acta Dermatovenerol Alp Pannonica Adriat* 2009;18(1):13–9.

25. Hamzavi IH, Lim HW, Syed ZU. Ultraviolet-based therapy for vitiligo: What's new? *Indian J Dermatol Venereol Leprol* 2012;78:42–8.

26. Leone G, Iacovelli P, Paro Vidolin A, and Picardo M. Monochromatic excimer light 308 nm in the treatment of vitiligo: A pilot study. *J Eur Acad Dermatol Venereol.* 2003;17(5):531–7.

OTHER THERAPIES FOR VITILIGO

Chapter 34

ALTERNATIVE MEDICINE IN VITILIGO INCLUDING HOME REMEDIES

Bela J. Shah

CONTENTS

INDIAN HISTORY OF VITILIGO

Vitiligo finds its place early in the history of human ailments, and most ancient civilizations and religions had some reference to lack of pigmentation. One of the earliest terms was "Kilas" in the *Rig Veda*, which means similar to a white spotted deer. The earliest known reference to Kilāsa (vitiligo) was in 2200 BC in the period of Aushooryan. In 1550 BC, information regarding vitiligo was noted in the *Ebers Papyrus*, where two forms of depigmentation are mentioned: one looking like that of leprosy and the other resembling vitiligo [1].

Atharvavĕda in 1400 BC also carries its description, where vitiligo spots were called Sveta khushtha. Japanese Shinto prayers in 1200 BC described depigmentation in the Amarakosa. Prognostic factors of depigmentation were explained in the *Ashtanga Hridaya* in 600 BC. Ayurvĕda used the word Kuṣṭa for all types of skin diseases. Kilāsa and Switra have similar etiology, so they are mentioned together in Ayurvĕda. Kilāsa is also called as Bāhya (external) Kuṣṭa. It is classified into three types based on three Dŏṣăs. Prognosis of the disease was also described in Ayurvĕda. This disease can be compared with vitiligo in modern medicine. In 200 BC, the Indian *Manusmriti* described "Sweta Kushtha," meaning "white disease," probably referring to vitiligo.

Throughout many centuries, vitiligo continued to be one of the most important depigmentation ailments worldwide, provoking discrimination or segregation in certain cultures (Indian), where affected individuals were unable to get jobs or even become married, probably based upon ancient religious beliefs.

AYURVEDIC MEDICATIONS IN VITILIGO

Herbal and mineral-based drugs are mainstays of Ayurvedic medicine. These act as blood purifiers and photosensitizers [2]. *Psoralea corylifolia*, *Ficus hispida*, and *Semecarpus anacardium* (marking nut) are some photosensitizing agents. They are given topically and/or systemically along with sun exposure 3 hours after drug administration. *Curcuma longa*, *Hemidesmus indicus*, *Acacia catachu*, *Eclipta alba*, *Acaranthus aspara*, and *Tinospora cordifolia* are among the variety of blood purifiers that are widely used [2].

PSORALEA CORYLIFOLIA

Commonly called babchi, *P. corylifolia* has been in use for a long time in traditional Ayurvedic and Chinese medicine for its excellent effects in treating a variety of skin disorders. Pharmacologically it has a role as an antimicrobial, antioxidant, anti-inflammatory, and chemoprotective agent. This plant grows throughout the plains of India, commonly in the semi-arid regions of Rajasthan and the eastern districts of Punjab, adjoining Uttar Pradesh [3,4], as well as in the tropical and subtropical regions of the world, especially southern Africa and China [5].

The furocoumarins promote pigmentation [6]. Traditional doctors use its powder internally for leprosy and vitiligo, and externally as an ointment and paste [7,8].

Its oil helps to repigment vitiligo and is also thought to have an inhibitory effect on the skin Streptococci [9]. Psoralen and isopsoralen, which are the major components, have inhibitory effects on tumors, bacteria, and viruses [10].

MECHANISM OF ACTION

P. corylifolia has a specifically local action on the arterioles of the subcapillary plexuses, which become dilated, increasing plasma in the area. The skin turns erythematous and the melanocytes become stimulated. In vitiligo, melanocytes function improperly, and their stimulation by the medication leads them to synthesize and exudate pigments that diffuse slowly into the vitiligo patches [5,12]. Covalent binding of the drug to pyrimidine bases, which is phytochemically induced, is also responsible for its therapeutic efficacy. Thymine dimer adducts on the opposite strands of DNA are involved in the photoconjunction. Psoralen intercalates into the DNA, forming mono- and di-adducts in the presence of UV light [13].

DOSAGE [14,6]
Oil: Topical application
Tincture: 3–15 mL/day
Seed powder: 1–3 gm

ADVERSE EFFECTS

After sun exposure, cutaneous damage and residual edema of the legs can occur. Acute dermatitis with edema and blistering with possible renal complications has also been seen in some cases. Other side effects include malaise, headache, nausea, vomiting, insomnia, loose stools or diarrhea, mental depression, and hepatotoxicity. Psoralen treatment and high-intensity long wavelength radiation have produced extensive chromosome damage in mammalian cells; hence it should be used cautiously because this may later lead to malignancy. Long-term therapy is seen to affect the liver, eyes, and immune system [9].

PRECAUTIONS

Caution is advised in pregnancy. Oral psoralen is contraindicated for use in pregnant and lactating women. It is contraindicated in patients with liver diseases, lupus erythematosus, or other diseases associated with photosensitivity. Avoiding a spicy diet, salt, and late nights during this treatment is advisable. Milk, butter, and ghee are to be taken in the diet. Seed oil should not be used on eyes and since it is thermogenic, it should be mixed with coconut oil before application [17].

SAFETY

Herb–drug interactions are unknown; the drug is considered safe in its prescribed doses [18,19].

CASSIA OCCIDENTALIS

The extracts of *C. occidentalis* were found to be effective in the induction of differentiation and migration of mouse melanocyte cell line. The drug induced tyrosinase activity and improved altered melanocyte cell morphology. Transwell migration assay showed the potential of the herbal drug induces direct migration of melanocytes to treat vitiligo at that site. [20].

CURCUMA LONGA

C. longa has been shown to exhibit an inhibitory effect on inflammation, microbes, oxidative stress, and tumors. There is growing evidence that curcumin, an active component of turmeric, may be used medically to treat many skin diseases. There is early evidence for the use of turmeric/curcumin products and supplements, oral as well as topical, and therapeutic benefits on skin health, especially vitiligo [21].

PICRORHIZA KURROA

P. kurroa is an Ayurvedic herb which may potentiate photochemotherapy due to its effects on the immune system. It can be used as a supplement to photochemotherapy in patients with vitiligo [22].

HERBS FOR TREATMENT OF VITILIGO

Herb treatments that may provide some benefit include immune tonics and adrenal tonics when these systems are weak. Because many skin problems are related to the liver, bowel function, and food allergies, liver-regulating herbs and bowel-strengthening herbs as well as a continuous course of probiotics may also be helpful [23].

Herbs used are *Plumbago indica* (Plumbaginaceae), *Semecarpus anacardium* (Anacardiaceae), *Ginkgo biloba* (Ginkgoaceae), *Nigella sativa* (Ranunculaceae), *Terminalia bellerica* (Combretaceae), *Ammi visnaga* (Apiaceae), *Picrorhiza kurroa* (Plantaginaceae), *Ammi majus* (Apiaceae), *Azadirachta indica* (Meliaceae), *Tribulus terrestris* (Zygophyllaceae), *Silybum marianum* (Asteraceae), and *Zingiber officinalis* (Zingiberaceae).

HOMEOPATHIC MEDICINES FOR VITILIGO

In homeopathy, the patient is analyzed on various aspects of mental, physical, and familial attributes, and a complete study is done on the psychological–environmental history of the patient. The homeopathic medicines are selected after a full individualized examination and case analysis, which includes the medical history of the patient, physical and mental constitution, etc. [16].

Homeopathic remedies include Arsenic sulfate, silicea, sepia, sulfur, Kali carbonicum, Nutricum acidum, falvus, Arsenic album, Baryta mur, Calcarea carb, Bacillinum, Graphites, Merc sol, Natrum muriaticum, Nitricum acidium, Nux vom, Phos. Sep, Sil, Sulph, Thuja, and Baryta carb are known to give good results.

TRADITIONAL SIDDHA MEDICINE FOR VITILIGO

Traditional Siddha medicine uses *Aristolochia indica*, *Tribulus terrestris*, and *Thespesia populnea* [23]. Among these, *Aristolochia indica* root contains aristolochic acid, which might cause renal failure or cancer [15].

UNANI MEDICINE FOR VITILIGO TREATMENT

Unani or Yunani medicine is based on the Greek disciplines by Hippocrates and Galen which believes that management of any disease lies upon its diagnosis. It postulates blood, phlegm, yellow and black bile as fluids to maintain equilibrium and their imbalance causes illness.

Safoof bars: The herbal powder is mixed with plain water and kept overnight. In the morning, the water is consumed and the remaining herbs are applied on patches.

Black seeds (kalonji) and fenugreek (methi) seeds: One pinch of black seeds and two pinches of fenugreek seeds are soaked in 1 cup of water and kept overnight. In the morning, the water and soaked seeds are consumed. Black seed oil is also found effective.

Itrifal Shahtra: 5 gm is consumed with water before bed.

Sharbat-e-Musaffi: One to two teaspoonful of herbal syrup mixed in water is consumed two times a day.

RESTRICTED FOOD ITEMS IN UNANI MEDICINE FOR VITILIGO TREATMENT

Beef, bananas, dairy products, fish, eggs, cashews, peanuts, most citrus fruits and vegetables (e.g., orange, lemon), fast foods, tamarind, processed foods, alcohol, sodas.

THE ROLE OF FOOD

A physician can consider the harmful effects of food additives, including dyes, defoaming agents, fungicides, emulsifiers, flavors, color retention agents, sweeteners, preservatives, thickeners, and chemicals in unstable and progressive vitiligo. Though food additives are generally considered harmful in vitiligo, medical evidence for these harmful effects is not established. The risk of a stress reaction is increased by consuming food additives in large amounts, and they may have a harmful effect on vitiligo.

VIRUDDHA AHARA

Shwitra is a dermatological disorder discussed in the Vedas, involving the skin only does not causing any pain or ulcerations. It can be corelated to vitiligo.

Shwitra is said to occur due to irregular dietary habits and lifestyle changes. Viruddha ahara (incompatible food) has been described to be a premise for many skin diseases including swithra (vitiligo) in Ayurveda, which believes that whatever food we eat affects the body and the mind. Therefore, to prevent disease incidence, eating incompatible food should be avoided [11].

Examples of viruddha ahara:

1. *Desha (place) viruddha*: To consume dry and unctous substances in dry and marshy regions respectively is incompatible. Consumption of cold and hot potency substances in combination is incompatible. Consuming cold and dry substances in winter, while taking hot and pungent substances in summer is incompatible.
2. *Veerya (potency) viruddha*: Cold potency substances in combination with those of hot potency.
3. *Kala (time) viruddha*: Intake of cold and dry substances in winter, pungent and hot substances in summer.
4. *Koshtha (bowel movements) viruddha*: To give less quantity with less potency and less stool-forming food to a person having constipation bowel, and vice-versa.
5. *Sampad viruddha (richness of quality against)*: Intake of substances that are not mature, overmatured, or purified.

REFERENCES

1. Prasad PVV, and Bhatnagar VK. Medico-historical study of "Kilasa" (vitiligo/leucoderma) a common skin disorder. 2003;33(2):113–27.
2. Srivastava RK. Vitiligo (leukoderma) Ayurvedic treatment. (August, 2011). 22/08/2011. Available from: http://ayurveda-foryou.com/treat/leucoderma.html.
3. Sah P, Agrawal D, and Garg SP. Isolation and identification of furocoumarins from the seeds of *Psoralea corylifolia* L. *Indian J Pharma Sci* 2006;68:768–71.
4. Sharma PC, Yelne MB, and Dennis TJ. *Database on Medicinal Plants Used in Ayurveda*. Vol. 2. New Delhi: Central Council for Research in Ayurveda and Siddha; 2001, pp. 89–93.
5. Krishnamurthi AK, Manjunath BL, Sastri BN, Deshaprabhu SB, and Chadha YR. *The Wealth of India: Raw Materials*. Vol. 7. New Delhi: CSIR; 1969, pp. 295–8.
6. Sebastian P. *Ayurvedic Medicine: The Principles of Traditional Practice*. Vol. 2. New York: Elsevier Health Sciences; 2006, pp. 135–6.
7. Panda H. *Herbs, Cultivation and Medicinal Uses*. New Delhi: National Institute of Industrial Research; 2000, pp. 479–81.
8. Nadkarni KM. *Indian Materia Medica*. Vol. 1. Mumbai: Popular Prakashan Pvt. Ltd; 1976, pp. 1019–22.
9. Rajpal V. *Standardization of Botanicals*. Vol. 2. New Delhi: Eastern Publishers; 2005, pp. 284–95.
10. Liu R, Li A, Sun A, and Kong L. Preparative isolation and purification of psoralen and isopsoralen from *Psoralea corylifolia* by high-speed counter-current chromatography. *J Chromatogr A* 2004;1057:225–8.
11. Kumari B, and Gharge A. The Role of Viruddha Ahara In Shwitra W.S.R To Leucoderma. *Int J Ayurvedic and Her Med* 2016;6(2):2172–7.
12. William B. *New Manual of Homeopathic Materia Medica and Repertory*, 9th ed. New Delhi: B. Jain Publishers Pvt. Ltd; 2002, p. 1129.
13. Vaidya AD. Reverse pharmacological correlates of Ayurvedic drug actions. *Indian J Pharmacol* 2006;38:311–5.
14. Kapoor LD. *Handbook of Ayurvedic Medicinal Plants*. Boca Raton, Florida: CRC Press; 2001, pp. 274–5.
15. Arlt VM, Stiborova M, and Schmeiser HH. Aristolochic acid as a probable human cancer hazard in herbal remedies: A review. *Mutagenesis*. July 2002;14(4):265–77.
16. Sharma V. 5 Best Homeopathic Medicines for Vitiligo. Available at: http://drhomeo.com. May 28, 2016.
17. Seth A. *The Herbs of Ayurveda*, 1st ed. Vol. 4. Gujarat: Hi Scan Pvt. Ltd; 2005, p. 950.
18. Chopra RN, and Chopra IC. *Indigenous Drugs of India*, 2nd ed. Kolkata: Academic Publishers; 1958, pp. 391–4.
19. Gupta AK, Neeraj T, and Madhu S. *Quality Standards of Indian Medicinal Plants*. Vol. 3. New Delhi: ICMR; 2005, pp. 290–8.
20. Babitha S, Shin JH, Nguyen DH et al. A stimulatory effect of *Cassia occidentalis* on melanoblast differentiation and migration. *Arch Dermatol Res* 2011;303:211. doi:10.1007/s00403-011-1127-y
21. Vaughn AR, Branum A, and Sivamani RK. Effects of turmeric (*Curcuma longa*) on skin health: A systematic review of the clinical evidence. *Phytother Res* 2016;30:1243–64.
22. Bedi KL, Zutshi U, Chopra CL, and Amla V. *Picrorhiza kurroa*, an Ayurvedic herb, may potentiate photochemotherapy in vitiligo. *J Ethnopharmacol* 1989 Dec 1;27(3):347–52.
23. Soni P, Patidar R, Soni V et al. A review on traditional and alteranative [sic] treatment for skin disease "vitiligo". *Int J Pharm Biol Arch* 2010;1(3):220–7.

Chapter 35

DEPIGMENTING AGENTS

Rashmi Kumari

CONTENTS

INTRODUCTION

Vitiligo, referred to as "ven kushtam" in India, translates to "white leprosy" [1]. It has a significant impact on the patient's quality of life, especially in dark-skinned individuals [2,3]. There is a marked contrast in vitiligo macules as compared to surrounding normal skin in those with extensive and resistant vitiligo. In such patients, repigmentation following therapy may result in patchy, cosmetically disfiguring pigmentation, and hence the patient may prefer to completely depigment the unaffected pigmented skin. The ultimate goal of depigmentation therapy is to give the patient a uniform skin color.

The cytotoxic potential of various chemicals, lasers, cryogen, allergens, vaccines, etc. is used to depigment normal skin in vitiligo patients. In this chapter, we discuss various established and potential depigmentation agents and emerging therapies.

An ideal depigmenting agent should have a potent, rapid, and selective effect on melanocytes, should lead to permanent removal of pigment, and should be nontoxic with minimal side effects [4]. Although an ideal agent for depigmentation is currently not available, Table 35.1 highlights the various depigmenting agents in use.

British guidelines in 2008 stated that depigmentation with monobenzyl ether of hydroquinone (MBEH) or 4MP should be reserved for adults severely affected by vitiligo who cannot or choose not to seek repigmentation and who can accept the permanence of never tanning. The grade of recommendation was level D, and the level of evidence for its use was level 4 [5]. Depigmentation therapy is carried out in a small minority of patients who fulfill the criteria and are mentally prepared for it (Table 35.2). It is important to discuss various aspects of this therapy with the patient, such as the cost, treatment time, course, risk of depigmentation at distant body sites, stress upon probable permanency of depigmentation, side effects such as contact dermatitis, and the possibility of repigmentation [5].

Also, results of depigmentation should be socially and culturally acceptable after depigmentation therapy. The individual and their family should be involved in the decision-making process. As this process is mostly irreversible, usually older patients are selected who have failed repigmentation in spite of the best approaches and have waited a few years. Depigmentation therapy should be avoided in

children less than 12 years of age [6]. Younger patients should be given the option of repigmentation in spite of greater social pressure [7]. A list of relative contraindications is provided in Table 35.3.

MONOBENZYL ETHER OF HYDROQUINONE

MBEH, a hydroquinone derivate also known as monobenzone or by its chemical name, p-(benzyloxy) phenol, is the most potent depigmenting agent and the mainstay of depigmentation therapy.

In the late 1930s, McNally [8] and Oliver and colleagues [9] reported that MBEH used to reduce the deterioration of rubber resulted in patches of depigmentation in areas of contact with rubber, primarily in tannery workers [10]. This was very similar to acral vitiligo, which on prolonged contact became generalized. It was attributed to sites of contact with the gloves while perspiring. Analysis of the gloves demonstrated the presence of an antioxidant known as agerite alba, or MBEH, and when this compound was removed from the gloves, repigmentation was reported. Though it initially sparked enthusiasm for use of MBEH in all types of hypermelanosis [11], presently its use is restricted to vitiligo universalis for depigmentation therapy [12].

MECHANISM OF ACTION

Various theories as to how MBEH causes depigmentation have been proposed. These include the following: [10,13]

- MBEH reacts with tyrosinase enzyme to form a reactive quinone product. This quinone metabolite in turn binds covalently to cysteine residues in tyrosinase proteins through the sulfhydryl (-SH) group to form hapten-carrier complexes, i.e., generation of neo-antigens in the tyrosinase peptide chain occurs which excites a systemic, melanocyte destructive, inflammatory response.

- MBEH induces cellular oxidative stress in exposed pigmented cells by producing reactive oxygen species (ROS) such as peroxide. This induces lysosomal degradation of melanosomes by autophagy, in addition to disruption of melanosomal membranes and melanosome structure. This is followed by increased surface expression of melanosomal antigens by both major histocompatibility complex (MHC) class I and II routes and initiation of melanocyte Ag-specific T-cell responses.

Table 35.1 Depigmenting agents

First-line agents	Second-line agents	Experimental agents
MBEH (monobenzyl ether of hydroquinone) MEH (monomethyl ether of hydroquinone) Mequinol Phenol Cryotherapy	Imatinib Imiquimod Diphencyprone (DPCP)	Hydroquinone Catechol 4-ethoxyphenol 4-tert-butylcatechol Monobenzone Ether IFN gamma Busulfan Vaccines against melanoma antigens

Table 35.2 Indications for depigmenting therapy

- Patients with extensive disease, i.e., BSA >50% who desire permanent matching of skin color and where the chance of repigmentation with other therapies is low. Usually patients with 60%–80% involvement.
- Those with 30%–50% involvement with progressive disease or resistance to standard therapies.
- Those involving cosmetically sensitive areas of face and hands where cosmetics are ineffective, although patch treatment is rarely carried out.
- Vitiligo of hands and malar areas that are resistant to complete repigmentation.

Table 35.3 Relative contraindications to depigmenting

- Young patients presenting for the first time to clinic
- Patients with limited body surface involvement
- Those not likely to adhere to strict photoprotection regime
- Those who are emotionally unstable
- Those not willing to accept inability to tan
- Those who have not taken repigmenting therapies

- ROS generation also results in release of tyrosinase and MART-1 antigen containing exosomes which further contributes to immune response.
- Rapid and persistent innate immune activation also occurs in MBEH-exposed skin. MBEH is a contact-sensitizer inducing a type IV delayed type hypersensitivity response against the quinone hapten mentioned earlier. This depends on the production of pro-inflammatory cytokines such as interleukin (IL)-1b and IL-18 by the Langerhans cells or keratinocytes.

TREATMENT PROCEDURE
The procedure can be carried out in the privacy of one's home and not necessarily in the hospital. First, an open-use test should be performed on pigmented skin of the forearm. If no contact dermatitis develops, the cream can be applied to the face or areas chosen by the patient as top priority. Most patients do not treat all areas with residual pigment at once, but rather in stages, moving from the highest to the lowest priority. Different concentrations of MBEH can be used at one time, for example, 5% on the neck, 10% on the face, and 20% on the arms and legs. If there is no response in some areas even with 20%, it can be increased to 30% and then 40%, especially over the extremities like the elbows and knees [7]. For stable vitiligo of long duration, higher concentrations of MBEH may be required to be applied for a longer duration [7].

This topical therapy causes gradual lightening of skin, which occurs over a period of 4 to 12 months [7]. MBEH causes irreversible depigmentation by loss of melanosomes and melanocytes [4]. A 35-g tube

of commercially prepared 20% MBEH costs around 30–40 USD to the patient. The shelf life of the compounded product is about 6 months, and it should always be kept refrigerated [7].

PRECAUTIONS
While using MBEH, a few precautions need to be kept in mind. Application of MBEH at one site can lead to loss of pigment at distant body sites, i.e., application of MBEH to the arm may result in loss of pigment on the face [6]. In the majority of patients, the pigment loss is permanent. Application of MBEH on the eyelids and areas close to the eye should be avoided [7]. After application of MBEH, close skin contact with other people is not advisable. To prevent repigmentation and sunburn, a sunscreen with higher than 30 SPF has to be used throughout the year [6]. Time to repigment may vary from as soon as therapy is discontinued [14] to months and years [7]. Recurrence usually starts in a perifollicular distribution in exposed areas after sun exposure or spontaneously. Repigmentation occurs in MBEH as follicular melanocytes may not be destroyed. One theory is that there is a lack of penetration of the MBEH to the level of the hair matrices, while a second theory is that two populations of melanocytes exist in the skin, the population more resistant to vitiligo as well as to depigmentation therapy residing in the hair follicle. Hair, eyebrows, and eyelashes may be resistant to depigmentation for the same reason [7].

SIDE EFFECTS
Contact dermatitis, irritant more than allergic, can develop mainly in areas of pigmented rather than vitiliginous skin [15]. If irritation develops, topical steroids and wet dressings are used until it subsides and MBEH is withheld. MBEH can be reconstituted at a lower concentration of 5% and restarted later when dermatitis subsides. Frequency of application is also reduced and gradually advanced as tolerated. Irritant reactions may also be decreased by mixing MBEH with emollients at the time of application [7]. Other side effects include exogenous ochronosis [16], unmasking of telangiectasias and phlebectasias on the lower extremities [7], pruritus, xerosis, erythema, rash, edema, conjunctival melanosis, and distant depigmentation [6]. Risk of carcinogenesis cannot be ruled out and hence it has been banned from the European Union since 2001 in cosmetics [5]. Two cases of alopecia and premature graying in patients using excessive quantities of MBEH have been reported [17]. Rare cases of corneal and conjunctival melanoses have also been reported [18]. Showers or baths should be taken before intimate physical contact [17].

HOW TO INCREASE THE EFFICACY OF MONOBENZYL ETHER OF HYDROQUINONE
MBEH alone may need to be used occasionally even beyond 1 year to maintain depigmentation. There have been reports of MBEH therapy combined with all-trans retinoic acid (ATRA) which enhances its depigmenting and melanocytotoxic effects via inhibition of enzyme glutathione S-transferase in melanocytes. This way, we can overcome the problem of using high concentrations of 40% MBEH, which can be harsh on the skin. Furthermore, retinoic acid may be substituted in the future with less irritant retinoids like retinaldehyde or retinol. However, it is important to note is that even ATRA-MBEH combination did not affect hair pigmentation in animal studies [19]. The depigmenting efficacy of MBEH has been demonstrated in the black guinea pig model to be synergistically enhanced by the addition of retinoic acid (RA), which can inhibit glutathione-s transferase protection of melanocytes, increasing melanocyte susceptibility to depigmenting agents. When 10% MBEH was combined with RA 0.025%, the combination produced complete depigmentation in four of six treated

areas, and moderate depigmentation in two areas after 10 days of treatment, which was significantly better than that achieved with MBEH alone (P <0.002). Unlike with the latter, the depigmentation that occurred with the combination was almost always uniform and reduced the average number of melanocytes to 6±6 per field versus 42± 6 per field with MBEH alone [19].

MEQUINOL

This compound is a phenol derivative and is also known as p-hydroxyanisole (HA) or mequinol [4].

MECHANISM OF ACTION

The mechanism of action is similar to that of MBEH. Through a dose-dependent response manner, melanocytes in the hair follicles may also be affected by 4-methoxyphenol (4-MP), but because of their deeper localization, these melanocytes are less susceptible to the compound compared with the epidermal melanocytes [4].

In a recent study, the depigmenting properties of a 4-MP and ATRA combination versus 2% 4-MP or 0.01% ATRA alone were studied on swine skin and it was found that the former produced moderate hypopigmentation in contrast to the latter, which did not produce any significant hypopigmentation. However, skin treated with both returned to normal color within 7–12 weeks. ATRA also caused hypopigmentation by decreasing transport of melanin into keratinocytes while leaving the melanocytes intact. Hence, 4-MP and ATRA affect two different stages, synthesis as well as transport of melanin. Blocking two different targets in the pigmentary process leads to synergistic activity [20]. ATRA is more active in the inhibition of melanin synthesis and tyrosinase activity of stimulated cells than non-stimulated cells; thus, hyperactive melanocytes in ultraviolet (UV)-exposed skin have a greater sensitivity to the cytotoxic and inhibitory effects of 4-MP and ATRA [20].

Njoo et al. [21] in their study demonstrated total depigmentation in 69% of cases using the 4-MP cream after 4–12 months. In those patients who do not respond to 4-MP or who relapse after depigmenting successfully, Q-switched ruby (QSR) laser can give an additional option for complete depigmentation [21]. The advantage with 4-MP is that it can be applied on all skin types, is inexpensive, and is easy to apply.

For resistant cases, 20% 4-MP can be used after initial depigmentation with cryotherapy. Further repigmentation, if it occurs, can be removed by a single session of spot cryosurgery. Another advantage of this method is that sequential application of melanocytotoxic compounds might prevent subsequent colonization of interfollicular epidermis [22].

TREATMENT PROCEDURE

Similar to MBEH, an open patch test is done on a normal pigmented test spot (as big as 5 cm [2]) with 4-MP 20% in an oil/water cream base. Patients with a negative allergic reaction after 48 hours are allowed to apply the cream on the remaining pigmented skin areas twice daily until complete depigmentation is observed [21]. The effectiveness of 4-MP has been correlated with the duration of use of the cream; the longer the cream was used, the better the results [4].

SIDE EFFECTS

Like MBEH, 4-MP also produces side effects like mild burning or itching, irregular leukoderma, contact dermatitis, and ochronosis;

risk of carcinogenesis cannot be ruled out [5]. Protection from sunlight is necessary to prevent high risk of repigmentation [4,5].

4-METHOXYPHENOL VERSUS MONOBENZYL ETHER OF HYDROQUINONE

4-MP is as effective as MBEH, but the side effects like skin irritation are less common and less severe. The melanocytotoxic properties of 4-MP are comparable with those of MBEH. However, compared with MBEH cream, a disadvantage of 4-MP is the longer time required prior to the onset of visible depigmentation [4].

PHENOL

Phenol is inexpensive and has been used for full-depth chemical peeling. A non-occluded 88% phenol application is applied in a small area (<20% of face or neck area). This 88% phenol coagulates the epidermis, preventing further penetration and absorption, whereas Baker-Gordon's phenol formula (40%−50%), being more dilute, needs more care as the risk of systemic absorption is higher [23].

MECHANISM OF ACTION

All phenol compounds have toxicity over melanocytes. Transient or definite hypopigmentation is a feature of phenol cauterizing. Phenol does not cause melanocyte destruction; rather, it compromises its activity [23]. On the other hand, other depigmenting agents, such as hydroquinone and MBEH, destroy melanocytes. Protein coagulation is observed in the epidermis immediately after application of 88% phenol solution. Phenol should not be reapplied, as risk of scarring increases because depth will be greater, with the capacity of reaching reticular dermis [4].

TREATMENT PROCEDURE

Before the application, the skin is cleaned with gauze soaked with alcohol. A swab moistened with 88% phenol is used to treat small areas until cutaneous frosting occurs. The patient feels a burning sensation for approximately 60 seconds, which gradually decreases in intensity and can last from minutes to hours. After two sessions, 45 days apart, total elimination of residual pigmented areas is noticed. No signs of repigmentation have been seen until after one and a half years of therapy [23].

POSTPROCEDURE CARE

Delicate cleaning with saline, antibiotic ointment with steroids of mild-to-moderate potency, and sun blocks should be used. Acyclovir prophylaxis is to be given in those who have a history of herpes simplex.

SIDE EFFECTS

In inexperienced hands, 88% phenol solution may produce complications such as non-aesthetic scar formation, dyschromia, and development of herpetic eczema. High-dose phenol usage is toxic, so it should not be applied over large areas. Phenol exerts a marked corrosive action on any tissue it comes in contact with, whether upon ingestion, inhalation, or direct contact with the skin. Its cellular uptake is both rapid and passive because of its lipophilic character, and signs of systemic toxicity develop soon after exposure. Phenol's main target organs are the liver, kidney, and respiratory and cardiovascular systems. Cardiovascular shock, cardiac arrhythmias, and bradycardia as well as metabolic acidosis have been reported within 6 hours of skin-peeling procedures with phenol. Repigmentation may occur if patients do not protect themselves properly from UV radiation [23].

88% PHENOL VERSUS MONOBENZYL ETHER OF HYDROQUINONE

With phenol, the side effects are fewer. It can be used in areas where MBEH is not available. It is cheap and practical, with no complications in experienced hands [23].

LASERS

Recently, many reports have suggested the use of various lasers for depigmentation therapy in vitiligo. Lasers are known to induce selective photothermolysis of pigmented lesions because their wavelengths are between 600 nm and 800 nm, which are absorbed easily by melanin. Because the duration of the energy pulse is shorter than the thermal relaxation time of melanosomes, no energy (i.e., heat) will be transduced into the surrounding tissue [4].

The main advantages include that they are an effective, fast, and safe method with short treatment duration. They are more effective in vitiligo patients with a positive Koebner phenomenon [24]. Lasers can be used in cases with failure to MBEH/other bleaching agents and for areas like the face where rapid depigmentation is required within days. Lasers also overcome the disadvantages of topical therapies, such as redness, burning, itching, etc. Topical therapy takes a long time, approximately 10 months, to depigment, with the possibility of only partial depigmentation and a relatively high failure rate and risk of repigmentation. With lasers, large areas can be depigmented in one sitting, as opposed to depigmentation performed using a bleaching agent. An additional advantage is that the risk of scar formation is lower due to controlled damage [21].

Q-SWITCHED RUBY LASER (694 NM)

Successful use of Q-switched ruby (QSR) laser (694 nm) was shown by Njoo et al. [21] for depigmentation in vitiligo. Bigger confluent areas of pigment on the extremities can first be treated with topical therapy. Combination therapy was seen to give better results than with any of the methods alone. Depigmentation is rapid and starts by 1 to 2 weeks. With a 5-mm spot at 1 Hz with energy varying between 1–10 J/cm [2], a 5-cm [2] area test spot is done. Results are evaluated at 8 weeks. If depigmentation is evident, a maximum size of 80 cm [2] can be treated in each session at an interval of 2–4 weeks under topical anesthesia. If no sign of depigmentation is seen, further laser treatment is withheld [21]. QSR laser therapy after tanning can induce permanent damage in activated melanocyte-containing structures. In a study by Kim et al. [25], no repigmentation was seen until 1 year, when tanning was employed prior to using QSR laser.

Q-SWITCHED ALEXANDRITE LASER (755 NM)

Rao and Fitzpatrick [26] reported the use of an alexandrite laser in a 68-year-old woman in whom 18 sessions of QSR laser over 5 years along with 20% MBEH application had failed in clearing residual pigmentation. Within 3 months after each laser session, most treated areas would begin to repigment. Subsequently, Q-switched alexandrite (QSA) laser (755 nm, 50–100 ns) was tried. A total of 10 treatment sessions (mean per session, 3.4–6.0 J/cm [2], 3–4 mm, 484–1636 pulses) were administered to the recalcitrant pigmented patches. Topical MBEH therapy was discontinued on the laser-treated sites. Within 22 months, the patient was nearly clear of all pigment within the treated sites. At 12 months of follow-up, she had only minimal recurrence of pigment.

The QSA laser is advantageous over the QSR laser because it has a faster pulse frequency, which allows for more rapid therapy. In addition, it also has a higher wavelength of 755 nm, as compared with the 694 nm QSR laser, which facilitates greater tissue penetration and improves results [26].

A retrospective study included 27 patients with widespread vitiligo who were treated with QSR depigmentation. After a mean follow-up time of 13 months, 48% showed greater than 75% depigmentation. Patients with active disease (63%) showed significantly greater depigmentation than those with stable disease ($P < 0.05$) [27].

Majid and Imran reported the use of Q-switched Nd:YAG laser for depigmentation of residual patches in 15 patients with vitiligo universalis [28]. Treatment was carried out with a frequency-doubled Q-switched Nd:YAG laser at 532-nm wavelength, with a fluence of range of 1–2 J/cm^2 and a spot size of 2–3 mm. Thirteen patients achieved excellent response, with 90% resolution of pigmentation.

SIDE EFFECTS

The main disadvantage is that local anesthesia may be required for these are side effects of both laser therapies extensive areas, as the procedure is painful and treatment is only possible in the clinic, rendering it an expensive therapy. Follicular repigmentation may develop due to migration of perifollicular melanocytes to the epidermis, indicating that these are not destroyed by the laser therapy. Chances for relapse are higher with stable patients than those with active vitiligo [21].

CRYOTHERAPY

When rapid depigmentation is desirable, physical agents like cryotherapy and lasers work faster than bleaching agents. Radmanesh [29] has demonstrated the use of cryosurgery for cost-effective rapid depigmentation that is permanent and has an excellent cosmetic result but can be done only over limited areas in each session.

MECHANISM OF ACTION

Intracellular ice formation leads to irreversible damage; melanocytes are particularly more sensitive to cryodamage in comparison with other epidermal cells. Inflammation develops within 24 hours of treatment, further contributing to destruction of lesions through immunologically mediated mechanisms. Mild freezing leads to a dermo-epidermal separation, which is useful in treating epidermal lesions.

TREATMENT PROCEDURE

Spot testing by a single freeze–thaw cycle is performed, and when the edema and erythema subside, the next session usually takes 3–6 weeks later. Either CO_2 or liquid nitrogen can be used. A 2-cm flat-topped and round cryoprobe is held approximately 40 mm from the skin surface. The whole patch can be frozen with a single freeze–thaw cycle from the periphery and then by forming successive rows inward. Procedure should be terminated when a narrow (<1 mm) frost rim forms around the periphery of the cryoprobe. The rim can develop within 10–20 seconds by a cryogun connected to a container with barometric pressure above 80 kg/cm [2]. For lesions around the orbits or uneven areas of the nose, cryoprobes with smaller diameters may be required. No more than one freeze–thaw cycle is advised [22].

After a week, a depigmented, unscarred, slightly atrophic, and erythematous smooth area appears. The best cosmetic result is obtained 4 weeks after cryotherapy. The depigmentation is permanent, although multiple sessions may be required for partially depigmented lesions, with 4- to 6-week intervals [29]. Spot cryotherapy can be used for areas which repigment.

ADVANTAGES

Cryotherapy has been suggested to depigment MBEH-resistant skin. The procedure requires no anesthesia and can be performed as an outpatient service. No dressing is required, and most dermatologists are familiar with the technique. Preparation time is short and inexpensive. The risk of infection is low and wound care is minimal. Depigmentation developed by cryotherapy is permanent and without scarring if performed by an experienced dermatologist. Many patients prefer a single short-term procedure to applying an expensive compound for 10 months or more with unpredictable effects and a considerable failure rate. A recent retrospective study that compared depigmentation in 22 patients with generalized vitiligo who had previously been treated with cryotherapy or alexandrite 755-nm laser therapy found no significant difference in depigmentation activity after one treatment [30].

DISADVANTAGES

Cryotherapy cannot be used by patient on themselves. Also, cryotherapy is suitable for small lesions, and a single sitting cannot be utilized for depigmenting extensive areas, unlike lasers.

SIDE EFFECTS

Immediate side effects include edema, pain, and bulla formation. If cryotherapy is performed aggressively, it can lead to permanent scarring. Cryotherapy should be used by an experienced individual.

SECOND-LINE AGENTS

Anecdotal reports occurring with use of other agents include imatinib, imiquimod, and diphencyprone (DPCP). These agents have the potential to cause depigmentation but have not been used in vitiligo treatment (Table 35.4).

Leong et al. [31] first reported 13 patients with chronic myeloid leukemia receiving imatinib mesylate for 2–3 months who gradually developed skin depigmentation (whitening/generalized hypopigmentation). The skin became darker during the discontinuation period and began lightening again once imatinib mesylate treatment was resumed. Imatinib mesylate, being a tyrosine kinase inhibitor, may interfere with the production of melanin. It is difficult to define the onset exactly, because the change is gradual within 12 weeks. An ethnic and/or genetic basis has also been considered [31]. Imatinib mesylate can also induce local or generalized hyperpigmentation.

Imiquimod is a novel imidazoquinolinone immune response modifier frequently used for topical treatment of anogenital warts and basal cell carcinomas [32]. Imiquimod increases production of proinflammatory cytokines, mainly interferon (IFN)-α, tumor necrosis factor (TNF)-α, and IL-6, IL-8, IL-10, and IL-12, all of which augment the type 1 helper T-cell (TH1) response which is found to be prominent in the pathogenesis of vitiligo [4]. Imiquimod also stimulates CD8 cells to become cytotoxic, and enhances antigen

presentation [33]. Recently, it was reported that human melanocytes express toll-like receptor 7 (TLR7). When applied topically, imiquimod binds to TLR7, followed by stimulation of various cytokines which induce the previously-mentioned T lymphocytic response [34]. Imiquimod also has a direct action on melanocytes via apoptosis of melanocytes. This action is related to reduction of expression of Bcl-2 and/or an increase in the proapoptotic stimulus (cytotoxic T lymphocytes, natural cytotoxic T cells/killer cells, granzyme B, Fas, TNF, Bax, etc.) [35]. Imiquimod (5%) application may be followed by erythema, which gradually turns to depigmented patches over a period of 3 months. No repigmentation has been seen until 6 months after the depigmentation. Also, depigmentation did not extend to areas that had not been treated with imiquimod [36]. The most common side effects of imiquimod are burning, itching, pain, erythema, erosions, and scabbing/crusting at the target site, which occur more frequently with twice-daily application [4].

Topical application of diphencyprone (DPCP) when used for the treatment of alopecia areata was found to produce depigmentation as part of its side effect profile. Duhra and Foulds [37] reported a case of alopecia totalis in which DPCP treatment resulted in appearance of hypopigmented patches that remained unchanged for 2 years after discontinuing DPCP therapy. Electron microscopy and incubation with dopa in the affected skin revealed an absence of melanosomes and melanocytes. DPCP-induced vitiligo is rare and may represent a Koebner phenomenon in predisposed individuals. Vitiligo can develop even with DPCP concentrations as low as 0.0001% [37].

The depigmenting effects of imatinib and imiquimod have only been reported in few studies, and randomized control trials are lacking. Hence, further studies are required on these agents and other similar molecules before they can be used as mainstream depigmenting agents.

EXPERIMENTAL THERAPIES

A huge number of phenolic compounds have been tested as inhibitors of melanin synthesis. In one animal study, eight compounds were selected on the basis of their known depigmenting effects, including hydroquinone (H), 4-ethoxyphenol (4-EP), 4-methylcatechol (4-MC), 4-tert-butylcatechol (4-t-BC), monobenzone (M), hydroquinone bis (2-hydroxyethyl)-ether (HHEE), and catechol (C). These compounds were injected into animal skin as 10% and 20% solutions dissolved in 95% ethanol. Six of the eight compounds tested showed positive depigmenting effects at 10% except C and HHEE. Compounds showed increased necrosis at a concentration of 20% [10,38].

Both 4-MC and 4-MP were also applied topically in a cream (liposome) base, failed to penetrate the horny layer of the skin, and

Table 35.4 Second-line depigmenting agents

	Imiquimod	Diphencyprone	Imatinib
Mechanism proposed	Induction of innate and cellular immunity via toll receptors, release of cytokines, and cell cytotoxicity resulting in melanocyte apoptosis	Immunomodulation and melanosome and melanocyte absence	Tyrosine kinase inhibition
Concentration/dose	5% cream	0.0001%	800 mg/day for 6 months
Onset of action	3 months	10 months	4 weeks
Side effects	Local burning, itching, pain	Irritation, blistering, pain, regional lymphadenopathy	Nausea, diarrhea, periorbital edema, fluid retention, myelosuppression
Remarks	Depigmentation does not spread to normal areas	Can occur over untreated normal areas as Koebner phenomenon	Not reported in Indian patients

showed low absorption rates due to drug remaining in the liposome, and hence failure of therapy.

Vaccines using melanoma-associated antigen were reported by many authors to produce depigmentation by eliciting an autoimmune response directed against malignant but also normal melanocytes. 4-(p-hydroxyphenyl)-2-butanone and 4-n-butylresorcinol not only inhibit tyrosinase but also act as cytotoxic agents as they are oxidized to their quinonic forms, leading to a double effect. Hydroquinone in higher concentrations of more than 4%, IFN-gamma, and alkylating agent busulfan should be further investigated as topical depigmenting agents for use in human beings with vitiligo universalis. Some compounds like N-acetyl-4-S-cysteaminylphenol, N-2,4-acetoxyphenyl thioethyl acetamide, and N-hydroxycinnamoyl-phenalkylamides have been proposed as anti-melanoma drugs as well as for use as hypopigmenting agents. Ethanolic extracts of *Myrica rubra* dried leaves have shown good depigmenting effects in vitro and pseudo superoxide dismutase activity. They contain quercetin, myricetin, and some 3-O-rhamnoside derivatives. In vivo studies have been recommended to evaluate their potential use as depigmenting agents [39]. Taking into consideration recent findings on the possible role of immune adjuvants such as imiquimod, CpG oligonucleotides, and heat shock proteins in melanocyte destruction, supplementing the depigmenting effect of MBEH with such adjuvants has been suggested [40].

CONCLUSION

Depigmentation therapies are the last resort for extensive vitiligo cases. A major lacuna still exists in this area and a great deal more research is desirable to give satisfactory cosmesis. Combination of topical agents like MBEH and 4-MP and lasers and cryotherapy for resistant and failure cases are the best approach to take. In the future, some of these new experimental agents may be safer and become mainstay of depigmentation therapies.

REFERENCES

1. Grimes PE. White patches and bruised souls: Advances in the pathogenesis and treatment of vitiligo. *J Am Acad Dermatol* 2004;51(S1):S5–7.

2. Ongenae K, Beelaert L, Van Geel N, and Naeyaert JM. Psychosocial effects of vitiligo. *J Eur Acad Dermatol Venereol* 2006;20:1–8.

3. Parsad D, Dogra S, and Kanwar AJ. Quality of life in patients with vitiligo. *Health Qual Life Outcomes* 2003;1:58.

4. Alghamdi KM, and Kumar A. Depigmentation therapies for normal skin in vitiligo universalis. *J Eur Acad Dermatol Venereol* 2011;25:749–57.

5. Gawkrodger DJ, Ormerod AD, Shaw L et al. Guideline for the diagnosis and management of vitiligo. *Br J Dermatol* 2008;159:1051–76.

6. Drake LA, Dinehart SM, Farmer ER et al. Guidelines of care for vitiligo. *J Am Acad Dermatol* 1996;35:620–6.

7. Bolognia JL, Lapia BK, and Somma S. Depigmentation therapy. *Dermatol Ther* 2001;14:29–34

8. McNally W. A depigmentation of the skin. *Industrial Med* 1939;8:405–10.

9. Oliver EA, Schwartz L, and Warren LH. Occupational leukoderma: Preliminary report. *JAMA* 1939;113:927.

10. Gupta D, Kumari R, and Thappa DM. Depigmentation therapies in vitiligo. *Indian J Dermatol Venereol Leprol* 2012;78:49–58.

11. Lerner AB, and Fitzpatrick TB. Treatment of melanin hyperpigmentation. *JAMA* 1953;152:577–82.

12. Mosher DB, Parrish JA, and Fitzpatrick TB. Monobenzylether of hydroquinone: A retrospective study of treatment of 18 vitiligo patients and a review of the literature. *Br J Dermatol* 1977;97:669–81.

13. Van doon Boorn JG, Melief CJ, and Luiten RM. Monobenzone induced depigmentation: From enzymatic blockade to autoimmunity. *Pigment Cell Melanoma Res* 2011;24:673–9.

14. Oakley A. Rapid repigmentation after depigmentation therapy: Vitiligo treated with monobenzyl ether of hydroquinone. *Australas J Dermatol* 1996;37:96–8.

15. Lyon CC, and Beck MH. Contact hypersensitivity to monobenzyl ether of hydroquinone used to treat vitiligo. *Contact Dermatitis* 1998;39:132–56.

16. Charlin R, Barcaui CB, Kac BK, Soares DB, Rabello Fonseca R, and Azulay-Abulafia L. Hydroquinone-induced exogenous ochronosis: A report of four cases and usefulness of dermoscopy. *Int J Dermatol* 2008;47:19–23.

17. Grimes PE, and Nashawati R. Depigmentation therapies for vitiligo. *Dermatol Clin.* 2017 Apr;35(2):219–27.

18. Hedges TR, Kenyon KR, Hanninen LA et al. Corneal and conjunctival effects of monobenzone in patients with vitiligo. *Arch Ophthalmol* 1983;101(1):64–8.

19. Kasraee B, Fallahi MR, Ardekani GS et al. Retinoic acid synergistically enhances the melanocytotoxic and depigmenting effects of MBEH in black guinea pig skin. *Exp Dermatol* 2006;15:509–14.

20. Nair X, Parab P, Suhr L, and Tramposch KM. Combination of 4-hydroxyanisole and all-trans retinoic acid produces synergistic skin depigmentation in swine. *J Invest Dermatol* 1993;101:145–9.

21. Njoo MD, Vodegel RM, and Westerhof W. Depigmentation therapy in vitiligo universalis with topical 4-methoxyphenol and the Q-switched ruby laser. *J Am Acad Dermatol* 2000;42:760–9.

22. Di Nuzzo S, and Masotti A. Depigmentation therapy in vitiligo universalis with cryotherapy and 4-hydroxyanisole. *Clin Exp Dermatol* 2010;35:215–6.

23. Zanini M. Depigmentation therapy for generalized vitiligo with topical 88% phenol solution. *An Bras Dermatol* 2005;80:415–6.

24. Thissen M, and Westerhof W. Laser treatment for further depigmentation in vitiligo. *Int J Dermatol* 1997;36:386–8.

25. Kim YJ, Chung BS, and Choi KC. Depigmentation therapy with Q-switched ruby laser after tanning in vitiligo universalis. *Dermatol Surg* 2001;27:969–70.

26. Rao J, and Fitzpatrick RE. Use of the Q-switched 755 nm alexandrite laser to treat recalcitrant pigment after depigmentation therapy for vitiligo. *Dermatol Surg* 2004;30:1043–5.

27. Komen L, Zwertbroek L, Burger SJ et al. Q-switched laser depigmentation in vitiligo, most effective in active disease. *Br J Dermatol* 2013;169:1246–51.

28. Majid I, and Imran S. Depigmentation therapy with Q-switched Nd:YAG laser in universal vitiligo. *J Cutan Aesthet Surg.* 2013;6:93–6.

29. Radmanesh M. Depigmentation of the normally pigmented patches in universal vitiligo patients by cryotherapy. *J Eur Acad Dermatol Venereol* 2000;14:149–52.

30. Van Geel N, Depaepe L, and Speeckaert R. Laser (755 nm) and cryotherapy as depigmentation treatments for vitiligo: A comparative study. *J Eur Acad Dermatol Venereol* 2015;29:1121–7.

31. Leong KW, Lee TC, and Goh AS. Imatinib mesylate causes hypopigmentation in the skin. *Cancer* 2004;100:2486–7.

32. Halder RM, Taliaferro SJ. Vitiligo. In: Wolff K, Goldsmith LA, Katz SI, Gilchrest BA, Paller AS, and Lefell DJ, eds. *Fitzpatrick's Dermatology in General medicine*, 7th ed, 1. New York: McGraw Hill; 2008, pp. 616–22.

33. Zirvi TB, Costarelis G, and Gelfand JM. Vitiligo-like hypopigmentation associated with imiquimod treatment of genital warts. *J Am Acad Dermatol* 2005;52:715–6.

34. Kang HY, Park TJ, and Jin SH. Imiquimod, a toll-like receptor 7 agonist, inhibits melanogenesis and proliferation of human melanocytes. *J Invest Dermatol* 2009;129:243–6.

35. Kim CH, Ahn JH, Kang SU et al. Imiquimod induces apoptosis of human melanocytes. *Arch Dermatol Res* 2010;302:301–6.

36. Senel E, and Seckin D. Imiquimod-induced vitiligo-like depigmentation. *Indian J Dermatol Venereol Leprol* 2007;73:422–3.

37. Duhra P, and Foulds IS. Persistent vitiligo induced by diphencyprone. *Br J Dermatol* 1990;123:415–6.

38. Schwartzkopf KS, Stookey JM, Hull PR, and Clark EG. Screening of depigmenting compounds for the development of an alternative method of branding beef cattle. *J Anim Sci* 1994;72:1393–8.

39. Solano F, Briganti S, Picardo M, and Ghanem G. Hypopigmenting agents: An updated review on biological, chemical and clinical aspects. *Pigment Cell Res* 2006;19:550–71.

40. Webb KC, Eby JM, Hariharan V, Hernandez C, Luiten RM, and Le Poole IC. Enhanced bleaching treatment: Opportunities for immune-assisted melanocyte suicide in vitiligo. *Exp Dermatol* 2014;23:529–33.

SURGICAL TREATMENT OF VITILIGO

Chapter 36

SURGICAL TREATMENT
Patient Evaluation and Expectation Assessment

Venkataram Mysore, Madhulika Mhatre, and Revanta Saha

CONTENTS

INTRODUCTION

Vitiligo is a pigmentary disorder of the skin associated with considerable social stigma. Patients seek treatment for improving aesthetic appeal. Treatment aims at stabilization of pigmentation and repigmentation of involved areas. This leads to improvement in the cosmetic appearance and skin tolerance to sunburns [1]. There are a great number of treatments available for vitiligo. Surgery for vitiligo forms one of the cornerstones of treatment. The principle of surgery for vitiligo is to obtain cosmetically acceptable repigmentation of vitiliginous lesions. Patients with vitiligo suffer psychologically and are often desperate to seek relief due to the stigma attached to the disease. Hence, proper evaluation of not only the clinical but also the psychological aspects is required. Counseling of the patients with respect to the disease, treatments, and outcomes is vital in order for patients to have realistic expectations.

PATIENT EXPECTATIONS

Patients expect that they will be completely cured of the disease with respect to both regaining color and stopping fresh lesions from occurring. Regaining color should be complete, and the treated skin should merge with the surrounding skin imperceptibly. Hence anything less than 100% pigmentation, while it may be impressive and significant to the doctor, may not satisfy the patient. However, such complete recovery is possible only in a minority of patients. Surgically grafted areas may look normal, hyperpigmented, or even hypopigmented post-intervention. In most patients, even after surgery, other modalities such as topical therapy and phototherapy may need to be continued.

Patients also need to be told about how the donor area will look after surgery—some hyperpigmentation is common after grafting. Koebnerization may occur, and this needs to be addressed.

Patients also need to be told about postoperative recovery—need for immobilization, pain, dressing, visits to the clinic, etc. A detailed instruction sheet may be given to the patient.

ASSESSMENT OF SUITABILITY OF A PATIENT FOR VITILIGO SURGERY

To date, none of the medical or surgical therapeutic choices can assure guaranteed success for all cases of vitiligo. This is primarily because of the obscure etiopathogenesis and elusive activity profile of the disease. Not only with medical therapy but also with any of the surgical modalities deployed, proper selection of cases is of paramount importance.

THE CONCEPT OF STABILITY
Stability of vitiligo is the most important parameter before opting for any transplantation technique [1]. The commonly accepted guidelines for clinical stability are:

- No new lesions should appear
- Existing lesions should remain the same size
- Absence of Koebnerization
- Spontaneous repigmentation
- Positive minigraft test, especially when minigrafting is performed

Various authors have added additional parameters to these criteria of evaluation of stability prior to undertaking surgery, such as consideration of induced versus spontaneous stability, the concept of cellular stability, overall stability versus regional stability versus lesional stability, etc. There has been no consensus regarding these additional factors and their importance; however, we will discuss these aspects in detail in this chapter.

Duration: Despite many studies, there is no consensus regarding the minimum required period of stability. The recommended period of stability in different studies has varied from 4 months to 3 years (Table 36.1) [2]. The Indian Association of Dermatologists, Venereologists and Leprologists (IADVL) Task Force recommends a period of stability of 1 year before undertaking surgery.

TEST GRAFTING
Due to lack of consensus on the duration of stability, Falabella et al. in 1995 introduced the concept of undertaking a test grafting before selecting a patient for surgery [3]. In the original suggested procedure, a few grafts (1.0–1.2 mm) were placed in the center of

Table 36.1 Period of stability recommended in various studies

Author	Year	Period of stability
Das SS, Pasricha JS	1992	4 months
Boersma BR, Westerhof W	1995	6 months
Jha AK, Pandey SS, Shukla VK	1992	1 year
Savant SS	1992	2 years
Falabella R	2003	2 years
Falabella R	1995	2 years
Falabella R	1992	3 years
Mulekar S	2004	1 year
IADVL Task Force	2009	1 year

Source: Majid I et al. *J Cutan Aesthet Surg* 2016;9:13–9.

the depigmented lesion to be scrutinized. The test was considered positive if unequivocal repigmentation took place beyond 1 mm from the border of the implanted grafts. On the other hand, if less than 1 mm or no repigmentation was observed, the test was considered negative. Over the years, this "test" had been acknowledged as a powerful tool for detecting stable vitiligo, which anticipates the repigmentation success in vitiligo when surgery becomes a therapeutic option. However, recently there has been much skepticism regarding its reliability, and Falabella himself expressed his doubts about the comprehensiveness of the test [4].

Koebner phenomenon: Koebner phenomenon (KP), also called the "isomorphic response," has been defined as "the development of lesions at sites of specifically traumatized uninvolved skin of patients with cutaneous diseases" [5,6]. In vitiligo, KP is responsible for the onset of so-called isomorphic depigmented lesions. These depigmented macules may correspond to traumatized areas (scratches) and are easily recognizable by their shape [7]. In some cases, KP has been described with a border of intermediate pigmentation, also termed "trichrome vitiligo" [8]. The incidence of KP in NSV has been reported to be from 15% to 70% by El-Nasr and El-Hefnawi

[9], Ormsby and Montgomery [10], Ortonne [11], Schallreuter et al. [12], and Sweet [13]. The occurrence of KP in segmental vitiligo (SV) is controversial; in these patients, whether KP is present or not inside or even outside the related segment is still a matter of debate. The Vitiligo Global Issues Consensus Conference (VGICC) unanimously endorses the Vitiligo European Task Force (VETF) KP classification system (history-based, clinical observation-based, and experimentally induced [Figure 36.1]).

VIDA SCORE

A set of objective criteria, the Vitiligo Disease Activity (VIDA) score, was suggested by Njoo et al. [16] to follow patient progress. It is a 6-point scale on which the activity of the disease is evaluated by the appearance of new vitiligo lesions or the enlargement of preexisting lesions gauged during a period ranging from <6 weeks to 1 year (Table 36.2). The VETF Task Force recommends that surgery for vitiligo should be performed only in patients with VIDA scores of −1 or 0.

LESIONAL VERSUS OVERALL DISEASE STABILITY

We do not have clear-cut guidelines about whether stability refers to the lesion that needs to be surgically treated or to the patient as a whole. There are clinical and experimental studies that have attempted to assess the stability of a lesion on the basis of biochemical and immunological parameters. In a landmark study on the issue of stability, investigators have shown cluster of differentiation (CD)8+ T-cell counts to be associated with the stability of the disease process. Lesional and perilesional CD8+ T-cell count has been shown to have a positive correlation with disease activity in vitiligo [15].

A multicentric study—ASSIST—was conducted on this issue as well. The most important observation was that patients with a disease stability of just above 6 months but a lesional stability of >1 year achieved comparable results to those patients in whom the disease stability was of >1-year duration. These observations hold a great deal of practical importance because any resistant vitiligo lesion stable over a period of 1 year becomes amenable to surgical treatment,

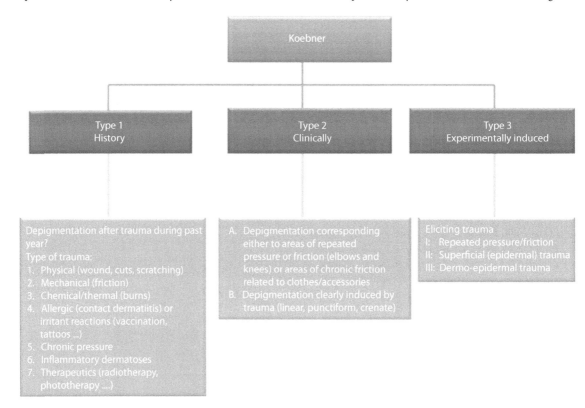

Figure 36.1 Classification of Koebner phenomenon as proposed by the Vitiligo European Task Force in 2011 [14].

Table 36.2 VIDA 6-point score

Disease Activity	VIDA Score
Active in past 6 weeks	+4
Active in past 3 months	+3
Active in past 6 months	+2
Active in past 1 year	+1
Stable for at least 1 year	0
Stable for at least 1 year and spontaneous repigmentation	−1

Source: Njoo MD et al. *Arch Dermatol* 1999;135:407–13.

even if the total duration of disease stability in the patient is only 6–12 months. Thus lesional stability seems to be as important as disease stability in contemplating surgical intervention in vitiligo. These findings are important in patients who are desperate for surgical intervention for their non-responding vitiligo lesions because of social or other reasons. Such cases need not wait for surgical treatment just because their disease has not been stable for >1 year [2].

INDUCED VERSUS SPONTANEOUS STABILITY

Stability can be induced, albeit temporarily, by treatment with steroids and phototherapy. However, evidence on this topic is lacking and further studies are needed to validate the practice of inducing stability and then undertaking surgery.

PATIENT SELECTION

Once stability has been established, certain other factors have to be taken into consideration in order to achieve a satisfactory surgical outcome. These include age of the patient, location of lesion, and type of vitiligo:

a. *Age*: No uniformly accepted opinion exists concerning the minimum age for surgery; however, due thought must be given when performing surgery in children, especially if general anesthesia is to be used. Injecting local anesthesia may be a difficult task in younger children, and this factor should also be considered. However, studies have shown that the surgical outcome is better in younger patients than older [17].

b. *Location*: Palms and soles respond poorly to surgery, and surgery by any method is not recommended for these areas.

c. *Type of vitiligo*: Surgery is generally preferred for individuals with localized patches or for segmental vitiligo, as these have superior outcome compared to vitiligo vulgaris or acral vitiligo. However, this is not a contraindication and can be done for stable cases. It has also been noted that individuals having any subtype of vitiligo with associated acral vitiligo respond poorly.

Keeping all these factors in consideration, it is important to assess each case on its own merit and counsel the patient in detail, with emphasis on the unpredictable nature of the disease. It must be stressed that surgery does not change the overall prognosis of the disease in the case of nonsegmental vitiligo (NSV). When a surgical treatment is conducted for NSV, it should be combined with other medical and/or UV-light treatment for the best outcome and long-term stability [18].

PSYCHIATRIC EVALUATION TO DETERMINE SUITABILITY FOR SURGERY

Vitiligo leads to little physical handicap but can be a potential source of psychiatric morbidity leading to poor self-esteem, poor body image, and feelings of stigmatization and guilt. Severe depression and suicidal tendencies have also been reported in these patients [19,20].

Patients opting for vitiligo surgery are highly motivated but also have high expectations regarding the outcome. A study demonstrated that patients with high Dermatology Life Quality Index (DLQI) scores responded less favorably to a given therapeutic modality, thereby suggesting that additional psychological approaches may be particularly helpful in these patients [21]. In some patients, failure of surgery may exacerbate underlying stress. We therefore recommend that before undertaking any surgery, patients should be asked to fill out a DLQI form to assess their psychological status and for appropriate counseling and treatment.

Studies have shown that counseling can help to improve body image, self-esteem, and quality of life of patients with vitiligo, and can also have a positive effect on course of the disease. It is important to recognize and deal with the psychological components of this disease to improve patient quality of life and to obtain a better treatment response [22].

Points to include in counseling:

- Nature of the disease
- Unpredictable progression of the disease
- Available treatment options
- Details of the procedure to be undertaken
- Expected outcome
- Possible complications
- Need for concomitant medical therapy
- Variability of results
- Duration of results

Patients should be provided with an adequate opportunity to seek all information through books, brochures, computer presentations, and face-to-face discussions with the doctor.

A detailed consent form (see Appendix 1) describing the procedure and possible complications should be signed by the patient. The consent form should specifically state the limitations of the procedure, possible future disease progression, and whether more procedures will be needed for optimal outcome [2].

CONCLUSION

Patient selection and expectation management are two of the most crucial steps in managing any type of vitiligo, and these should be given adequate importance and consideration.

APPENDIX 1

CONSENT FOR VITILIGO SURGERY

I named _____, aged_____ years, have been advised to undergo leucoderma surgery (Test Graft/ Miniature Punch Grafting/ Split-thickness skin Grafting/ Epidermal cell suspension/ Follicular cell suspension) for my skin condition, Vitiligo.

I hereby give my consent after being explained about the procedure by Dr._____.

I also state that I have understood the following information:

I have understood that Vitiligo is a disease with chronic, recurrent course.

I am aware that surgery is only a cosmetic procedure and other medical treatments may be essential. Also surgery will not alter the course of the disease or prevent any recurrence.

My lesions have been stable for the last one year. They have not increased or no new lesions have appeared during this period. I also do not have any tendency of keloids.

I am aware that the exact course of the disease cannot be predicated and though the disease is stable at present, flare-ups and relapse may occur later, in any part of the body.

I have been explained the procedure of the operation as follows:

1. The procedure will be done under local anesthesia.
2. The donor area is from back/thigh/gluteal area.
3. The donor graft will be taken by punch/suction blister/grafting knife.
4. Recipient area will be abraded by a dermabrader and then the graft applied, sealed by dressing.
5. I am aware that avoiding movements and care of the recipient are is essential for optimum results.
6. I am aware that I may experience some pain post operatively and may need to take analgesics.
7. I may need dressing to be done after 7 days: the donor area may need follow-up treatment during this period.
8. I am aware that for optimum cosmetic results, it may take up to 2–3 months. I may need follow up treatment during this period.
9. I am also aware that the grafted area may be different from normal, in texture and appearance. A perfect matching with surrounding normal skin may not always be possible.

I have fully understood the above information after reading it/being translated the same by _____.

I hereby give consent for Dr._____ to perform the procedure and other medical service that may become necessary during the procedure.

The consent form has been signed by when I was not under the influence of any drug. I hereby give consent to take my photographs which will not be used for publicity.

Signature of the Doctor   Signature of the Patient

CASE SHEET FOR VITILIGO SURGERY

                                                                    Date

Name: Age: Sex:

Address:

                                                     Phone no:

Email ID:

Clinical diagnosis: Subtype of vitiligo:

Duration of the disease: Duration of stability:

Treatment history:

Associated other medical conditions:

History of allergy to any medication:

Family history:

Preop medication: Lignocaine test dose / EMLA/ Inj Kenacort

Operative notes:

Total amount of Lignocaine injected:

Procedure done: Test graft/ Miniature punch grafting/ Split-thickness skin graft/ Epidermal cell suspension

Surgeons:

Type of anaesthesia:

Duration of the surgery: Starting: Ending:

Area operated: Total size of operated area:

Donor area:

Postoperative Instructions:

1. Do not soil the dressing, keep it dry
2. Do not move the operated part much, give rest to the bandaged area
3. Cap. Droxyl 500 mg 1–1–1 for 5 days
4. Cap Proxyvon 1–1–1 for 2–3 days
5. Dressing will be removed on day 7
6. Phototherapy to be restarted after 2–3 weeks

REFERENCES

1. Olsson MJ, and Juhlin L. Long-term follow-up of leucoderma patients treated with transplants of autologous cultured melanocytes, ultrathin epidermal sheets and basal cell layer suspension. *Br J Dermatol* 2002;147:893–904.

2. Majid I, Mysore V, Salim T, Lahiri K, Chatterji M, Khunger N, Talwar S, Sachhidanand S, and Barua S. Is lesional stability in vitiligo more important than disease stability for performing surgical interventions? Results from a multicentric study. *J Cutan Aesthet Surg* 2016;9:13–9.

3. Falabella R, Arrunategui A, Barona MI, and Alzate A. The minigrafting test for vitiligo: Detection of stable lesions for melanocyte transplantation. *J Am Acad Dermatol* 1995;32:228–32.

4. Falabella R, Escobar C, and Borrero I. Treatment of refractory and stable vitiligo by transplantation of *in vitro* cultured epidermal autografts bearing melanocytes. *J Am Acad Dermatol* 1992;26:230–6.

5. Koebner H. Zur aetiologie der psoriasis. *Vrtljscher Dermatol Syphil* 1876;8:559–61.

6. Miller RA. The Koebner phenomenon. *Int J Dermatol* 1982;21:192–7.

7. Dupré A, and Christol B. Cockade-like vitiligo and linear vitiligo: A variant of Fitzpatrick's trichrome vitiligo. *Arch Dermatol Res* 1978;262:197–203.

8. Gauthier Y, and Benzekri L. Vitiligo. In: Picardo M, and Taieb A, eds. *The Koebner's Phenomenon*. Heidelberg: Springer Verlag; 2010, pp. 167–73.

9. El-Nasr HS, and El-Hefnawi H. Koebner's phenomenon in dermatology. A study and report of some unusual stigmata of this phenomenon. *J Egypt Med Assoc* 1963;46:1067–86.

10. Ormsby OS, and Montgomery H. *Koebner's Phenomenon in Dermatology: A Study and Report of Some Unusual Stigmata of this Phenomenon*. Philadelphia, PA: Lea and Febiger; 1948, p. 306.

11. Ortonne JP. Vitiligo. In: Ortonne JP, Mosher DB, and Fitzpatrick TB, eds. *Vitiligo and Other Hypomelanosis of Hair and Skin*. New York: Plenum Medical Books; 1983, pp. 163–310.

12. Schallreuter KU, Lemke R, Brandt O, Schwartz R, Westhofen M, Montz R, and Berger J. Vitiligo and other diseases: Coexistence or true association? Hamburg study on 321 patients. *Dermatol (Basel)* 1994;188:269–75.

13. Sweet RD. Vitiligo as a Köbner phenomenon. *Br J Dermatol* 1978;99:223–4.

14. Van Geel N, Speeckaert R, Taieb A et al. and on behalf of the other VETF members. Koebner's phenomenon in vitiligo: European position paper. *Pigment Cell Melanoma Res* 2011;24:564–73.

15. Rao A, Gupta S, Dinda AK et al. Study of clinical, biochemical and immunological factors determining stability of disease in patients with generalized vitiligo undergoing melanocyte transplantation. *Br J Dermatol* 2012;136:1230–6.

16. Njoo MD, Das PK, Bos JD, and Westerhof WW. Association of the Koebner phenomenon with disease activity and therapeutic responsiveness in vitiligo vulgaris. *Arch Dermatol* 1999;135:407–13.

17. Gupta S, and Kumar B. Epidermal grafting for vitiligo in adolescents. *Pediatr Dermatol* 2002;19:159–62.

18. Taieb A, Alomar M, Böhm ML et al. *Guidelines for the management of vitiligo: The European Dermatology Forum Consensus. Br J Dermatol*. 2013;168(1):5–19.

19. Papadopoulos L, Bor R, Legg C, and Hawk JL. Impact of life events on the onset of vitiligo in adults, preliminary evidence for psychological dimension in aetiolgy. *Clin Exp Dermatol* 1998;23(6):243–8.

20. Porter J, Beuf AH, Lerner A, and Nordlund J. Response to cosmetic disfigurement: Patients with vitiligo. *Cutis* 1987;39(6):493–4.

21. Parsad D, Pandhi R, Dogra S, Kanwar AJ, and Kumar B. Dermatology Life Quality Index score in vitiligo and its impact on the treatment outcome. *Br J Dermatol* 2003;148:373–4.

22. Papadopoulos L, Bor R, and Legg C. Coping with the disfiguring effects of vitiligo: A preliminary investigation into the effects of cognitive-behaviour therapy. *Br J Med Psych* 1999;72:385–96.

TISSUE GRAFTING TECHNIQUES
Minigrafting

Koushik Lahiri

CONTENTS

HISTORICAL PERSPECTIVE

Vitiligo is the most significant form of cutaneous achromia, which has been an elusive, if not enigmatic, problem through the ages. In all the ancient civilizations and religions, there is some reference to vitiligo. In the *Rigveda*, it was referred to as "Kilas," meaning a white spotted deer. It is interesting to note that as per a Vedic myth, the anthropomorphic adoration of the sun, Bhagavantam, developed vitiligo after being gazed upon by his illegitimate son [1]. The disease was mentioned in *Tarkh-e-Tibbl-e-Iran* in the period of the *Aushooriyan*, as early as 2200 BC. In 1550 BC, information regarding vitiligo was noted in the Ebers Papyrus [2]. Unfortunately, in some of the prominent ancient texts, the disease was confused with leprosy and also other skin diseases like psoriasis. This was referred to as *Swethakushtha* (white leprosy) in the *Atharba Veda* (1400 BC) [3]. An accurate description also exists in a collection of Japanese Shinto prayers, Amarakosa, dating from 1200 BC [4]. In the Old Testament, the white spots were also described in Verse 2 of Chapter 13 of Leviticus under the Hebrew word *Zora at* or *Tzaraat/Tzoraath*. *Tsoraath* was translated using the Greek word "Lepros," which means a scale or scales. Along with this the phonetic resemblance of the word *Tsoraath* (which in Ashkenazi pronunciation would read *tsoraas*) led to the belief that "leprosy" was psoriasis. In truth, in all likelihood, most cases of biblical "leprosy" were achromic or hypochromic disorders that would include vitiligo, some cases of psoriasis, cases of pityriasis alba, probably albinism, and also leprosy. The word got translated as "lepra" in the Greek and English translations of the Bible. Also, the theory of vitiligo as a dirty/polluted/contaminated disease was initiated, as the word *Tzaraat* refers to a group of skin diseases, which according to the Old Testament renders one ritually unclean [5]. The exact word "vitiligo" may have been derived from the Latin word *vitium*, meaning "blemish," or possibly *vitulum*, meaning "small blemish" [5]. Another theory is that the Latin derivation is from the white, glistening flesh of calves (vitelius). Others believe that the actual word was first used by Celsus in his tome De Medicina in the first century AD [4,6,7]. References to this disease can also be found in the ancient Koran and Buddhist scripts [7]. The

treatment has undergone an enormous evolutionary change from the Vedic days of *Vasuchika* to the most modern transplantation techniques. However, the ultimate goal remains the same, which is replenishment of lost pigment.

Many patients respond to standard medical treatment options, but some remain recalcitrant or respond only partially. Any attempt at repigmentation of these resistant patches with conventional medicinal modalities is often unsuccessful and sometimes exasperating, indicating the absence of a melanocyte reservoir to induce repigmentation. Under these circumstances, the melanocyte repopulation of the achromic areas is not possible unless a new source of pigment cells is placed via surgical methods within the depigmented lesion(s) [8].

Various corrective surgical methods have evolved during the last four decades, including the thin Thiersch's graft [9], epidermal grafting by suction blister [10], punch grafting [11], minipunch grafting [12,13], cultured melanocyte grafting [14,15], grafting of cultured epidermis [16], autografting and PUVA [17,18], transplantation of autologous cultured melanocytes [19], single-hair transplant [20], ultrathin epidermal sheets and basal cell layer suspension [21], and minigrafting and NB-UVB [22]. Among these, minipunch grafting is the easiest, fastest, least aggressive, and least expensive method.

THE PUNCH INSTRUMENT

The skin punch or surgical punch is an instrument used almost solely by dermatologists. It is interesting to note that it was originally used as a trephine to cut through the skull bone. Its use was documented in abscess removal from tibia as early as in 1852 [25]. In 1878, Watson described its use in the correction of accidental gunpowder disfigurement [26], but the importance of the cutaneous punch instrument in dermatology was first established by Keyes in 1887 [27].

The Keyes punch (Figure 37.1.1) has been used in dermatology since then for diagnostic purposes. Its rounded sharp cutting end and thick handle make it ideal for small skin biopsies. Because of the thick walls

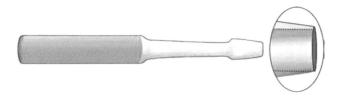

Figure 37.1.1   Keyes punch.

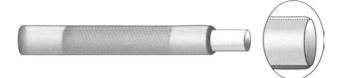

Figure 37.1.2   Loo trephine.

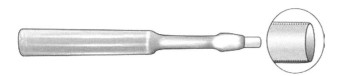

Figure 37.1.3   Disposable punch.

with angled sides above the cutting edge, tissue leans to be pushed away as the punch is made, causing less dermis to be cut through (in diameter) than overlying epidermis. This is also a function of the bevel, which is outside the barrel of the Keyes punch [28]. To overcome these difficulties other punches have been developed [29].

The walls of the Loo trephine (Figure 37.1.2) are thinner and less slanted than those of the Keyes punch, making it advantageous to use on depressed scars or minor autotransplants (where a straight vertical incision is needed), which is difficult to do with the Keyes punch.

The newer disposable punches (Figure 37.1.3) are excellent for punch biopsies or excisional work on cysts. The razor-sharp edge is a great benefit. The punch is made in a number of different dimensions.

EVOLUTION OF MINIPUNCH GRAFTING

In the history of skin grafting, a few observations can be mentioned as a preamble to further discussion on punch grafting.

The first documented successful result of experimental skin grafting was described in sheep by Baronio in 1804 [30], but it took another almost one-and-a-half centuries to get the first recorded autograft response of dark-skinned autografts when transplanted to light areas in spotted Guinea pigs by Lewin and Peck in 1941 [31].

In 1972, Norman Orentriech first reported autograft repigmentation in humans. He treated a black woman with long-standing leukoderma that followed a chemical burn many years previously, when she was treated with home remedy that included a copper penny dipped in vinegar for a presumptive tinea infection on her cheek. Orentriech deployed nine 1- and 2-mm diameter normal skin autografts and observed the "pigment spread phenomenon." He reported a maximum of 1-mm pigment spread from both 1- and 2-mm grafts [11]. In 1976, Labuono and Shatin made a similar observation after transplanting hair bulbs with hair punch grafting within the leucodermic scars of DLE [12].

Falabella, in 1978, reported a novel method of repigmenting leukoderma. With the help of a power-driven dermabrasion unit, he

used dental burrs to create abrasion 2–3 mm in diameter and less than 1 mm in depth and 5 mm apart. In the donor area, skin was raised by means of a curved needle, and was snipped off just below it to harvest 1–2 mm size minigrafts. He reported about a 3-mm perigraft pigment spread by this technique. Three patients, one with piebaldism, another with chemical leukoderma, and a third with post-burn depigmentation, were treated by this method [13]. He observed that these superficial split-thickness grafts provided a much better outcome than the full-thickness hair punch grafting by Labuono. In the same article, interestingly, it was concluded that "… true vitiligo is not treatable by transplantation of grafts of normally pigmented, autologous skin" [13].

Miniature punches of 1.5 mm diameter were used by Falabella while repigmenting three cases of segmental vitiligo in 1983 [34]. Behl (1985) expressed some reservation while commenting on Falabella's work on minigrafting, and claimed better results with thin Thiersch grafting. In a rejoinder, Falabella reiterated his faith in miniature punch grafting and countered with his sets of reasons and logics in favor of punch grafting [35,36].

In the following years, Falabella reported success with minipunch grafting in chemical leukoderma, post-dermabrasion leukoderma, and focal and segmental vitiligo [37–39].

While repigmenting stable leukoderma with autologous minigrafting, Falabella made an important observation regarding the relationship between the donor graft area and the area of surgical repigmentation, and found that a 1-mm donor graft can originate a pigmented spot 25 times larger than its size [37].

In 1995, it was Falabella again who combined epidermal grafting and minigrafting in treating vitiligo and piebaldism [40].

Westerhof, in 1994, reported success with punch grafting in stable vitiligo and observed a maximum of 5 mm of pigment spread [41]. In the subsequent year (1995) Boersma stressed the importance of proper selection of cases before minigrafting [42].

Various studies delineate the effectiveness of the procedure [43–46]. An assortment of different evaluation parameters of minipunch grafting has also evolved over the years [47–50].

Minipunch grafting has been combined with NB-UVB (311 nm) and documented encouraging results [22].

TEST GRAFTING

Before embarking upon any surgical intervention in vitiligo, proper assessment of the stability status is of paramount importance.

Clinically, stability can be judged by three simple indicators:

- *History*: Lack of progression of old lesions and absence of development of any new lesion within a specified period (6 months to 2 years).
- *Koebner phenomenon (Kp)*: Absence of a recent Kp either from history (Kp-h) or experimentally induced (Kp-e).
- *Test grafting*: On the backdrop of pervasive incongruity about the minimal period of stability, an attempt was made for the first time by Falabella in 1995 to fathom stability before surgery by introducing the minigrafting test [50]. The objective of this test vowed to serve several purposes, noted in the following.

In the original suggested procedure, a few grafts (1.0–1.2 mm) were placed in the center of the depigmented lesion to be scrutinized. Dressing was done by Micropore® adhesive tape and kept for a couple of weeks. After removal of the tape, the area was exposed to sunlight for 15 minutes daily for a period of 3 months. No treatment was permitted during this test period.

All test sites are visualized under Woods light. The test was considered positive if unequivocal repigmentation took place beyond 1 mm from the border of the implanted grafts. On the other hand, if less than 1 mm or no repigmentation was observed, the test was considered negative.

Some of the largest studies termed this evaluation *test grafting* (TG), and found it to be a more reliable exercise than the unjustified dependence on the period of stability alone [22,44,45]. Over the years this "test" has been vindicated and acknowledged as a powerful tool for detecting stable vitiligo, which anticipates the repigmentation success in vitiligo when surgery becomes a therapeutic option.

MINIGRAFTING PROCEDURE [13,43–45]

After proper assessment of the stability status and routine physical examination and investigations an informed consent is taken from the patient. The donor and recipient areas are surgically prepared.

1. The instruments required are 1.5- or 1.2-mm punches, a small jeweler's or graft-holding forceps, and small curved-tip scissors (Figures 37.1.4 and 37.1.5).

2. The recipient area is prepared first. Two percent lignocaine with or without adrenaline is infiltrated as a local anesthetic.

3. To minimize the chance of developing any perigraft halo, the initial recipient chambers are made on or very close to the border of the lesion. The punched-out chambers are spaced according to the result of test grafting or at a gap of 5–10 mm from each other.

4. The donor area is the upper lateral portion of either the thigh or gluteal area. Punch impressions are made very close to each other so that a maximum number of grafts can be taken from a small area.

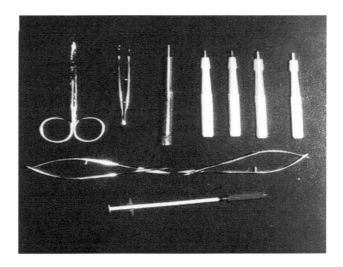

Figure 37.1.5   Instruments needed for minigrafting.

5. The same sized punches are used for both donor and recipient areas.

6. The grafts are placed directly from donor (buttock/upper thigh) to the recipient areas. This speeds up the procedure and lessens the chance of infection. Care is taken that the graft edges are not folded and the tissue is not crushed or placed upside-down. The needle of the syringe or the tip of the scissors is used for proper placement of grafts in the recipient chambers.

7. Hemostasis is achieved by pressing a saline-soaked gauze piece over the area.

8. For the recipient area, the three layers of dressing from the inside out are paraffin-embedded non-adherent sterile gauze (Gelonet®), sterile Surgipad®, and bioocclusive Micropore (Figure 37.1.6).

9. For the donor area only Surgipad and Micropore are used.

10. The recipient area may be immobilized if necessary. Proper instructions for special areas like lips are necessary. To secure the recipient area, these patients are advised to take a liquid diet for the first 24 hours, preferably with a straw. Patients are allowed a normal diet after that.

11. Dressings are sometimes opened after 24 hours to look for any dislodgement of grafts, and if found they are replaced.

12. After 4–7 days the dressings are removed.

FOLLOW-UP AND COURSE OF EVENTS

Post-surgically, patients are exposed to PUVA [17,18], PUVAsol (psoralen plus UVA from sunlight) [44,45], or NB-UVB [22] or even kept as such in some studies [31]. The patients are followed up fortnightly for the initial 2 months and then monthly until complete repigmentation is achieved.

In the donor site, after healing with secondary intention, minimal superficial scarring is expected and acceptable.

Scabs may fall off from the recipient site within 7–14 days, though in many instances there may not be any scab formation. Perigraft repigmentation is expected to start in around 3–4 weeks [22,44–46].

The entire depigmented and grafted area is expected to be completely repigmented within 3–6 months, based on the area of grafting and body part involved. Minigrafting can be deployed on any part of the body (Figures 37.1.7 through 37.1.11).

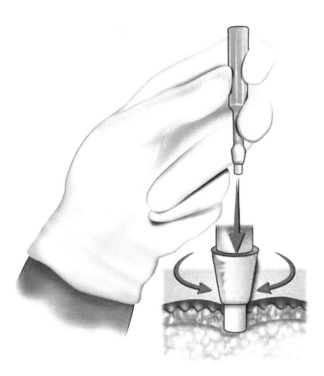

Figure 37.1.4   Correct positioning of the hand while taking grafts with a miniature punch.

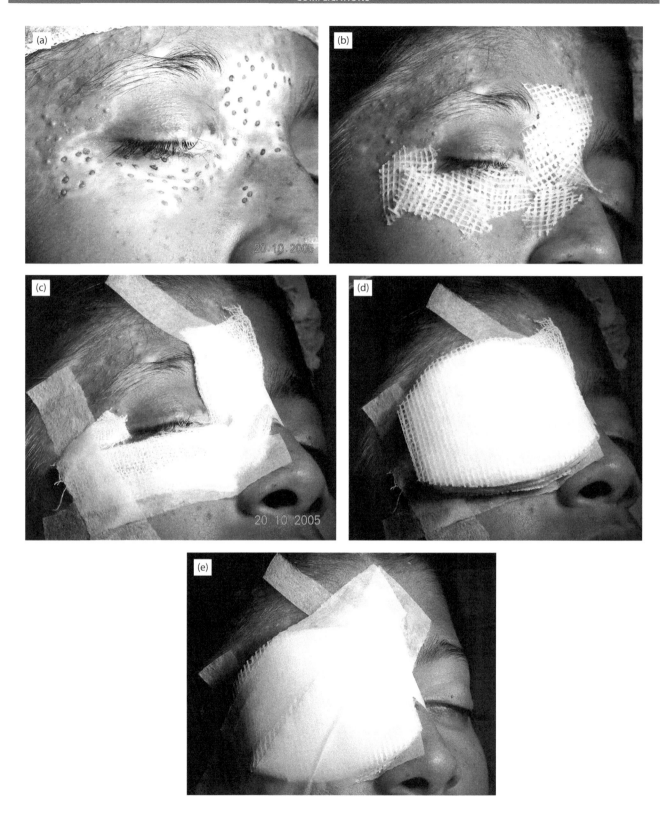

Figure 37.1.6 (a–e) Three layers of dressing from inside out. Paraffin-embedded nonadherent sterile gauze (Jelonet®), sterile Surgipad, and bio-occlusive Micropore.

COMPLICATIONS

Complications are seen in punchgrafting (PG) frequently and are enumerated in Table 37.1.2 [22,43–45]. By proper selection of cases and with proper technique, most of these complications are entirely avoidable. Cobblestoning (Figure 37.1.12) is regarded as the most common [22,44,45,51]. It was observed that with time cobbleston-ing was corrected in most cases [41]. In resistant cases, corrective electrofulguration may be needed [52]. It can be avoided by avoid-ing punches more than 1.5 mm in diameter. On the face and lips, punches should be even smaller (1.2 or 1 mm) [22]. Rejection of grafts is another complication, particularly seen in herpes labialis–induced lip leukoderma [53–56]. By proper selection of cases, most of these complications are entirely avoidable.

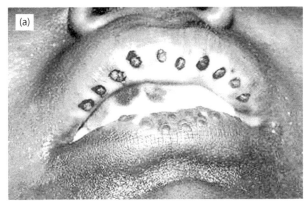 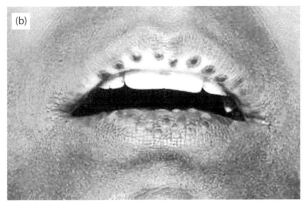

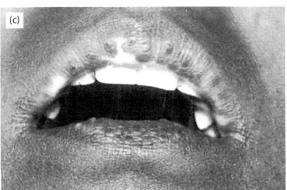 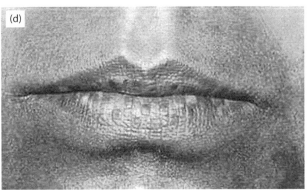

Figure 37.1.7 (a–d) Minigrafting on lips. Upper lip showing gradual repigmentation. Lower lip showing resolving of cobblestoning.

DISCUSSION AND ANALYTICAL PERSPECTIVE

Surgical correction of vitiligo and other cutaneous achromia has come a long way in the last four decades, but among all methods, autologous miniature punch grafting has already established its place as the easiest, fastest, least aggressive, and one of the most effective means of vitiligo therapy.

When the graft is removed, the piece of tissue is completely detached from the donor site and is then placed on the vascular bed in the recipient holes. From this vascular bed it derives its blood supply. Initially the graft adheres to its new bed by fibrin. There is diffusion of nutrients through this fibrinous layer which keep the graft alive initially. Within 2–3 days, capillary linkage occurs with vascularization of the graft. The thinner the graft, the denser the capillary network in the superficial dermis and thus the earlier is the process of vascularization [57].

Several aspects of PG need special consideration.

MECHANISM OF PIGMENTATION OF GRAFTING PROCEDURES

The mechanism of pigmentation of grafting procedures has been the subject of several studies. Melanocytes have been shown to spread centrifugally from the infundibulum of the hair follicle to the basal cell layer and recolonize the epidermis with active and functional melanocytes [58,59]. However, the presence of pilosebaceous apparatus within the minigrafts is not necessary for the repigmentation process because in suction blister grafts only epithelial cells present in the grafts are enough to induce repigmentation [60]. In 1970, Billingham and Silvers demonstrated the phenomenon of melanocyte migration from the graft's edge within the achromic skin to recolonize and replenish the area with functional and active melanocytes [61].

RELAPSE AFTER GRAFTING

The major limitation of all grafting techniques is lack of specific criteria for defining stability [62–64]. It is often hard to predict how long the disease will remain stable. Similarly, it is difficult to foresee when it will start to become unstable [32,68]. This has made assessment of results difficult. Treatment of relapsed cases is considered difficult. However, repigmentation has been successfully induced in previous graft failure cases under NB-UVB (311 nm) phototherapy [22]. Even after recognizing the significance of stability and after three decades of experience in vitiligo surgery, it is ironic to note the lack of consensus regarding the optimal required period of stability. This lack of unanimity can be glaring in some cases (Table 37.1.3). In one study, the minimal period of stability as a prerequisite for grafting was mentioned to be as little as 4 months [62], while in another study it was reported to be 3 years [13,14]. Other variable figures like 6 months, 1 year, and 2 years have been reported as well [12,13,54].

Even the same author has taken different periods of stability into consideration in different articles [16,35].

The curious reverse-Koebner phenomenon after PG and spontaneous repigmentation of distant non-grafted vitiligo patches after PG have been reported [23,24,33]. This was attributed to possible release of cytokines from grafts.

The size of the grafted lesions varied from 15–144 cm² in different studies (Table 37.1.4). Likewise, the size of the punch instrument differed among studies (Table 37.1.5). Now the consensus is toward using smaller punches like 1.2 or 1.5 mm. Falabella even recommends 1-mm grafts for the facial region and 1.2 mm for other body parts [65]. In this way, the most common complication of punch grafting can also be avoided. Although the rate of cobblestoning was substantial in most of the studies, it was found that with time it was corrected. In resistant cases, electrofulguration is helpful [52].

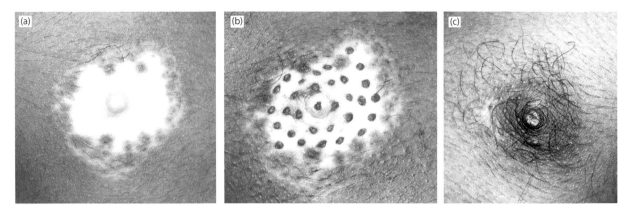

Figure 37.1.8 (a–c) Minigrafting on male nipple, without any glue or stay suture, showing graft take-up and repigmentation.

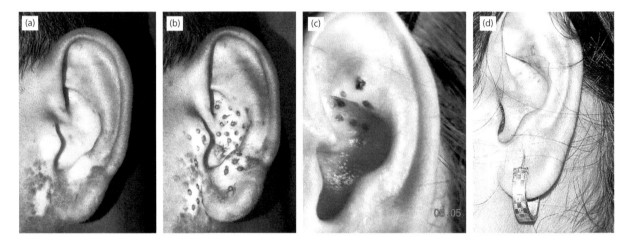

Figure 37.1.9 (a–d) Minigrafting on inner part of the external ear.

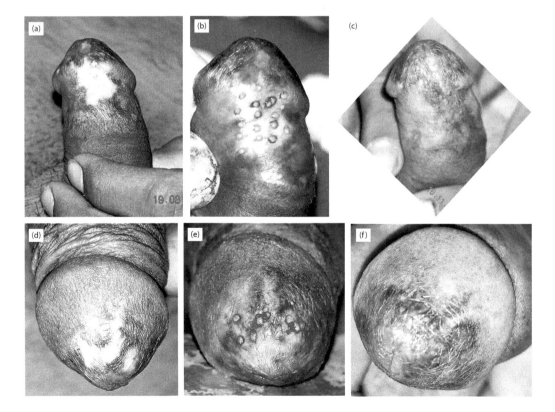

Figure 37.1.10 (a–f) Minigrafting on ventral and dorsal aspect of glans penis.

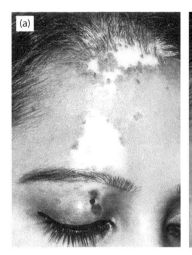
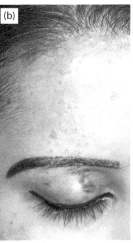

Figure 37.1.11 (a) Segmental vitiligo with leukotrichia. (b) Complete repigmentation with resolving cobblestoning and repigmentation of leukotrichia.

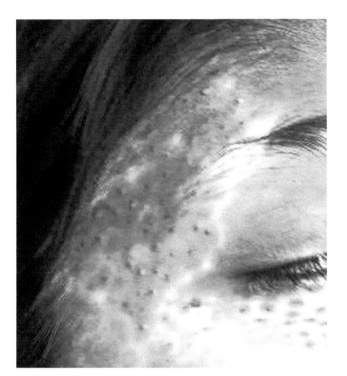

Figure 37.1.12 Cobblestoning and perigraft halo.

Table 37.1.1 Advantages and disadvantages of minigrafting

Advantages
• Easiest, fastest, and least expensive method
• Can be performed anywhere on any site (except angle of the mouth)
• Particularly suitable for areola
• It is perhaps the only suitable method for palm, though results may not be fully satisfactory
Disadvantages
• Side effects are common, particularly cobblestoning
• Phototherapy is always necessary after grafting
• Perfect match may not occur

Table 37.1.2 Complications of minigrafting

Recipient site	Donor site
Cobblestoning (Figure 37.1.12)	Keloid
Polka dot	Hypertrophic scar
Variegated appearance and color mismatch	Superficial scar
Static graft (no pigment spread)	Depigmentation/spread of disease
Depigmentation of graft	Contact dermatitis to adhesive tapes
Perigraft halo (Figure 37.1.12)	
Graft dislodgement/rejection	
Hypertrophic scar and keloid formation	

Table 37.1.3 Minimum period of stability in different studies

Author [Ref]	Year	Period of stability
Das SS, Pasricha JS [62]	1992	4 months
Boersma BR, Westerhof W [41]	1995	6 months
Jha AK, Pandey SS, Shukla VK [63]	1992	1 year
Savant SS [42]	1992	2 years
Falabella R [39]	1995	2 years
Falabella R [16]	1992	3 years

Table 37.1.4 Maximum grafted area in different studies

Author [Ref]	Year	Maximum grafted area (cm²)
Jha AK, Pandey SS, Shukla VK [63]	1992	15
Das S, Pasricha JS [62]	1992	80
Boersma BR, Westerhof W [41]	1995	96
Malakar S, Dhar S [45]	1999	>100
Falabella R [38]	1988	110
Lahiri K, Sengupta SR [44]	1997	144

Table 37.1.5 Size of graft in different studies

Author [Ref]	Year	Size of punch (diameter in mm)
Das S, Pasricha JS [62]	1992	4
Jha AK, Pandey SS, Shukla VK [63]	1992	3 and 4
Boersma BR, Westerhof W [41]	1995	2
Lahiri K, Sengupta SR [44]	1997	2
Malakar S, Dhar S [45]	1999	2
Malakar S, Lahiri K [51]	2004	1.5
Falabella R [38]	1988	1.2
Orentriech N, Selmanwitz VJ [11]	1972	1 and 2

Repigmentation of leukotrichia with PG and NB-UVB was noticed [22] (Figure 37.1.11). The same was also observed and documented before with PUVAsol and PG [67].

TIME TO APPEARANCE OF REPIGMENTATION

Another important parameter is the post-graft appearance of repigmentation (AOR) time. This was found to be between 2–6 weeks in different studies (Table 37.1.6).

After PG and PUVAsol, AOR time in different regions varied between 14 and 39 days, with an overall average of approximately 21.6 days, as shown in one study [44]. With the deployment of NB-UVB along with PG, AOR time in different regions varied between 14 and 32 days, with an overall average of approximately 20.6 days [22].

Table 37.1.6   Appearance of repigmentation time in different studies

Author [Ref]	Year	Earliest AOR (in days)
Lahiri K, Malakar S et al. [22]	2005	14
Lahiri K, Sengupta SR [44]	1997	14
Malakar S, Dhar S [45]	1999	16
Savant SS [42]	1992	30–45

Table 37.1.7   Maximum pigment spread (MPS) in different studies

Author [Ref]	Year	MPS (in mm)
Orentriech N, Selmanwitz VJ [11]	1972	1
Falabella R [12]	1978	2–3
Falabella R [38]	1988	3–4
Westerhof W, Boersma M [40]	1994	5
Savant SS [42]	1992	5–15
Lahiri K, Sengupta SR [44]	1997	1–10
Lahiri K, Malakar S et al. [22]	2005	12

MAXIMUM PIGMENT SPREAD

Orentriech, in his original article (1972), observed that whether 1- or 2-mm grafts were employed, the pigment spread was consistently 1 mm [11].

Various other results can be found in the literature (Table 37.1.7). Falabella, in establishing a relationship between donor graft and the area of surgical repigmentation, found that a 1-mm donor graft can repigment an area 25 times larger than the graft itself [36]. In a later study with 1.5-mm grafts and NB-UVB in type IV and V skin type subjects, this value was found to be more than double of that (56.21 times) [22]. In a previous study with PUVAsol, this relationship was found to be 42 times [46]. Larger grafts, darker skin types, and deployment of NB phototherapy all may have accounted for this high statistical value.

CONCLUSION

Considering all the indicators and parameters, it can be concluded that minigrafting is an easy, inexpensive, effective method of treating stable and recalcitrant vitiligo [66]. The advantages and disadvantages are summarized in Table 37.1.1.

REFERENCES

1. Millington GW, and Levell NJ. Vitiligo: The historical curse of depigmentation. *Int J Dermatol* 2007;46(9):900–5.

2. Ebbel B. *The Papyrus Ebers*. Copenhagen: Levin and Muntisgaard; 1937.

3. Whitney MD. *Atharvaveda Samhita (Translation and notes)*. Harvard Oriental series, Vol 7, Lannman, Cambridge: Harvard University Press; 1905.

4. Nair BK. Vitiligo—A retrospect. *Int J Dermatol* 1978;17(9):755–7.

5. Freilich AR. Tzaraat—Biblical leprosy. *J Am Acad Dermatol* 1982;6(1):131–4.

6. Mercurialis H. *De morbidis cutaneis et omnibus corporis humani excrementis tractatus*. Venezia. Paulus et Antonium Meietos; 1572.

7. Sutton RL. On definition of vitiligo. *Arch Dermatol* 1965;91:288.

8. Ortonne JP, Mosher DB, and Fitzpatrick TB. *Vitiligo and Other Hypomelanoses of Hair and Skin*. New York: Plenum Medical; 1983.

9. Behl PN. Homologous thin Thiersch's grafts in treatment of vitiligo. *Curr Med Pract* 1964;8:218–21.

10. Falabella R. Epidermal grafting: An original technique and its application in achromic and granulating areas. *Arch Dermatol* 1971;104(6):592–600.

11. Orentriech N, and Selmanwitz VJ. Autograft repigmentation of leucoderma. *Arch Dermatol* 1972;105(5):734–6.

12. Falabella R. Repigmentation of leukoderma by minigrafts of normally pigmented, autologous skin. *J Dermatol Surg Oncol* 1978:4:916–9.

13. Falabella R. Repigmentation of segmental vitiligo by autologous minigrafting. *J Am Acad Dermatol* 1983;9:514–21.

14. Lerner AB, Halaban R, Klaus SN et al. Transplantation of human melanocytes. *J Invest Dermatol* 1987;89:219–24.

15. Lerner AB. Repopulation of pigmented cells in patients with vitiligo. *Arch Dermatol* 1988;124(11):1701–2.

16. Falabella R, Escobar C, and Borrero I. Treatment of refractory and stable vitiligo by transplantation of *in vitro* cultured epidermal autografts bearing melanocytes. *J Am Acad Dermatol* 1992;26(2 Pt 1):230–6.

17. Skouge JW, Morison WL, Diwan RV et al. Autografting and PUVA. A combination therapy for vitiligo. *Dermatol Surg Oncol* 1992;18(5):357–60.

18. Hann SK, Im S, Bong HW et al. Treatment of stable vitiligo with autologous epidermal grafting and PUVA. *J Am Acad Dermatol* 1995;32(6):943–8.

19. Olsson MJ, and Juhlin L. Repigmentation of vitiligo by transplantation of cultured autologous melanocytes. *Acta Derm Venereol (Stockh)* 1993;73:49–51.

20. Malakar S, and Dhar S. Repigmentation of vitiligo patches by transplantation of hair follicles. *Int J Dermatol* 1999;38(3):237–8.

21. Olsson MJ, and Juhlin L. Long-term follow-up of leucoderma patients treated with transplants of autologous cultured melanocytes, ultrathin epidermal sheets and basal cell layer suspension. *Br J Dermatol* 2002;147(5):893–904.

22. Lahiri K, Malakar S, Sarma N et al. Repigmentation of vitiligo with punch grafting and narrow-band UV-B (311 nm)—A prospective study. *Int J Dermatol* 2006;45(6):649–55.

23. Malakar S, and Dhar S. Spontaneous repigmentation of vitiligo patches distant from the autologous skin graft sites: A remote reverse Koebner's phenomenon? *Dermatology* 1998;197(3):274.

24. Malakar S, and Lahiri K. Spontaneous repigmentation in vitiligo: Why it is important. *Int J Dermatol* 2006;45(4):478–9.

25. Watson BA. Gunpowder disfigurements. *St Luis Med Surg J* 1878;35:145.

26. Keyes EL. The cutaneous punch. *J Cutan Geniturin Dis* 1887;5:98.

27. Hagerman D, and Wilson H. The skin biopsy punch: Evolution and modification. *Cutis* 1970;6:1139.

28. Stegman SJ. Commentary: The cutaneous punch. *Arch Dermatol* 1982;118:943.

29. Baronio G. Degli innesti animali, Milano, 1804, Stamperia e Fonderia del genio. https://www.sophiararebooks.com/pages/books/4516/giuseppe-baronio/degli-innesti-animali

30. Lewin ML, and Peck SM. Pigment studies in skin grafts on experimental animals. *J Invest Dermatol* 1941;4:504.

31. Labuono P, and Shatin H. Transplantation of hair bulbs and melanocytes into leucodermic scars. *J Dermatol Surg Oncol* 1976;2:53–5.

32. Lahiri K, Malakar S, Banerjee U et al. Clinico-cellular stability of vitiligo in surgical repigmentation: An unexplored frontier. *Dermatology* 2004;209:170–1.

33. Malakar S. Spontaneous repigmentation of vitiligo patches other than the grafted site. *Indian J Dermatol.* 1997;47(2):68–70.

34. Behl PN. Repigmentation of segmental vitiligo by autologous minigrafting. *J Am Acad Dermatol* 1985;12:118–9.

35. Falabella R. Reply. (Article 34 published by Behl) *J Am Acad Dermatol* 1985;12:119.

36. Falabella R. Repigmentation of stable leucoderma by autologous minigrafting. *J Dermatol Surg Oncol* 1986;12:172–9.

37. Falabella R. Post dermabrasion leucoderma. *J Dermatol Surg Oncol* 1987;13:44–8.

38. Falabella R. Treatment of localized vitiligo by autologous minigrafting. *Arch Dermatol* 1988;124:1649–55.

39. Falabella R. Barona M. Escobar C et al. Surgical combination therapy for vitiligo and piebaldism. *Dermatologis Surgery* 1995;21(10):852–7.

40. Westerhof W, Boersma B et al. *Grafting techniques in leucoderma.* Book of Abstracts. 7th International Congress of Dermatology. 1994, New Delhi. India.

41. Boersma BR, Westerhof W et al. Repigmentation in vitiligo vulgaris by autologous minigrafting: Results in nineteen patients. *J Am Acad Dermatol* 1995;33(6):990–5.

42. Savant SS. Autologous miniatures punch grafting in vitiligo. *Indian J Dermatol Venereol Leprol* 1992;58:310–4.

43. Malakar S (ed.). Punch grafting. In: *An Approach to Dermatosurgery.* 1st ed. Calcutta: A Paul; 1996, pp. 44–6.

44. Lahiri K, and Sengupta SR. Treatment of stable and recalcitrant depigmented skin conditions by autologous punch grafting. *Indian J Dermatol Venereol Leprol* 1997;63:11–4.

45. Malakar S, and Dhar S. Treatment of stable and recalcitrant vitiligo by autologous miniature punch grafting: A prospective study of 1,000 patients. *Dermatology* 1999;198:133–9.

46. Lahiri K, and Sengupta SR. A regionwise comparative study of post punch graft appearance of repigmentation (AOR) time in cutaneous achromia, *Indian J Dermatol* 1998;43(1), 13–5.

47. Lahiri K, and Sengupta SR. A clinico-microscopic corroboration of surgical repigmentation-a study of 30 cases. *IJD Dermatol.* 1998;43(3):99–101.

48. Lahiri K, and Sengupta SR. A regionwise comparative study of the extent of post punchgraft surgical repigmentation in cutaneous achromia. *Indian J Dermatol Venereol Leprol* 1998;64(4):173–5.

49. Lahiri K, and Sengupta SR. Relationship between donor graft area and area of surgical repigmentation. *Indian J Dermatol* 1999;44(1)11–14.

50. Falabella R, Arrunategui A, Barona MI, and Alzate A. The minigrafting test for vitiligo: Detection of stable lesions for melanocyte transplantation. *J Am Acad Dermatol* 1995;32:228–32.

51. Malakar S, and Lahiri K. Punch grafting for lip leucoderma. *Dermatology* 2004;208(2):125–8.

52. Malakar S, and Lahiri K. Electrosurgery in cobblestoning. *Indian J Dermatol* 2000;45(1):46–7.

53. Malakar S, and Dhar S. Rejection of punch grafts in three cases of herpes labialis induced lip leucoderma, caution and precaution. *Dermatology* 1997;195:414.

54. Malakar S, and Dhar S. Acyclovir can abort rejection of punch grafts in herpes-simplex induced lip leucoderma. *Dermatology* 1999;199:75.

55. Malakar S, and Lahri K. Successful repigmentation of six cases of Herpes labialis induced lip leucoderma by micropigmentation. *Dermatology* 2001; 03:194.

56. Lahiri K, and Malakar S. Herpes simplex induced lip leucoderma: Revisited. *Dermatology* 2004;208:182.

57. Burge S, and Rayment R. (eds). Free skin grafts. In: *Simple Skin Surgery.* 1st ed. Bombay: Blackwell Scientific Publications; 1986, pp. 71–84.

58. Parrish JA, Fitzpatrick TB, Shea C et al. Photochemotherapy of vitiligo: Use of orally administered psoralen and a high-intensity long-wave ultraviolet light system. *Arch Dermatol* 1976;112:1531–4.

59. Ortonne JP, Schmnitt D, Thivolet J et al. PUVA induced repigmentation of vitiligo, scanning electron microscopy of hair follicles. *J Invest Dermatol* 1980;74:40–2.

60. Suvanprakorn P, Dee-Analap S, Pongsomboon CH et al. Melanocyte autologous grafting for treatment of leukoderma. *J Am Acad Dermatol* 1985;13:968–74.

61. Billingham RE, and Silvers WK. Studies on the migratory behaviour of melanocytes in guinea pig skin. *I J Exp Med* 1970;131:101–17.

62. Das SS, and Pasricha JS. Punch grafting as a treatment for residual lesions in vitiligo. *Indian J Dermatol Venereol Leprol* 1992;58:315–19.

63. Jha AK, Pandey SS, and Shukla VK. Punch grafting in vitiligo. *Indian J Dermatol Venereol Leprol* 1992;58:328–30.

64. Singh KG, and Bajaj AK. Autologous miniature skin punch grafting in vitiligo. *Indian J Dermatol Venereol Leprol* 1995;61:77–80.

65. Falabella R. Surgical treatment of vitiligo: Why, when and how. *(Editorial) J Eur Acad Dermatol Venereol* 2003;17:518–20.

66. Malakar S, and Lahiri K. Mini grafting for vitiligo. In: Gupta S, Olsson MJ, Kanwar AJ, and Ortonne JP, eds. *Surgical Management of Vitiligo,* 1st ed. Oxford: Blackwell Publishing; 2007, pp. 87–95.

67. Malakar S, and Dhar S. Repigmentation of leukotrichia over vitiligo patches after punch grafting. *Indian J Dermatol Venereol Leprol* 1998;64(5):252–3.

68. Malakar S, and Lahiri K. How unstable is the concept of stability in surgical repigmentation of vitiligo? *Dermatol* 2000;201:182–3.

TISSUE GRAFTING TECHNIQUES
Ultrathin Skin Grafting

Imran Majid and Tasleem Arif

CONTENTS

INTRODUCTION

Ultrathin skin grafting (UTSG) is a special type of split-thickness skin grafting where the skin graft is extremely thin (epidermal) and almost devoid of any dermal tissue, a result of which the harvested graft is translucent in nature. The basic difference between ultrathin and conventional split-thickness skin grafting is the thickness of the graft. Accordingly, split-thickness skin grafts can be of various types (Table 37.2.1) depending upon the thickness of the graft [1]. Though there are many surgical techniques for repigmenting vitiliginous areas, UTSG is simple, with the most rapid onset of pigmentation, in addition to being the most cost-effective procedure. In addition to vitiligo, it can be employed for piebaldism, halo nevi, and for other secondary leukodermas such as post-herpetic, post-burns, post-discoid lupus erythematosus, and contact leukoderma.

HISTORICAL BACKGROUND

Ollier (1872) and Thiersch (1874) introduced thin split-thickness skin grafts that now bear their names (Table 37.2.2). In 1947, Haxthausen transplanted Ollier-Thiersch grafts from normal to vitiliginous skin in three patients, though pigmentation persisted in only one patient. Later, Behl in 1964 treated 107 vitiligo patients surgically employing Ollier-Thiersch grafts. In 70% of the treated patients, he got good results, while a complication rate of 19% was observed [2]. Kahn et al. (1993), using ultrathin epidermal sheets (also called ultrathin skin grafts), successfully repigmented vitiligo lesions [3]. At present, UTSG is being employed in a good number of dermatosurgery centers as a means of surgical management of recalcitrant vitiligo.

BASIC PRINCIPLES AND BIOLOGY OF SKIN GRAFTING

The basic principle in split-thickness skin grafting is that a section of the skin having epidermis and a variable amount of dermis (in UTSG the graft is almost devoid of dermis) is detached from its blood supply from the donor site and placed on a new recipient site. The outcome of skin grafts depends on their thickness. However, in vitiligo, the primary aim is to get repigmentation in the depigmented lesion rather than filling the anatomical defect, as is the case with most plastic surgeons. This is why in the surgical management of vitiligo, thin split-thickness (Ollier-Thiersch) grafts or ultrathin grafts (also called epidermal sheets or epithelial grafts) are preferred.

Before going into detail, it is important to understand that UTSG for vitiligo differs from conventional split-thickness skin grafting in some aspects (Table 37.2.3). First, the graft in ultrathin grafting is very thin (0.08–0.15 mm) and devoid of any dermal tissue, as can be noted by the translucent nature of the graft. The absence of whitish tissue on the dermal side of the graft is the hallmark of the ultrathin skin graft [4]. Second, the behavior of the ultrathin skin graft differs from that of conventional split-thickness skin graft in the sense that the former is not permanent and falls off within 10–14 days after procedure [5]. There are three biological changes (Table 37.2.4) that follow skin grafting [6]:

1. *Graft take and adherence*: This is the first and the most crucial phase, as the fate of graft success is dependent on it. It begins with placement of the graft and continues for 72 hours. During this phase, the adherence of the graft to the recipient site is due to fibrin bonding and a process of plasmatic imbibitions nourishing the transplanted tissue. At this stage, the graft appears pink. After fibrin bonding, there occurs vascular anastomosis and fibrovascular growth. The transplanted graft imbibes the dermabraded/wound exudates by capillary action via the sponge-like structure of the graft dermis and through the blood

Table 37.2.1   Types of split-thickness skin grafts according to thickness

Type of graft	Thickness (in inches)	Thickness (in mm)
Thick	0.018–0.030	0.45–0.75
Medium	0.012–0.018	0.3–0.45
Thin	0.008–0.012	0.2–0.3
Ultrathin	0.003–0.006	0.08–0.15

Table 37.2.2   Historical background of vitiligo surgery

Author	Year	Detail
Ollier	1872	First introduced thin split-thickness grafting
Thiersch	1874	First introduced thin split-thickness grafting
Brown	1944	Developed electric dermatome to harvest thin homogenous grafts
Haxthausen	1947	Transplanted thin split-thickness skin grafts from normal to vitiliginous skin in three cases
Behl	1964	From India was the first to describe the surgical treatment of vitiligo in a large study of 107 patients
Falabella	1971	Described the suction blister technique for repigmentation of vitiligo
Falabella	1978	Described miniature punch grafting technique
Falabella et al.	1989	Described the use of in vitro cultures of melanocyte-bearing epidermis for the treatment of vitiligo
Gauthier and Surleve-Bazeille	1992	Described use of epidermal suspensions obtained by trypsinization
Olsson and Juhlin	1995	Modified the Surleve-Bazeille technique by adding a melanocyte culture medium
Kahn and Cohen	1998	Utilized the motorized dermatome to obtain ultrathin grafts
Kahn et al.	1996	Reported the use of a short-pulse carbon dioxide laser to dermabrade the recipient area

Table 37.2.3   How ultrathin skin grafting is different from conventional split-thickness grafting

The ultrathin skin graft is very thin, ranging in size from 0.08 to 0.15 mm
Its devoid of dermal tissue
Appears translucent when harvested, lacking the whitish tissue on dermal side
Graft contracture is not observed in an ideal ultrathin graft
It is not a permanent graft and falls off within 10–14 days after transplantation

Table 37.2.4   Biological changes during skin grafting

Graft take and adherence
The most crucial phase for graft survival
Begins with placement of the graft and continues for 72 hours
The adherence of the graft to the recipient site is due to fibrin bonding and a process of plasmatic imbibitions nourishing the transplanted tissue
The graft imbibes the wound exudates by capillary action
Factors like bleeding, infection, and mechanical movement due to improper immobilization can lead to graft failure
Graft revascularization
Formation of endothelial buttons
Establishment of direct anastomosis between recipient site blood vessels and graft
Insufficient vascular proliferation; formation of a thick fibrin layer or hematoma or seroma can adversely affect graft revascularization
Contracture
Contracture in the graft can occur immediately (after harvesting) or after placement of the graft
Contraction of the elastin fibers due to myofibroblasts has been suggested
Perigraft halo and achromic fissures are the results of contracture
In an ultrathin skin graft lacking a dermal component, contracture should be absent
Applying 1 to 2 mm larger graft than the vitiligo patch and overlapping of graft edges at the recipient site is recommended for optimal results

3. *Contracture*: Contracture in the graft can occur immediately (after harvesting) or after placing the graft at the recipient site. Contraction of the elastin fibers has been incriminated for graft contracture. Myofibroblasts are said to be responsible for this. The contracture of a graft is more in thicker grafts with more dermal component which leads to the inhibition of myofibroblast function by some unknown mechanism. This implies that chances of success in a thinner graft are better compared to the thicker one. As a result of contracture, perigraft halo and achromic fissures can follow the grafting procedure. However, if a uniform ultrathin skin graft has been harvested lacking a dermal component, then contracture should be absent since elastin fibers are lacking in the graft. Applying a 1–2 mm larger graft than the recipient vitiligo patch and overlapping of graft edges at the recipient site can prevent such complications.

PATIENT SELECTION

Important points to consider in selecting a patient for grafting procedure in vitiligo are given next. These are not unique for UTSG but can apply to any surgical procedure meant for repigmentation in vitiligo (Table 37.2.5).

STABILITY OF VITILIGO

The concept of stability in vitiligo has been a topic of debate. Researchers have defined it in different ways. Authors have recommended different time durations that vary widely from as low as 4 months (Das and Pasricha, 1992), 6 months (Boersma and Westerhof, 1995), 1 year (Jha et al., 1992) and 2 years (Savant, 1992 and Falabella, 2003) to 3 years (Falabella, 1992) [7]. To resolve this question, the IADVL task force defined stability as "a patient with no new lesions, no progression of existing lesions and absence of Koebner phenomenon during the last one year" [8]. However, Falabella proposed some

vessels of the dermis. This provides nourishment to the graft, maintains graft vascular patency, and prevents desiccation of the graft. Certain factors such as bleeding, infection, and mechanical movement due to improper immobilization at this stage can lead to graft failure. Hence for the first 3 days, strict immobilization is mandatory.

2. *Graft revascularization*: Revascularization of the transplanted graft occurs during this phase. There is formation of endothelial buttons and then capillaries that rapidly penetrate into the deeper part of the graft. This stage is characterized by establishment of direct anastomosis between recipient site blood vessels and graft, a process called *inoculation*. At this stage, some factors can adversely affect graft uptake, including insufficient vascular proliferation, formation of a thick fibrin layer, or hematoma or seroma. This explains why compression dressing in the postoperative period is advised.

Table 37.2.5 Factors affecting selection of a patient for grafting procedure in vitiligo

Stability of vitiligo in the patient
VIDA score
Age of the patient
Morphological type of vitiligo
Area of depigmentation
Anatomical site of vitiligo

criteria to assess the stability of the disease which include (i) lack of progression of old lesions within the past 2 years (in unilateral vitiligo this may be shorter, and in bilateral vitiligo, stability establishes after several years); (ii) no new lesions developing within the same period; (iii) absence of a recent Köbner phenomenon (either from history or experimentally produced); (iv) repigmentation of depigmented areas by medical treatment or sometimes spontaneous repigmentation; (v) a positive minigrafting test; and (vi) lack of Köbnerization at donor site [7]. Another unsolved question regarding stability of vitiligo is the concept of lesional versus disease (global) stability. Studies have shown that while the grafted lesions are showing repigmentation, the other untreated lesions are still progressing in depigmentation. Conversely, after grafting, depigmentation has occurred at the recipient site while the donor area has spontaneously repigmented. This implies that in the same patient different lesions can be in different states of stability. However, results from a multicenter study have shown that lesional stability is as relevant as disease stability for surgical management of vitiligo [9].

VIDA SCORING METHOD
Researchers have proposed a system called Vitiligo Disease Activity (VIDA) to measure disease activity on a 6-point scale from −1 to +4 and therapy-induced repigmentation grade. If the disease is active in past 6 weeks, the score is +4; in past 3 months, +3; 6 months, +2; 1 year, +1; stable for at least 1 year, 0; stable for at least 1 year and spontaneous pigmentation, −1. The patient is considered for vitiligo surgery only if VIDA score is less than or equal to zero [10]. However, the applicability of VIDA score has been questioned.

AGE OF THE PATIENT
Since grafting procedure is performed under local anesthesia, carrying out the procedure in children is always an additional challenge for the surgeon. However, there is as yet no consensus on the lower age limit for performing grafting. Grafting procedures have been successfully performed in children with good results. It should be mentioned that nonsegmental vitiligo developing in an early age is regarded as immunologically more unstable.

MORPHOLOGICAL TYPE OF VITILIGO
The best results of vitiligo grafting are seen in stabilized segmental or focal vitiligo. Acral vitiligo, on the contrary, is reported to give the worst results following grafting comparing to other types.

AREA OF DEPIGMENTATION
Nonsegmental vitiligo involving more than 30% of the body surface area should not be selected for grafting, as it is most likely to be immunologically unstable.

ANATOMICAL SITE OF VITILIGO
Certain anatomical regions are considered difficult to treat, including the skin overlying joints, lips, dorsum of hands and feet especially fingers and toes, eyelids, genitals, and body folds. In skin folds, eyelids, etc., the difficulty is primarily with regard to grafts holding on to the dermabraded recipient skin. On the contrary, in areas like acral parts, fingers, toes, etc., the chances of repigmentation are lower because of a decreased number or absence of melanocyte

reservoirs present in hair follicles. Studies have shown that UTSG has resulted in slight hyperpigmentation in the treated lesion compared to the initial shade of pigmentation [11]. This means that one has to be cautious while using this procedure for the face. This aspect will be discussed in detail later in the chapter.

COUNSELING
Before employing any surgical technique, proper counseling of the patient is very important. Certain issues should be clearly mentioned to the patient like that grafting is not universally effective in all patients; progression of the disease cannot be stopped by grafting; disease may recur even after surgical intervention at the same site; getting exactly the same color shade is not guaranteed; and obtaining cosmetically acceptable results can take up to 1–6 months or longer.

TECHNIQUE

PREOPERATIVE PREPARATION
Shaving of the donor and recipient sites before the procedure is important. However, if the recipient area has thick terminal hair, as the transplanted graft starts to grow the hair tends to lift up the graft, which can adversely affect the results. Hence some authors recommend plucking the hair with forceps after administerng anesthesia instead of shaving, as it delays hair growth, thus preventing the graft from being lifted up [12]. Chemical depilation of the hair is another alternative for getting rid of hair prior to the procedure.

PREMEDICATION
For attaining success in the surgical procedure, a still and calm patient is a prerequisite. In an anxious patient, 5 mg diazepam can be given the previous night and 2 hours before the procedure. At some centers its customary to give 5–10 mg of diazepam and/or 10 mg of ketobemidone orally 60–90 minutes before the procedure plus 500–1000 mg paracetamol 40–50 minutes before the transplantation [13].

HARVESTING THE GRAFT

DONOR SITE PREPARATION AND ANESTHESIA
The gluteal region and anterior surface of the thigh are the most preferred sites, for cosmetic reasons. However, posterior, lateral, and medial surfaces of the thigh can also be used. Other sites include arms, abdomen, etc. Taking an ultrathin skin graft from a curved surface like the gluteal region requires expertise; hence for beginners an even surface is recommended by authors. An area slightly larger than the size of the recipient patch(es) is marked with a sterile surgical marking pen.

Topical anesthesia using a mixture of lidocaine and prilocaine (EMLA[R], AstraZeneca, Sweden) or lidocaine and tetracaine (Tetralid[R] Ajanta Pharma, India) under occlusion for 1–2 hours before the procedure is usually sufficient [14,15]. In certain cases, the anesthesia attained may not be satisfactory. In such cases, field block with 1% lignocaine at the margins of the donor area should be given. It must be noted that infiltration of anesthesia into the marked area must be avoided, as it can result in an uneven surface of the skin, making it difficult to harvest a uniform ultrathin epidermal sheet for grafting.

INSTRUMENTS
The choice of instrument for taking an ultrathin skin graft depends upon surgeon expertise, availability of instruments, etc. The various instruments that can be employed to take a uniform graft are

Table 37.2.6   Instruments used for taking a uniform skin graft

| A sterile razor blade mounted on a Kochers forceps |
| Humby's skin grafting knife |
| Zimmer motor-driven dermatome |
| Padget's or Davol's dermatome or a hand dermatome |
| Silvers razor blade holding knife |
| Any straight-tipped forceps (e.g., Kelly or Rochester Pean forceps) fitted with a razor blade |

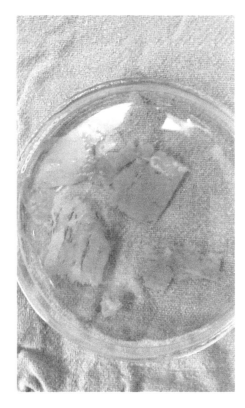

Figure 37.2.1   Thin, translucent skin grafts used in UTSG.

noted in Table 37.2.6. The Humby knife has a roller mechanism that provides larger size grafts of uniform thickness. By adjusting the distance between the roller and the blade, the thickness of the graft can be easily controlled. However, the Humby knife can only be used on convex surfaces [16]. Very thin epidermal sheets can be harvested by motor-driven Zimmer dermatome [13].

METHOD

Normal saline or mineral oil or xylocaine jelly (which is readily available in theaters) can be used to hydrate and lubricate the skin, which can aid in stabilizing the skin during graft harvesting. The procedure is commenced by an assistant stretching the skin firmly at one end by applying downward and outward traction with the help of the flat of his hand while the treating surgeon provides outward traction at the other end. The importance of this traction is that it flattens the skin and thus decreases the drag felt during harvesting of the graft. While harvesting the graft, the cutting blade (employing any of the previously mentioned instruments) is held tangential to the skin surface, and a sliding to-and-fro movement is employed to cut through the uppermost part of dermis. The thickness of the graft depends on the angle with which the blade is introduced into the skin, which comes with practice.

The harvested skin is immediately submerged in normal saline in a sterile Petri dish or moistened with s-MEM (Joklik's modified minimal essential medium [GIBCO BRL, Life Technology, Gaithersburg, MD, USA]) so that it does not dry up before transplanting it to the recipient site (Figure 37.2.1). The graft is examined for its translucency and presence of any whitish dermal tissue on the dermal side. An ideal ultrathin skin graft is translucent and devoid of any dermal tissue. In addition, it floats on the saline solution and does not curl on itself due to lack of dermal component. The pattern of bleeding on the donor site also reflects the thickness of the harvested graft. A thin graft produces closely placed fine bleeding points, while a thicker graft produces sparsely placed, coarse bleeding points.

DRESSING OF THE DONOR AREA

Many types of dressings are currently available for dressing the donor site, including occlusive dressings (hydrocolloid dressing; Duoderm™), semiocclusive dressings (Tegaderm™), semi-open dressings (Vaseline gauze) and even no dressing [17]. Among these, semiocclusive dressings are considered superior due to favorable properties such as lowest infection rates, lowest subjective pain scores, and fastest healing rates [18]. The authors use a semiocclusive dressing, and a pressure dressing is applied using a strapping tape (Leukoband ™, BSN Medical, India).

RECIPIENT SITE
PREPARATION

After proper surgical cleansing and marking of vitiliginous lesion, topical anesthetic cream (EMLA or Tetralid) is applied for 2–3

hours before the procedure, which suffices in most cases [14]. Alternatively, local anesthetic in the form of 1% lignocaine is infiltrated into four quadrants, the deep dermis as well as subcutaneous tissue involving the lesional skin and 4–5 cm of surrounding perilesional normal skin [19]. Freezing spray such as ethyl chloride or fluor-ethyl (Gebauer Pharmaceutical Preparations, Cleveland, OH, USA) can also be employed as local anesthetic immediately prior to the dermabrasion. This spray gives some anesthesia but is not sufficient to give complete pain relief. Its advantage is that when skin is chilled it becomes firmer and therefore easier to dermabrade. It also makes it easier for a beginner to detect remaining epidermal remnants on the chilled dermabraded recipient surface [13]. Only in rare cases when the disease is extensive is general anesthesia required.

DERMABRASION

Various instruments can be employed for dermabrasion of the recipient site, including manual metallic dermabrader, electric dermabrader with a diamond fraise endpiece, Er:YAG laser, UltraPulse carbon dioxide (CO_2) laser, etc. Using a high-speed dermabrader (20,000 rpm) which has been fitted with a diamond fraise, the skin is dermabraded down to the dermal–epidermal junction. Diamond fraises can be of various types such as wheel, pear, and/or cone, depending upon the site to be used on. Generally, a 6-mm-wide regular fraise wheel is used, but on rough skin such as knees one might need a coarse wheel. In delicate areas such as around the nostrils, corners of the mouth, and on the eyelids, a small pear-shaped fraise may be preferred. At some centers, a specially made hand tool fitted with a regular cone is used for eyelids, which ensures that no damage is done to the eyelid or eye during the procedure [13]. However, the authors routinely use Manekshaw's metallic dermabraders (of various sizes depending upon the site to be dermabraded) with good results. Dermabrasion should be done uniformly all over the depigmented area and the additional 2–3 mm of the perilesional surrounding normal skin to prevent the development of postoperative perigraft depigmented halo. Visibility of uniform punctate capillary bleeding from the dermal papilla marks the stopping point of further dermabrasion. At this stage, light freezing with fluor-ethyl spray can reveal the presence of any islands of epidermis left at the denuded site. The recipient site can also be prepared using a pulsed Er:YAG laser or UltraPulse CO_2 laser. However, the UltraPulse CO_2 laser is preferred over Er:YAG because it achieves better hemostasis and causes an epidermal–dermal split in a single pass [20]. The dermabraded areas are washed with saline solution or phosphate buffered saline (PBS) and kept under moistened gauze until the donor area is harvested and grafts ready for transplantation.

TRANSPLANTING THE GRAFT

The graft is placed over the dermabraded area ensuring that the dermal surface is facing down. There should be no wrinkling in the graft. The free edges of the graft should be stretched evenly at the periphery employing a spatula or a graft spreading rod or non-traumatizing ring forceps to ensure that no bubbles or fluid are left within between the dermabraded bed and the graft. If a graft is larger, small fenestrations can be made on the graft surface with a 22-gauge needle or a No. 11 blade to allow drainage of the exudates. Ideally, the graft should be larger than the actual size of denuded area and should extend 3–5 mm beyond the edges of the recipient area to prevent perigraft halo.

SECURING THE GRAFT AND IMMOBILIZATION

Securing and immobilization of the graft are considered most important criteria to obtain a successful result. Octyl-2-cyanoacrylate adhesive has been used to secure the graft. It also has antimicrobial properties against Staphylococci, *Pseudomonas*, and *Escherichia coli*. It is effective in immobilizing the grafts even over mobile areas, and prevents graft wrinkling. It is quick to act, easy to apply, and can be removed easily by peeling with forceps. It is applied in an interrupted manner at the edges of the graft and in the center over mobile areas such as eyelids to prevent wrinkling of the graft [2]. This is followed by a non-adherent dressing, such as paraffin dressing, silicone netting (Mepitel, Molnlycke AB, Molnlycke Sweden), or framycetin tulle (Soframycin® tulle, Aventis, Mumbai, India) and then covered with saline-moistened sterile gauze pads and bandaged with a Leukoband. Ideally, the patient should stay at least for 4 hours in a hospital bed after the procedure has been completed to maintain strict immobilization, but in practice this is rarely done. For grafting involving hands, they should be splinted, and if legs or feet have been treated the patient should be transported in a wheelchair to the car for home transportation.

POSTOPERATIVE CARE AND FOLLOW-UP

The dressing at the recipient site is usually removed after 7–8 days. However, some surgeons inspect the dressing at 24 hours to observe for any serous collection or hematoma, which if found is drained. The dressing at the donor site is also removed on 8th day; by that time the healing is almost complete. Prophylactic oral antibiotics are given for 1 week starting from the day of surgery to prevent postoperative infection. After removal of the dressings, an ultrathin graft is expected to be shed within a few days. Gradual repigmentation is seen within a few weeks, and repigmentation is complete within 2–3 months, or may take longer. To hasten the repigmentation process, supplementary narrowband UVB (NB-UVB) or targeted phototherapy can be used [21].

A slight hyper- or hypopigmentation in some of the treated lesions is not uncommon during the first year. However, gradually the color matches with the shade of the surrounding skin and most often blends in well in about 1–2 years. Long-lasting hyperpigmentation can occur [13] (Figures 37.2.2–37.2.4).

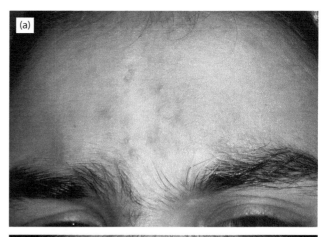
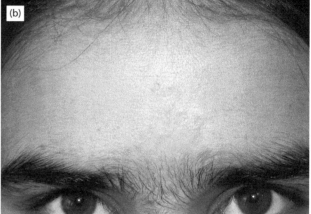

Figure 37.2.2 (a, b) Segmental vitiligo on forehead with excellent response to UTSG.

MODIFICATIONS NEEDED AT DIFFICULT-TO-TREAT SITES

Certain sites that are considered difficult to treat need some modifications, as explained next.

EYELIDS

Dermabrasion has to be done very gently at this site as the skin is extremely thin. A special form of hand tool fitted with a regular cone, a type of manual dermabrader, is used by some surgeons [13]. The authors use a smaller size and finer manual dermabrader rather than a motorized one for this purpose. For graft uptake, strict immobilization of the upper eyelid is required, which can be achieved by spreading a thin layer of cyanoacrylate adhesive, which secures the graft and also prevents wrinkling. Most authors suggest neomycin eye ointment to be applied before closing the eye to prevent dryness [2]. The eye is then bandaged firmly.

BEARD AREA, EYEBROWS, AND HAIRY AREAS

As noted earlier, it has been observed that plucking the hair with forceps after giving anesthesia delays hair growth and prevents the graft from being lifted up. Hence plucking the hairs instead of shaving them to avoid graft displacement is recommended [22]. Chemical epilation is an alternative to plucking of hair [23].

LIPS

Lip vitiligo poses a difficult challenge for the dermatosurgeon. UTSG has been carried out with excellent results over lips. Maintaining strict immobilization of the graft, especially of the lower lip, is the

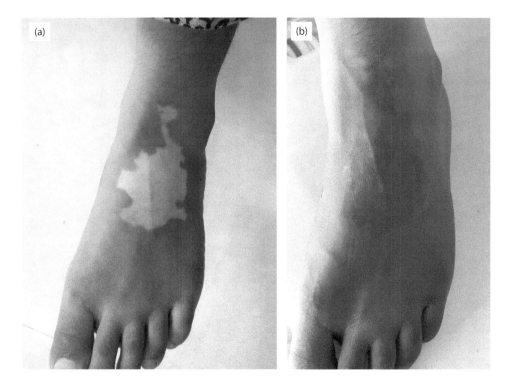

Figure 37.2.3   (a, b) UTSG on acral areas (foot).

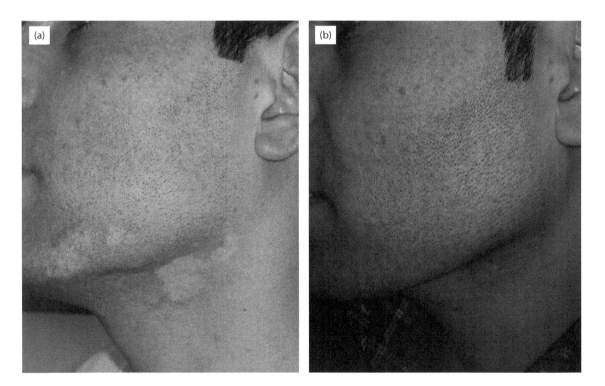

Figure 37.2.4   (a, b) UTSG on beard area.

key to success. When the inner mucosa of the lower lip is involved, it can be everted with a suture. To prevent contamination of the graft during food intake, the patient should be advised to take a liquid diet using a straw for 1 week. The literature regarding the treatment of lip vitiligo with thin split-thickness skin grafts is scarce. A study of 14 patients with lip vitiligo (9 patients with lower lip and 5 patients with upper lip involvement) demonstrated excellent response (75%–100%) in 7 patients; good response (50%–75%) in 2 patients; fair response (25%–50%) in 2 patients, and poor response (<25% repigmentation) in 3 patients [24].

AREOLAE

When an areola is involved, researchers have recommended that entire areola should be grafted (even if small area is affected) to prevent color mismatch at this site. It is fortunate for patients that the color of the graft is recipient-dominant in a majority of cases, probably because of local factors that play a role in regulating melanocyte activity [25].

ACRAL AREAS

Acral areas, especially fingers, can be surgically treated with UTSG but the results are poorer compared to other sites. Maintaining graft immobilization is relatively difficult at this site, and splints may be needed. In addition, dermabrasion poses difficulty even with a motorized dermabrader, which can be explained by the inherent thickness of the skin and prior use of psoralens at these sites.

COMPLICATIONS

Complications can occur at the recipient or donor site, as described next (Table 37.2.7).

RECIPIENT SITE
GRAFT REJECTION

Various factors that can cause graft rejection include seroma, hematoma, or accumulation of air bubbles between the graft and dermabraded surface; improper immobilization; technical error, where the graft is placed with dermal surface facing upward; and traumatized grafts.

HYPERPIGMENTATION

A study of leukoderma patients treated with transplants of autologous cultured melanocytes, ultrathin epidermal sheets, and basal cell layer suspension showed that the ultrathin epidermal sheet method resulted more often in slight hyperpigmentation. In 70%, the shade was hyperpigmented; it was the same shade in 25% and a somewhat lighter shade in 5% [11]. Before carrying out the procedure on the face, patients should be informed about the risk of hyperpigmentation. This can be treated with topical retinoids or with laser resurfacing.

PERIGRAFT HALO

Peripheral depigmentation (halo) and achromic fissures may be seen at the edges of the graft because of graft contraction. The graft should extend 3–5 mm beyond the abraded area to prevent this complication. Perigraft halos can be managed with topical or systemic psoralens, NB-UVB, or excimer laser (308 nm).

HYPERTROPHY

Hypertrophy is usually encountered with thicker grafts and is ideally not seen in true ultrathin skin grafts. Topical retinoids or midpotent topical steroids can be used to treat this complication.

Table 37.2.7   Complications of ultrathin skin grafting

Recipient site
Graft rejection
Hyperpigmentation
Perigraft halo
Achromic fissures
Hypertrophy
Milia formation
Secondary infection
Donor site
Scarring
Postinflammatory hyperpigmentation
Koebnerization

MILIA FORMATION

In the first 6 months, milia-like cysts can occur at the recipient site, especially on the face and neck. Many authors believe that milia develop due to remnants of epithelial cells following the dermabrasion, but a more plausible explanation for their development is occlusion of the sweat ducts where the outflow is blocked, in collaboration with rapid proliferation of the epithelial cells at the ends of the ducts [13]. A uniform dermabrasion and thorough cleansing of the dermabraded site before applying the graft can reduce this complication. Once developed, these can be managed easily by puncturing them with a fine needle and expressing out the contents. However, the authors have rarely encountered milia in clinical practice.

SECONDARY INFECTION

Under strict aseptic precautions and systemic antibiotic prophylaxis, this complication is rarely seen.

DONOR SITE
SCARRING

Superficial scarring can occur at the donor site if thicker grafts have been harvested. Ideally, if ultrathin epidermal sheets are harvested lacking a dermal component, then scarring at donor site is only a theoretical concept.

POST-INFLAMMATORY HYPERPIGMENTATION

This is common in darker skin types. It can be treated with topical retinoids.

KOEBNERIZATION

Vitiligo lesions can appear at the donor site which can be explained by Koebnerization or emergence of vitiligo at the donor site. Avoiding treatment of patients with active disease (positive Koebnerization) can prevent this complication.

EFFICACY OF ULTRATHIN SKIN GRAFTING

A recent study employing UTSG followed by NB-UVB has showed that 83% patients achieved >90% repigmentation of the grafted lesions. Cosmetic matching was graded on a visual analog scale as good to excellent in 90% of the cases. The average time for the onset of repigmentation in the treated lesions was 11 days after the start of NB-UVB therapy [4]. The predicted long-term outcome with the ultrathin sheet transplantation method is as good as with other methods. Excellent results have been seen with UTSG in most patients at 6-month follow-up. In one study, at a mean follow-up time of 4.5 years, patients with segmental vitiligo and piebaldism retained all repigmentation [11]. A follow-up study of resistant stable vitiligo patients treated with UTSG from Kashmir Valley involving 554 lesions in 370 patients showed excellent response (≥90% repigmentation) in 78.9% lesions, whereas only 8.67% lesions demonstrated poor results. Pigmentation was retained in >98% patients over a follow-up of 4 years [26].

ADVANTAGES AND DISADVANTAGES OF ULTRATHIN SKIN GRAFTING

The various advantages and disadvantages of UTSG are summarized in Tables 37.2.8 and 37.2.9.

Table 37.2.8 Advantages of ultrathin skin grafting

Excellent color matching
Does not require any specialized laboratory, expensive equipment, reagents, or technicians
In comparison to miniature punch grafting, complications like cobblestone appearance, or polka dot appearance are not seen
Simple, easy, and cost-effective
Difficult areas like eyelids, lips, areolae, etc., can be treated with relatively successful results
Takes less time in comparison to other procedures like suction blister grafting, melanocyte suspension methods, punch grafting
Hypertrophy at the recipient site is very rare since the graft is extremely thin, which greatly decreases the chances of hypertrophy
Lacking a dermal (elastin) component, the ultrathin grafts undergo very minimal contracture
The chances of scarring are minimal at the recipient site as the grafts are devoid of dermal tissue
The same area of the donor site can be used repeatedly for future sessions

Table 37.2.9 Disadvantages of ultrathin skin grafting

Multiple sittings are required for larger areas
Surgical skill of harvesting an ultrathin skin graft is required
The yield provided is 1:1, while melanocyte suspension/culture methods can give much higher ratios
Hyperpigmentation is a common occurrence, especially over photo-exposed areas and face

CONCLUSION

Ultrathin epidermal grafting is a simple, safe, and cost-effective treatment modality in stable vitiligo that is unresponsive to medical therapy. With this technique, the outcome at both the donor and recipient sites has improved. When performed in carefully selected patients with proper technique, excellent cosmetic results can be yielded. This procedure does not require any laboratory, chemical reagents, expensive equipment, or technicians, though expertise of harvesting an ultrathin skin graft is a prerequisite.

ULTRATHIN SKIN GRAFTING

- UTSG is a special type of split-thickness skin grafting where the skin graft is extremely thin and is devoid of any dermal tissue.
- It can be used for vitiligo, piebaldism, halo nevi, other secondary leukodermas like post-herpetic, post-burns, post-discoid lupus erythematosus, and contact leukoderma.
- Ultrathin skin graft differs from the conventional split-thickness skin graft in the sense that the former is not permanent and falls off within 10–14 days after transplantation.
- It leads to slight hyperpigmentation in the treated lesion. One has to be cautious while using this procedure for the face.

- Certain areas that are considered difficult to treat require some modifications.
- Supplementary NB-UVB can be used to hasten the repigmentation process.
- Ultrathin epidermal grafting is a simple, safe, cost-effective treatment modality in stable vitiligo that is unresponsive to medical therapy.
- Advantages are that it does not require any laboratory, chemical reagents, expensive equipment, or technicians, though expertise in harvesting an ultrathin skin graft is needed.

REFERENCES

1. Gupta DK. Thin and ultra thin split thickness skin grafts (STSG-UT, STSG-T). In: Gupta DK, ed. *Microskin Grafting for Vitiligo*, 1st ed. London: Springer Ltd; 2009, pp. 15–8.

2. Khunger N. Thin split-thickness skin grafts for vitiligo. In: Gupta S, Olsson MJ, and Kanwar AJ eds. *Surgical Management of Vitiligo*, 1st ed. London: Blackwell Publishing Ltd; 2007, pp. 108–13.

3. Kahn AM, Cohen MJ, and Kaplan L. Vitiligo: Treatment by dermabrasion and epithelial sheet grafting—A preliminary report. *J Am Acad Dermatol* 1993;28:773–4.

4. Majid I, and Imran S. Ultrathin split thickness skin grafting followed by narrowband UVB therapy for stable vitiligo: An effective and cosmetically satisfying treatment option. *Indian J Dermatol Venereol Leprol Halder* 2012;78:159–64.

5. Kahn AM, and Cohen MJ. Repigmentation in vitiligo patients-melanocytes transfer via ultra-thin grafts. *Dermatol Surg* 1998;24:365–7.

6. McCarthy JG. *Plastic Surgery*. Philadelphia, PA: WB Saunders, 1990.

7. Majid I, Mysore V, Salim T, Lahiri K, Chatterj M, Khunger N, Talwar S, Sachhidanand S, and Barua S. Is lesional stability in vitiligo more important than disease stability for performing surgical interventions? results from a multicentric study. *Journal of Cutaneous and Aesthetic Surgery*. 2016 Jan;9(1):13.

8. Parsad D, and Gupta S. Standard guidelines of care for vitiligo surgery. *Indian J Dermatol Venereal Leprol* 2008;74:S37–45.

9. Majid I, Mysore V, Salim T, Lahiri K, Chaaterji M, Khunger N, Talwar S, Sachhidanand S, and Barua S. Is lesional stability in vitiligo more important than disease stability for performing surgical interventions? Results from a multicentric study. *J Cutan Aesthet Surg* 2016;9:13–9.

10. Njoo MD, Das PK, Bos JD, and Westerhof W. Association of the Köbner phenomenon with disease activity and therapeutic responsiveness in vitiligo vulgaris. *Arch Dermatol* 1999;A135:414.

11. Olsson MJ, and Juhlin L. Long-term follow-up of leukoderma patients treated with transplants of autologous cultured melanocytes, ultra-thin epidermal sheets and basal cell layer suspension. *Br J Dermatol* 2002;147:893–904.

12. Van Geel N, Ongenae K, de Mil M, and Naeyaert JM. Modified technique of autologous noncultured epidermal cell transplantation for repigmentating vitiligo: A pilot study. *Dermatol Surg* 2001;27:873–6.

13. Olsson MJ. Treatment of leukoderma by transplantation of ultra-thin epidermal sheets In: Gupta S, Olsson MJ, Kanwar AJ, and Ortonne JP, *Surgical Management of Vitiligo*, 1st ed. London: Blackwell Publishing Ltd; 2007, pp. 115–22.

14. Juhlin L, and Olsson MJ. Optimal application times of eutectic mixtures of local anaesthetics (EMLA) cream before derm-abrasion of vitiliginous skin. *Eur J Dermatol* 1995;5:365–70.

15. Majid I. Can injectable lignocaine be replaced by topical anesthesia in melanocyte transplant or ultrathin skin grafting? *J Cutan Aesthet Surg* 2013;6:127–8.

16. McGregor IA, and McGregor AD. *Fundamental Techniques of Plastic Surgery*. Edinburgh: Churchill Livingstone, 1995.

17. Kilinc H, Sensoz O, Ozdemir R, Unlu RE, and Baran C. Which dressing for split-thickness skin graft donor site? *Ann Plast Surg* 2001;46:409–14.

18. Terill PJ, Goh RC, and Bailey MJ. Split thickness skin graft donor sites: A comparative study of two absorbent dressings. *J Wound Care* 2007;16:433–8.

19. Savant SS. *Textbook of Dermatosurgery and Cosmetology*. Mumbai: ASCAD, 2005.

20. Oh CK, Cha JH, Lim JY, Jo JH, Kim SJ, Jang HS, and Kwon KS. Treatment of vitiligo with suction epidermal grafting by the use of an UltraPulse CO_2 laser with a computerised pattern generator. *Dermatol Surg* 2001;27:563–8.

21. Yaar M, and Gilchrest BA. Vitiligo. The evolution of cultured epidermal autografts and other surgical treatment modalities. *Arch Dermatol* 2001;137:348–9.

22. Khunger N. Vitiligo surgery at difficult sites. Paper presented at *The 5th Biennial Conference of Association of Cutaneous Surgeons of India*, Chandigarh, India, November 22–24, 2002, Book of Abstracts, p. 40.

23. Kim CY, Yeon TJ, and Kim TH. Epidermal grafting after chemical epilation in the treatment of vitiligo. *Dermatol Surg* 2001;27:855–6.

24. Khunger N, and Misra RS. Refractory vitiligo on the lips: Surgical treatment by split thickness skin grafting. Paper presented at *The 2nd National Conference of Association of Dermatological Surgeons of India*, January 25–26, 1998, Book of Abstracts, p. 30.

25. Khunger N, Kapoor S, Pall A, and Jain RK. Cosmetic results of surgical treatment of vitiligo of the nipple–areolar complex. A clinical study of melanocyte activity. Paper presented at *The 1st Conference of Asian Society for Pigm Cell Research*, February 1–2, 2005, Book of Abstracts, p. 31.

26. Majid I, and Imran S. Ultrathin skin grafting in resistant stable vitiligo: A follow-up study of 8 years in 370 patients. *Dermatol Surg* 2017;2:219–25.

TISSUE GRAFTING TECHNIQUES
Suction Blister Grafting

Somesh Gupta and Sanjay Singh

CONTENTS

INTRODUCTION

Vitiligo is a common acquired pigmentary disorder of skin characterized by localized loss of skin pigmentation secondary to melanocyte damage. While most of the patients with vitiligo are managed by medical means, there remains a group that is resistant to all non-surgical means of treatment. These patients require surgical replacement of the damaged melanocytes. Furthermore, there is a subgroup of vitiligo in which surgical therapy is considered to be more appropriate than medical means. The type of the surgical procedure depends upon the extent or size of the vitiligo lesion to be treated, the site of the lesion, the age of the patient, his/her expectations and social needs, and finally, the expertise of the operating surgeon. In general, grafting techniques in vitiligo are divided into two main groups: tissue grafting and cellular grafting procedures [1]. The former group encompasses the different techniques of transferring skin tissue grafts as a whole to the involved recipient skin, while the latter involves further separation of these skin grafts into cellular components. As a whole, tissue grafting procedures are simpler and easier to perform than the cellular transplantation methods. Surgical treatments are among the most effective interventions but are limited by their invasive nature as well as the training and expertise needed to perform specific procedures. An important factor to be considered in the workup of patients prior to surgical therapy includes disease stability. The commonly accepted guidelines for the definition of disease stability are: (i) no new lesions in last 1 year; (ii) existing lesions should remain the same size; (iii) absence of Koebnerization; (iv) spontaneous repigmentation; and (v) positive minigraft test, especially when minigrafting is performed. The period for which these criteria are applied ranges from 6 months to 3 years.

SUCTION BLISTER GRAFTING

Suction blister grafting (SBG) is a procedure wherein epidermis is harvested from the donor site, i.e., the thigh, in the form of suction blister and then transferred to the dermabraded vitiliginous area (white patches). In SBG, cleavage occurs between the basal cells and the basal lamina of the basement membrane zone, and only the epidermal portion of the donor area is grafted [2]. Hence, the graft generally acquires the characteristics of the recipient site, thus leading to a better color match and cosmetic outcome [2].

TECHNIQUE

HARVESTING OF THE GRAFT SITE
The donor site can be anywhere from the flexor aspect of the arm or forearm, abdomen, or the anterolateral aspect of the thigh or leg (Figures 37.3.1–37.3.7). In a study by Laxmisha and Thappa, it was found that there was 100% success in raising blisters on the flexor aspect of the arm, and complete blisters were most often raised on the leg or flexor aspect of the forearm, although the number of patients was small [3]. However, covered sites such as the gluteal region or the thigh are preferred, as pigmentary changes can occur at the donor site.

PREPARATION OF THE DONOR SITE
After surgical cleansing, a topical local anesthetic may be applied, as the procedure is painful. Some prefer injecting the area with local anesthetic with saline as it reduces blister induction time.

RAISING OF BLISTERS
Blisters can be developed by using syringes or suction pump and suction cups, a modified conventional gastric or respiratory suction pump, or a negative-pressure cutaneous suction chamber

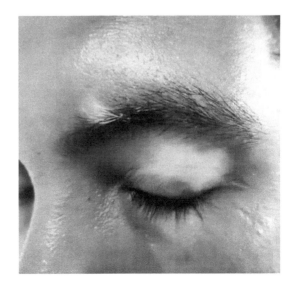

Figure 37.3.1 Stable vitiligo on left upper eyelid of a 20-year-old male. (Photograph courtesy: Dr. Vineet Relhan.)

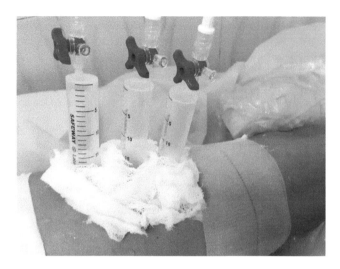

Figure 37.3.2   Bases of 20 mL syringes applied on the thigh and 30 mL air aspirated with the help of three-way canula to create negative pressure in the lumina of syringes. (Photograph courtesy: Dr. Vineet Relhan.)

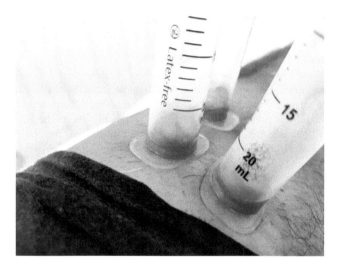

Figure 37.3.3   Formation of small blisters seen after approximately 2 hours of syringe placement. (Photograph courtesy: Dr. Vineet Relhan.)

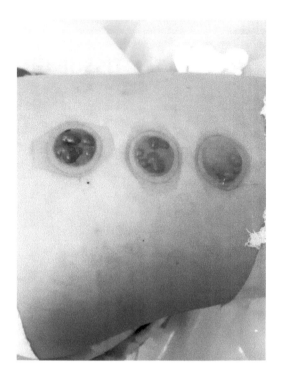

Figure 37.3.4   Multiple small hemorrhagic blisters seen after removal of syringes. (Photograph courtesy: Dr. Vineet Relhan.)

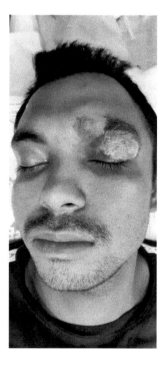

Figure 37.3.5   Recipient site is dermabraded after local anesthesia until pinpoint bleeding points are seen, and graft is placed in such a manner that the dermal side of the graft comes in contact with the dermabraded area. (Photograph courtesy: Dr. Vineet Relhan.)

system [4–7]. In India, syringes are most commonly used to create blisters. Vaseline is applied at the donor site and bases of 10 mL or 20 mL syringes are placed. Approximately 30−35 mL of air is aspirated using a 50-mL syringe with the help of a three-way-cannula to create negative pressure in the lumina of syringes. Larger syringes (>20 mL) take a longer time to create a blister, and smaller syringes (<10 mL) produce smaller blisters. It usually takes approximately 2 hours for the development of blisters. A single unilocular non-hemorrhagic blister is the desirable result. In the case of smaller blisters, one can inject saline or distilled water into lumen of the blister to expand it. Gupta et al. concluded that use of 10- or 20-mL syringes as suction cups and 300 mmHg pressure are appropriate choices for suction blister induction and produce blisters in about 1–2 hours [8]. Various modifications have been made in the conventional technique to accelerate the process of blister formation. Arora et al. used a hair dryer to increase the surface temperature of the skin to 44°C and found mean time taken for the formation of blister on the right thigh was significantly decreased to 69.6 ± 5.4 min compared to that conventional method which took 121.1 ± 6.2 min for blister formation [9]. Similarly, Woods lamp, ultraviolet radiation, and infrared lamp have been used for faster induction of suction blister formation [10].

FACTORS AFFECTING THE PROCEDURE

DIAMETER OF THE SUCTION CUP

Suction blister induction time is directly proportional to the diameter of the suction syringe. Large syringes (50 mL) take more time,

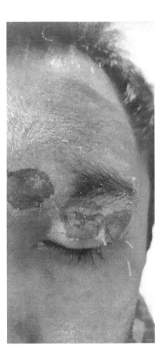

Figure 37.3.6 Follow-up after 5 days showing graft in situ expected to fall off anytime between 1 and 2 weeks. (Photograph courtesy: Dr. Vineet Relhan.)

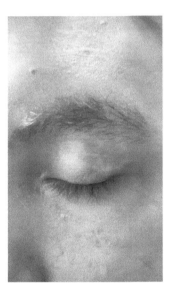

Figure 37.3.7 Follow-up after 6 months showing significant repigmentation at site of suction blister grafting. (Photograph courtesy: Dr. Vineet Relhan.)

but the large roof of the blister can be used for grafting of a single patch of 3.5–4 cm in size. Very small blisters (induced by 5-mL or 2-mL syringes) are difficult to handle but are useful in experiments and in grafting of smaller geographic extensions of achromic areas into the pigmented skin [8].

SITE OF SUCTION BLISTERING

Various body sites have seen used including the inner aspect of the thigh, inner portion of the arm, the abdomen, buttocks, and the extensor surface of the thigh. More rapid induction of blisters in the skin occurs over a hard or firm base, like the bony prominences [8]. The skin overlying the shin is a good site for rapid induction of suction blisters, because in addition to the close proximity to the bone, its distensibility and elasticity are also lower.

AGE OF THE SUBJECT

The dermo-epidermal junction (DEJ) weakens as a person grows older. There is a progressive decrease in vertical resistance at the DEJ. This results in easier and faster separation of the DEJ by means of suction in older individuals.

TEMPERATURE

Suction area temperature in the range of 40–50°C facilitates suction blister formation [8]. Various methods like a small light bulb inside the suction cup and a hair dryer have been used to increase suction area temperature [8,9,11].

PRETREATMENT WITH TOPICAL PUVA

Donor site pretreatment with topical psoralen plus ultraviolet A (PUVA) for about 2 weeks has been found to decrease the extensibility of skin by causing photosclerosis and making the base firm, thereby reducing suction blister induced trauma (SBIT) . Furthermore, topical PUVA also stimulates melanogenesis in the donor epidermis and helps to achieve better pigmentation at recipient site [8,12].

NEGATIVE PRESSURE

Various investigators have used a negative pressure ranging from −200 to −500 mmHg [8,12–14]. High negative pressure can lead to hemorrhagic blister formation.

INTRADERMAL INJECTION OF SALINE

The normal saline injected in the suction area leads to intradermal edema, which hastens the accumulation of fluid at the DEJ, subsequently reducing SBIT.

DEROOFING THE BLISTER

After blister formation, the roofs of the blisters are gently cut at the margins using iris scissors. The roof is inverted onto a glass slide such that the epidermal surface touches the glass slide while the dermal side faces upward. The graft is then cleaned, and dermal attachments are removed. It is spread to its maximum size and kept moist with normal saline. The donor site is cleaned and bandaged using nonadherent dressing such as paraffin chlorhexidine gauze (Bactigras®) followed by cotton pad dressing, which is further fixed with surgical adhesive tape (Micropore).

RECIPIENT SITE PREPARATION

The epidermis should be separated from the underlying dermis at approximately the DEJ, which can be recognized by pinpoint bleed. The recipient vitiligo lesion is surgically cleaned using spirit and povidone iodine and then anesthetized using injection lignocaine 2%. Alternatively, eutectic mixture of lignocaine and prilocaine under occlusion can be used to anesthetize the recipient area. The area is dermabraded using a manual dermabrader, motorized dermabrader, CO_2 laser, or an erbium laser until minute pinpoint bleeding spots are visible.

Brief details of the techniques used for recipient site preparation are as follows.

LIQUID NITROGEN

Liquid nitrogen freezing or suction blistering have also been used for the preparation of the recipient site [15–17]. Maleki et al., in two separate studies, developed blister formation by the application of liquid nitrogen via a cotton swab applicator for 15–20 seconds, two cycles with a 20-second thawing interval [17,18]. Similarly, Hann et al. produced blister formation at recipient sites within 24 hours after three to six freeze-thaw cycles with liquid nitrogen exposure times of 3–5 seconds per cycle [19]. In all three studies, grafting onto recipient sites was performed with suction blisters obtained from donor sites. There was good response in most of the patients in all three studies [17–20]. Various complications, i.e., peripheral hypopigmentation, hyperpigmentation, and hypertrophic scarring, can be seen on the recipient site [19,20].

SUCTION BLISTERS

The suction blister technique is not commonly used in India for recipient site preparation. This preparation method uses a negative pressure apparatus, such as a syringe, to generate a pressure of −200 to −500 mmHg and induce epidermal blister formation [20]. When compared to recipient-site preparation with CO_2 laser, suction blisters appear to yield a more favorable microenvironment for subsequent melanocyte grafting [15]. A hypothesis has been put forth that a more favorable microenvironment develops due to adequate serous drainage in areas prepared by suction blisters, whereas areas prepared by the CO_2 laser lead to an unfavorable, dry, and devitalized surface [21].

An important shortcoming of this method is a yield of only limited amounts of recipient skin, making suction blisters an inferior method of preparation for large vitiliginous lesions, as compared to other methods.

DERMABRASION

Recipient-site preparation with dermabrasion utilizes a manual dermabrader or rapidly rotating abrasive tools (diamond fraise, wire brush, or serrated wheel) to remove the epidermis and superficial dermis [20]. A diamond fraise generally creates a more uniform abrasion, which has been documented upon histologic examinations [20]. Silpa-Archa et al., in their study, found better results with dermabrasion compared to CO_2 laser for recipient site preparation [22]. A high-speed dermabrader is fitted with a diamond fraise steel wheel, set to 10,000 rpm, and applied to the vitiligo lesions, which are abraded until pinpoint bleeding is achieved [2,20,23].

There are many advantages of dermabrasion compared to recipient site preparation techniques. Compared to excisional procedures like split or full thickness grafting, scarring is a rare occurrence with dermabrasion. It is a relatively quicker method. Various studies have compared laser ablation to dermabrasion and have found similar to lower efficacy [20,22]. An important shortcoming of this technique is difficulty in performing this procedure on concave surfaces such as periorbital lesions and soft tissues such as genitalia [15].

PSORALEN AND ULTRAVIOLET A

The use of psoralen and ultraviolet A (PUVA) to de-epithelialize vitiliginous recipient sites are achieved through the induction of a phototoxic blister. This method is useful when a large recipient area is prepared, as the use of suction blisters, liquid nitrogen, or dermabrasion may be impractical. A few authors have raised concerns of carcinogenesis in Type 1 and 2 skin types [20].

CARBON DIOXIDE LASER

The carbon dioxide (CO_2) laser leads to rapid vaporization of the epidermis with easy depth control. Depth control is essentially required where skin is thin, delicate, and irregularly shaped, such as the mouth, eyes, and nose, where precise de-epithelialization is necessity [20]. Furthermore, short-pulsed CO_2 laser and UltraPulse CO_2 laser equipped with a computerized pattern generator allow more precise tissue ablation [24,25].

ERBIUM-DOPED YTTRIUM ALUMINUM GARNET LASER

The erbium-doped yttrium aluminum garnet (Er:YAG) laser works on the same principles as the CO_2 laser, with target chromophore as water, but compared to the CO_2 laser, its penetration is less and it leads to vaporization of the superficial layers of the epidermis. With the help of this laser, large recipient areas can be prepared within minutes with minimal injury to the papillary dermis. Many authors have used this laser without anesthesia.

TRANSFER OF GRAFT

The graft is placed in such a manner that the dermal side of the graft comes in contact with the dermabraded area. A nonadherent paraffin gauze dressing is placed over the graft followed by cotton gauze, and then it is bandaged using Tegaderm® or Dynaplast®. Recently, a few authors have used fibrin glue to secure the graft [26].

POSTOPERATIVE CARE

The dressing over the recipient site is kept in place for 7 days. To keep the graft secured, the patient is advised to keep the grafted area immobile. The dressing over the donor site is removed after 24 hours and area is kept clean and dry. Usually, the grafts fall off in 1 to 2 weeks, so essentially this is a technique of melanocyte transfer.

FOLLOW-UP

The patient can be started on oral or topical psoralen-UVA or PUVAsol from the day of removal of dressing. Uncommonly, leukotrichia also improves.

COMPLICATIONS

Complications such as hyperpigmentation, incomplete pigmentation, variegated discoloration, perigraft halo, infection, scarring/keloid formation, and graft rejection have been reported [27,28].

EFFICACY

A meta-analysis found efficacy of SBG similar to split-thickness grafting (87% of the patients achieved more than 75% repigmentation), but better than minigrafting (68%) and grafting of noncultured epidermal suspensions (31%) [29]. Gupta et al., in a retrospective study, assessed the efficacy of SBG and found generalized vitiligo has inferior response compared to segmental and focal vitiligo (53% vs 91% achieving >75% repigmentation, $P < 0.001$) [29]. There was no significant difference in repigmentation rates at different body sites [30]. Li et al., in their retrospective study on 1100 patients, found complete repigmentation in 227 patients (20.6%) and excellent repigmentation (>50%) in 568 (51.6%). No superficial scarring was observed at the grafted or donor sites, and no serious complications were encountered in this study [31].

ADVANTAGES

Epidermal grafts have many advantages over other conventional methods. It is a simple, easy to do, and inexpensive, with very good success rates. Multiple small grafts of 2–3 cm may be harvested simultaneously using several syringes. Graft uptake is rapid and complete in most instances. Repigmentation is faster and the color match is very good, especially over the lips, eyelids, and areolae [32,33]. Various complications such as scar/keloid formation, cobblestoning, sinking pits, thick margins, and milia formation are much fewer compared to punch grafting or split-thickness grafting [29].

DISADVANTAGES

SBG is not a good modality when larger areas need to be treated. Furthermore, it takes approximately 2 hours to create blisters, and the raising of blisters is painful. Rarely, placing epidermal side of graft to recipient area leads to failure of uptake of the graft.

REFERENCES

1. Majid I. Grafting in vitiligo: How to get better results and how to avoid complications. *J Cutan Aesthetic Surg* 2013 Apr;6(2):83–9.
2. Khunger N, Kathuria SD, and Ramesh V. Tissue grafts in vitiligo surgery - past, present, and future. *Indian J Dermatol* 2009 Apr 1;54(2):150.

3. Laxmisha C, and Thappa DM. Reliable site for suction blister induction and harvesting. *Indian J Dermatol Venereol Leprol* 2005 Oct;71(5):321–4.

4. Gupta S, Shroff S, and Gupta S. Modified technique of suction blistering for epidermal grafting in vitiligo. *Int J Dermatol* 1999 Apr;38(4):306–9.

5. Burm JS. Simple suction device for autologous epidermal grafting. *Plast Reconstr Surg* 2000 Oct;106(5):1225–6.

6. Alexis AF, Wilson DC, Todhunter JA, and Stiller MJ. Reassessment of the suction blister model of wound healing: Introduction of a new higher pressure device. *Int J Dermatol* 1999 Aug;38(8):613–7.

7. Rusfianti M, and Wirohadidjodjo YW. Dermatosurgical techniques for repigmentation of vitiligo. *Int J Dermatol* 2006 Apr;45(4):411–7.

8. Gupta S, and Kumar B. Suction blister induction time: 15 minutes or 150 minutes? *Dermatol Surg* 2000 Aug;26(8):754–6.

9. Arora S, and Kar BR. Reduction of blister formation time in suction blister epidermal grafting in vitiligo patients using a household hair dryer. *J Cutan Aesthetic Surg* 2016;9(4):232–5.

10. Kaliyadan F, Venkitakrishnan S, and Manoj J. Use of a Wood's lamp as an ultraviolet light source to improve the speed and quality of suction blister harvesting. *Indian J Dermatol Venereol Leprol* 2010 Aug;76(4):429–31.

11. Skouge JW, Morison WL, Diwan RV, and Rotter S. Autografting and PUVA. A combination therapy for vitiligo. *J Dermatol Surg Oncol* 1992 May;18(5):357–60.

12. Suga Y, Butt KI, Takimoto R, Fujioka N, Yamada H, and Ogawa H. Successful treatment of vitiligo with PUVA-pigmented autologous epidermal grafting. *Int J Dermatol* 1996 Jul;35(7):518–22.

13. Koga M. Epidermal grafting using the tops of suction blisters in the treatment of vitiligo. *Arch Dermatol* 1988 Nov;124(11):1656–8.

14. Yang JS, and Kye YC. Treatment of vitiligo with autologous epidermal grafting by means of pulsed erbium:YAG laser. *J Am Acad Dermatol* 1998 Feb;38(2 Pt 1):280–2.

15. Lee D-Y, Park J-H, Choi S-C, and Lee J-H. Comparison of recipient site preparations in epidermal grafting for vitiligo: Suction blister and CO2 laser. *J Eur Acad Dermatol Venereol* 2009 Dec;23(12):1448–9.

16. Pagliarello C, Calogero P, Paradisi A, and Andrea P. An effective way to perform suction-blister grafts: Using an insulin syringe as a sardine tin key. *Dermatol Surg* 2011 Apr;37(4):549–53.

17. Maleki M, Banihashemi M, and Sanjari V. Efficacy of suction blister epidermal graft without phototherapy for locally stable and resistant vitiligo. *Indian J Dermatol* 2012 Jul;57(4):282–4.

18. Masoud M, Javidi Z, Ebrahami-rad M, and Hamidi H. Treatment of vitiligo with blister grafting technique. *Iran J Dermatol* 2008 Jan 1;11(244):55–9.

19. Hann SK, Im S, Bong HW, and Park YK. Treatment of stable vitiligo with autologous epidermal grafting and PUVA. *J Am Acad Dermatol* 1995 Jun;32(6):943–8.

20. Al-Hadidi N, Griffith JL, Al-Jamal MS, and Hamzavi I. Role of recipient-site preparation techniques and post-operative wound dressing in the surgical management of vitiligo. *J Cutan Aesthetic Surg* 2015 Jun;8(2):79–87.

21. Kahn AM, Ostad A, and Moy RL. Grafting following short-pulse carbon dioxide laser de-epithelialization. *Dermatol Surg* 1996 Nov;22(11):965–7; discussion 967-968.

22. Silpa-Archa N, Griffith JL, Williams MS, Lim HW, and Hamzavi IH. Prospective comparison of recipient-site preparation with fractional carbon dioxide laser vs. dermabrasion and recipient-site dressing composition in melanocyte-keratinocyte transplantation procedure in vitiligo: A preliminary study. *Br J Dermatol* 2016 Apr;174(4):895–7.

23. Fioramonti P, Onesti MG, Marchese C, Carella S, Ceccarelli S, and Scuderi N. Autologous cultured melanocytes in vitiligo treatment comparison of two techniques to prepare the recipient site: Erbium-doped yttrium aluminum garnet laser versus dermabrasion. *Dermatol Surg* 2012 May;38(5):809–12.

24. Hasegawa T, Suga Y, Ikejima A et al. Suction blister grafting with CO(2) laser resurfacing of the graft recipient site for vitiligo. *J Dermatol* 2007 Jul;34(7):490–2.

25. Oh CK, Cha JH, Lim JY et al. Treatment of vitiligo with suction epidermal grafting by the use of an ultrapulse CO2 laser with a computerized pattern generator. *Dermatol Surg* 2001 Jun;27(6):565–8.

26. Kim H, Kang J-N, Hwang S-H, Seo J-K, and Sung H-S. Fibrin glue fixation for suction blister epidermal grafting in two patients with stable vitiligo. *Ann Dermatol* 2014 Dec;26(6):751–4.

27. Gupta S, Jain VK, and Saraswat PK. Suction blister epidermal grafting versus punch skin grafting in recalcitrant and stable vitiligo. *Dermatol Surg* 1999 Dec;25(12):955–8.

28. Babu A, Thappa DM, and Jaisankar TJ. Punch grafting versus suction blister epidermal grafting in the treatment of stable lip vitiligo. *Dermatol Surg* 2008 Feb;34(2):166–78; discussion 178.

29. Njoo MD, Westerhof W, Bos JD, and Bossuyt PM. A systematic review of autologous transplantation methods in vitiligo. *Arch Dermatol* 1998 Dec;134(12):1543–9.

30. Gupta S, and Kumar B. Epidermal grafting in vitiligo: Influence of age, site of lesion, and type of disease on outcome. *J Am Acad Dermatol* 2003 Jul;49(1):99–104.

31. Li J, Fu W-W, Zheng Z-Z, Zhang Q-Q, Xu Y, and Fang L. Suction blister epidermal grafting using a modified suction method in the treatment of stable vitiligo: A retrospective study. *Dermatol Surg* 2011 Jul;37(7):999–1006.

32. Gupta S, Sandhu K, Kanwar A, and Kumar B. Melanocyte transfer via epidermal grafts for vitiligo of labial mucosa. *Dermatol Surg* 2004 Jan;30(1):45–8.

33. Nanda S, Relhan V, Grover C, and Reddy BSN. Suction blister epidermal grafting for management of eyelid vitiligo: Special considerations. *Dermatol Surg* 2006 Mar;32(3):387–91; discussion 391–392.

TISSUE GRAFTING TECHNIQUES
The Epidermal Harvesting System (CelluTOME™) for Stable Vitiligo Surgery

Debdeep Mitra

CONTENTS

INTRODUCTION

Skin grafts have been used to achieve successful repigmentation in vitiligo patients. Traditional types of autografts include full-thickness and split-thickness skin grafts. Some disadvantages of autografts include the need for a surgical procedure with anesthesia, creation of a second wound at the donor site, difficulty in obtaining uniform graft thickness, pain, and challenges with graft take and graft rejection. Allografts and xenografts address some of these disadvantages. However, chances of graft rejection are greater with allografts and xenografts than autografts. Some of these treatment modalities are painful procedures, require long recovery times for the donor site, and may increase operating room costs and potential donor site complications, such as infection. The rates of donor site complications vary, depending on donor site location, comorbidities of the patient, and other risk factors, and can be as high as 28% [1,2].

Epidermal skin grafts offer an alternative to traditional autografts and use only a minimal amount of autologous tissue from the donor site. Epidermal skin grafts differ from full-thickness and split-thickness skin grafts in that they only contain the epidermal layer of the skin (Figure 37.4.1), which is comprised of five layers and four cell types. The cell types of most relevance to epidermal grafting are keratinocytes and melanocytes, which play an important role in re-epithelialization and repigmentation, respectively. The epidermal-melanocyte unit comprises of keratinocytes, melanocytes, and fibroblasts, and each cell plays a key role through intercellular signaling pathways to achieve melanocyte proliferation and sustenance.

Various methods of epidermal skin grafting have been developed and expanded throughout the years since Jacques-Louis Reverdin first used small, full-thickness skin pieces as grafts for wound healing in 1869 [3]. The Reverdin technique (i.e., epidermic grafting) consisted of removing the epidermis with a needle point and transplanting it to a granulating wound bed to assist with epithelialization [4]. Pinch grafting involves the harvesting of small areas of skin that will be used over a wound, enabling epithelialization from the wound edge to the graft. Patch/postage stamp grafts allow for more uniform skin islands to be created and involve removing donor pieces of skin and placing them (dermis side up) on sheets of sticky paper. The paper is then cut into strips, placed on another piece of paper, and then cut horizontally into small squares. In 1958, C. Parker Meeks introduced the dermatome, which creates skin pieces from small donor skin areas. A thin, standard split-thickness skin graft is placed dermal side down on a cork carrier, which is then placed on the cutting block of the microdermatome. Both the carrier and graft are passed

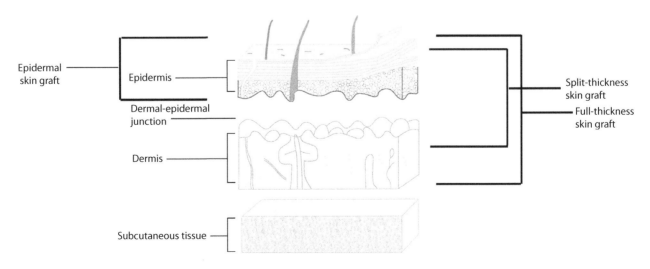

Figure 37.4.1 Schematic of skin layers showing skin graft thickness.

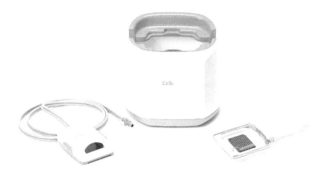

Figure 37.4.2   CelluTOME Epidermal Harvesting System.

Table 37.4.1   Benefits of epidermal skin grafting

1. Minimally invasive procedure
2. Autologous grafts
3. Keratinocytes are sufficient for graft acceptance
4. Provides consistent microdome spacing and proper graft orientation
5. Optimizes cosmesis of the donor site
6. Can be performed in the office/outpatient setting
7. Does not require anesthesia at the donor site
8. Minimal patient discomfort with procedure
9. Minimal scarring at donor site
10. Operation technique and postoperative care are simplified and convenient
11. Less expensive/cost-effective alternative to skin substitutes

through the dermatome. The carrier is then moved 90 degrees and passed through again to create the micrografts. Several studies have demonstrated successful use of epidermal skin grafting using suction blisters in pigmentation disorders, such as both non-dermatomal and segmental vitiligo [3,5–8] as well as for lesions of chronic discoid lupus erythematosus [9,10]. When treating pigmentation disorders using epidermal skin grafting, the recipient site is dermabraded mechanically (e.g., sandpaper) or chemically (e.g., lasers and liquid nitrogen) in order to remove the existing hypopigmented epidermis. This creates a superficial wound that is then covered with autologous transplanted epidermal skin grafts.

In addition, the previous harvesting methods were often tedious and time consuming. This has led to the development of a suction blister harvesting system that simplifies the harvesting process: the CelluTOME™ Epidermal Harvesting System (Figure 37.4.2). This is a minimally invasive tool for harvesting epidermal micrografts and is designed for use in the outpatient setting. This system combines suction and warmth and produces consistent thin sections of epidermal skin. The technology of the device involves splitting the dermal-epidermal junction to form microdomes (i.e., blisters), which are harvested into epidermal micrografts. These micrografts consist of undamaged epithelium with keratinocytes and melanocytes. The benefits of epidermal skin grafting using suction microdomes are listed in Table 37.4.1 [11–16].

CelluTOME EPIDERMAL HARVESTING SYSTEM

The CelluTOME Epidermal Harvesting System consists of a control unit, vacuum head, and a harvester. The system produces autologous epidermal microdomes for use as skin grafts. A 3M Tegaderm™ film is currently used to transfer the microdomes onto the recipient site. Table 37.4.2 describes the components of the CelluTOME Epidermal Harvesting System.

Table 37.4.2   CelluTOME Epidermal Harvesting System components

Name/Description	Picture
Control unit A reusable component of the system. Creates and regulates the suction (negative pressure: −400 to −500 mmHg) and warming (37°C–41°C) required to raise the epidermal microdomes.	
Vacuum head A reusable component of the system. Delivers the negative pressure and warming from the control unit to the harvester.	
Harvester A disposable component of the system. Provides the structure for formation of the microdomes. After insertion of the 3M Tegaderm film, microdomes are harvested into micrografts. The 3M Tegaderm film is used to both capture the microdomes prior to cutting and transfer the micrografts to the recipient site. In addition, it aids in maintaining proper graft orientation. A Tegaderm film is also placed on the donor site after harvesting of micrografts.	

TECHNOLOGY FOR THE CelluTOME EPIDERMAL HARVESTING SYSTEM

The development of the suction microdomes and the harvesting of the epidermal micrografts are automated, eliminating the need for physician handling of the grafts and resulting in proper graft orientation and simplified application. The film dressing is used to transfer the epidermal micrografts to the recipient site from the donor site (Figure 37.4.3). The microdomes form gradually over approximately 30–40 minutes. Visual observation is used to determine optimal harvesting time (Figure 37.4.4).

The placement of the harvester on the anterior aspect of the thigh is shown in Figure 37.4.5, and the illuminated microdome formation is shown in Figure 37.4.6.

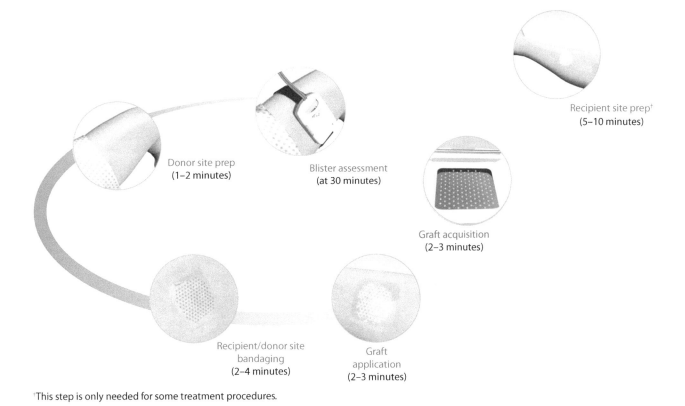

Donor site prep
(1–2 minutes)

Blister assessment
(at 30 minutes)

Recipient site prep†
(5–10 minutes)

Graft acquisition
(2–3 minutes)

Recipient/donor site
bandaging
(2–4 minutes)

Graft
application
(2–3 minutes)

†This step is only needed for some treatment procedures.

Figure 37.4.3 Harvesting procedure.

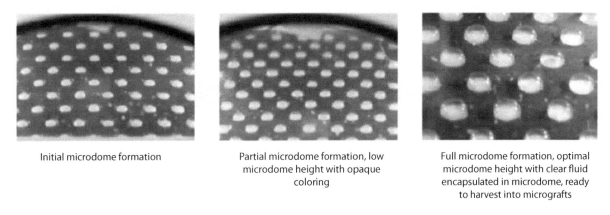

Initial microdome formation

Partial microdome formation, low
microdome height with opaque
coloring

Full microdome formation, optimal
microdome height with clear fluid
encapsulated in microdome, ready
to harvest into micrografts

Figure 37.4.4 Microdome formation.

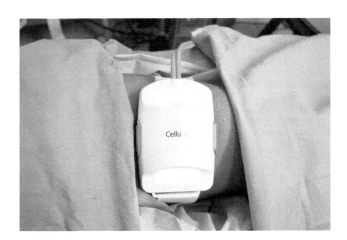

Figure 37.4.5 Epidermal harvester placed on anterior thigh.

DONOR SITE HEALING

Donor site healing after microblister harvesting was assessed using a Skin Appearance Scale and Dermal Response Score. After micrograft harvesting and through the follow-up visits, donor site skin appearance in comparison with its surrounding skin was summarized using percentages, and digital photographs were collected as shown in Figure 37.4.7. Pain during and after microblister harvesting was assessed using the Wong-Baker FACES Pain Rating Scale. The pain score was recorded as 0, No Hurt; 1, Hurts a Little Bit; 2, Hurts a Little More; 3, Hurts Even More; 4, Hurts a Whole Lot; and 5, Hurts Worst. Skin assessment results showed that the donor sites appeared to heal with minimal irritation during the follow-up period and showed that 76%–100% of donor sites were the same in appearance to the surrounding skin by 14 days after epidermal harvest (Figure 37.4.7). The pain results showed minimal discomfort from the subjects during microblister formation and the harvesting process, suggesting that no anesthesia is required at the donor

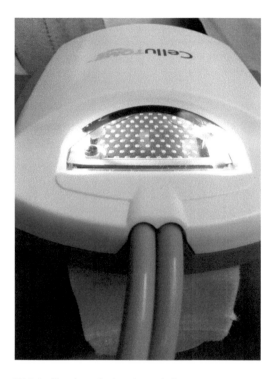

Figure 37.4.6   Illuminated microdome device.

site. The mean pain score was 1.3 (scale of 1–5) throughout the harvesting process.

CONCLUSION

The CelluTOME Epidermal Harvesting System is an automated and claimed to be precise, simplified, convenient, reproducible process of harvesting autologous and non-damaged epidermal tissue. The epidermal harvesting system is a minimally invasive tool for harvesting epidermal micrografts. The system combines suction and warmth and produces consistent thin sections of epidermal skin. The technology of the device involves splitting the dermal-epidermal junction to form microdomes (2-mm-wide blisters), which are harvested

into epidermal micrografts. These micrografts consist of undamaged epithelium with keratinocytes. This minimize donors site complications by harvesting epidermis at the dermal-epidermal junction. It allows skin harvesting without the need for donor site anesthesia.

Its advantages are that it is a minimally invasive, simplified, convenient, cost-effective, and office/outpatient-based procedure. It shows optimum cosmesis and minimal scarring without any anesthesia at the donor site.

REFERENCES

1. Kim PD, Fleck T, Heffelfinger R, and Blackwell KE. Avoiding secondary skin graft donor site morbidity in the fibula free flap harvest. *Arch Otolaryngol Head Neck Surg* 2008 December;134(12):1324–7.

2. Shindo M, Fong BP, Funk GF, and Karnell LH. The fibula osteocutaneous flap in head and neck reconstruction: A critical evaluation of donor site morbidity. *Arch Otolaryngol Head Neck Surg* 2000 December 1;126(12):1467–72.

3. Tang WY, Chan LY, and Lo KK. Treatment of vitiligo with autologous epidermal transplantation using the roofs of suction blisters. *Hong Kong Med J* 1998 June 1;4(2):219–24.

4. Biswas A, Bharara M, Hurst C, Armstrong DG, and Rilo H. The micrograft concept for wound healing: Strategies and applications. *J Diabetes Sci Technol* 2010 July 1;4(4):808–19.

5. Koga M. Epidermal grafting using the tops of suction blisters in the treatment of vitiligo. *Arch Dermatol* 1988 November 1;124(11):1656–8.

6. Gupta S, Jain VK, Saraswat PK, and Gupta S. Suction blister epidermal grafting versus punch skin grafting in recalcitrant and stable vitiligo. *Dermatol Surg* 1999 December 1;25(12):955–8.

7. Njoo MD, Westerhof W, Bos JD, and Bossuyt PM. A systematic review of autologous transplantation methods in vitiligo. *Arch Dermatol* 1998 December 1;134(12):1543–9.

8. Budania A, Parsad D, Kanwar AJ, and Dogra S. Comparison between autologous noncultured epidermal cell

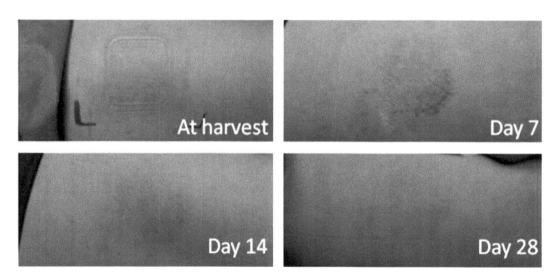

Figure 37.4.7   Donor site healing.

suspension and suction blister epidermal grafting in stable vitiligo: A randomized study. *Br J Dermatol* 2012 December 1;167(6):1295–301.

9. Gupta S. Epidermal grafting for depigmentation due to discoid lupus erythematosus. *Dermatology* 2001 January 1;202(4):320–3.

10. Yamaguchi Y, Yoshida S, Sumikawa Y et al. Rapid healing of intractable diabetic foot ulcers with exposed bones following a novel therapy of exposing bone marrow cells and then grafting epidermal sheets. *Br J Dermatol* 2004 November 1;151(5):1019– 28.

11. Yamaguchi Y, Sumikawa Y, Yoshida S, Kubo T, Yoshikawa K, and Itami S. Prevention of amputation caused by rheumatic diseases following a novel therapy of exposing bone marrow, occlusive dressing and subsequent epidermal grafting. *Br J Dermatol* 2005 April 1;152(4):664–72.

12. Ichiki Y, and Kitajima Y. Successful treatment of scleroderma-related cutaneous ulcer with suction blister grafting. *Rheumatol Int* 2008 January 1;28(3):299–301.

13. Hanafusa T, Yamaguchi Y, and Katayama I. Intractable wounds caused by arteriosclerosis obliterans with end-stage renal disease treated by aggressive debridement and epidermal grafting. *J Am Acad Dermatol* 2007 August 1;57(2):322–6.

14. Burm JS, Rhee SC, and Kim YW. Superficial dermabrasion and suction blister epidermal grafting for postburn dyspigmentation in Asian skin. *Dermatol Surg* 2007 March 1;33(3):326–32.

15. Costanzo U, Streit M, and Braathen LR. Autologous suction blister grafting for chronic leg ulcers. *J Eur Acad Dermatol Venereol* 2008 January 1;22(1):7–10.

16. Rusfianti M, and Wirohadidjodjo YW. Dermatosurgical techniques for repigmentation of vitiligo. *Int J Dermatol* 2006 April 1;45(4):411–7.

TISSUE GRAFTING TECHNIQUES
Flip-Top Transplantation Technique and Smash Grafting

Vineet Relhan and Sudhanshu Sharma

CONTENTS

INTRODUCTION

Vitiligo can be treated by both medical and surgical methods. The following surgical methods are commonly used for vitiligo:

- *Tissue grafts*: Includes thin and ultrathin split-thickness skin grafts (STSG), suction blister epidermal grafts (SBEG), mini-punch grafts (MPG), hair follicular grafts (HFG), flip-top transplants, and mesh grafts.
- *Cellular grafts*: Includes noncultured epidermal cell suspension (NCES), cultured pure melanocytes (CM), and cultured epithelial grafts (CE) [1–6].

FLIP-TOP TRANSPLANTATION TECHNIQUE

There is always a need for newer and more innovative techniques to treat vitiligo. McGovern et al. [7] devised a new technique, called the flip-top transplantation (FTT) technique, for the treatment of vitiligo. This procedure has distinct advantages as can be performed with speed and ease, with minimal clinical scarring. It does not require special equipment or a laboratory to culture melanocytes, so it has the added advantage of low cost.

In FTT, a normally pigmented donor site is marked in the inner aspect of the thigh or the retroauricular region. A 10- to 15-mm skin graft containing epidermis with minimal underlying dermis is obtained by a razor blade after injecting 1% lidocaine into the donor site (Figure 37.5.1). In the flip-top method, grafts consist of very thin dermo-epidermal slices bearing epidermis and minimal dermis, which makes a great deal of difference in terms of side effects when compared with large 4-mm "punch grafts" with 2- to 4-mm thickness. The graft is placed on gauze soaked with isotonic sodium chloride solution and divided into small pieces of 3–5 mm. At the recipient sites, one to five sites at 5- to 10-mm intervals are chosen. A flap of 6–8 mm containing epidermis with minimal papillary dermis is raised at the recipient site. The pieces of the graft from the donor site are placed juxtapositioning the dermis of the graft to the dermis of the recipient site (Figure 37.5.1). Both sites are dressed with Sofra-Tulle, and the patients are advised to keep it clean and not to wet the dressing.

The dressing is removed after 1 week and patients are assessed to see if the grafts have taken at the recipient site. The patients are further assessed by using clinical photography, mapping of the treated areas, and patient and physician's visual analog scale at weekly intervals for 1 month and then monthly intervals for the next 6 months. Repigmentation is graded as excellent with 91%–100% repigmentation of the treated area; very good, 76%–90%; good, 51%–75%; fair, 31%–50%; poor, <30% and no repigmentation.

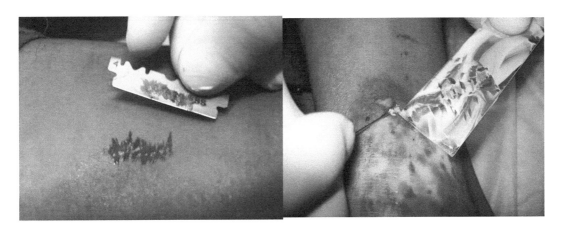

Figure 37.5.1   Separation of graft from the donor site with the help of razor blade and placement of the graft with elevated flap at recipient site in FTT procedure.

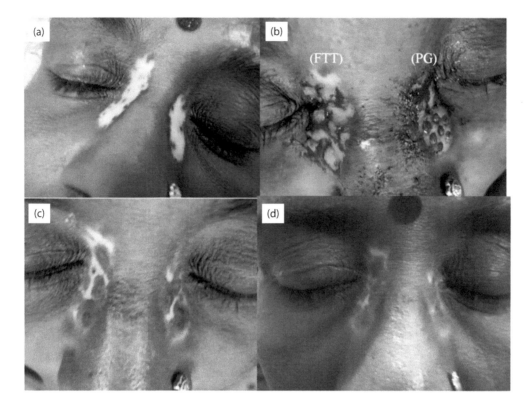

Figure 37.5.2 (a) Preoperative photograph. (b) Postoperative photograph. (c) After 1 month, perifollicular pigmentation is seen over graft sites. (d) After 6 months, diffuse pigmentation is seen over graft sites.

There are two studies available in the literature regarding FTT. The FTT procedure was first studied by McGovern et al. in 1999 [7]. Four patients with stable vitiligo and one patient with posttraumatic leukoderma were taken in the study. Repigmentation was noted in 22 (88%) of 25 grafts in the first three patients, and the grafts in patient four were not taken up [7].

In 2013, we conducted a study in MAMC and Lok Nayak Hospital, New Delhi, comparing FTT and minipunch grafting on 20 patients and concluded that FTT was equally effective to punch grafting (PG) for treating stable vitiligo. In the FTT group, the results were excellent in 13 (65%), very good in 3 (15%), good in 2 (10%), and fair in 2 (10%) (Figures 37.5.2 and 37.5.3). Graft uptake rate was higher;

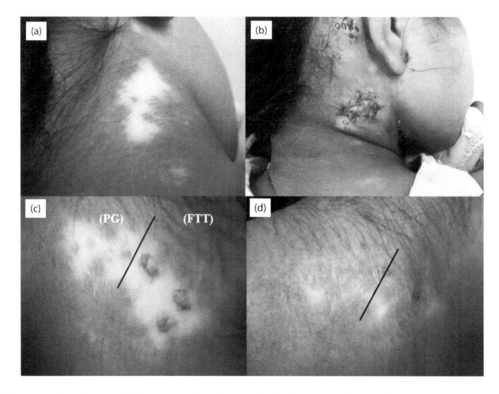

Figure 37.5.3 (a) Preoperative photograph. (b) Postoperative photograph. (c) After 3 months, mixed pigmentation is seen over graft sites. (d) After 6 months, diffuse pigmentation is seen over flip-top transplantation and punch grafting sites; cobblestoning present over punch grafting sites.

Table 37.5.1 Comparison in between flip-top transplantation and punch grafting

Feature	Punch grafting (PG)	Flip-top transplantation (FTT)
Graft uptake	86%	100%
Onset of pigment spread	15–20 days	20–25 days
Completion of pigment spread	16–20 weeks	20–23 weeks
Maximum pigment spread	3–4.50 mm	5–9.10 mm
Cobblestoning	More common	Less common
Hyperpigmentation	More common	Less common
Variegated appearance	Rare	Common
Cost	Punch = 80–90 INR (1.79111–2.01500 USD)	Razor-blade = 1 INR (0.02239 USD)

there was more pigment spread and cost of the procedure was low as compared to punch graft (Table 37.5.1) [8].

The high graft uptake rate in FTT is due to the flap, which covers the underlying graft and works as a biological dressing and retains the graft in the grafted site. The higher pigment spread in FTT is because of preservation of follicular reservoirs and melanocytes in the depigmented lesion, as we do not discard the skin over the recipient site [1–3]. Cobblestoning is slightly more common in PG compared to FTT, but it is seen in both procedures. A variegated appearance is mainly seen with FTT and usually this does not occur in PG.

The cost of razor blade, the main surgical instrument used in FTT, is 1.0 INR (0.02239 USD) as compared to the 85 times higher cost of punches (80–90 INR; 1.79111–2.01500 USD) used in PG. So FTT is a more economical method as compared to PG (Table 37.5.1).

SMASH GRAFTING TECHNIQUE

Smashed skin grafting, or smash grafting, is a modification of split-thickness grafting. In this procedure, the graft undergoes smashing before being applied to the recipient site. Although it is a simple and effective procedure, but very few people are doing it due to either lack of awareness or lack of published data (Figures 37.5.4 and 37.5.5).

In a study conducted by Kaur et al. on 30 cases, repigmentation was observed from 3 weeks on and continued to increase on subsequent follow-ups. At 12 weeks, 76.66% of patients achieved more than 50% repigmentation. Although the number of study cases was small and the follow-up period was short (only 12 weeks), smash grafting was found to be a simple, easy to learn, and cost-effective one-stage procedure with gratifying results for extensive areas of vitiligo with no surgical complications as compared to other surgical methods [9].

In another study by Krishan et al., smashed skin grafting helped to achieve more than 90% repigmentation of the vitiligo patches in 30 patients [18]. The authors concluded that smashed skin grafting is a

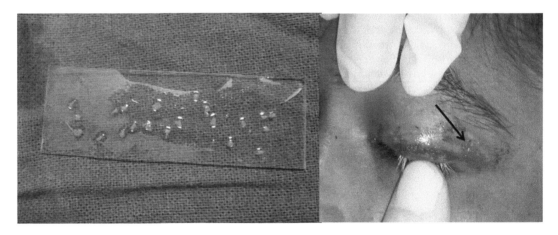

Figure 37.5.4 Smash grafts and graft in situ on recipient site (black arrow).

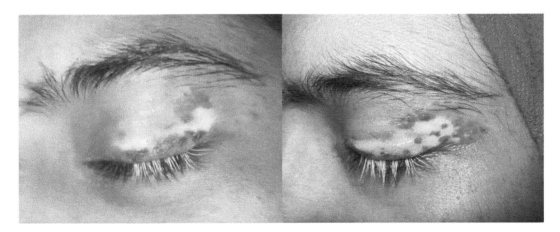

Figure 37.5.5 Pre- and postoperative photograph of smash grafting (after 6 weeks).

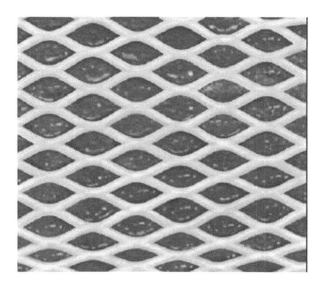

Figure 37.5.6   Mesh graft.

simple procedure with fewer side effects, better outcome, and high patient satisfaction, and can be considered as an alternative to various conventional surgical modalities such as PG and melanocyte cell culture methods [10].

MESH GRAFTING TECHNIQUE

The mesh grafting is a technique where the graft is expanded by making slits in it such that it appears like a mesh (Figure 37.5.6). The advantage of this technique is that it allows coverage of large body surface areas with a smaller graft. The donor site is cleaned and a split-thickness graft of 0.0252-inch thickness is obtained either manually or by using a Padgett or Duval dermatome. The graft is then meshed into any expansion size (1:1, 1:2, 1:4, 1:6). Meshing can also be done manually by making cuts in the graft using a sterile blade. Once the recipient site is cleaned and dermabraded, the graft is transferred and bandaged with saline soaked

dressing or Sofra-Tulle. The donor site is also dressed using aseptic precautions [11].

REFERENCES

1. Hann SK, and Nordlund J. *Vitiligo: Monograph on the Basic and Clinical Science*. Oxford: Blackwell Science; 2000, pp. 49–69.

2. King R, Nordlund J, Boissy R et al. *The Pigmentary System: Physiology and Pathophysiology*. Oxford: Oxford University Press; 1998, pp. 513–40.

3. Hann SK, Chun WH, and Park WH. Clinical characteristics of progressive vitiligo. *Int J Dermatol* 1997;36:353–5.

4. Sehgal VN. Evaluation of 202 cases of vitiligo cutis. *Ind J Dermatol Venereol Leprol* 1974;14:439–45.

5. Sarkar R, Mehta SD, and Kanwar AJ. Repigmentation after autologous miniature punch grafting in segmental vitiligo in North Indian patients. *J Dermatol* 2001;28:540–6.

6. Lahiri K. Evolution and evaluation of autologous mini punch grafting in vitiligo. *Ind J Dermatol Venereol Leprol* 2009;54:159–67.

7. McGovern TW, Bolognia J, and Leffell DJ. Flip-top pigment transplantation a novel transplantation procedure for the treatment of depigmentation. *Arch Dermatol* 1999;135:1305–7.

8. Sharma S, Garg VK, Sarkar R, and Relhan V. Comparative study of flip-top transplantation and punch grafting in stable vitiligo. *Dermatol Surg* 2013;39:1376–84.

9. Kaur M. Smash grafting in stable vitiligo: A case study of 30 cases in a tertiary care hospital in north India. *5th International Conference on Clinical and Experimental Dermatology* July 13–15, 2015, New Orleans, LA.

10. Krishnan A, and Kar S. Smashed skin grafting or smash grafting – a novel method of vitiligo surgery. *Dermatol Surg* 2012;36:1006–20.

11. Khunger N, Kathuria SD, and Ramesh V. Tissue grafts in vitiligo surgery - past, present, and future. *IJD Symposium* 2009; 54(2):150–8.

TISSUE GRAFTING TECHNIQUES
Hair Follicle Transplantation in Vitiligo

Kavish Chauhan

CONTENTS

INTRODUCTION

Vitiligo is an idiopathic acquired dermatosis characterized by circumscribed milky white patches and macules, with a tremendous psychological impact on society [1]. Over the past decades multiple treatment modalities comprising of topical/systemic immunosuppressives, phototherapy, excimer laser, and surgical grafting (split-thickness skin grafting, suction blister, punch grafting, follicular unit, and melanocyte transfer) have been successfully tried [2]. The pathogenesis of vitiligo has led us to understand that the destruction of the melanocytes of the epidermis and hair follicles leads to depigmented patches and leukotrichia, respectively. As we already know that a vitiliginous patch with leukotrichia is considered to have a poor prognosis, this finding suggests that repigmentation of vitiligo is linked to hair follicles, and this in turn is the principle of follicular unit transplantation in vitiligo.

HISTORICAL BACKGROUND

Staricco [3] in 1959 demonstrated two types of pigment cells in the hair follicle: active and inactive DOPA-negative melanocytes in the outer root sheath (ORS) of the normal hair follicle. Ortonne et al. [4] in 1980 proposed that the melanocyte reservoir in the hair follicles leads to repigmentation in vitiliginous patches. Cui et al. [5] in 1991 demonstrated that in vitiligo, there was destruction of only the active (DOPA-positive) melanocytes, whereas the inactive melanocytes in the ORS of the hair follicle were unaffected. These inactive melanocytes move up along regenerated epidermis, leading to perifollicular pigmentation, and downward toward the hair matrices where on maturation they synthesize melanin on activation by ultraviolet light or removal of epidermis following dermabrasion [3,6,7]. In 1992, noncultured melanocyte transfer was introduced by Gauthier and Surleve Bazeille [8]. In 1998, Na et al. [9] popularized the concept of follicular unit transplantation for repigmentation in vitiligo based on the existence of undifferentiated stem cells in the hair follicle.

FUTURE PERSPECTIVES

The epidermal stem cells evolve from the hair follicle melanocyte stem cells [10] and form a reservoir for skin and hair pigmentation [11]. These cells possess the ability to supply the hair matrix with transient amplifying cells and eventually mature into melanocytes producing melanin [11]. This reservoir of inactive melanocyte stem cells is present in the lesional epidermis of patients with vitiligo, even after disease of 25 years duration [12]. This melanocyte reservoir was also found in ORS of the white hair in lesional skin [13]. This concept lead to advancement of vitiligo surgery from epidermal melanocyte noncultured and cultured transfer to direct transfer of extracted follicular units, and finally noncultured extracted follicular ORS.

Follicular unit extraction (FUE) for repigmentation in vitiligo has been reported earlier with appearance of pigmentation between the 2nd and 8th week [14]. FUE circumvents the need for the tedious cultured or noncultured melanocyte suspension process [15]. On average, 15−25 follicular units provide approximately 3,00,000−20,00,000 cells, with a huge number of melanocytes, enough to treat a vitiliginous patch of up to 20 cm^2. There are several advantages of hair transplantation in treatment of vitiligo over other methods. The ORS of the hair follicle provides a larger melanocyte and stem cell reservoir than epidermal cells. The melanocyte to keratinocyte ratio in a follicular unit is 1:5, which is much higher than the epidermal melanin unit (1:36) [16,17]. Furthermore, anagen hair bulb melanocytes are larger, more dendritic, more active, have extensive Golgi and rough endoplasmic reticulum, and produce larger melanosomes [17]. These melanocytes also have an amazing replicative ability and potential for producing a larger quantity of melanin and are immunologically less susceptible to autoimmune destruction due to their protected localization [17]. The hair follicle is an immunologically privileged site not subject to immune surveillance besides follicular melanocytes below the arrector pili muscle, which show reduced expression of class I major histocompatibility molecules. For these reasons follicular melanocytes are more resistant to immune destruction. Although the appearance of pigmentation is delayed as compared to other modalities, the color match is much more acceptable due to stem cell migration from the graft and the specific location that amplifies cell proliferation. If the occiput is the donor area, we can completely avoid the complications of other grafting procedures such as scarring, pigmentation, and cobblestoning. In the case of body hair transplantation, the advantage is that hair does not require frequent trimming as is required with scalp hair. It can also be carried out in the non-glaborous areas of the face, e.g., angle of mouth, eyelash, and beard and moustache areas in males, where other epidermal grafting methods are difficult. Also, the tiny scars of FUE on the scalp are invisible, and as compared to follicular unit transplant (FUT), the healing time is less.

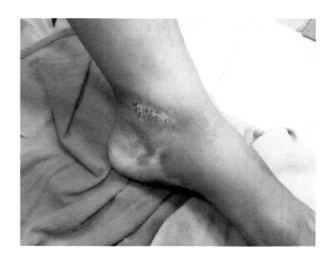

Figure 37.6.4   Implantation of the follicular units in the recipient area.

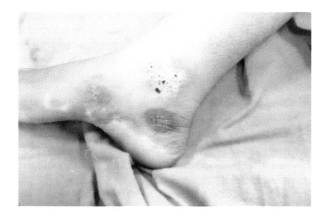

Figure 37.6.1   Baseline photograph.

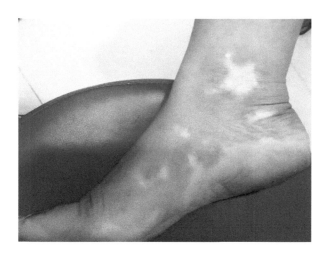

Figure 37.6.2   Slit making in the recipient area.

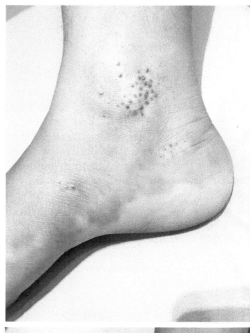

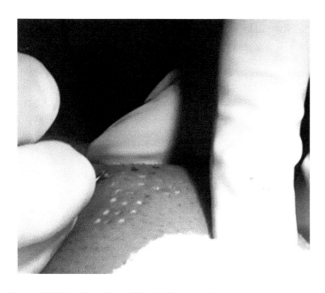

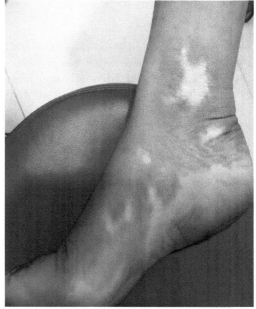

Figure 37.6.3   Extraction of the folbicular units.

Figure 37.6.5   After 1 week.

The disadvantage of this method is in achieving repigmentation in glaborous areas, technical limitations of extracting intact follicular units, and the procedure being cumbersome for larger areas. Vaenscheidt et al. [18] described plucking as a different method of follicular harvest, which is inferior to FUE. They found almost complete (>90%) repigmentation in three of five patients with vitiligo, around 50% repigmentation in one patient, and less than 10% repigmentation in one patient. Their technique is simple; however, the cell yield is less in the case of plucked hair follicles, and optimization of cell harvest from the hair follicular unit needs to be standardized for optimum yield.

In the era of cell-based therapies, the future may involve culturing melanocytes to treat a variety of pigment disorders, such as albinism and vitiligo. Cultivation of melanocytes in vitro can increase the cell number dramatically, and cells from a small piece of normal skin can be used to treat large depigmented areas. Since evidence from the previous literature has already concluded follicular melanocyte stem cells to be more robust than epidermal melanocyte stem cells, suspension prepared from extracted hair follicles ORS is the future strategy in vitiligo surgery [19]. Noncultured extracted hair follicular ORS cell suspension transplantation has successfully been tried with 65.7% repigmentation [20]. As compared to other methods like epidermal melanocyte culture, it is easy to obtain hair follicle ORS cell suspension as it does not require separation of the epidermis from the dermis. This method of obtaining hair follicle ORS cell suspension showed more CD200+ cells as compared to plucked cells [19].

Mesenchymal stem cells inhibit T-cell proliferation and induce T-cell apoptosis [21]. Studies have shown that dermal mesenchymal stem cells modulate the infiltration of perilesional CD8+ T-cells [22]. They inhibit CD8+ T-cell proliferation, induce their apoptosis, and regulate their cytokine/chemokine production. Thus they improve efficacy of transplantation in patients undergoing noncultured/cultured autologous melanocyte transplantation.

Theoretically, we should expect better repigmentation with follicular melanocytes due to the presence of more stem cells, a better melanocyte-keratinocyte ratio, and morphological properties of melanocytes in the hair follicle in comparison to epidermal stem cells. However, in the study by Singh et al. [23] the outcome of follicular stem cells was numerically inferior to the response seen with epidermal stem cells. It is proposed that the presence of keratinocytes in the suspension supplies essential growth factors for melanocyte growth [8]. Melanocyte proliferation, migration, dendricity, and differentiation are influenced by keratinocytes and fibroblasts as well as the melanocyte-derived growth factors and cytokines [24]. Therefore, a better pigmentation rate may be obtained by adding keratinocyte growth factors to follicular stem cells. This needs to be assessed in future studies.

PRACTICAL TIPS

Vital steps in hair transplantation in vitiligo are as follows:
Obtain informed consent, baseline photographs, and administer local anesthesia (after lignocaine sensitivity testing) in both recipient and donor area (Figure 37.6.1). Slits are created for hair grafting in the recipient area by use of either CTS blades (0.9 mm) or needles (19 or 20 G) (Figure 37.6.2).
Hair follicles are extracted by FUE/FUT from scalp or body hairs (Figure 37.6.3). Grafts are simultaneously planted in recipient sites without damaging the lower one-third of the graft (Figure 37.6.4). No dressing is required in the recipient

area. The donor area dressing is removed after 48 hours, followed by topical antibiotic application. Phototherapy can be started after 10 days with NB-UVB to expedite repigmentation. Perifollicular repigmentation in the vitiligo patch is usually seen by 4–8 weeks, and complete pigmentation is achieved at 12–20 weeks (Figures 37.6.5 through 37.6.7).

CONCLUSION

FUE is a safe, efficient, and inexpensive method of surgical repigmentation without requiring sophisticated equipment. Small and stable lesions on non-glaborous areas with leukotrichia can be easily and effectively treated by this method [25]. As compared to the other surgical modalities available, complications of this procedure are minimal, and the color match is excellent.

This procedure can serve as a novel, minimally invasive, scar-less technique with good yield of melanocyte stem cells and other stem cells, which may serve as a good source for restoration of other tissues like cornea and nerves. Further research is required in this arena.

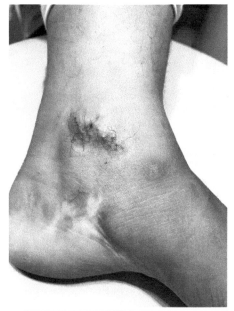
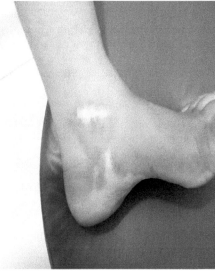

Figure 37.6.6   Left ankle at 12 weeks.

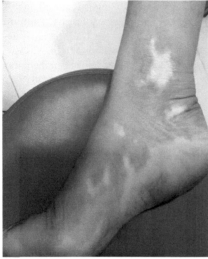

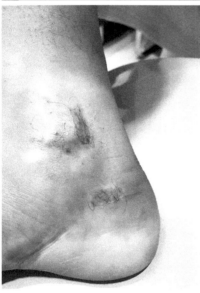

Figure 37.6.7   Right ankle at 12 weeks.

REFERENCES

1. Pichaimuthu R, Ramaswamy P, Bikash K, and Joseph R. A measurement of the stigma among vitiligo and psoriasis patients in India. *Indian J Dermatol Venereol Leprol* 2011;77:300–6.

2. Birlea SA, Spritz RA, and Norris DA. Vitiligo. In: Goldsmith LA, ed. *Fitzpatrick's Dermatology in General Medicine*. New York: McGraw Hill Medical; 2012, pp. 792–803.

3. Staricco RG, and Miller-Milinska A. Activation of amelanotic melanocytes in the outer root sheath of the human hair follicle following ultraviolet rays exposure. *J Invest Dermatol* 1962;39:163–4.

4. Ortonne JP, Schmitt D, and Thivolet J. PUVA-induced repigmentation of vitiligo: Scanning electron microscopy of hair follicles. *J Invest Dermatol* 1980;74:40–2.

5. Cui J, Shen L, and Wang G. Role of hair follicles in the repigmentation of vitiligo. *J Invest Dermatol* 1991;97:410–6.

6. Staricco RG. Amelanotic melanocytes in outer sheath of the human hair follicle. *J Invest Dermatol* 1959;33:295–7.

7. Staricco RG. Mechanism of migration of the melanocytes from the hair follicle into the epidermis following dermabrasion. *J Invest Dermatol* 1961;36:99–104.

8. Gauthier Y, and Surleve-Bazeille JE. Autologous grafting with noncultured melanocytes: A simplified method for treatment of depigmented lesions. *J Am Acad Dermatol* 1992;26:191–4.

9. Na GY, Seo SK, and Choi SK. Single hair grafting for the treatment of vitiligo. *J Am Acad Dermatol* 1998;38:580–4.

10. Plonka PM, Passeron T, Brenner M et al. What are melanocytes really doing all day long? *Exp Dermatol* 2009;18:799–819.

11. Nishimura EK, Jordan SA, Oshima H et al. Dominant role of the niche in melanocyte stem-cell fate determination. *Nature* 2002;416:854–60.

12. Tobin DJ, Swanson NN, Pittelkow MR, Peters EM, and Schallreuter KU. Melanocytes are not absent in lesional skin of long duration vitiligo. *J Pathol* 2000;191:407–16.

13. Song HJ, Choi GS, and Shin JH. Preservation of melanoblasts of white hair follicles of segmental vitiligo lesions: A preliminary study. *J Eur Acad Dermatol Venereol* 2011;25:240–2.

14. Chouhan K, Kumar A, and Kanwar AJ. Body hair transplantation in vitiligo. *J Cutan Aesthet Surg* 2013 Apr;6(2):111–2.

15. Mou Y, Jiang X, Du Y, and Xue L. Intelligent bioengineering in vitiligo treatment: Transdermal protein transduction of melanocyte-lineage-specific genes. *Med Hypotheses* 2012;79:786–9.

16. Tobin DJ. Aging of the hair follicle pigmentation system. *Int J Trichology* 2009;1:83–93.

17. Tobin DJ, and Paus R. Graying: Gerontobiology of the hair follicle pigmentary unit. *Exp Gerontol* 2001;36:29–54.

18. Vanscheidt W, and Hunziker T. Repigmentation by outer-root-sheath-derived melanocytes: Proof of concept in vitiligo and leucoderma. *Dermatology* 2009;218:342–3.

19. Kumar A, Gupta S, Mohanty S, Bhargava B, and Airan B. Stem cell niche is partially lost during follicular plucking: A preliminary pilot study. *Int J Trichology* 2013;5(2):97–100.

20. Mohanty S, Kumar A, Dhawan J, Sreenivas V, and Gupta S. Noncultured extracted hair follicle outer root sheath cell suspension for transplantation in vitiligo. *Br J Dermatol* 2011 Jun;164(6):1241–6.

21. Plumas J, Chaperot L, Richard MJ, Molens JP, Bensa JC, and Favrot MC. Mesenchymal stem cells induce apoptosis of activated T cells. *Leukemia* 2005;19:1597–604.

22. Van Geel N, Goh BK, Wallaeys E, De Keyser S, and Lambert J. A review of non-cultured epidermal cellular grafting in vitiligo. *J Cutan Aesthet Surg* 2011;4:17–22.

23. Singh C, Parsad D, Kanwar AJ, Dogra S, and Kumar R. Comparison between autologous noncultured extracted hair follicle outer root sheath cell suspension and autologous noncultured epidermal cell suspension in the treatment of stable vitiligo: A randomized study. *Br J Dermatol* 2013;169:287–93.

24. Zhou MN, Zhang ZQ, Wu JL et al. Dermal mesenchymal stem cells (DMSCs) inhibit skin-homing CD8+T cell activity, a determining factor of vitiligo patients' autologous melanocytes transplantation efficiency. *PLOS ONE* 2013;8:e60254.

25. Lee BW, Schwartz RA, Hercogová J, Valle Y, and Lotti TM. Vitiligo road map. *Dermatol Ther* 2012;25(Suppl 1):S44–56.

TISSUE GRAFTING TECHNIQUES
Jodhpur Technique

Dilip Kachhawa

CONTENTS

INTRODUCTION

Vitiligo surgeries have provided excellent repigmentation. One of their limitations is cost. In developing countries like India with a significant population still living below the poverty line, affordable health care remains a challenge, especially for cosmetic concerns. Vitiligo is a disease surrounded in misconceptions and myths, with a significant psychosocial impact.

In 2008, Kacchawa and Kalla had a new idea for vitiligo surgery while performing dermabrasion on a facial scar. They introduced noncultured, non-trypsinized melanocytes keratinocytes epidermal cell suspension known as the Jodhpur technique, named after the city in which it was first conceptualized [1].

INDICATIONS

1. Stable vitiligo
2. Chemical leukoderma

CONTRAINDICATIONS

1. Active lesion
2. Skin atrophy
3. Associated with secondary infection, keloidal tendency, bleeding, and inflamed skin

PROCEDURE [1,2]

1. The patient is informed about the procedure, its various steps and probable outcome, and consent is signed.
2. Both donor and recipient areas are shaved.

3. Each white patch is numbered with proper charting of each patch size, shape, and site. Then a photograph is taken of both donor and recipient site.
4. The donor site area to be used as graft is roughly calculated as being one-third of recipient size.

RECIPIENT SITE
1. *Preparing the area:* Mark the recipient area and include an additional 2–3 mm of normal skin beyond the vitiligo margin. Clean the area with ethyl alcohol and povidone iodine.
2. *Dermabrasion of area:* Using either manual or electrical dermabrader, remove the epidermis up to the dermo-epidermal junction and further still until pinpoint bleeding occurs. Take special care to include the previously marked margin, in order to prevent perigraft halo. Wait until hemostasis occurs and then cover the site with gauze moistened with normal saline or isotonic sodium chloride.

DONOR AREA
1. *Site*: Any region of body with appropriate melanocytes can be used as a donor site. In practice, the gluteal region is preferred due to its lower cosmetic significance.
2. *Preparation of site*: Clean the donor site with povidone iodine and ethyl alcohol. Mark the site to be dermabraded. The marked area is locally anesthetized with 2% xylocaine given as a four-quadrant-deep dermal infiltration.
3. *Procedure*
   a. *Abrasion of skin*: Apply 2% mupirocin on the surface of the donor area. Use either a manual or electrical dermabrader with a disc diamond fraise endpiece. Hold the dermabrader in a safety razor grip. Roll the fraise all over the donor site in a smooth back-and-forth motion in all directions. For proper dermabrading of the donor site, ensure the skin is taut by stretching it, and initiate the dermabrasion from the peripheral border of the donor site along the markings.
   b. *Collection of melanocytes*: Just before finishing the dermabrasion, rotate the dermabrader clockwise in small circles so as to blend the mupirocin ointment with abraded epidermal particles containing the desired melanocytes and keratinocytes. This helps to decrease spraying of particles and increases collection of melanocytes.
   c. The donor site is then dressed in ointment-soaked dressing to speed up the recovery, and pressure gauze is placed over that to achieve the required hemostasis.

ADVANTAGES OF PREPARING THE RECIPIENT SITE BEFORE THE DONOR SITE

1. This negates the need to harvest the graft, as it is transferred directly to the already-prepared recipient site.
2. By the time the graft is collected, the oozing is reduced in the recipient site.
3. The desired hemostasis is also achieved during that time, which further reduces the of graft and provides better imbibing of the paste (graft).

TRANSFER OF GRAFT

1. Remove the wet gauze in the recipient area and transfer the previously made paste into this newly dermabraded area. Spread it evenly over the surface with a spatula.
2. Cover this newly grafted area with collagen dressing on the bottom followed by a sterile gauze piece and supported by Tegaderm transparent dressing or cotton dressing.
3. The patient is discharged within an hour of the procedure.

POSTOPERATIVE CARE AND FOLLOW-UP [4,6]

1. The patient is discharged with advice to take proper care of the wound and follow aseptic precautions. Further oral antibiotics and analgesics are given for 8–10 days.
2. The donor site dressing is changed after 1 day and removed after 12–15 days.
3. At the recipient site, the dressing is changed after 1 week and removed after 10–15 days. After removing the dressing, a black/brown crusted collagen sheet remains partially attached to the site. It will fall off on its own within 2–3 days, leaving behind an erythematous patch.

TIME FOR REPIGMENTATION [3,5]

1. Repigmentation is observed after 4–6 weeks of the procedure, and significant pigmentation is seen after 16–20 week.
2. A concurrent method for pigmentation can be used to achieve faster and more uniform pigmentation.
3. Use of natural sunlight, phototherapy with psoralen and UVA (topical/systemic PUVA, PUVAsol), NB-UVB, or excimer lamp after 10–15 days of procedure for at least 3–6 months.
4. Oral and topical steroid and tacrolimus can also be prescribed to accelerate repigmentation.

COMPLICATIONS AND SIDE EFFECTS

The surgery is associated with very few side effects, if any. Side effects can include the following.
1. Mismatch of color.
2. Hypo/hyperpigmentation with or without scarring at the recipient or donor site.
3. Secondary infection with edema, erythema, pain.
4. Persistent erythema.

LIMITATIONS [7,8]

1. Only useful for stable vitiligo.
2. Pigmentation requires at least 4–6 months.
3. Achronic/hypochromic skip area may be left behind.
4. May require another round of surgery for a larger vitiligo patch.

ADVANTAGES [9,10]

1. Safe, simple procedure, requires minimal surgical expertise, and can be easily adopted for an outpatient procedure.
2. Provides a cosmetically acceptable result with relatively few, if anys side effects.
3. Multiple areas can be treated at the same time.
4. Large areas can be treated either in the same sitting or in multiple sittings.

5. It is an autologous, noncultured, epidermal cell suspension method, hence requires no special grafting equipment for either cell suspension or for cell culture.
6. It is also useful for treating non-healing ulcers.

JODHPUR TECHNIQUE FROM PERILESIONAL VITILIGO SKIN

The main purpose of vitiligo surgery is to improve the cosmetic appearance of the patient. It is a comparatively safe surgery with few side effects or complications. In the commonly chosen vitiligo surgery, e.g., split-thickness grafting (STG)/punch/micro punch graft, one site is chosen as the donor site (commonly the lateral side of the thigh) and the vitiligo patch is the recipient site.

One of the side effects most commonly observed in these surgeries is hyper/hypopigmentation of the donor site with or without scarring. Newer techniques of STG/ noncultured epidermal cell suspension/suction blister grafting have perilesional hypopigmentation as a known complication. Further pain and trauma may occur in both sites during and after the procedure.

Using the perilesional skin of the vitiligo patch as a donor site theoretically minimizes the side effects seen in two-site grafting surgery.

PROCEDURE

1. Patient consent is taken prior to the procedure.
2. Vitiligo patch along with its surrounding skin is shaved and photographic documentation is accomplished.
3. Recipient site: The site is prepared as previously mentioned
4. Donor area: Under aseptic precautions, the donor area is prepared (perilesional skin) and anesthetized using 2% lignocaine.
5. Collection and grafting of melanocytes: Using either a Manekshaw manual dermabrader or electrical dermabrader, dermabrade the epidermis of both the vitiligo patch (recipient site) and its perilesional skin (donor site) until there is pinpoint bleeding, indicating that the papillary dermis has been reached. This means that the recipient area is now ready to accept the graft.

Apply 2% mupirocin ointment in the donor perilesional skin before starting dermabrasion. Application of mupirocin ointment helps to reduce the splattering of abraded epidermis and helps to lock in the melanocytes and keratinocytes. Now collect the paste (graft) from the perilesional skin and apply it onto the previously abraded vitiligo patch with the help of a spatula (grafting). The area is dressed with dry collagen and antibiotic-soaked gauze in layers followed by dressing with dry gauze. The patient is prescribed antibiotics and analgesics and followed up on the seventh day. Figures 37.7.1–37.7.4 illustrate a patient with vitiligo on right upper eyelid treated with the Jodhpur technique.

ADVANTAGES

1. Cost, time, and labor effective
2. Ideal for perilesional halo of previous surgeries
3. Hypo/hyperpigmentation of donor area is minimized
4. Perilesional melanocytes are hypothetically hyperfunctional than normal melanocytes

JODHPUR TECHNIQUE IN NON-HEALING ULCERS [5]

Chronic non-healing ulcer is defined as a loss of skin and soft tissue which takes more than 6 weeks to heal. Chronic non-healing ulcer can be due to various reasons, e.g., leprosy, diabetes, peripheral

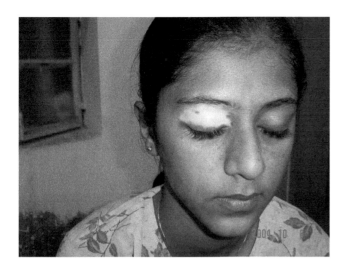

Figure 37.7.1 Preprocedural picture showing depigmented patch over right eyelid extended to the ipsilateral inferior eyebrow region, with white eyebrow hairs.

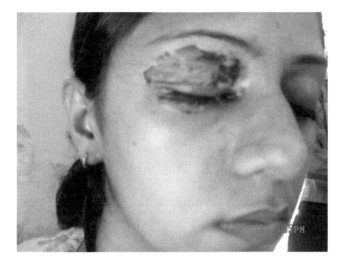

Figure 37.7.2 Image at 14th day post-surgery showing graft uptake in the lateral side versus beginning of repigmentation through perilesional Jodhpur technique in medial region. Note: Eyelashes remain depigmented at this stage.

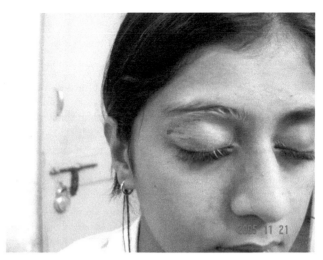

Figure 37.7.3 Image at week 12 post-surgery showing repigmentation on the lateral side along with stuck-on appearance over the region, while repigmentation is diffuse and almost complete on the medial side through the perilesional Jodhpur technique. Note: Lashes and brows remain depigmented, indicating delay or resistance in follicular repigmentation.

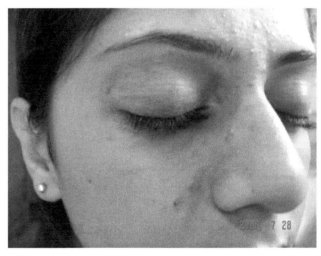

Figure 37.7.4 Image at week 20 post-surgery showing complete repigmentation on the lateral side and medial side with repigmentation of lashes and brow hairs on the medial side, indicating the superiority of the perilesional Jodhpur technique over split-thickness grafting.

vascular disease, or pressure sores. The most common site is the leg, which also poses a therapeutic challenge. Management of the ulcer begins with finding the primary etiology and treating it. The challenge is to treat those ulcers that fail to respond to existing management strategies. One conjecture is the lack of necessary growth factor causing the persistence of ulcer.

Since the graft retrieved in the Jodhpur technique is known to have abundant growth factors in the melanocytes and keratinocytes, it can be helpful in healing the chronic non-healing ulcer.

PROCEDURE

1. The lateral side of the thigh is used as a donor site in this technique. The area to be abraded is calculated using one-third of recipient ulcer area. Under aseptic conditions, the donor area is anesthetized and 2% mupirocin ointment is evenly spread. Using an electrical dermabrader at 4000–5000 rpm, scrape the epidermis until pinpoint bleeding occurs. Rotate the dermabrader in small clockwise circles to apply the ointment uniformly all over the site. This helps to entrap the epidermal and dermal particles containing the melanocytes, keratinocytes, and plenty of growth factors.

2. The dermabraded paste is the skin graft and is collected in a spatula. Carboxymethylcellulose can be used to homogenize the paste and help to spread the paste. This paste is then applied over the ulcer area.

3. Post-procedure, non-absorbable dressing will be placed and the bandage is left on for 7 days. The patient is prescribed oral antibiotics and analgesics. In addition, vitamin C, zinc, and a multivitamin for 4 months is given. Postoperative follow-up is done weekly until 8 weeks post-procedure.

ADVANTAGES

1. Higher probability of healing in less time with minimal chance of infection

2. Inexpensive, simple, and convenient approach

REFERENCES

1. Kachhawa D, Rao P, and Kalla G. Simplified non-cultured non-trypsinised epidermal cell graft technique followed by psoralen and ultraviolet A light therapy for stable vitiligo. *J Cutan Aesthet Surg* 2017;10(2):81–5.

2. Sidharth S, and Dilip K. Jodhpur technique. (Updated 2019 Oct 28). In: *StatPearls* (Internet). Treasure Island, FL: StatPears Publishing; 2020. http://www.ncbi.nlm.nih.gov/books/NBK549891/#_NBK549891_pubdet_

3. Kachhawa D, and Kalla G. Keratinocyte-melanocyte graft technique followed by PUVA therapy for stable vitiligo. *Indian J Dermatol Venereol Leprol* 2008 Nov-Dec;74(6):622–4.

4. Parsad D, Gupta S. IADVL Dermatosurgery Task Force. Standard guidelines of care for vitiligo surgery. *Indian J Dermatol Venereol Leprol* 2008 Jan;74(Suppl):S37–45.

5. Kachhawa D, Bhansali S, Kachhawa N et al. Jodhpur technique for chronic non-healing leg ulcer. *Dermatol Res* 2019; 1(1):1–3.

6. Gauthier Y, and Surleve-Bazeille JE. Autologous grafting with non-cultured melanocytes: A simplified method for treatment of depigmented lesion. *J Am Acad Dermatol* 1992;26:191–4.

7. Parsad D, Dogra S, and Kanwar AJ. Quality of life in patients with vitiligo. *Health Qual Life Outcomes* 2003;1:58.

8. Lahiri K, and Malakar S. The concept of stability of vitiligo: A reappraisal. *Indian J Dermatol* 2012;57(2):83–9.

9. Verma R, Grewal RS, Chatterjee M, Pragasam V, Vasudevan B, and Mitra D. A comparative study of efficacy of cultured versus non cultured melanocyte transfer in the management of stable vitiligo. *Med J Armed Forces India* 2014;70:26–31.

10. Falabella R. Surgical treatment of vitiligo: Why, when and how. *J Eur Acad Dermatol Venereol* 2003;17:518–20.

CELLULAR GRAFTING TECHNIQUES
Noncultured Epidermal Cell Suspension

Thurakkal Salim

CONTENTS

INTRODUCTION

Vitiligo is a common depigmenting dermatosis affecting approximately 0.5%–1% of the general population [1,2]. Medical treatment modalities for vitiligo vary from PUVA, NB-UVB, and excimer lasers to topical steroids and topical immunomodulators. While medical therapies are the primary forms of treatment, they are effective only in 60%–70% of patients. Surgical methods can always be an alternative therapeutic option, especially in cases of stable vitiligo. These surgical techniques have been devised over the years and have come a long way from tissue grafting techniques to cellular grafts.

Surgical therapy of vitiligo is the gold standard in the management of resistant areas and residual lesions. Certain types of vitiligo such as segmental, mucosal, acral, and leukotrichia fail to respond well to medical treatments at all, and in those cases that do respond, resistant lesions persist. Cellular grafting techniques—noncultured epidermal cell suspension (NCES) and hair follicle cell suspension (HFCS) have revolutionized the management of vitiligo. It is possible to treat very large areas using small donor areas. It yields faster, uniform, normal textured, natural pigmentation. This chapter focuses on the procedure and modifications of NCES.

HISTORY

The first noncultured epidermal cellular grafting was performed under experimental conditions on piebald guinea pig skin by Billingham and Medawar [3]. In 1992, Gauthier and Surleve-Bazeille used this technique for the treatment of stable vitiligo [4]. The donor sample was obtained from the scalp and treated with 0.25% trypsin solution for 18 hours. Liquid nitrogen was used to raise blisters at the recipient site into which the suspension was inoculated. This technique was then modified by Olsson and Juhlin in 1998, where the donor skin

was taken from the gluteal region and the trypsinization time was reduced to 60 minutes, and the suspension was applied directly on the dermabraded vitiligo lesion [5]. A limiting factor of this technique was fixation of the liquid suspension at the recipient area. To overcome this hurdle, further modification in the technique was introduced by Van Geel et al. in 2001 [6] with the use of hyaluronic acid to increase the viscosity of the suspension and to prevent runoff.

PREREQUISITES FOR PERFORMING NCES

Proper case selection is of paramount importance for any surgical method to yield good results. Stability of vitiligo should be the primary consideration while opting for any transplantation methods. Proper counseling is essential; the nature of the disease, procedure, expected outcome, and possible complications should be clearly explained to the patient. As per the literature, vitiligo is labeled as being "stable" when progression of old lesions and/or development of new lesions is absent for 1 year [7]. Segmental vitiligo stabilizes spontaneously usually within the first year of onset, hence this remains the best surgical treatment indication. Before performing the treatment in patients with generalized vitiligo, it has to be highlighted that the procedure will not alter the underlying patho-etiology and despite the treatment, the natural course of the disease will remain the same. A history of keloids, hypertrophic scars, or signs of Koebner phenomenon must be ruled out, as these factors may have a negative impact on the surgical results [6].

PRINCIPLE OF NONCULTURED EPIDERMAL CELL SUSPENSION

All grafting techniques rely on the basic principle of repopulating depigmented lesions with functional melanocytes arising from normal epidermis or outer root sheath (ORS) and bulge areas of the hair follicle. The transplanted melanocyte will establish and function as an epidermal melanin unit, and the cells survive and function if stability has been achieved. NCES is based on extraction of the basal cell layer followed by concentration of these cells by centrifugation. The basal cell extraction is carried out by enzymatic separation of the intercellular bridges and dermo-epidermal junction using the proteolytic enzyme trypsin. Trypsin separates the basal keratinocytes and melanocytes. These separated cells are concentrated in suspending media and further transplanted over the recipient area. Figure 38.1.1 explains the principle of NCES.

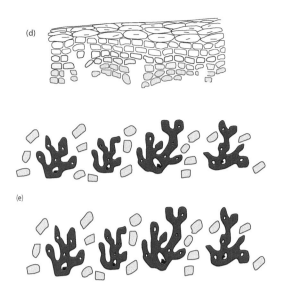

Figure 38.1.1 (Continued) Principle of NCES. (d) Basal melanocytes and keratinocytes separated. (e) Basal cells are concentrated in the suspending media and the epidermal and dermal components are discarded.

PROCEDURE

INSTRUMENTS AND CONSUMABLES
A skin grafting knife in the form of Hamby's knife, Silver's knife, straight artery forceps with razor blade, or Padget's, Zimmer's, or Davol's dermatome can be used for harvesting. The consumables and instruments required for NCES are given in Table 38.1.1 and Figure 38.1.2.

TECHNIQUE
The technique involves three steps:
1. Preparation of the donor area and harvesting of donor skin
2. Preparation of autologous noncultured epidermal cell suspension
3. Dermabrasion followed by application of the cells over the recipient area

STEP 1: PREPARATION OF THE DONOR AREA AND HARVESTING THE DONOR SKIN
The lateral aspect of the gluteal region is usually selected as the donor site. Hair at the donor site is shaved off. After cleansing the

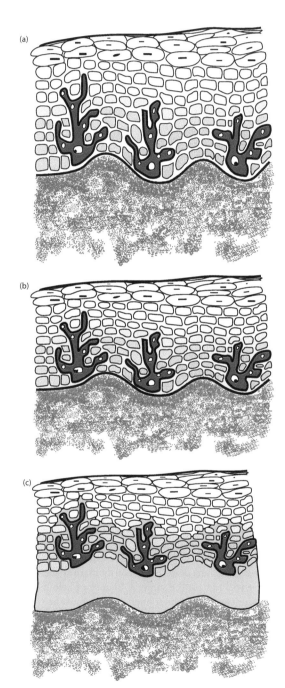

Figure 38.1.1 Principle of NCES. (a) Cross-section of normal skin showing dermis, epidermis, and dermo-epidermal junction with basal melanocytes and keratinocytes. (b) Trypsin entering through the intercellular bridges and dermo-epidermal junction. (c) Cells getting separated due to the action of trypsin. (Continued)

Table 38.1.1 Consumables and equipment for NCES

Consumables
0.25% Trypsin-0.8% EDTA solution
Trypsin inhibitor, to neutralize excess trypsin
Dulbecco's modified Eagle's medium (DMEM)
Equipment
Centrifuge
Aerobic incubator
Micromotor diamond fraise dermabrader or a CO_2 laser
A manual or electric dermatome
Two pairs of fine pointed non-toothed forceps
Pasture pipette or calibrated micropipette
Centrifuge tubes, petri dishes
Dressings
Collagen dressings
Tulle dressings

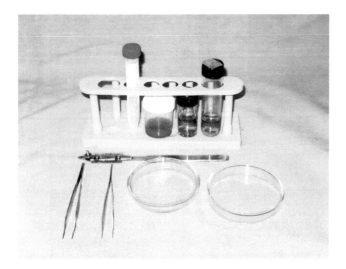

Figure 38.1.2   Reagents and instruments required for NCES.

area with povidone iodine and alcohol, local or topical anesthesia is administered. Using a skin grafting knife, a superficial skin sample is obtained. Usually, one-fifth to one-tenth the size of the recipient area is harvested from the donor site.

STEP 2: PREPARATION OF AUTOLOGOUS NONCULTURED EPIDERMAL CELL SUSPENSION

The skin sample obtained is immediately transferred into a petri dish holding 8 mL of 0.25% trypsin EDTA solution. The skin sample has to be completely immersed in the solution and is placed with the epidermis facing upward. The sample is then incubated in an aerobic incubator at 37°C for 50 minutes. After incubation, the grafts are transferred to a petri dish containing about 5 mL of trypsin inhibitor to neutralize the action of trypsin-EDTA. Epidermis and dermis are then separated using a pair of non-toothed forceps. Following this, the epidermis is transferred into a petri dish containing the melanocyte nourishment medium, i.e., Dulbecco's modified Eagle's medium (DMEM). The dermal tissue is discarded. The epidermal pieces are then gently teased to separate the melanocytes that fall into the medium. The epidermis is teased until no pigment is left on its surface. The transparent epidermal pieces are discarded and the remaining DMEM solution with the melanocytes is transferred into a centrifuge tube. The media along the cells are centrifuged at 2000 rpm for 10 min. A cell pellet rich in melanocytes is formed at the bottom of the tube. After discarding the supernatant, the pellet is re-suspended in 0.8 mL of fresh medium in a 1-mL syringe.

STEP 3: TRANSPLANTATION

The recipient area is cleaned with povidone iodine and alcohol. Under local anesthesia, using a high-speed diamond fraise dermabrader or CO_2 laser, the recipient area is abraded down to the dermo-epidermal junction. The cell suspension is evenly applied with the syringe and spread out with its tip over the recipient area. Cells are covered with a thin transparent collagen film. This is then covered with a sterile pad and finally with Tegaderm (3M) dressing.

POSTOPERATIVE CARE

All patients are advised to take complete rest and avoid vigorous physical activities. All cases with area treated less than 150 square centimeters can be managed as daycare. The patient is sent home under antibiotic coverage and the dressings are removed after a week; anti-inflammatory medicines are prescribed to manage the postoperative pain.

SURGICAL OUTCOME

The pigmentation usually begins in about 3–6 weeks and is almost complete in about 2–6 months. The pigmentation attained has good texture and cosmetic color match with uniformity (Figures 38.1.3–38.1.5).

IMPACT OF PATIENT-ASSOCIATED FACTORS ON THE RESPONSE TO NCES

1. *Duration of disease stability.* Strict selection of patients with stable vitiligo is the most important factor for a successful outcome. Disease activity is defined as the appearance of new lesions/enlargement of old ones observed in the past year and/or the presence of Koebner phenomenon [6]. Other indications of disease activity include hypomelanotic color of the vitiligo lesions, poorly defined hazy borders, confetti lesions, and trichrome vitiligo [8]. Early studies by Mulekar which included cases with a minimum of 6 months disease stability showed that ≤95% repigmentation occurred in 36/43 cases of segmental vitiligo cases with 1-year stability [9]. Hence disease stability should be considered in both segmental and nonsegmental vitiligo, and whenever in doubt, a longer pretreatment observation period is required, documented with photography.

2. *Type of vitiligo.* Gauthier and Surleve-Bazeille, in 1992, described that NCES was used in the treatment of localized vitiligo areas of ≤50cm² in three segmental vitiligo and eight focal vitiligo cases [10]. The response was found to be better in segmental vitiligo cases, with an average repigmenting rate of 92% versus 41% in focal vitiligo cases and 4/7 cases failing to repigment. A few other studies also documented better response in segmental vitiligo, and certain immunological factors probably interfered with the outcome in generalized vitiligo. Acrofacial type vitiligo is usually resistant to surgical therapy. The lip-tip type was also associated with a poor outcome when NCES was performed at other sites in the same patient [11]. Mixed vitiligo cases also responded less favorably than segmental and generalized vitiligo cases to NCES [12].

3. *Size of the treated lesion and extent of vitiligo.* The majority of the authors used NCES in the treatment of lesions <100cm² with a favorable outcome. Several authors excluded cases with widespread vitiligo involving >30% of the BSA [13].

4. *Skin type.* Similar repigmentation rates were observed in different ethnic groups, and the majority of the reports did not comment on the skin type of treated cases [11].

5. *Gender.* No significant difference was found in the repigmentation rates between males and females [7].

6. *Age.* Several studies showed that age per se did not affect the percentage of repigmentation. A study conducted by Mulekar et al. involving 25 children and adolescents showed ≥95% repigmentation on 7/12 focal vitiligo and 8/13 segmented vitiligo cases [14]. The major concern involving children was their level of pain tolerance and fidgeting during the procedure. In cooperative children, the concentration of the topically applied anesthetic cream can be increased to keep them comfortable.

7. *Duration of the disease.* A few studies assessed the impact of this variable and found no correlation [7].

8. *Site of the lesion.* On literature review, the sites that showed the best response were the head and neck regions. The response rates over these areas ranged from 70%–100% with more than half of the lesions achieving ≥95% repigmentation [4,15,16]. The next sites in line to show a good response were lesions over the limbs (excluding elbows, knees, ankles) and

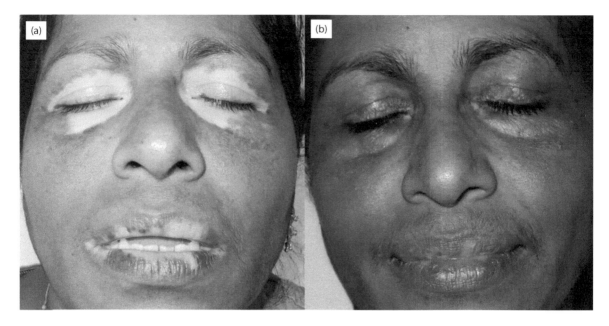

Figure 38.1.3 (a and b) Vitiligo periorbital and lips before NCES and after.

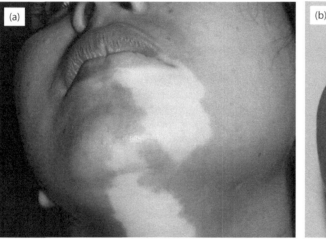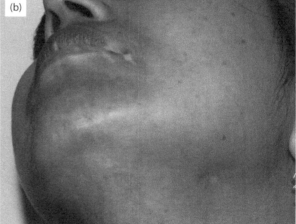

Figure 38.1.4 (a) Segmental vitiligo before NCES. (b) After 3 months.

the trunk. Acral skin tended to respond the least; among the acral lesions, those over the dorsum of the hands and feet responded better than those over fingers and toes, as per few conducted studies. Manual dermabrasion or diamond fraise wheel at a low speed of 5000 rpm was used to yield a good response in difficult-to-manage sites like the eyelids, nipples, and genital skin.

EFFECT OF TECHNIQUE-RELATED FACTORS ON THE RESPONSE TO NCES

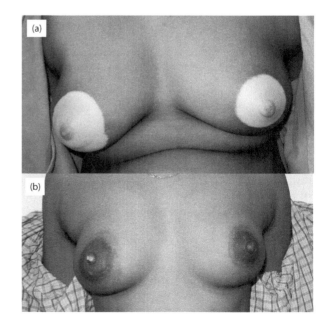

1. *Type of tissue used.* A few studies compared the technique of NCES to suction blister epidermal grafting (SBEG). More cases achieved excellent repigmentation (≥90%) in the NCES group ($p=0.002$). The level of patient satisfaction and DLQI score reduction were also significantly higher in the NCES group [17].
2. *Donor site.* The thigh or the gluteal region is the usually chosen site. No significant difference in the melanocyte cell count was found between both sites.

Figure 38.1.5 (a and b) Vitiligo vulgaris before NECS and after.

Table 38.1.2 Summarizes the advantages and disadvantages of NCECS

Advantages
A large area can be treated using a small skin sample. Donor recipient ratio 1:10
Can be used in difficult areas like joints, pressure sites, mucosa, etc.
Faster, uniform pigmentation matching with adjoining skin
Does not need laboratory, as the cell separation can be done in operating room
Daycare procedure
Donor site pigments with minimal scarring

Disadvantages
Requires specific cell culture grade biochemicals and media
The operating room has to be equipped with incubator, centrifuge, and equipment for preparation of cell suspension
Surgical skill required to harvest adequate-sized, thin grafts
Perilesional halo seen in a few cases

3. *Preparation of the recipient skin.* Several methods can be used for preparing such as dermabrasion, laser resurfacing, or cryo. Dermabrasion is relatively safe and produces pinpoint bleeding, which denotes reaching the ideal level. Uniform resurfacing can be attained with CO_2 ablative resurfacing; however, the technique is expensive and does not denote pinpoint bleeding points. A pilot study demonstrated that dermabrasion using a high-speed dermabrader fitted with a diamond fraise wheel produced better repigmentation than fractional CO_2 laser resurfacing [18]. According to the experience of a few authors, laser resurfacing showed greater efficacy in improving repigmentation following NCES over acral areas [19].

   One study compared cryoblebbing over laser resurfacing. Cryoblebbing produced $\geq 75\%$ repigmentation in significantly more lesions, probably due to a good response achieved over distal areas [20].

4. *Donor-to-recipient area ratio.* The usual dictum is that NCES can be performed using donor tissue that is one-tenth the recipient area treated, but a further search into the literature revealed that in the majority of the cases, a donor area of one-third to one-fifth recipient size was used. A study conducted by Olson and Juhlin suggested that a melanocyte count of 190/mm² was the lower limit capable of producing repigmentation [15].

   Another study assessed the effect of the donor-to-recipient area ratio variable on repigmentation and found a significant difference in the extent of repigmentation between cases with a 1:3 and those with a 1:5 donor-to-recipient ratio. It was then concluded by the authors that the minimum number of melanocytes in epidermal cell suspension required to produce satisfactory repigmentation was in the range of 210–250 cells/mm² (Table 38.1.2) [21].

MODIFICATIONS OF THE PROCEDURE

There is ongoing research to simplify the procedure of noncultured cellular grafting, and modifications with respect to safety of the procedure and to reduce the cost of treatment. These modifications have significantly helped in reducing the cost of treatment and enabling its use in resource-limited settings. The methods are being revised rapidly to achieve a concentrated pigment cell population for transplantation.

NCES WITHOUT DMEM

Phosphate-buffered saline (PBS) is a buffer solution commonly used in biological research. The osmolarity and ion concentrations of the solution usually match those of the human body (isotonic), and it is nontoxic to cells. With this, the cost of the procedure can be reduced since there is no need for melanocyte media and there are no concerns of mitogenesis due to the melanocyte medium [22].

AVOIDING THE USE OF TRYPSIN INHIBITOR IN THE PROCESS OF PREPARATION OF NONCULTURED EPIDERMAL SUSPENSION

Trypsinized skin graft can be washed with PBS instead of treating with a trypsin inhibitor solution so as to prevent further action of the enzyme. The treatment outcome is comparable with that of the original technique. As trypsin inhibitor is one of the costliest reagents used in NCES, and this modification reduces the cost of the procedure [22].

INCUBATION UNDER ROOM TEMPERATURE

The graft is placed in EDTA solution and followed by incubation at 37°C using an incubator for 50 minutes in conventional technique. This is thought to be important for trypsin activation and subsequent separation of the epidermis from the dermis. Al Jasser et al. found that incubation at room temperature is as effective as using an incubator and shows that the use of an incubator may not be necessary to separate the dermis from epidermis in order to prepare epidermal cell suspension [23].

USE OF HYALURONIC ACID/METHYLCELLULOSE TO INCREASE VISCOSITY

A crucial limiting factor of this grafting technique, at least in our experience, was the fixation of the liquid suspension at the recipient area. Significant runoff of the suspension from the recipient site was associated with the high fluidity of the suspension. Van Geel et al. used hyaluronic acid as a biodegradable cell carrier to increase the viscosity of the suspension [6]. We have used methylcellulose gel as well as hyaluronic acid for the same purpose.

CRYO-SEPARATION OF RECIPIENT EPIDERMIS

Liquid nitrogen is commonly used in cryosurgery as a method of selective tissue destruction through the rapid formation of intracellular and extracellular ice crystals. This selective destruction can be utilized in recipient site preparation to induce blister formation. The patient is called in on the day before the surgery and the recipient area is prepared using liquid nitrogen spray. Blisters will be formed in the treated area. The blister fluid is removed, and cellular suspension is injected into this pocket (Figure 38.1.6).

This method is very useful in treating palmer and acral areas. Repigmentation is better compared with conventional dermabrasion or laser abrasion. It has to be restricted to the recipient site, as cryo-separation at the donor site for harvesting the blister roof will destroy the melanocytes.

RE-CELL KIT AND WELL PLATES

A commercial Re-Cell kit (Clinical Cell Culture, Cambridge, UK) (Figure 38.1.7) has also been devised, which is a portable battery-operated cell-harvesting device, aiming to eliminate the need for either a separate laboratory setup or equipment such as a centrifuge or incubator to process the cell suspension preparation. Mulekar et al. evaluated this device vis-à-vis conventional melanocyte-keratinocyte transfer and showed slightly better results in Re-Cell–treated lesions, though not statistically significant [24]. Goh et al. devised a "6-well plate" technique where the graft is successively processed

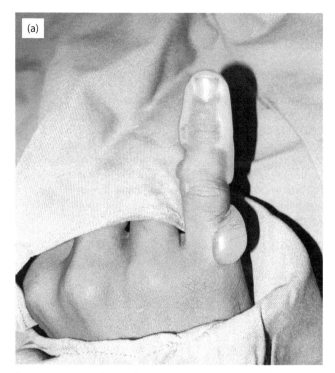

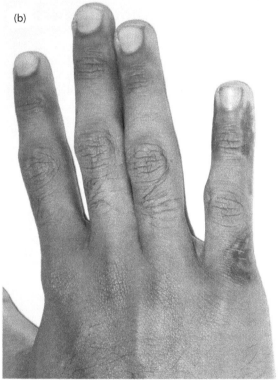

Figure 38.1.6 (a) Acral vitiligo cryo-blistering done. (b) Two months after NCES.

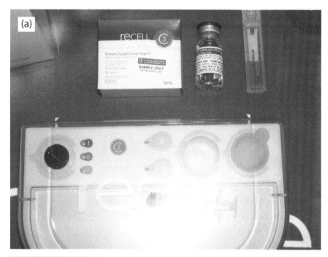

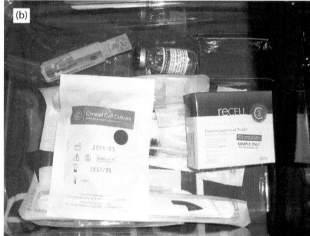

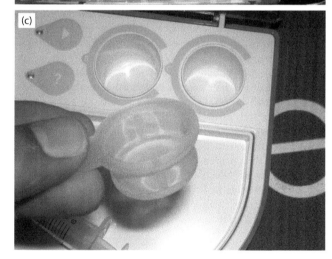

Figure 38.1.7 (a–c) Commercial Re-Cell kit.

in six wells filled with reagents arranged in a plate to obtain basal cell−enriched suspension [25]. They successfully used this technique to achieve good to excellent repigmentation in four vitiligo patients. Mrigpuri et al. at PGIMER, Chandigarh, modified it further to a four-compartment method, simplifying the process even more. They compared their new technique with the conventional laboratory-based method in a randomized controlled trial done on anatomically matched lesions (41 pairs) in 30 patients and found it to be equally efficacious [26].

CONCLUSION

It is evident that the world of NCES transfer in vitiligo is abuzz with innovation and research. Gone are the days when doing this procedure required a sophisticated laboratory setup. Due to consistent attempts at simplification of this procedure, it has been shown by workers from around the world that it can be successfully performed in a small clinic setup with inexpensive reagents and equipment.

REFERENCES

1. Gauthier, Y. and Benzekri, L. Non-cultured epidermal suspension in vitiligo: From laboratory to clinic. *Indian J Dermato, Venereol Leprol* 2012;78(1):59.

2. Taieb A, and Picardo M. The definition and assessment of vitiligo: A consensus report of the Vitiligo European Task Force. *Pigment Cell Res* 2007;20:27–35.

3. Billingham RE, and Medawar PB. Pigment spread in mammalian skin: Serial propagation and immunity reaction. *Heredity* 1950;4:141–64.

4. Gauthier Y, and Surleve-Bazeille JE. Autologous grafting with non cultured melanocytes: A simplified method for treatment of depigmented lesions. *J Am Acad Dermatol* 1992;26:191–4.

5. Olsson MJ, and Juhlin L. Repigmentation of vitiligo by transplantation of cultured autologous melanocytes. *Acta Derm Venereol* 1993;73:49–51.

6. Van Geel N, Ongenae K, De Mil M, Haeghen YV, Vervaet C, and Naeyaert JM. Double-blind placebo-controlled study of autologous transplanted epidermal cell suspensions for repigmentingvitiligo. *Arch Dermatol* 2004;140:1203–8.

7. Van Geel N, Wallaeys E, Goh BK, De Mil M, and Lambert J. Long term results of non cultured epidermal cellular grafting in vitiligo, halo nevi, piebaldism and nevus depigmentosus. *Br J Dermatol* 2010;163(6):1186–93.

8. Benzekri L, Gauthier Y, Hamada S, and Hassam B. Clinical features and histological findings are potential indicators of activity in lesions of common vitiligo. *Br J Dermatol* 2013;168(2):265–71.

9. Mulekar SV. Long-term follow-up study of 142 patients with vitiligo vulgaris treated by autologous, non-cultured melanocyte-keratinocyte cell transplantation. *Int J Dermatol* 2005;44(10):841–5.

10. Gauthier Y, and Surleve-Bazeille JE. Autologous grafting with noncultured melanocytes: A simplified method for treatment of depigmented lesions. *J Am Acad Dermatol* 1992;26(2 Pt 1):191–4.

11. Huggins RH, Henderson MD, Mulekar SV et al. Melanocyte-keratinocyte transplantation procedure in the treatment of vitiligo: The experience of an academic medical center in the United States. *J Am Acad Dermatol* 2012;66(5):785–93.

12. Vinay K, Dogra S, Parsad D et al. Clinical and treatment characteristics determining therapeutic outcome in patients undergoing autologous non-cultured outer root sheath hair follicle cell suspension for treatment of stable vitiligo. *J Eur Acad Dermatol Venereol* 2015;29(1):31–7.

13. Mulekar SV. Melanocyte-keratinocyte cell transplantation for stable vitiligo. *Int J Dermatol* 2003;42(2):132–6.

14. Mulekar SV, Al Eisa A, Delvi MB, Al Issa A, and Al Saeed AH. Childhood vitiligo: A long-term study of localized vitiligo treated by noncultured cellular grafting. *Pediat rDermatol* 2010;27(2):132–6.

15. Olsson MJ, and Juhlin L. Leucoderma treated by transplantation of a basal cell layer enriched suspension. *Br J Dermatol* 1998;138(4):644–8.

16. Van Geel N, Ongenae K, de Mil M, and Naeyaert JM. Modified technique of autologous noncultured epidermal cell transplantation for repigmenting vitiligo: A pilot study. *Dermatol Surg* 2001;27(10):873–6.

17. Budania A, Parsad D, Kanwar AJ, and Dogra S. Comparison between autologous noncultured epidermal cell suspension and suction blister epidermal grafting in stable vitiligo: A randomized study. *Br J Dermatol* 2012;167(6):1295–301.

18. Silpa-Archa N, Griffith JL, Williams MS, Lim HW, and Hamzavi IH. Prospective comparison of recipient-site preparation with fractional carbon dioxide laser vs. dermabrasion and recipient-site dressing composition in melanocyte–keratinocyte transplantation procedure in vitiligo: A preliminary study. *Br J Dermatol* 2016;174:895–89.

19. Bassiouny D, and Esmat S. Autologous non-cultured melanocyte–keratinocyte transplantation in the treatment of vitiligo: Patient selection and perspectives. *Clin Cosmet Investig Dermatol* 2018;11:521–40.

20. El-Zawahry BM, Esmat S, Bassiouny D et al. Effect of procedural-related variables on melanocyte-keratinocyte suspension transplantation in nonsegmental stable vitiligo: A clinical and immunocytochemical study. *Dermatol Surg* 2017;43(2):226–35.

21. Tegta GR, Parsad D, Majumdar S, and Kumar B. Efficacy of autologous transplantation of noncultured epidermal suspension in two different dilutions in the treatment of vitiligo. *Int J Dermatol* 2006;45(2):106–10.

22. Holla AP, Kumar R, Parsad D, and Kanwar A. Modified procedure of noncultured epidermal suspension transplantation: Changes are the core of vitiligo surgery. *J Cutan Aesthet Surg* 2011;4:44–5.

23. AlJasser MI, Mulekar SS, and Mulekar SV. Epidermal cell suspension: Achieved by incubation at room temperature. *J Cutan Aesthet Surg* 2013;6:126.

24. Mulekar SV, Ghwish B, Al Issa A, and Al Eisa A. Treatment of vitiligo lesions by ReCell vs. conventional melanocyte-keratinocyte transplantation: A pilot study. *Br J Dermatol* 2008;158:45–9.

25. Goh BK, Chua XM, Chong KL, de Mil M, and van Geel NA. Simplified cellular grafting for treatment of vitiligo and piebaldism: The "6-well plate" technique. *Dermatol Surg* 2010;36:203–7.

26. Mrigpuri S, Razmi T M, Sendhil Kumaran M, Vinay K, Srivastava N, and Parsad D. Four compartment method as an efficacious and simplified technique for autologous noncultured epidermal cell suspension preparation in vitiligo surgery: A randomized, active-controlled study. *J Eur Acad Dermatol Venereol* 2019;33:185–90.

CELLULAR GRAFTING TECHNIQUES
Cultured Melanocyte Grafting

Ravinder Kumar, Seema Rani, Naveed Pervaiz, and Davinder Parsad

CONTENTS

INTRODUCTION

Vitiligo is an acquired hypopigmentary disorder characterized by the progressive loss of epidermal melanocytes and sometimes hair follicle melanocytes [1,2]. It is a disease with no mortality but significant psychosocial effects [3], especially in dark-skinned races, that greatly impacts quality of life [4]. Several hypotheses have been put forward to describe the pathogenesis of vitiligo—autoimmune, biochemical, self-destructive, genetic, and neural hypotheses are noteworthy. However, the etiology of vitiligo seems to be multifactorial, with all the factors playing significant roles in the pathogenesis [5].

To date, there is no complete cure for vitiligo, but many treatments are available that can prevent disease progression and help in repigmentation. Common therapeutic options include camouflage products [6], potent topical corticosteroids [7], oral and topical psoralen with ultraviolet A (PUVA) radiation [8], and broadband and narrowband UVB phototherapy [9,10]. Surgical methods represent an alternative therapeutic approach to treating patients with stable vitiligo [11,12]. The surgical techniques used for repigmenting vitiligo lesions are broadly classified in two types: tissue grafting and cellular grafting, based on the nature of the grafts.

Tissue grafting includes transferring of whole skin tissue grafts containing epidermis and dermis to the depigmented recipient skin [11,13]. Cellular grafts, on the other hand, employ the autologous melanocyte rich cell suspension (noncultured technique) [14,15] or the cultured melanocyte (culture technique) to the recipient skin [16]. Both these methods are based on the same principle of selective refilling of melanocytes at the recipient stable vitiligo lesions.

PROCEDURE OF MELANOCYTE CULTURE

The autologous transplantation of cultured melanocyte is performed by following the trypsinization method delineated here.

- *Collection of skin graft*: A shaved biopsy of normal pigmented skin was used as the source for culture of epidermal melanocyte. Skin grafts were obtained under aseptic conditions in phosphate buffer saline (PBS) with added antibiotics (penicillin, streptomycin, gentamycin).

- *Trypsinization*: The graft was cut into small pieces and incubated with a 0.25% trypsin and 0.02% EDTA solution at 4°C overnight (cold trypsinization) or at 37°C for 45 minutes to 1 hour (hot trypsinization). The duration of incubation depends upon the thickness of graft. After trypsinization, trypsin inhibitor in the ratio of 1:1 was added to neutralize the activity of trypsin, and it was then replaced by PBS solution.

The epidermis and dermis were detached from each other with the help of sterile forceps. Thorough pipetting was done to detach the cells from epidermis to prepare the single-cell suspension. The acquired suspension of cells was centrifuged for 5 minutes at 1000 rpm and the obtained cell pellet was used for the culturing of melanocytes.

- *Melanocyte culture*: After centrifugation, the cell pellet was resuspended in serum and *12-O*-tetradecanoylphorbol-13-acetate (TPA) free melanocyte basal media added with growth supplements. The culture was established and maintained in the CO_2 incubator at 37°C, 5% CO_2%, and 95% humidity. Cultures were routinely examined for the contamination, and every 2 days the medium was changed. The melanocyte culture became confluent in 15–20 days (Figures 38.2.1 and 38.2.2).

The epidermal cell suspension technique by trypsinization for vitiligo transplantation was first reported by Gauthier and Surleve-Bazeille in 1992 [17]. The technique of transplantation of cultured autologous melanocytes was reported by Olsson and Juhlin in 1993 [16]. Autologous cultured pure melanocyte suspension is an efficacious therapy for stable vitiligo patients who have failed to respond to clinical treatments, particularly for patients with stable localized vitiligo [18]. Transplantation of cultured melanocytes is a complex, but it provides the best donor-to-recipient size ratio of greater than 1:10 to up to 1:60 [19]. A study [20] demonstrated progressive repigmentation of depigmented skin by both methods of epidermal cell suspension and the cultured melanocyte method. Another study was conducted to determine the relative effectiveness of the autologous transplant of noncultured cell suspension technique and the melanocyte culture technique in the repigmentation of stable vitiligo, which revealed an outstanding response in 62.17% and 52% cases, respectively [21]. In another comparative study, the efficacy of noncultured epidermal cell suspension transplantation, cultured melanocytes transplantation and blister roof grafting in the repigmentation of macules in stable vitiligo was checked [22]. A satisfactory response (450% repigmentation) was accomplished in 81%, 82%, and 92% of the 83 patients with the noncultured epidermal cell suspension transplantation, cultured melanocyte transplantation,

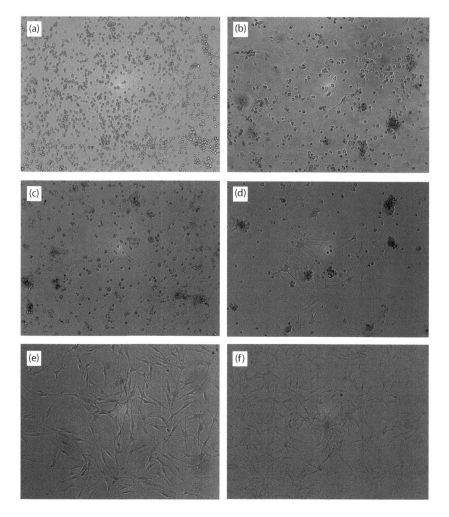

Figure 38.2.1 Representative pictures of the cultured primary melanocytes at day 1 (a), day 5 (b), day 7 (c) day 10 (d), day 14 (e), and day 18 (f). (Original magnification X100.)

and blister roof grafting procedures, correspondingly. A variance in the time of beginning of repigmentation was also witnessed, with repigmentation initially appearing after 430 days, 20–30 days, and 10 days in the noncultured epidermal cell suspension transplantation, cultured melanocyte transplantation, and blister roof grafting groups, respectively. From the studies conducted on transplantation technique, it has been observed that patients are in general satisfied and pleased with the results of both cultured and noncultured techniques [21].

Therefore, it can be concluded that each of the transplantation approaches is efficient and can be utilized according to the dimensions and locations of the lesions. Choice of transplantation

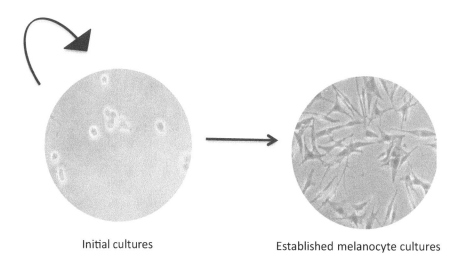

Initial cultures   Established melanocyte cultures

Figure 38.2.2 Figure depicting initial melanocyte cultures and established melanocyte culture. (Courtesy of Dr. Vivek Natrajan, Sr. Scientist IGIB, Delhi.)

technique also depends upon the available laboratory resources. To record long-term repigmentation status and other complications, patients must be monitored for an extended period. However, there is still the need for large-scale patient studies on autologous cultured melanocyte transplant techniques to confirm their relative efficacy.

ADVANTAGES OF AUTOLOGOUS TRANSPLANTATION OF CULTURED MELANOCYTES TECHNIQUE

- It is a clinically efficient method that can be accomplished as outpatient treatment.
- A major advantage is that the melanocytes achieved from skin biopsy are expanded in vitro to treat large depigmented skin, i.e., this method provides the highest donor-to-recipient size ratio.
- The technique has probably the best efficiency in terms of color match [21].
- Repigmentation is likely to remain for an extended period.
- The procedure does not leave any scars at either donor or recipient site.
- No side effects are associated with this transplant technique.
- This technique is a state-of-art novel surgery in vitiligo, and the obtained outcomes specify that the approach can be beneficial in motivated stable vitiligo patients, with affected area not exceeding 30% of the total body surface area [21].

DISADVANTAGES OF AUTOLOGOUS TRANSPLANTATION OF CULTURED MELANOCYTES TECHNIQUE

- The major disadvantage of culturing techniques that it is a time-consuming procedure—it takes several weeks to grow the melanocyte culture.
- Culturing and transfer of melanocytes need highly skilled personnel and well-furnished laboratories.
- Several complications are associated with minor surgical procedures, including infections, graft failures, and bleeding problems.
- Some safety concerns are associated with the use of growth factors, e.g., TPA in the culture medium [23–26].
- The mechanism of vitiligo pathogenesis is still not fully understood, so even after the surgical procedures the stability and reactivation of disease cannot be predicted.

REFERENCES

1. Bilal A and Anwar I. Guidelines for the management of vitiligo. *J Pak Assoc Derma* 2014;24(1):68–78.
2. Zhang Y, Mooneyan-Ramchurn JS, Zuo N, Feng Y, and Xiao S. Vitiligo nonsurgical treatment: A review of latest treatment researches. *Dermatol Ther* 2014;27(5):298–303.
3. Wu J, Zhou M, Wan Y, and Xu A. CD8+ T cells from vitiligo perilesional margins induce autologous melanocyte apoptosis. *Mol Med Rep* 2013;7(1):237–41.
4. Parsad D, Dogra S, and Kanwar AJ. Quality of life in patients with vitiligo. *Health Qual Life Outcomes* 2003;1:58.
5. Njoo MD and Westerhof W. Vitiligo pathogenesis and treatment. *Am J Clin Dermatol* 2001;2(3):167–81.
6. Al-Otaibi SR, Zadeh VB, Al-Abdulrazzaq AH, Tarrab SM, Al-Owaidi HA, Mahrous R, Kadyan RS, and Najem NM. Using a 308-nm excimer laser to treat vitiligo in Asians. *Acta Dermatovenerol Alp Panonica Adriat* 2009;18(1):13–9.
7. Chang HC, Hsu YP, and Huang YC. The effectiveness of topical calcineurin inhibitors compared with topical corticosteroids in the treatment of vitiligo: A systematic review and meta-analysis. *J Am Acad Dermatol* 2020;82(1):243–5.
8. Handa S, Pandhi R, and Kaur I. Vitiligo: A retrospective comparative analysis of treatment modalities in 500 patients. *J Dermatol* 2001;28(9):461–6.
9. Scherschun L, Kim JJ, and Lim HW. Narrow-band ultraviolet B is a useful and well-tolerated treatment for vitiligo. *J Am Acad Dermatol* 2001;44(6):999–1003.
10. Njoo MD, Bos JD, Westerhoff W. Treatment of generalized vitiligo in children with narrow-band (TL01) UVB radiation therapy. *J Am Acad Dermatol* 2000;42(2 Pt 1):245–53.
11. Bahadoran P, and Ortonne JP. Classification of surgical therapies for vitiligo. In: Gupta S, Olsson MJ, Kanwar AJ, and Ortonne JP, eds. *Surgical Management of Vitiligo*. Blackwell Publishing Ltd; 2007, pp. 69–79.
12. Gupta S, Narang T, Olsson MJ, and Ortonne JP. Surgical management of vitiligo and other leukodermas: Evidence-based practice guidelines. In: Gupta S, Olsson MJ, Kanwar AJ, and Ortonne JP, eds. *Surgical Management of Vitiligo*. Massachusetts: Blackwell Publishing Ltd; 2007, pp. 69–79.
13. Majid I. Grafting in vitiligo: How to get better results and how to avoid complications. *J Cutan Aesthet Surg* 2013;6(2):83–9.
14. El-Zawahry BM, Zaki NS, Bassiouny DA, Sobhi RM, Zaghloul A, Khorshied MM, and Gouda HM. Autologous melanocyte-keratinocyte suspension in the treatment of vitiligo. *J Eur Acad Dermatol Venereol* 2011;25(2):215–20.
15. Mulekar SV. Melanocyte-keratinocyte cell transplantation for stable vitiligo. *Int J Dermatol* 2003;42(2):132–6.
16. Olsson MJ and Juhlin L. Long-term follow-up of leukoderma patients treated with transplants of autologous cultured melanocytes, ultrathin epidermal sheets and basal cell layer suspension. *Br J Dermatol* 2002;147(5):893–904.
17. Gauthier Y and Surleve-Bazeille JE. Autologous grafting with non-cultured melanocytes: A simplified method for treatment of depigmented lesions. *J Am Acad Dermatol* 1992;26(2 Pt 1):191–194.
18. Chen YF, Yang PY, Hu DN, Kuo FS, Hung CS, and Hung CM. Treatment of vitiligo by transplantation of cultured pure melanocyte suspension: Analysis of 120 cases. *J Am Acad Dermatol* 2004;51(1):68–74.
19. Hong WS, Hu DN, Qian GP, McCormick SA, and Xu AE. Ratio of size of recipient and donor areas in treatment of vitiligo by autologous cultured melanocyte transplantation. *Br J Dermatol* 2011;165(3):520–5.
20. Issa CMBM, Rehder J, and Taube MBP. Melanocyte transplantation for the treatment of vitiligo: Effects of different surgical techniques. *Eur J Dermatol* 2003;13(1):34–9.
21. Verma R, Grewal RS, Chatterjee M, Pragasam V, Vasudevan B, and Mitra D. A comparative study of efficacy of cultured versus non cultured melanocyte transfer in the management of stable vitiligo. *Med J Armed Forces India* 2014;70(1):26–31.

22. Bao H, Hong W, Fu L, Wei X, Qian G, and Xu A. Blister roof grafting, cultured melanocytes transplantation and non-cultured epidermal cell suspension transplantation in treating stable vitiligo. A mutual self-control study. *J Dermatolog Treat* 2015;26(6):571–4.

23. Van Geel N, Ongenae K, De Mil M, and Naeyaert JM. Modified technique of autologous noncultured epidermal cell transplantation for repigmenting vitiligo: A pilot study. *Dermatol Surg* 2001;27(10):873–6.

24. Van Geel N, Ongenae K, De Mil M, Haeghen YV, Vervaet C, and Naeyaert JM. Double-blind placebo-controlled study of autologous transplanted epidermal cell suspensions for repigmenting vitiligo. *Arch Dermatol* 2004;140(10): 1203–8.

25. Pandya V, Parmar KS, Shah BJ, and Bilimoria FE. A study of autologous melanocyte transfer in treatment of stable vitiligo. *Indian J Dermatol Venereol Leprol* 2005;71(6):393–7.

26. Szabad G, Kormos B, Pivarcsi A, Szell M, Kis K, Kenderessy Szabo A, Dobozy A, Kemeny L, and Bata-Csorgo Z. Human adult epidermal melanocytes cultured without chemical mitogens express the EGF receptor and respond to EGF. *Arch Dermatol Res* 2007;299(4):191–200.

Chapter 39

MANAGEMENT OF DIFFICULT VITILIGO (ACRAL, GENITAL, LIPS, PALMS, AND SOLES)

Sanjeev Gupta and Swetalina Pradhan

CONTENTS

INTRODUCTION

Vitiligo is an acquired and the most common disorder of hypopigmentation, characterized by progressive loss of melanocytes. The estimated prevalence of vitiligo in world is 0.5%–1% in most populations. In almost half of patients, vitiligo starts before the age of 20 years, and it affects males and females equally [1]. Although vitiligo is not a life-threatening disease, it has been associated with concomitant occurrence of a number of other autoimmune diseases, as well as a wide range of psychosocial difficulties, significantly impacting quality of life, and hence needs to be treated [2–4].

Two treatment modalities exist for vitiligo, medical therapy and surgical therapy.

- *Medical therapy*: Always considered as the first line of therapy for vitiligo. The mechanism of action of various medical therapies is to:
  - Enhance epidermal melanocyte accumulation, both by stimulating recovery of damaged melanocytes in situ and by reactivating residual melanocytes or stimulating melanocyte in-migration from neighboring skin or hair follicles.
  - Inhibit the immune response in vitiligo, thereby reducing melanocyte destruction.
- *Surgical therapy*: This can be considered for stable vitiligo that is refractory or only partially responsive to medical therapy, and in general limited in extent.

The mechanism of action of various surgical procedures varies according to the type of surgical modality. The basic principle is to introduce active melanocytes to the lesion sites, which will then establish and function as epidermal melanin units. Transfer of active melanocytes can be done through either tissue grafts or cellular grafts.

However, surgical modalities cannot be performed in resource-poor settings, and experienced physicians are needed to perform them effectively. Side effects like secondary infections and scarring have also been observed. The appoach to a case of vitiligo depends on certain factors:

- Extent of involvement
- Stability of the vitiligo

- Site of involvement
- Response to medical treatment
- Patient compliance to both medical and surgical treatment
- Experience of the treating physician
- Plausibility of the surgical procedure

Difficult sites for vitiligo include:

- Areas with low density of melanocytes (due to absence of hair follicles), e.g., below the ankles, genitalia, lips, distal ends of fingers, and palms.
- Areas like genitals and areolae where phototherapy is not an acceptable option.
- Lesions over joints like wrists and ankles, where response to surgical therapy is poor due to movement of the area, uneven surfaces, and increased chance of loss of transplanted cells [5,6].

LIP VITILIGO

Before considering any treatment modality, the stability of vitiligo should be ascertained. First aim is to make the disease stable by immunosuppressive therapy.

MEDICAL TREATMENT
TOPICAL TREATMENT

Topical corticosteroids are the first-line therapy for localized vitiligo. High-potency fluorinated corticosteroid (e.g., clobetasol propionate ointment, 0.05%) are given for 1–2 months. Treatment can be gradually tapered to a lower potency corticosteroid (e.g., hydrocortisone butyrate cream, 0.1%). It is very important to observe the side effects of topical steroids during treatment.

Calcineurin inhibitors: Calcineurin inhibitors have the capacity to restore the altered cytokine network. Tacrolimus inhibits T cell activation by downregulating transcription of genes encoding proinflammatory cytokines IL-2, IL-3, IL-4, IL-5, interferon-γ (IFN-γ), tumor necrosis factor-α (TNF-α), and granulocyte macrophage colony-stimulating factor (GM-CSF) in T cells. In addition to this, it has a direct effect on melanocyte growth and migration [7,8]. Topical calcineurin inhibitors (e.g., tacrolimus ointment 0.03%–0.1%, pimecrolimus ointment 1%) are generally preferred.

Topical vitamin D analogs: Vitamin D analogs—calcipotriol ointment (0.005%) and tacalcitol ointment (20 µg/g)—restore pigmentation in vitiligo by inducing skin immunosuppression, which halts the local autoimmune process, and via direct activation of melanocytic precursors and melanogenic pathways. However, their efficacy when used alone has been found to be low in various studies and randomized controlled trials. Nevertheless, they have been found to decrease the "mean repigmentation time" when used in combination therapy with potent topical steroids, narrow-band UVB, and PUVA, though the quality of evidence is not high.

PHOTOTHERAPY

Ultraviolet (UV) light therapy is another treatment option with both innate and cellular immunosuppressive as well as mitogenic and melanogenic properties that promote melanocyte proliferation and melanin synthesis [9]. UVA light therapy combined with psoralen (PUVA) helps to reverse melanocyte and keratinocyte degeneration in and around lesions of vitiligo. The sun can also be the source of UVA light in PUVA—a technique termed PUVAsol—which utilizes fewer healthcare resources. UVB therapy is classified as narrowband (NB-UVB, 311–313 nm) or broadband (BB-UVB, 280–320 nm). Although published data suggest that BB-UVB stimulates repigmentation more effectively than NB-UVB, use of the latter predominates due to its exclusion of more harmful wavelengths [10].

SURGICAL TREATMENT
AUTOLOGOUS MINIPUNCH GRAFTING

This is the easiest, fastest, least aggressive, and minimally expensive technique [11]. The procedure is as follows.

After preparing the recipient area, 2% lignocaine (with/without adrenaline) is infiltrated for local anesthesia. The recipient chambers are made on or very close to the border of the lesion. The punched-out chambers are spaced at a gap of 5–10 mm from each other. The donor area is either the upper lateral portion of the thigh or the gluteal area. Punches sized 3 mm are used for both the donor and recipient areas; however, the punch size is not standard—it depends on size of lesion and site. A small-size punch gives better results as far as cosmesis is concerned.

Ideally, the donor site punch should be 0.5 mm bigger than that of recipient site punch. The grafts are placed directly from the donor area to the recipient area. Dressings are removed after 4–7 days. Antibiotics and anti-inflammatory drugs are administered for 8–10 days. PUVA/PUVAsol or NB-UVB are usually given for 3–6 months to enhance repigmentation.

SUCTION BLISTER GRAFTING

This is the best method for lip vitiligo involving a small area. The procedure is as follows.

After raising the blisters on patient's thigh, with the use of syringes/ suction pump/suction cups or a negative pressure cutaneous suction chamber system [12,13], deroofing of the blister is done with the help of iris scissors. The graft is then placed on a glass slide with the dermal side facing upward. The recipient area is then dermabraded using a manual dermabrader, motorized dermabrader, microdermabrader, or a CO_2 laser until minute pinpoint bleeding spots are visible. The grafts are then placed in such a way that the dermal side of the graft comes in contact with the dermabraded area. Graft fixation is done with a sterile moist gauze, giving firm pressure over the graft. The recipient area is then dressed with a double layer of framycetin tulle, moist gauze, followed by sterile gauze and elasto crepe bandage. The dressings over the donor site and recipient site are removed after 24 hours and 7 days, respectively. The patient is advised to keep the area immobile. Some authors advocate removing the dressing on 7th day only.

SPLIT-THICKNESS GRAFTING

Thin split-thickness grafts give a good cosmetic outcome on lip vitiligo involving large areas.

The epidermis and often the uppermost part of superficial dermis is transferred into dermabraded patch of vitiligo, thereby achieving the transfer of melanocytes and keratinocytes from the donor graft to the recipient area. The thickness of the graft ranges from 0.1 mm to 0.7 mm [14]. The gluteal area, anterolateral aspect of the thigh, abdomen, and arms are preferred as donor sites [15,16]. After anesthesia, the area is stretched, and a thin, even split-thickness graft is harvested using either a sterile razor blade mounted on a Kochers forceps or a blade-holding instrument. The grafts thus obtained are transferred to a petri dish containing normal saline. The recipient area is dermabraded until pinpoint hemorrhages are seen uniformly all over the lesion. The grafts obtained are then placed upside down on the sterile glass slides. The slide is then placed on the recipient area and pressed against the skin. The graft is immobilized by using surgical adhesive, octyl-2-cyanoacrylate, and pressure dressing. Patients are advised to avoid excessive movement of the grafted area.

TATTOOING

Tattooing or micropigmentation is defined as uniform implantation of minute inert pigment granules into the dermis so as to artistically create a permanent cosmetic camouflage [17,18]. A thick layer of pigment paste is applied to the site under local anesthetic agent lignocaine 2%. The site is stretched with the thumb and index finger, while the tattooing machine, held in the pen-holding manner, makes repeated vertical movements of needles up and down on the surface of the skin. Tattooing is done in the entire area in an overlapping manner. Follow-up at 4–6 weeks and 6 months may require touch-up tattooing for the areas of pigment that have shed off.

THERAPEUTIC WOUNDING

This is a modality suitable for small and stable vitiligo patches where superficial wounding of epidermis is done to achieve repigmentation. Various modalities like dermabrasion, CO_2 laser, and Er:YAG laser ablation, cryosurgery, needling, spot chemical peeling with 88% phenol solution, or tricolor acetic acid 30%–50% have been used for wounding the vitiligo and thereby to induce repigmentation [19–25].

ACRAL VITILIGO

MEDICAL TREATMENT

Medical treatment is always the first option in any type of vitiligo. However due to inadequate hair density, medical therapy usually fails to achieve complete repigmentation in acral vitiligo, and hence surgical procedures are chosen as second-line treatment modality to achieve repigmentation of remaining stable vitiligo patches.

SURGICAL TREATMENT
PUNCH GRAFTING

Punch grafting is preferred for acral vitiligo and is the best option to treat vitiligo involving the palms and soles.

Mechanism of pigmentation after grafting: The graft of the donor area produces active melanin, and the melanocytes from infundibulum of hair follicles present in the graft spread centrifugally to the basal cell layer and thereby recolonize the epidermis of recipient area with active and functional melanocytes leading to perigraft pigmentation [26].

Advantages:

- Simple, safe, and inexpensive office procedure
- Needs no special training for a dermatologist

- High success rate and excellent cosmetic results
  - Areas of residual vitiligo between grafts or rejected can be re-grafted

SUCTION BLISTER GRAFTING

This method is suitable for vitligo on the dorsal aspects of acral areas.

Principle of suction blister grafting: In suction blister grafting, only the epidermal portion of the donor area is grafted, so the graft generally acquires the characteristics of the recipient site rather than the donor site, resulting in a better color match and cosmetic outcome [27]. The melanocytes are transferred within 48–72 hours from the graft to the recipient site.

Advantages:

- Safe, easy, and inexpensive
- Very good success rates
- Repigmentation is faster
- Very good color match

SPLIT-THICKNESS GRAFTING

Split-thickness grafting is suitable for vitligo on the dorsal aspects of the acral areas.

Advantages:

- Pigmentation can instantly cover larger areas over a short period of time
- Pigmentation achieved is uniform [28]
- Repigmentation of leukotrichia is also possible [29,30]

CELLULAR GRAFTING

Noncultured epidermal cellular grafting is described here [31].

The graft is harvested from the medial aspect of the thigh or the lateral aspect of the gluteal region of size about one-tenth the size of the recipient area. After anesthetizing the area, a very superficial sample of skin is obtained using Silver's skin grafting knife. The graft is then trypsinized and incubated at 37°C for 50 min. The grafts are then transferred into a petri dish containing 8 mL of melanocyte nourishment medium, i.e,. Dulbecco's modified Eagle's medium (DMEM)/F-12. The epidermis is further broken into smaller pieces in a petri dish and washed with the DMEM/F-12 medium and finally transferred to a test tube containing the DMEM/F-12 medium. The test tube is then centrifuged for 6 minutes at 3000 rpm and the pellet at the bottom is suspended in a 1 mL insulin syringe after discarding the supernatant. The cell suspension is then applied evenly on the dermabraded recepient area, which is then covered with dressing. The dressing is removed after 1 week. Phototherapy can be initiated after 3 weeks.

Advantages:

- Tenfold large areas can be treated at a time
- Excellent cosmetic results
- Excellent texture and color matching
- No stuck-on look
- No cobblestoning

CULTURED MELANOCYTE TRANSPLANTATION

After the formation of cell suspension pellet, the cell suspension is cultured in tissue culture flasks along with 05 mL of M2 medium which is F12 medium supplemented with bFGF (20 ng/ml), isobutyl methyl xanthine (0.1 mM), cholera toxin (10 ng/mL), glutamine 2 mM and 10% fetal bovine serum (serum free tetradecanoylphorbol acetate) to attain a density of 1000–2000 melanocytes/mm [2]. The cultured grafts are transferred to a petridish, containing 8 mL of DMEM media and then centrifuged at 3000 rpm for 6 min. The melanocyte cell suspension pellet is obtained and is transplanted to the recipient area [32,33].

Advantages:

- A very small donor graft is adequate to cover a very large area
- The cells can be cryopreserved for future use

Disadvantages:

- This method is not very user friendly
- It requires a skilled staff and good infrastructure
- This method is more of academic interest
- It is not very feasible in a private setup

GENITAL VITILIGO

Treatment of genital vitiligo is difficult, as hair follicles are absent in glabrous skin of genitalia [34]. There have been reports of genital vitiligo treated with topical pimecrolimus and other various surgical procedures like melanocyte transplantation (cultured and noncultured melanocytes) [35–38]. However, other procedures like suction blister grafts, thin split-thickness skin grafts, and minipunch grafts can be tried in genital vitiligo depending on the size of the vitiligo patch and the expertise of the surgeon. Before undertaking surgical treatment of vitiligo, a history of genital herpes should be ruled out, and in all such cases long-term prophylaxis with acyclovir should be given and the prognosis should be explained to the patient [39].

AREOLAE

Just like genitalia and the palms and soles, treatment of vitiligo in areolae is challenging due to absence of hair folicles in this region. Surgical treatment is the best mode of treatment in vitiligo involving the areolae. Both tissue grafting and cellular grafting can be tried in such cases, however the procedure obtaining most uniform color should be tried. Various procedures such as suction blister grafting, split-thickness grafting, and autologous melanocyte suspension (both cultured and noncultured) achieve good results in areola vitiligo resulting in uniform color.

SCALP

MEDICAL TREATMENT
TOPICAL

There are no specific studies on the use of topical steroids and topical tacrolimus in scalp vitiligo. Both of these can be used in lotion formulation in stable localized vitiligo involving the scalp, as in other areas.

Topical melagenine: In one study, topical melagenine−infrared combination treatment was used in treatment of scalp vitiligo in children and was found to be effective in 45% cases [40].

PHOTOTHERAPY

PUVAsol: After removing the hair on the vitiligo patch either by shaving, plucking, or chemical epilation, the patient can be given PUVAsol treatment.

Comb phototherapy: After taking oral psoralen, the patient can have exposure to UVA or UVB through a comb that emits UVA/UVB light.

Turban PUVA: This can be used as a treatment modality for scalp vitiligo. The hair on the affected area needs to be removed. An absorbent cotton cloth is soaked for 30 seconds in a 3.75 mg/L solution of

8-methoxypsoralen and is gently squeezed to remove excess water and wrapped around the head for 5 minutes. This is repeated four times (i.e., a total of 20 minutes) and the area is then exposed to UVA or sunlight. If sunlight is used as the source of UVA, exposure starts with 5 minutes, increased by 1 minute with each exposure up to a maximum of 15 minutes. The treatment is given three to four times/week.

SURGICAL TREATMENT
There are reports of successful treatment of leukotrichia and vitiligo scalp with transplantation of autologous cultured pure melanocyte and epidermal grafting [41,42].

SUMMARY OF PREFERRED TREATMENT MODALITY

Area	Method of choice	Alternative method
Lip	Suction blister, epidermal cell suspension	Split-thickness grafts, punch grafting
Acral areas	Punch grafts	
Genital	Suction blister, epidermal cell suspension	Split-thickness grafts, punch grafting
Areola	Suction blister grafting, split-thickness grafting, epidermal cell suspension	Punch grafting

REFERENCES

1. Ezzedine K, Eleftheriadou V, Whitton M, and van Geel N. Vitiligo. *Lancet* 2015;386(9988):74–84.
2. Kostopoulou P, Jouary T, Quintard B, Ezzedine K, Marques S, Boutchnei S, and Taieb A. Objective vs. subjective factors in the psychological impact of vitiligo: The experience from a French referral centre. *Br J Dermatol* 2009;161:128–33.
3. Mashayekhi V, Javidi Z, Kiafar B, Manteghi AA, Saadatian V, Esmaeili HA, and Hosseinalizadeh S. Quality of life in patients with vitiligo: A descriptive study on 83 patients attending a PUVA therapy unit in Imam Reza Hospital, Mashad. *Indian J Dermatol Venereol Leprol* 2010;76:592.
4. Wang KY, Wang KH, and Zhang ZP. Health-related quality of life and marital quality of vitiligo patients in China. *J Eur Acad Dermatol Venereol* 2011b;25:429–35.
5. Holla AP, and Parsad D. Vitiligo surgery: Its evolution as a definite treatment in the stable vitiligo. *G Ital Dermatol Venereol* 2010; 145: 79–88.
6. Mutalik S. Surgical management of acral vitiligo. In: Gupta S, Olsson MJ, Kanwar AJ, and Ortonne JP, eds. *Surgical Management of Vitiligo*, 1st ed. Massachusetts: Blackwell Publishing Ltd.; 2007, pp. 225–8.
7. Lan CC, Chen GS, Chiou MH, Wu CS, Chang CH, and Yu HS. FK506 promotes melanocyte and melanoblast growth and creates a favourable milieu for cell migration via keratinocytes: Possible mechanisms of how tacrolimus ointment induces repigmentation in patients with vitiligo. *Br J Dermatol* 2005;153:498–505.
8. Wong R, and Lin AN. Efficacy of topical calcineurin inhibitors in vitiligo. *Int J Dermatol* 2013;52:491–6.
9. Anbar TS, El-Sawy AE, Attia SK et al. Effect of PUVA therapy on melanocytes and keratinocytes in non-segmental vitiligo: Histopathological, immuno-histochemical and ultrastructural study. *Photodermatol Photoimmunol Photomed* 2012;28:17–25.
10. El-Mofty M, Mostafa W, Youssef R et al. BB-UVA vs. NB-UVB in the treatment of vitiligo: A randomized controlled clinical study (single blinded). *Photodermatol Photoimmunol Photomed* 2013;29:239–246.
11. Malakar S, and Lahiri K. Punch grafting for lip leucoderma. *Dermatology* 2004;208(2):125–8.
12. Gupta S, Shroff S, and Gupta S. Modified technique of suction blistering for epidermal grafting in vitiligo. *Int J Dermatol* 1999;38:306–9.
13. Gupta S. Double syringe blistering by adding a three-way connector. *J Dermatolog Treat* 2001;12:219.
14. Robinson JK. *Surgery of the Skin: Procedural Dermatology.* Philadelphia, PA: Elsevier Mosby; 2005.
15. Behl PN, Azad O, Kak R et al. Autologous thin Thiersch's grafts in vitiligo: Experience of 8000 cases, 50,000 grafts (1959–98) with modified technique in 198 cases in the year 1997–98. *Indian J Dermatol Venereol Leprol* 1999;65:117–21.
16. Khunger N. Thin split-thickness skin grafts for vitiligo. In: Gupta S et al., eds. *Surgical Management of Vitiligo*. Blackwell Publishing Ltd; 2007, pp. 108–14.
17. Savant SS. Tattooing. In: Savant SS, Shah RA, and Gore D, eds. *Textbook and Atlas of Dermatosurgery and Cosmetology*. AS CAD Publishers Mumbai (India); 1998, pp. 222–6.
18. Roberts TA, and Ryan SA. Tattooing and high-risk behavior in adolescents. *Pediatrics* 2002;110:1058–63.
19. Savant SS. Therapeutic spot and regional dermabrasion in stable vitiligo. *Indian J Dermatol Venereol Leprol* 1996;62:139–45.
20. Savant SS. Therapeutic spot dermabrasion. Study of 197 sites in 11 skin conditions. *Indian J Dermatol Surg* 1999;1:6–15.
21. Savant SS. Therapeutic wounding. In: Savant SS, ed. *Textbook and Atlas of Dermatosurgery and Cosmetology*, 2nd ed. Mumbai: ASCAD; 2005, pp. 370–7.
22. Savant SS. Cryosurgery with liquid nitrogen in stable vitiligo. *Indian J Dermatol Venereol Leprol* 1999;65:246–7.
23. Ahmad TJ, Rashid T, and Rani Z. Needling: An adjunct to narrowband ultraviolet B therapy in localized fixed vitiligo. *J Pak Assoc Derma* 2008;18:149–53.
24. Savant SS, and Shenoy S. Chemical peeling with phenol for the treatment of stable vitiligo and alopecia areata. *Indian J Dermatol Venereol Leprol* 1999;65:93–8.
25. Savant SS. Surgical therapy of vitiligo: Current status. *Indian J Dermatol Venereol Leprol* 2005;71:307–10.
26. Falabella R. Treatment of localized vitiligo by autologous minigrafting. *Arch Dermatol* 1988;124:1649–55.
27. Khunger N, Kathuria SD, and Ramesh V. Tissue grafts in vitiligo surgery—past, present, and future. *Indian J Dermatol* 2009;54(2):150–158.
28. Khandpur S, Sharma VK, and Manchanda Y. Comparison of minipunch grafting versus split-skin grafting in chronic stable vitiligo. *Dermatol Surg* 2005;31:436–41.
29. Agrawal K, and Agrawal A. Vitiligo: Surgical repigmentation of leukotrichia. *Dermatol Surg* 1995;21:711–5.
30. Bose SK. Is there any treatment of leukotrichia in stable vitiligo? *J Dermatol* 1997;24:615–7.

31. Gauthier Y, and Surleve-Bazeille JE. Autologous grafting with non-cultured melanocytes: A simplified method for treatment of depigmented lesions. *J Am Acad Dermatol* 1992; 26:191–4.

32. Eisinger M, and Marko O. Selective proliferation of normal human melanocytes *in vitro* in the presence of phorbol ester and cholera toxin. *Proc Natl Acad Sci U S A* 1982;79:2018–22.

33. Lerner AB, Halaban R, Klaus SN, and Moellmann GE. Transplantation of human melanocytes. *J Invest Dermatol* 1987;89:219–24.

34. Olsson MJ, and Juhlin L. Transplantation of melanocytes in vitiligo. *Br J Dermatol* 1995;132(4):587–591.

35. Mulekar SV, Al Issa A, Al Eisa A, and Asaad M. Genital vitiligo treated by autologous, noncultured melanocyte–keratinocyte cell transplantation. *Dermatol Surg* 2005;31(12):1737–1739.

36. Souza Leite RM, and Craveiro Leite AA. Two therapeutic challenges: Periocular and genital vitiligo in children successfully treated with pimecrolimus cream. *Int J Dermatol* 2007;46(9):986–989.

37. Redondo P, del Olmo J, García-Guzman M, Guembe L, and Prósper F. Repigmentation of vitiligo by transplantation of autologous melanocyte cells cultured on amniotic membrane. *Br J Dermatol* 2008;58(5):1134–1173.

38. Anbar T, Hegazy R, Picardo M, and Taieb A. Beyond vitiligo guidelines: Combined stratified/personalized approaches for the vitiligo patient. *Exp Dermatol* 2014;23(4):219−23.

39. Mulekar SV, Al Issa A, Al Eisa A, and Asaad M. Genital vitiligo treated by autologous, noncultured melanocyte-keratinocyte cell transplantation. *Dermatol Surg* 2005;31:1737–40.

40. Xu AE, and Wei XD. Topical melagenine for repigmentation in twenty-two child patients with vitiligo on the scalp. *Chin Med J (Engl)* 2004 Feb;117(2):199–201.

41. Wu XG, and Xu AE. Successful treatment of vitiligo on the scalp of a 9-year-old girl using autologous cultured pure melanocyte transplantation. *Pediatr Dermatol* 2017;34(1):e22–3.

42. Kim CY, Yoon TJ, and Kim TH. Epidermal grafting after chemical epilation in the treatment of vitiligo. *Dermatol Surg* 2001;27(10):855−6.

Chapter 40

MICRONEEDLING IN VITILIGO

Vijay Zawar and Gayatri Karad

CONTENTS

INTRODUCTION

Vitiligo is a chronic acquired depigmenting disorder affecting approximately 1%–2% of the world's population [1]. Various theories are proposed for its etiology, including genetic, autoimmune, autocytotoxic, and neuronal theories. There is also a well-known association with thyroid and diabetes mellitus, which makes treatment challenging. Therapeutic success also varies, depending on the activity, association, and site of lesions [1,2]. Various therapies such as medical treatment with corticosteroids (oral and topical), immunosuppressants such as azathioprine, and oral or topical psoralens plus ultraviolet A (PUVA) are used as primary modes of therapy to achieve repigmentation [1,2]. For those not responding to medical treatment alone and phototherapy (narrowband ultraviolet B [NB-UVB] therapy and UVA), various surgical modalities (autologous transplantation, split-thickness epidermal grafting, suction blister grafting, melanocyte cell transfer) are successful used either alone or in conjunction with medical treatment to achieve repigmentation [1–3]. Despite numerous recent advances in the form of new modalities, treatment of vitiligo remains an unsolved problem. Needling is relatively recent addition, especially for those who are not responding to medical measures, phototherapy, and denies undergoing surgical procedure [4].

The process of pushing of needle into the epidermis is called needling. Its application is in the vitiligo patch, where multiple sites are penetrated by a needle from pigmented area to depigmented area. This micro-pushing drags the epidermal cells with melanocytes, leading to micro-inoculation of melanocyte in the vitiligo patch [2].

MECHANISM OF ACTION

The mechanisms postulated for the action of microneedling inducing pigmentation in vitiligo (Figure 40.1) [2–4].

Penetrating trauma of the epidermis is the primary mode of action of needling, as it leads to perforation of epidermis, creating multiple mini-pores over the stratum corneum and consecutively inciting a strong inflammatory reaction of wound healing locally, leading to inflammatory cascade as described in Figure 40.1.

Microneedling also enhances the transdermal drug delivery of topical therapies through the microchannels by bypassing the stratum corneum barrier in adequate concentration, and stimulates melanocyte proliferation and migration (Table 40.1) [5].

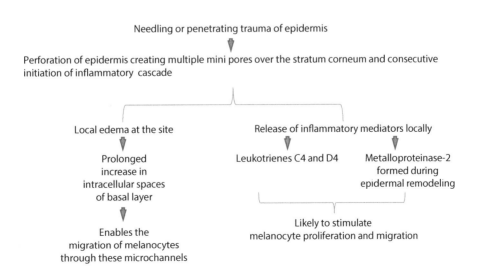

Figure 40.1 Conglomeration of the events which facilitate melanocyte activation and enables its migration from the pigmented periphery of the vitiligo patch or outer root sheath of pigmented hair to the depigmented epidermis [2–4].

Table 40.1   Studies of needling with combination of various therapies

Author	Studies	Response
Ahmad et al. [6]	Needling with narrowband ultraviolet B (NB-UVB)	90% Showed excellent response
Stanimirovic et al. [7]	Microneedling, NB-UVB, topical latanoprost against topical latanoprost and NB-UVB	Microneedling combination therapy Showed 26%–50% repigmentation in 20.8% >50 Repigmentation in only 8.8%, suggesting modification of microneedling technique
Song et al. [8]	Fire needling therapy	79.8% Showed repigmentation compared to control (<0.05)
Santosh et al. [3]	Microneedling with topical 5-FU (26-gauge needle)	60% Showed repigmentation at 3 months
Sheikh [2]	Needle with NB-UVB (30 gauge)	90% Showed repigmentation

PROCEDURE

- Detailed counseling about the procedure and results should be done followed by written informed consent.
- Apply local anesthetic cream (2.5% lidocaine and 2.5% prilocaine) over the vitiligo patch 1 hour before the procedure [4].
- The area to be surgically cleansed with betadine followed by Sterillium (1-propanol and 2-propanol with 75% mecetronium methyl sulfate).
- *Size of the needle*: 20 gauge (various studies have used different sizes such as 26- and 30-gauge). A 20-gauge needle is inserted at an angle of 45° into the pigmented skin on the rim of a vitiligo patch and then moved gradually toward the depigmented zone with multiple insertions at several places.

The appearance of pinpoint bleeding is taken as an endpoint (Figure 40.2).

Post-procedure: Topical mupirocin and anti-inflammatory tablet SOS is given following the procedure.

Number of sittings: Three to four sittings 2 weeks apart depending on the size and response.

Follow-up: We observed improved peripheral as well perifollicular pigmentation in the patch after first sitting, which gradually showed excellent repigmentation after three sittings (Figures 40.3 and 40.4).

Indications:

- Stable localized vitiligo not responding to medical measures or NB-UVB and denies undergoing surgical procedure
- Post grafting achromic borders

Contraindications:

- Active vitiligo
- Viral or bacterial infection at the site
- Pregnancy (insufficient data available for its safety)

Advantages:

- Simple, inexpensive office-based procedure

Disadvantages:

- Not effective for larger patches
- Multiple sittings required

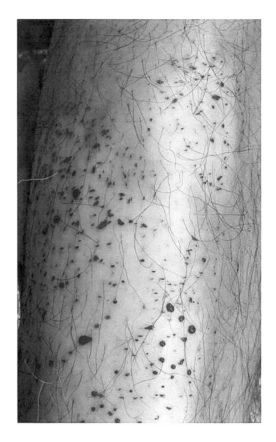

Figure 40.2   Appearance of pinpoint bleeding taken as an endpoint for microneedling.

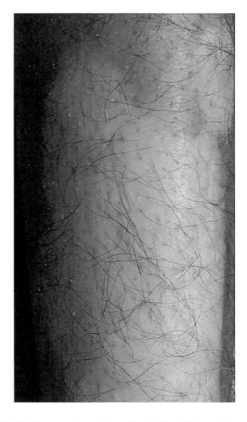

Figure 40.3   Preoperative picture of a stable vitiligo patch on leg not responding to medical management.

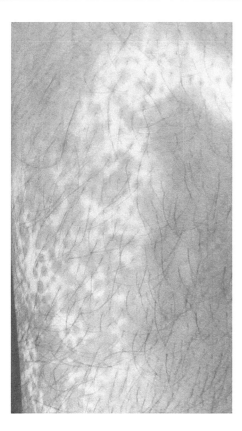

Figure 40.4 Postoperative pictures after the first sitting. Peripheral as well perifollicular pigmentation are noted; the response improved further after three sittings.

MODIFICATION OF NEEDLING

There are various studies where needling is used in combination with topical therapies, shown in Table 40.1. Combination therapies such as NB-UVB, topical application of 5-fluorouracuil, tacrolimus, and latanaprost are successfully used. Fire needling was used by Song et al. by heating the needle before the procedure [8]. NB-UVB can be used in combination with needling for vitiligo unresponsive to medical measures. Malik et al. used Dermaroller with topical 0.1% tacrolimus for extensive vitiligo [5].

CONCLUSION

Localized unresponsive vitiligo to medical measures after treatment with needling achieves repigmentation, and if combined with other topical measures used in vitiligo or NB-UVB, further enhances a favorable response in previously unresponsive vitiligo.

REFERENCES

1. Vedamurthy M, Moorthy A, and Samuel S. Successful treatment of vitiligo by needling with topical 5-fluorouracil. *Pigment Disord* 2016;3:242.

2. Sheikh MI. Needle sheikhing treatment of vitiligo, a study of needling + UVB for vitiligo. *Cosmetol J* 2017;1(1):000101.

3. Santosh SK, Sushantika, Mohan L, Gupta AK, Mohammad A, and Kumar N. Treatment of vitiligo with 5-Fluorouracil after microneedling of the lesion. *Int J Sci Stud* 2018;5(11):125–7.

4. Zawar VP, and Karad GM. Needling in unresponsive vitiligo. *J Am Acad Dermatol* 2016;75(5):e199–200.

5. Malik N, Singh Y, and Goyal T. A simple office-based procedure for patients with extensive vitiligo. *J Am Acad Dermatol* 2016;75(5):e195-7.

6. Ahmad TJ, Rashid T, and Rani Z. Needling: An adjunct to narrowband ultraviolet B therapy in localized fixed vitiligo. *J Pak Assoc Dermatol* 2008 July;18:49–153.

7. Stanimirovic A, Kovacevic M, Korobko I, Šitum M, and Lotti T. Combined therapy for resistant vitiligo lesions: NB-UVB, microneedling, a topical latanoprost, showed no enhanced efficacy compared to topical latanoprost and NB-UVB. *Dermatol Ther* 2016;29(5):312–6.

8. Song X, Tang S, Jiang W, Wang Q, Xu R, and Xie S. Observations on the efficacy of fire needling therapy for vitiligo. *Shanghai J Acupuncture Moxibustion* 2017;36:983–5.

Chapter 41

PRP IN VITILIGO

Rajesh Kumar and Neetu Bhari

CONTENTS

INTRODUCTION

Platelet-rich plasma (PRP) refers to a high concentration of platelets that are concentrated into a small volume of plasma. The concept was first popularized by Whitman in 1997 and Marx et al. in 1998 in oral and maxillofacial surgery for regenerative medicine [1,2]. PRP is currently widely used in various fields of dermatology, from chronic ulcer management to trichology and aesthetics, due to its role in wound healing.

WHAT IS PRP?

PRP is defined as the volume of the plasma that has a platelet concentration above the baseline value [3]. For therapeutic effectiveness, a platelet count of 4–5 times above the baseline should be present in the concentrate. A platelet concentration of at least 1,000,000 platelets/μL in 5 mL of plasma is required in PRP with a three- to fivefold increase in growth factor concentrations.

MECHANISM OF ACTION

PRP contains various growth factors contained in alpha granules and dense granules of platelets. Alpha granules contain various growth factors as platelet-derived growth factors (PDGFaa, PDGFbb, and PDGFab), transforming growth factor beta (TGFb1 and 2), epithelial growth factor (EGF), and vascular endothelial growth factor (VEGF) [4]. In an analysis of PRP prepared from 10 healthy individuals, in comparison to the whole blood as compared with platelet-rich plasma, the platelet-derived growth factor-BB concentration increased from 3.3 +/− 0.9 ng/mL to 17 +/− 8 ng/mL, TGFb1 concentration increased from 35 +/− 8 ng/mL to 120 +/− 42 ng/mL, VEGF concentration increased from 155 +/− 110 pg/mL to 955 +/− 1030 pg/mL, and EGF concentration increased from 129 +/− 61 pg/mL to 470 +/− 320 pg/mL [5].

These cytokines play important roles in cell proliferation, chemotaxis, cell differentiation, and angiogenesis. Platelet-derived growth factor has a significant role in the formation of blood vessels (angiogenesis) that induces proliferation of various cells as epithelial cells, collagen tissue, and smooth muscle cells. VEGF is another chemical signal stimulating the growth of new blood vessels and tissue growth. Dense granules of platelet contain serotonin, histamine, dopamine, calcium, and adenosine. These bioactive factors have fundamental effects on the biologic aspects of wound healing [6].

PREPARATION OF PRP

PRP is prepared either manually or by the use of automated devices. The process must be carried out under strict aseptic conditions as well as optimum temperature regulations; that is, 20–22°C. In order to inhibit platelet aggregation, it is prepared with an anticoagulant, commonly using anticoagulant citrate dextrose solution formula A (ACD-A) or sodium citrate [7].

Two centrifugation steps are required to separate platelet-rich plasma from whole blood. The first step is "light-spin" centrifugation, which separates red blood cells (RBCs) from the rest of the plasma, and subsequently the platelets are concentrated by "heavy-spin" centrifugation with removal of the supernatant plasma.

The basis of this centrifugation process is separation of the blood components owing to their different specific gravities, RBCs being the heaviest, precipitates first followed by other cells. The first centrifugation is slow and results in separation of RBCs at the bottom of the tube. Platelets are mostly concentrated right on top of the buffy coat layer.

Subsequent centrifugation is faster so that platelets are spun down and separate as a pellet at the bottom of the tube from platelet-poor plasma (PPP) above. Approximately 3/4 of the supernatant is discarded, and the platelet-rich pellet is resuspended in the remaining plasma. PRP is usually activated by adding $CaCl_2$ (250 μL per 1 mL of plasma) just before its injection. The viability of the platelets is assured by carrying out the process in a refrigerated centrifuge at 20°C. Trypan blue staining can confirm the viable state of the platelet concentrate obtained by the aforementioned method.

The active secretion of prepackaged growth factors begins within 10 minutes of clot initiation and most of the secretion is completed within first hour. Hence, PRP must be used within 10 minutes of activation to achieve maximum concentration of growth factors.

CLASSIFICATION OF PRP

Ehrenfest et al. proposed a classification of platelet concentrates into four categories, depending upon their leucocyte and fibrin content as follows [8].

LEUCOCYTE-POOR OR PURE PLATELET-RICH PLASMA (P-PRP)

After the first slow spin centrifugation, three layers are obtained as RBC base, buffy coat (BC) and acellular plasma. Acellular plasma contains plasma poor in growth factors (PPGF) and plasma rich in growth factors (PRGF). The PPGF layer (1 mL) is discarded, and the PRGF, just above the BC, is collected by careful pipetting. PRGF from all sample tubes is collected into one tube and calcium chloride is added for clotting.

LEUCOCYTE- AND PLATELET-RICH PLASMA (L-PRP)

After the first centrifugation, the blood components are separated into three layers of RBCs, BC, and acellular plasma. The plasma and BC layers are then carefully transferred to another tube and are subjected to a second centrifugation step at high speed. After the second centrifugation step, PPP is discarded, and the PRP concentrate obtained with this method is composed of a high quantity of platelets, leucocytes, and circulating fibrinogen.

PURE PLATELET-RICH FIBRIN (P-PRF)

Blood is collected with anti-coagulant and is centrifuged at high speed. Blood separates in three layers of RBCs, BC, and plasma. BC and plasma are transferred to a second tube containing $CaCl_2$ which triggers the clotting process and a platelet-rich fibrin matrix (PRFM) clot is obtained after centrifugation.

LEUCOCYTE- AND PLATELET-RICH FIBRIN (L-PRF)

Blood is collected without any anticoagulant and immediately centrifuged in slow spin. A natural coagulation process results in separation of blood is into three components with the formation of a strong fibrin clot in the middle of the tube. This clot acts as a plug that traps most light blood components, such as platelets and leucocytes, as well as circulating molecules, such as growth factors and fibronectin.

DERMATOLOGICAL INDICATIONS OF PRP

PRP has been tried with varying results in a vast array of indications in dermatology:

1. Androgenetic alopecia
2. Alopecia areata
3. Skin rejuvenation
4. Acne scars and contour defects
5. Wound ulcers, connective tissue disease—associated ulcers
6. Leprosy neuropathy
7. Striae distensae
8. Lipodermatosclerosus
9. Lichen sclerosus
10. Vitiligo

PRP IN VITILIGO

In view of limited response to the existing therapies in vitiligo, there is a continuous search for better treatment options in the management of vitiligo. It has shown its efficacy in augmenting the repigmentation in two case studies so far [9,10]. It was used as intradermal injections for localized disease as a monotherapy in the first study while, its use in the second study was an adjunct therapy to narrowband ultraviolet B.

The exact mechanism of action of PRP in vitiligo in unknown. The proposed mechanisms of action are as follows:

1. Deficiency in growth factors may be responsible for the weak attachment of melanocytes to the basal layer of keratinocytes leading to melanocytorrhagy and their transepidermal elimination [11]. PRP may improve the melanocyte—keratinocyte interaction by providing growth factors stabilizing their bond.

2. PRP treatment—induced accelerated proliferation and migration of fibroblasts through upregulation of cyclin E and CDK4 may help in improving the stabilization of melanocytes fibroblast interaction [12].

3. Growth factors in PRP are known to suppress proinflammatory cytokine release, thus limiting inflammation and promoting tissue regeneration [13]. Studies have shown that inflammatory cytokines play an important role in the pathogenesis of vitiligo. Vitiligo patients have shown significantly higher concentration of proinflammatory cytokines as IL-6 and IL-2 with a lower concentration of anti-inflammatory cytokine as IFNγ compared to control population [14]. The role of cellular immunity in vitiligo was also substantiated by a study involving 45 patients with vitiligo and 45 healthy controls, showing higher levels of IL-2, IL-4, and IL-17 ($P < 0.001$) and lower levels of TGF-b ($P < 0.001$) in patients as compared with control subjects [15]. Thus, growth factors in PRP may halt the progression of vitiligo by virtue of their anti-inflammatory properties.

4. Angiogenic factors in PRP as VEGF and fibroblast growth factor enhances proliferation of undifferentiated mesenchymal stem cells [16]. These stem cells may contribute to the proliferation and differentiation of epidermal and dermal cells as keratinocytes, melanocytes, and fibroblasts. Proliferation of melanocytes will result in repigmentation of the vitiligo lesions, and proliferation of the other two cells will result in stabilization of melanocytes in the epidermis.

CONCLUSION

Although existing evidence favors the use of PRP in the management of vitiligo as a stand-alone or an adjunct therapy, future studies are warranted to explore this use of PRP in dermatology.

REFERENCES

1. Whitman DH, Berry RL, and Green DM. Platelet gel: An autologous alternative to fibrin glue with applications in oral and maxillofacial surgery. *J Oral Maxillofac Surg* 1997;55:1294–9.

2. Marx RE, Carlson ER, Eichstaedt RM, Schimmele SR, Strauss JE, and Georgeff KR. Platelet-rich plasma: Growth factor enhancement for bone grafts. *Oral Surg Oral Med Oral Pathol Oral Radiol Endod* 1998;85:638–46.

3. Marx RE. Platelet-rich plasma (PRP): What is PRP and what is not PRP? *Implant Dent* 2001;10:225–8.

4. Lubkowska A, Dolegowska B, and Banfi G. Growth factor content in PRP and their applicability in medicine. *J Biol Regul Homeost Agents* 2012;26(2 Suppl 1):3s–22s.

5. Eppley BL, Woodell JE, and Higgins J. Platelet quantification and growth factor analysis from platelet-rich plasma: Implications for wound healing. *Plast Reconstr Surg* 2004;114:1502–8.

6. Foster TE, Puskas BL, Mandelbaum BR, Gerhardt MB, and Rodeo SA. Platelet-rich plasma: From basic science to clinical applications. *Am J Sports Med* 2009;37:2259–72.

7. Arshdeep, and Kumaran MS. Platelet-rich plasma in dermatology: Boon or a bane? *Indian J Dermatol Venereol Leprol* 2014;80:5–14.

8. Dohan Ehrenfest DM, Rasmusson L, and Albrektsson T. Classification of platelet concentrates: From pure platelet-rich plasma (P-PRP) to leucocyte- and platelet-rich fibrin (L-PRF). *Trends Biotechnol* 2009;27:158–67.

9. Lim HK, Sh MK, and Lee MH. Clinical application of PRP in vitiligo: A pilot study. *Official 1st International Pigment Cell Conference*, Bordeaux, France 2011.

10. Ibrahim ZA, El-Ashmawy AA, El-Tatawy RA, and Sallam FA. The effect of platelet-rich plasma on the outcome of short-term narrowband-ultraviolet B phototherapy in the treatment of vitiligo: A pilot study. *J Cosmet Dermatol* 2016;15:108–16.

11. Kumar R, and Parsad D. Melanocytorrhagy and apoptosis in vitiligo: Connecting jigsaw pieces. *Indian J Dermatol Venereol Leprol* 2012;78:19–23.

12. Cho JW, Kim SA, and Lee KS. Platelet-rich plasma induces increased expression of G1 cell cycle regulators, type I collagen, and matrix metalloproteinase-1 in human skin fibroblasts. *Int J Mol Med* 2012;29:32–6.

13. El-Sharkawy H, Kantarci A, Deady J, Hasturk H, Liu H, Alshahat M, and Van Dyke TE. Platelet-rich plasma: Growth factors and pro- and anti-inflammatory properties. *J Periodontol* 2007;78:661–9.

14. Singh S, Singh U, and Pandey SS. Serum concentration of IL-6, IL-2, TNF-α, and IFNγ in vitiligo patients. *Indian J Dermatol* 2012;57:12–4.

15. Khan R, Gupta S, and Sharma A. Circulatory levels of T-cell cytokines (interleukin [IL]-2, IL-4, IL-17, and transforming growth factor-β) in patients with vitiligo. *J Am Acad Dermatol* 2012;66:510–1.

16. Rubio-Azpeitia E, and Andia I. Partnership between platelet-rich plasma and mesenchymal stem cells: *In vitro* experience. *Muscles, Ligaments Tendons J* 2014;4:52–62.

Chapter 42

DERMABRASION IN VITILIGO

Bharat Bhushan Mahajan, Shweta Sethi, and Shashank Tyagi

CONTENTS

INTRODUCTION

Vitiligo is a cumbersome pigmentary disorder characterized by loss of melanocytes from the skin and subsequent development of depigmented patches of variable sizes that may enlarge and coalesce to form extensive areas of leukoderma [1]. There are many forms of treatment available for vitiligo. Up to 80% of patients suffering from vitiligo respond to medical treatment [2,3]. However, when the disease becomes stable and refractory to medical treatment, surgical treatment may be the only viable option to replenish the lost melanocytes. Dermabrasion is an extensively used surgical modality for treating many cutaneous problems like facial scars, acne, stable vitiligo, hyperkeratotic lesions, pigmentation, tumors, actinic lesions, and removal of tattoos [4].

Dermabrasion consists of sequential planing of areas from the epidermis through the superficial and midpapillary dermis to the junction of the upper and mid-reticular dermis with electrical or manual abrader and allowing the wound to heal by secondary intention. Dermabrasion achieves a resurfacing effect and makes the lesion appear less conspicuous. Re-epithelialization takes place from remnants of dermal appendages like sebaceous glands, hair follicles, and sweat glands. The process of re-epithelialization begins within 24 hours and takes about 10 days to complete. The process of re-epithelialization after dermabrasion has been confirmed by histopathological examination of the lesion after 10 days [5].

INDICATIONS

Stable vitiligo is one of the main indications for dermabrasion. Stability in vitiligo has been defined as no progression in the form of appearance of new lesions or enlargement of existing lesions for at least 12 months [6].

Apart from vitiligo, dermabrasion is used for many other dermatological conditions, which are summarized in Table 42.1.

CONTRAINDICATIONS

1. Active progressive disease and positive Koebner phenomenon
2. Infection at the site of transplantation
3. Keloid diathesis
4. Bleeding diathesis

PROCEDURE

EQUIPMENT

1. Mechanical (manual) (Figure 42.1)
   a. Sandpapers (Water paper No. 80,110)
   b. Hand-held metallic dermabraders (Dr. Maneksha's)
2. Electrical (Figures 42.1–42.2)
   a. Wire brushes and diamond fraises (various sizes and shapes)
   b. Cable unit or hand machine (average 15000 rpm)

Table 42.1 Indications for dermabrasion

1. Stable vitiligo	Stability has been defined as no progression in the form of appearance of new lesions or enlargement of existing lesions for at least 12 months
2. Facial scars	Post acne scars, post varicella scars
3. Acne	Chronic resistant acne
4. Hyperkeratotic lesions	Hypertrophic lichen planus, lichen simplex chronicus
5. Pigmentation	Tattoos, postinflammatory pigmentation
6. Tumors	Syringomas, trichoepitheliomas, seborrheic keratosis, Adenoma sebaceum, Darier disease
7. Others	Fine wrinkling, rejuvenation

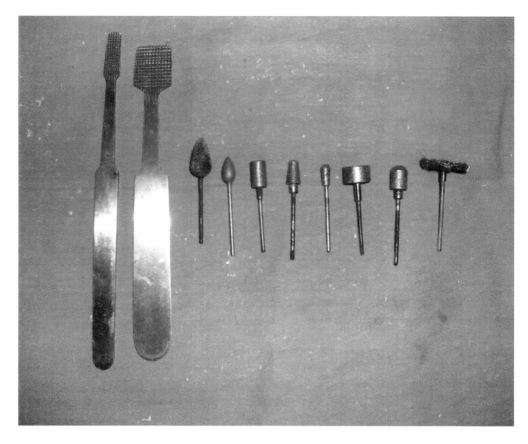

Figure 42.1 Manual dermabrader and diamond fraises of different sizes and shapes used for dermabrasion.

TECHNIQUE

1. Anesthesia
   a. Topical application of eutectic mixture of local anesthetics (EMLA) patch 60 minutes preoperatively.
   b. If the topical anesthesia achieved by EMLA is not sufficient, tumescent anesthesia with 1% xylocaine infiltration.
2. Electrical and/or mechanical abrasion
   a. With wire brush or diamond fraise attached to handpiece, abrade the skin until multiple pinpoint bleeding is observed, as shown in Figure 42.3. Give multiple parallel side-to-side above downward strokes to cover the lesion.

   b. Feather 1 cm from the border of the lesion into the surrounding normal skin boundary followed by mechanical abrasion.
3. Mechanical (manual metallic) abrasion
   a. Select an appropriate size of dermabrader. Give side-to-side, longitudinal, and horizontal (crisscross) strokes so as to smoothen out the firmness (depth until whitish pink parallel lines and rapidly bleeding larger points are observed).
   b. Feather gently into surrounding 1 cm of normal skin border.
   c. Hemostasis is achieved and dressing of double-layer framycetin tulle pressure is applied.

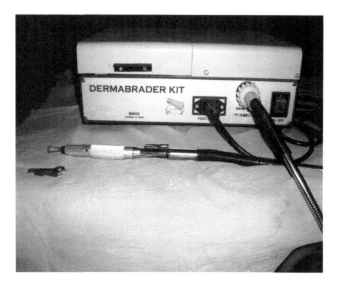

Figure 42.2 Electrical dermabrader kit.

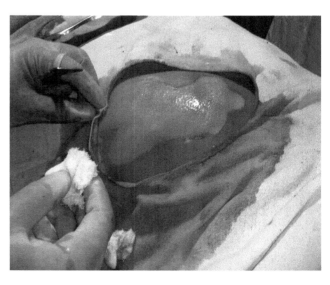

Figure 42.3 Vitiligo patch immediately after dermabrasion.

POSTOPERATIVE CARE

1. Oral antibiotics and nonsteroidal anti-inflammatory drugs for 10 days.
2. Dressing to be removed after 10 days.

MECHANISM OF REPIGMENTATION

The mechanism of migration of melanocytes from the remaining and undamaged portion of the hair follicles into the epidermis following dermabrasion was first reported by Staricco. In 1959, he found that there were some DOPA-negative amelanotic melanocytes in the outer sheaths of normal hair follicles which showed light cytoplasm and dark blue nuclei by DOPA Toluidine blue stain [7]. These melanocytes did not synthesize melanin under normal circumstances but became active to produce melanin when stimulated by ultraviolet (UV) light or by the removal of the epidermis and the upper part of follicles by dermabrasion. It was concluded that these amelanotic melanocytes could move up along the regenerated epidermis and mature morphologically and functionally. This process is divided into five phases [8].

1. Amelanotic migration mostly due to passive transport by the epidermal regenerative flow.
2. Division of amelanotic melanocytes in the middle hair follicles.
3. Pigmentation and formation of juvenile melanocytes (premelanocytes).
4. Tansformation of the premelanocytes into the normal melanocytes and later into hypertrophic melanocytes.
5. Migration of the hypertrophic melanocytes from the infundibulum into the basal layer of the epidermis.

Clabough further noticed that there was peripheral perilesional pigmentation in non-hairy areas of stable vitiligo as well [4]. Therapeutic spot or regional dermabrasion was found to be useful by itself in stimulating patches of stable vitiligo [9].

Repigmentation in stable vitiligo requires proliferation and migration of melanocytes from the reservoir into depigmented skin. The melanocytes migrate only a few millimeters from the pigmented edge toward the center. The lesional hair follicles are the mainstem reservoirs of the melanocytes required for repigmentation. Also, during the wound healing process, the inflammatory reaction and the re-epithelialization phase stimulate the follicular and perilesional melanocytes and thereby perifollicular and perilesional pigmentation [10].

On histopathological examination after dermabrasion, characteristic spindle cells were demonstrated. The cells looked flattened, oriented vertically on basement membrane or swarming near follicular infundibular compartment [5]. The spindle form of detected non-melanized cells with light cytoplasm and dark nuclei were the main descriptive terms provided by many authors describing melanocyte precursors [11–15]. Those cells were reported to mature during migration from outer root sheath to epidermis as result of several signaling pathways.

Removal of excessive keratotic layer is another way by which dermabrasion plays a role in stable vitiligo. Hyperkeratosis is a well-known pathological finding in vitiliginous patches [16,17]. The thickness of stratum corneum is known for its protective power against the effects of UV light, and subsequent hyperkeratosis can have a sun blocking effect [18]. This hyperkeratosis can prevent the known beneficial effect of the UV light in stimulating melanocyte

proliferation and melanization in the epidermis or melanocyte stem cell maturation in the outer root sheath [19]. The dermabrasion procedure here was able to eradicate these unwanted keratotic layers and subsequently allowed the heliotherapy to provide the preceding favorable effects.

COMBINATION THERAPY

To enhance the repigmentation after dermabrasion, various combination therapies have been used with good results.

1. Topical steroids
2. Narrowband UVB therapy
3. Placentrex gel
4. 5-Fluorouracil (5-FU) application

Placental extract promotes melanin synthesis by supplying the amino acid tyrosine, which is a precursor of melanin, and also by promoting copper tyrosinase linkage. The mechanism by which 5-FU induces the repigmentation of vitiligo may possibly be by the overstimulation of follicular melanocytes, which migrate to the surface during epithelialization, resulting in hyperpigmentation.

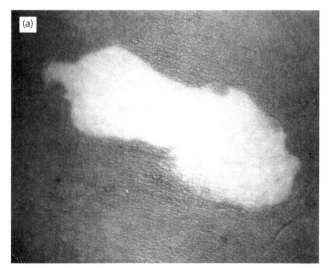

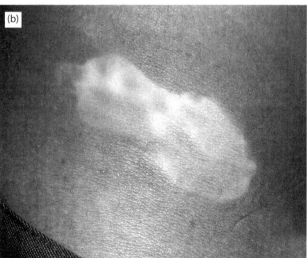

Figure 42.4 (a) Preoperative vitiligo patch on right lumbar area treated with dermabrasion alone. (b) Excellent pigmentation at 6 months of follow-up in the patch treated with dermabrasion.

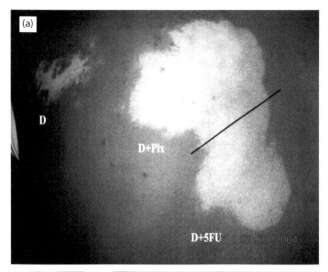

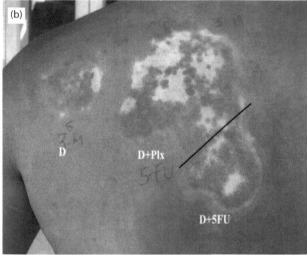

Figure 42.5 (a) Preoperative vitiligo patches on left upper back. (b) Excellent repigmentation at 6 months of follow-up in patches treated with dermabrasion and dermabrasion with 5-fluorouracil application.

The author has personal experience in the use of dermabrasion and combination therapies in vitiligo. Thirty patients with localized stable vitiligo (at least three lesions each) were treated. After dermabrasion, a Soframycin tulle dressing was placed on the first lesion, a topical 5% 5-fluorouracil dressing on the second, and a topical placentrex gel dressing on the third for 7 days after the procedure, and the patients were followed up for 6 months. The efficacy of treatment was highest (73.33%) and most rapid in lesions treated with dermabrasion combined with 5-FU. Dermabrasion alone and dermabrasion combined with placentrex gel showed similar efficacy in localized stable vitiligo (Figures 42.4 and 42.5).

CONCLUSION

Dermabrasion holds an important place in the current scenario of management of stable vitiligo. It is easy, inexpensive, and effective and its effects can be further enhanced with various combination therapies.

REFERENCES

1. Kovacs SO. Vitiligo. *J Am Acad Dermatol* 1998;38:647–66.
2. Bleechen SS, and Anstey AV. Disorders of skin colour. In: Burns T, Breathnach S, Cox N, and Griffiths C, eds. *Rook's Textbook of Dermatology.* 7th ed. London: Blackwell; 2004, pp. 39–13.
3. Mosher DB, Fitzpatrick TB, and Ortonne JP. Hypomelanosis and Hypermelanosis. In: Freedberg IM, Eisen AZ, Wolff K et al. eds. *Fitzpatrick's Dermatology in General Medicine.* 5th ed. New York: Mcgraw-Hill; 1999, pp. 950–4.
4. Clabough W. Removal of tattoos by superficial dermabrasion. *Arch Dermatol* 1968;98:515–21.
5. Awad SS. Dermabrasion may repigment vitiligo through stimulation of melanocyte precursors and elimination of hyperkeratosis. *J Cosmet Dermatol* 2012 Dec 1;11(4):318–22.
6. Parsad D, and Gupta S. IADVL Dermatosurgery Task Force. Standard guidelines of care for vitiligo surgery. *Indian J Dermatol Venereol Leprol* 2008;74:537–45.
7. Starrico RG. Amelanotic melanocytes in the outer root sheath of the human hair follicle. *J Invest Dermatol* 1959;33:295–7.
8. Starrico RG. Mechanism of migration of the melanocytes of the hair follicle into the epidermis following dermabrasion. *J Invest Dermatol* 1961;36:99–104.
9. Savant SS. Therapeutic spot dermabrasion. Study of 197 sites in 11 skin conditions. *Indian J Dermatol Surg* 1999;1:5–15.
10. Savant SS. Therapeutic spot and regional dermabrasion in stable vitiligo. *Indian J Dermatol Venerol Leprol* 1996;62:139–45.
11. Tobin DJ, and Bystryn JC. Different populations of melanocytes are present in hair follicles and epidermis. *Pigment Cell Res* 1996;9:304–10.
12. Nishikawa-Torikai S, Osawa M, and Nishikawa S. Functional characterization of melanocyte stem cells in hair follicles. *J Invest Dermatol* 2011;131:2358–67.
13. Bennett DC, Cooper PJ, Dexter TH et al. Cloned mouse melanocyte lines carrying germline mutations albino and brown: Complementation in culture. *Development* 1989;105:379–85.
14. Hirobe T. Control of melanocyte proliferation and differentiation in the mouse epidermis. *Pigment Cell Res* 1992;5:1–11.
15. Peters EM, Tobin DJ, Botchkareva N et al. Migration of melanoblasts into the developing murine hair follicle is accompanied by transient c-Kit expression. *J Histochem Cytochem* 2002;50:751–66.
16. Kim YC, Kang HY, Seonghyang S, and Lee ES. Histopathologic features in vitiligo. *Am J Dermatopathol* 2008;30:112–5.
17. Awad SS, Abdel-Raof H, Hosam El-Din W, and El-Domyati M. Epithelial grafting for vitiligo requires ultraviolet A phototherapy to increase success rate. *J Cosmet Dermatol* 2007 Jun 1;6(2):119–24.
18. Gniadecka M, Wulf HC, Mortensen NN, and Poulsen T. Photoprotection in vitiligo and normal skin. A quantitative assessment of the role of stratum corneum, viable epidermis and pigmentation. *Acta Derm Venereol* 1996;76:429–32.
19. Ortonne JP, Schmitt D, and Thivolet J. PUVA-induced repigmentation of vitiligo: Scanning electron microscopy of hair follicles. *J Invest Dermatol* 1980;74:40–2.

Chapter 43

ROLE OF DIET IN VITILIGO

Rachita Misri and Khushbu Mahajan

CONTENTS

INTRODUCTION

The importance of diet in skin disorders has often been a subject of debate among dermatologists. Patients are often anxious about what foods to consume and what to avoid. No matter how impractical it may be, patients believe that following a certain diet will cure their disease. Dietary modifications have been advocated by practitioners of alternative medicine in India and in other parts of the world to deal with commonly encountered disorders. The word diet itself is derived from the Latin word *diaeta*, meaning "prescribed way of life," and from the Greek word *diaita,* meaning "way of life, regimen, dwelling" [1]. Though the literature support for dietary modifications may be controversial in our system of medicine, knowing and explaining the relatively beneficial or harmful dietary products helps build the patient's confidence, especially in the Indian population where diet is believed to be a cure for many diseases.

ROLE OF DIET IN VITILIGO

There is an uncertain relationship of diet in vitiligo. In fact, in a review by Kaimal et al. on diet in dermatology, vitiligo has been classified under "Miscellaneous Disorders with an Uncertain Relationship to Diet" [2]. There are few reports in the published literature of dietary interventions for vitiligo as a treatment modality.

Vitiligo is an autoimmune disorder that involves the interplay between oxidative stress and the immune system. Over the years, neural, biochemical, autoimmune, and genetic aspects of the pathogenesis have been proposed. Vitiligo has a multifactorial etiology characterized by an increase of external or internal phenol/catechol concentrations and reactive oxygen species (ROS) [3,4]. It has recently been suggested that ROS can alter melanocyte-specific factors to produce neo-antigens and can also amplify antigen presentation and autoimmune destruction of melanocytes [4]. Furthermore, estrogen has also been implicated in the development of autoimmunity [5]. Considering the contribution of reactive oxygen species, estrogen, and phenol-containing agents in the pathophysiology of vitiligo, it makes sense to assess the role of diet.

AGGRAVATING FACTORS IN DIET

Oxidative stress plays a pivotal role in the pathogenesis of vitiligo. Thus, food contaminants/additives/preservatives and cosmetic products could aggravate vitiligo because they can produce oxidative stress in the skin [6]. In some countries, such as India, patients with vitiligo are cautioned to avoid sour food items, milk, and fish; however, this has not been proved in controlled studies.

There are certain general dietary recommendations based on the antioxidant and micronutrient composition of foods. For example, vegetable oils that are high in omega-6 fatty acids (sunflower oil, wheat germ oil, grapeseed oil, soybean oil, margarine, corn oil) may increase the production of ROS and proinflammatory cytokines that may play a role in vitiligo. They could also exacerbate autoimmune disease by increasing the free radical formation through decreasing the antioxidant enzyme mRNA levels. In contrast, omega-3 lipid intake has a beneficial role in vitiligo as discussed next.

A recent study examined the relationship between exposure to a number of thyroid disruptors and toxins and the presence of thyroid hormone antibodies to T3 and T4 in 70 patients with vitiligo. It was found that 95.7% of the subjects had thyroid hormone antibodies and most had both T3 and T4 antibodies. A significant association was noted between intake of foods containing nitrates (leafy green vegetables), thiocyanate (broccoli, cabbage, and other brassicas), and soy isoflavones and the presence of T3 antibodies [7]. This study underlined a possible influence of diet and environment in vitiligo patients in eliciting thyroid antibodies, and suggested evaluation of thyroid function in the event of a positive exposure to thyroid disruptors in these patients.

Some products containing phenol and polyphenolic compounds (tannins), which may aggravate vitiligo, are cashew, oak, raspberry, cassava, mango, areca nut, pistachio, cherry, cranberry, blackberry, red chilies, and tea. Phenol molecules induce the release of interleukin-1α (IL-1α) and tumor necrosis factor-α (TNF-α) from keratinocytes. Increased TNF-α and IL1-α levels in the lesional skin of patients with nonsegmental vitiligo has been recently reported and it is suggested that these cytokines play important roles in the pathophysiology of vitiligo [8]. In addition, tannins induce apoptosis in vitro, inhibit cellular enzymes, bind to cell membrane and make it fragile, and chelate metal ions [9]. All these effects can aggravate vitiligo. The high phenol and tannin content of the foods widely consumed in India could explain the highest incidence of vitiligo in this country [10].

BENEFICIAL FOODS IN VITILIGO

Foods rich in omega-3 fatty acids (flaxseed oil, canola oil, fish oil, walnuts, oysters, soybeans, and spinach) in the presence of an antioxidant supplement appears to have a beneficial role in vitiligo through various mechanisms, as postulated next:

- Enhancing antioxidant enzymes and transforming growth factor-β mRNA levels, thus protecting against autoimmunity [11].
- Inhibition of proinflammatory cytokines such as TNF-α [12].
- Enrichment of cell membranes with omega-3 polyunsaturated fatty acids has been reported to increase the glutathione (GSH) peroxidase activity [13].
- The organic compound indole-3-carbinol, found in omega-3 fatty acids, induces CYP1A1, which hydroxylates estrogens into 2-hydroxyestrone [14].
- Omega-3 fatty acids play a critical role in the development and function of the central nervous system and may favorably influence the outcome in depressive disorders [12]. This fact points further to the beneficial effect in vitiligo, as 20% of the vitiligo patients are reported to be depressed about their illness [14].

It is therefore advisable that vitiligo patients avoid omega-6 fatty acids and use omega-3 fatty acids.

Carotenoids (carrots, plums, apricots, sweet potatoes, spinach, pumpkins) can also be beneficial in vitiligo because of their free radical scavenging properties.

Foods rich in vitamin B_{12}, folic acid, vitamin C, D, E, and zinc have also proved beneficial in various studies.

Folates are needed for DNA repair, synthesis, and methylation of DNA and thus are crucial for cell growth and division. However, they are not synthesized in the human body and hence must be obtained via diet (green leafy vegetables, asparagus, broccoli, citrus fruits, okra). Montes and colleagues reported diminished blood levels of vitamin B_{12}, folic acid, and ascorbic acid in a group of 15 patients with vitiligo. Prolonged supplementation with oral folic acid, parental B_{12}, and oral ascorbic acid was associated with repigmentation of vitiliginous patches in these patients [15]. However, several other studies found no association between serum B_{12} and folate levels and vitiligo [16,17]. Thus the evidence for vitamin B_{12} and/or folic acid supplementation, either alone or as an adjuvant, is mixed. The rationale for their use is their possible role in melanin synthesis and also the possible association of vitiligo with pernicious anemia, in which vitamin B_{12} is insufficiently absorbed [18].

There is a common belief that foods rich in vitamin C (oranges, strawberries, guava, red peppers, grapefruit) should be avoided in vitiligo because of their skin-lightening activity. However, Yoon et al. suggested that the antioxidant benefits of vitamin C might override this risk [19]. In an Indian study, 188 patients of vitiligo were divided into 3 groups: 75 patients avoided vitamin C products, 113 patients consumed vitamin C daily in their diet and/or medicinal products, and a third group of 12 patients ingested vitamin C 1000 mg daily for 6 months. Statistical analysis of the three groups showed no difference in the progression of the disease [20]. Thus though the beneficial role of vitamin C cannot be fully established, there is definitely no harm in consuming it as commonly believed.

Amla (*Phyllanthus emblica*) or Indian gooseberry, has antioxidant, anti-inflammatory, antimicrobial, and antiviral properties. It contains vitamin C, tannins, and polyphenols [21]. Colucci et al. have suggested its beneficial efficacy in vitiligo patients. They treated 65 subjects (group A) with one tablet of an oral supplement containing *P. emblica* (100 mg), vitamin E (10 mg), and carotenoids (4.7 mg) three times a day for 6 months and compared with a control group (group B, 65 patients), which was not treated with antioxidants. Both groups were simultaneously treated with a comparable topical therapy and/or phototherapy. After a 6-month follow-up, a significantly greater number of patients in group A had higher repigmentation, fewer signs of inflammation, and more stable disease, thus suggesting a positive contribution of antioxidant supplementation to other vitiligo treatments [22].

Melanocytes are believed to express 1-alpha-dihydroxyvitamin D3 receptors, which may have a role in stimulating melanogenesis [23]. Vitamin D exerts immunomodulatory effects by inhibiting the expression of proinflammatory and proapoptotic cytokines. Although it is not clear whether vitamin D deficiency plays a role in vitiligo, it may be useful as an immunomodulator in this disorder. Some studies have investigated the association between vitiligo and 25(OH)D levels. In the study by Silverberg et al. [24], decreased levels of 25(OH)D were found in patients with vitiligo with additional autoimmune diseases, and in another study by Li et al. [25], statistically significantly decreased levels of 25(OH)D were seen in patients with vitiligo as compared to controls, suggesting that a deficiency in 25(OH)D may be a contributing factor in the development of vitiligo. Thus food rich in vitamin D (cod liver oil, salmon, tuna, egg yolk, raw milk, mushrooms) may be beneficial in vitiligo patients to reduce the disease activity [26].

Vitamin E is a potent scavenger of free radicals. Ramadan et al. found low levels of vitamin E in patients with vitiligo compared with controls [27]. Thus foods rich in vitamin E such as almonds, spinach, sweet potato, and avocado might be beneficial in vitiligo patients.

Zinc, as a trace element, is a cofactor for the antioxidant defense system, has a role as an antiapoptotic factor, and plays an important role in the process of melanogenesis. Thus zinc-rich foods (spinach, kidney beans, flax seeds, pumpkin seeds, oysters, beef) may be effective in prevention and treatment of vitiligo and may be beneficial when combined with other therapies [28].

Quercetin has been found to have strong cytoprotective effects against hydrogen peroxide–induced oxidative stress [29]. Thus the foods rich in quercetin (onion and apple) can be of benefit to vitiligo patients. Onions also have abundant thiols, which exert an antioxidant activity toward ROS and also block electrophilic metabolites and modulate several xenobiotic-metabolizing pathways [30].

Mushrooms also seem to have a beneficial effect in vitiligo. Cremini mushrooms and brown mushrooms are excellent sources of selenium, riboflavin, pantothenic acid, niacin, and copper, which act as free-radical scavengers [31]. Mushrooms also contain a powerful antioxidant L-ergothioneine (a sulfur-containing amino acid, synthesized by soil bacteria in fungal substrates) which scavenges superoxide and singlet oxygen and suppresses TNF-α [32]. L-ergothioneine is not destroyed when mushrooms are cooked.

Celiac disease (CD) and vitiligo may share similar genetic risks. Studies suggest that both CD and vitiligo may be triggered by a common immune system signal associated with a high-gluten diet [33]. Thus, in patients who have both conditions, a gluten-free diet can be considered. Two case reports in patients with vitiligo who were unresponsive to topical agents and phototherapy showed some degree of repigmentation with a gluten-free diet [34,35]. Gluten-free diets (corn, rice, amaranth, arrowroot, buckwheat, flax, millet, quinoa, sorghum, soy, tapioca, flours made from gluten-free grain) are easily available.

Table 43.1 The aggravating and beneficial food constituents in vitiligo along with their sources

Aggravating foods	Food contaminants/additives/preservatives	
	Vegetable oils high in omega-6 fatty acids	Sunflower oil, wheat germ oil, grape seed oil, soybean oil, margarine, corn oil
	Foods containing nitrates, thiocyanate, and soy isoflavones	Leafy green vegetables, broccoli, cabbage
	Phenol and polyphenolic compounds (tannins)	Cashews, oak, raspberry, cassava, mango, areca nut, pistachio, cherry, cranberry, blackberry, red chili, tea
Beneficial foods	Omega-3 fatty acids	Flaxseed oil, canola oil, fish oil, walnuts, oysters, soybeans, spinach
	Carotenoids	Carrots, plums, apricots, sweet potatoes, spinach, pumpkins
	Vitamin B_{12}, folic acid	Green leafy vegetables, asparagus, broccoli, citrus fruits, okra
	Vitamin C	Amla, oranges, strawberries, guava, red peppers, grapefruit
	Vitamin D	Cod liver oil, salmon, tuna, egg yolk, raw milk, mushrooms
	Vitamin E	Almonds, spinach, sweet potato, avocado
	Zinc	Spinach, kidney beans, flax seeds, pumpkin seeds, oysters, beef
	Quercetin	Onion, apple
	Mushrooms	Cremini mushrooms, brown mushrooms
	Whey protein	

Whey, a protein complex derived from milk, has a number of health benefits and can help vitiligo patients in following ways:

- It is a potent antioxidant and contributes cysteine-rich proteins that aid in the synthesis of GSH. Thiols (sulfhydryl) present in cysteine serve as active reducing agents in preventing oxidation and further tissue damage.
- Lactoferrin, an iron-binding glycoprotein found in whey, is a non-enzymatic antioxidant and anti-inflammatory agent [31]. It decreases the levels of TNF-α and IL-6, involved in the pathogenesis of vitiligo [36].
- Lactoperoxidase, also found in whey, catalyzes certain molecules, including the reduction of hydrogen peroxide.
- Alpha-lactalbumin, another enzyme in whey, can chelate heavy metals and reduce oxidative stress due to its iron-chelating properties.
- Whey also has GSH peroxidase activity [36].
- Whey protein also causes a rise in serotonin, which helps in improved cognitive function and stress coping abilities. Tryptophan available in whey is a substrate for serotonin [37]. Considering the role of stress both as an aggravator and result of the disease, whey can be of further benefit to the vitiligo patient.

CONCLUSION

Though diet does not have a definite role in the management of vitiligo, there are certain food items that can aggravate the disease, and some that can be beneficial adjuvants to other treatment modalities. Thus knowing about diet in vitiligo can help a clinician give a judicious advice to patients who believe that diet forms a major part of treatment of any disease, especially the chronic ones. Table 43.1 summarizes the aggravating and beneficial food constituents along with their sources.

REFERENCES

1. Harper D. *Online Etymology Dictionary*. 2001 [cited 2009 January 31]. Available from: http://www.etymonline.com (Accessed on 31 May 2017.)

2. Kaimal S, and Thappa DM. Diet in dermatology: Revisited. *Indian J Dermatol Venereol Leprol* 2010 Mar-Apr;76(2):103–15.

3. Westerhof W, and d'Ischia M. Vitiligo puzzle: The pieces fall in place. *Pigment Cell Res* 2007;20:345–59.

4. Namazi MR. Neurogenic dysregulation, oxidative stress, autoimmunity, and melanocytorrhagy in vitiligo: Can they be interconnected? *Pigment Cell Res* 2007;20:360–3.

5. Ackerman LS. Sex hormones and the genesis of autoimmunity. *Arch Dermatol* 2006;142:371–6.

6. Bickers RD, and Athar M. Oxidative stress in the pathogenesis of skin disease. *J Invest Dermatol* 2006;126:2565–75.

7. Colucci R, Lotti F, Arunachalam M et al. Correlation of serum thyroid hormones autoantibodies with self reported exposure to thyroid disruptors in a group of nonsegmental vitiligo patients. *Arch Environ Contam Toxicol* 2015;69:181–90.

8. Birol A, Kisa U, Kurtipek GS, Kara F, Kocak M, Erkek E, and Caglayan O. Increased tumor necrosis factor alpha (TNF-alpha) and interleukin 1 alpha (IL1-alpha) levels in the lesional skin of patients with nonsegmental vitiligo. *Int J Dermatol* 2006;45:992–3.

9. Tur E, and Brenner S. The role of the water system as an exogenous factor in pemphigus. *Int J Dermatol* 1997;36:810–6.

10. Sehgal VN, and Srivastava G. Vitiligo: Compendium of clinico-epidemiological features. *Indian J Dermatol Venereol Leprol* 2007;73:149–56.

11. Fernandez G. Dietary lipids and risk of autoimmune disease. *Clin Immunol Immunopathol* 1994;72:193–7.

12. Logan AC. Omega-3 fatty acids and major depression: A primer for the mental health professional. *Lipids Health Dis* 2004;3:25.

13. Joulain C, Prigent AF, Nemoz G, and Lagarde M. Increased glutathione peroxidase activity in human blood mononuclear cells upon *in vitro* incubation with n-3 fatty acids. *Biochem Pharmacol* 1994;47:1315–23.

14. Namazi MR. Prescribing cyclic antidepressants for vitiligo patents, which agents are superior, which are not? *Psychether Psychosom* 2003;72:361–2.

15. Montes LF, Diaz ML, Lajous J et al. Folic acid and vitamin B12 in vitiligo: A nutritional approach. *Cutis* 1992;50(1):39–42.

16. Gonul M, Cakmak SK, Soylu S et al. Serum vitamin B12, folate, ferritin, and iron levels in Turkish patients with vitiligo. *Indian J Dermatol Venereol Leprol* 2010;76:448.

17. Balci DD, Yonden Z, Yenin JZ et al. Serum homocysteine, folic acid, and vitamin B12 levels in vitiligo. *Eur J Dermatol* 2009;19:382.

18. Kim SM, Kim YK, and Hann S-Y. Serum levels of folic acid and vitamin B12 in Korean patients with vitiligo. *Yonsei Med J* 1999;40:195–8.

19. Yoon J, Kim TH, and Sun YW. Complementary and alternative medicine for vitiligo. In: Park KK, and Murase JE, eds. *Vitiligo: Management and Therapy*. INTECH Open Access Publisher; 2011.

20. Bhattacharya SK, Dutta AK, Mandal SB et al. Ascorbic acid in vitiligo. *Indian J Dermatol* 1981;26(3):4.

21. Rehman HU, Yasin KA, Choudhary MA et al. Studies on the chemical constituents of Phyllanthus emblica. *Nat Prod Res* 2007;21(9):775–81.

22. Colucci R, Dragoni F, Conti R et al. Evaluation of an oral supplement containing Phyllanthus emblica fruit extracts, vitamin E, and carotenoids in vitiligo treatment. *Dermatol Ther* 2015;28(1):17–21.

23. Grimes PE. New insights and new therapies in vitiligo. *JAMA* 2005;293(6):730–5.

24. Silverberg JI, Silverberg AI, Malka E, and Silverberg NB. A pilot study assessing the role of 25 hydroxy vitamin D levels in patients with vitiligo vulgaris. *J Am Acad Dermatol* 2010;62:937–41.

25. Li K, Shi Q, Yang L et al. The association of vitamin D receptor gene polymorphisms and serum 25-hydroxyvitamin D levels with generalized vitiligo. *Br J Dermatol* 2012;167:815–21.

26. AlGhamdi K, Kumar A, and Moussa N. The role of vitamin D in melanogenesis with an emphasis on vitiligo. *Indian J Dermatol Venereol Leprol* 2013;79(6):750.

27. Ramadan S, Tawdy A, Hay RA et al. The antioxidant role of paraoxonase 1 and vitamin E in three autoimmune diseases. *Skin Pharmacol Physiol* 2013;26:2–7.

28. Bagherani N, Yaghoobi R, and Omidian M. Hypothesis: Zinc can be effective in treatment of vitiligo. *Indian J Dermatol* 2011;56(5):480.

29. Jeong YM, Choi YG, Kim DS et al. Cytoprotective effect of green tea extract and quercetin against hydrogen peroxide-induced oxidative stress. *Arch Pharm Res* 2005;28: 1251–6.

30. De Flora S, Izzotti A, D'Agostini F, and Cesarone CF. Antioxidant activity and other mechanisms of thiols involved in chemoprevention of mutation and cancer. *Am J Med* 1991;91:122S–30S.

31. Namazi MR, and Chee Leok G. Vitiligo and diet: A theoretical molecular approach with practical implications. *Indian J Dermatol Venereol Leprol* 2009;75:116–8.

32. Obayashi K, Kurihara K, Okano Y, Masaki H, and Yarosh DB. L-Ergothioneine scavenges superoxide and singlet oxygen and suppresses TNF-alpha and MMP-1 expression in UV-irradiated human dermal fibroblasts. *J Cosmet Sci* 2005;56:17–27.

33. Grimes PE, and Nashawati R. The role of diet and supplements in vitiligo management. *Dermatol Clin.* 2017 Apr;35(2):235–43.

34. Rodríguez-García C, González-Hernández S, Pérez-Robayna N, Guimerá F, Fagundo E, and Sánchez R. Repigmentation of vitiligo lesions in a child with celiac disease after a gluten-free diet. *Pediatr Dermatol* 2011;28:209–10.

35. Khandavala BN, and Nirmalraj MC. Rapid partial repigmentation of vitiligo in a young female adult with a gluten-free diet. *Case Rep Dermatol* 2014;6:283–7.

36. Marshal K. Therapeutic applications of whey protein. *Altern Med Rev* 2004;2:136–56.

37. Marcus CR, Olivier B, and de Haan EH. Whey protein rich in alpha-lactalbumin increases the ratio of plasma tryptophan to the sum of the other large neutral amino acids and improves cognitive performance in stress-vulnerable subjects. *Am J Clin Nutr* 2002;75:1051–6.

SECTION IX

MISCELLANEOUS

Chapter 44

TATTOOING IN VITILIGO

Gurvinder P. Thami

CONTENTS

INTRODUCTION

Vitiligo or leukoderma is an asymptomatic, cosmetically unacceptable loss of melanin pigment from the skin due to malfunctioning of melanocytes. Various medical and surgical modalities aim to replace natural melanin pigment by stimulating existing melanocytes or alternatively by transplanting melanocytes from normal skin to vitilignous skin [1–3]. Treating melanin-devoid lesions of vitiligo using extraneous pigments is the basis of camouflage therapy, which can be temporary or permanent. Micropigmentation or dermatography is a technique used for permanent camouflaging of various medical conditions of cosmetic importance, including vitiligo. Scientific use of the age-old art of tattooing in a medical framework to produce cosmetic camouflage is called micropigmentation. Tattoos have probably been used for medical purposes since 3000 BC or more, but the term *micropigmentation* came into fashion in the 1980s, and its use in vitiligo also started in the same time period [4,5].

Tattooing is a process of uniform implantation of minute, metabolically inert, pigmented chemical particles or microscopic granules into the dermis through a multiple puncture technique using manually or electrically driven, closely held needles. It may be used to camouflage the depigmented skin in a lesional pattern or to create designs [2,4].

BASIC CONCEPTS

The main purpose of tattooing or micropigmentation in vitiligo is to conceal the depigmented white spots with external pigments which can be introduced into skin layers where they reside permanently and give a darker appearance to the skin. Traditional tattooing implants pigment at the level of the mid dermis where the pigment particles are initially engulfed by macrophages and mononuclear cells and remain intercellular for the initial few years. Gradually the pigment becomes both intercellular and extracellular and lays in the deep dermis and superficial supporting tissue and collagen fibers. Some pigment is also taken by hair follicle, blood vessels, and

regional lymph nodes as well. The leaching out of the pigment to lymph nodes and deeper tissues is responsible for gradual fading of the pigment over a period of few years. The deeper pigment lying within tissue microphages is also responsible for the Tyndall effect, whereby the pigment of different colors and shades eventually looks bluish gray after years. The pigments used are mostly inert, non-allergenic, and usually lie in the tissue without causing any foreign body granuloma or dermatitis [2–5].

TATTOO DYES AND INSTRUMENTS

The most commonly used tattoo pigment is iron oxide, which can give different shades of light brown, dark brown, camel yellow and black, depending upon the shades of the constitutional skin tone and complexion of the normal skin to which it needs to be matched. However, good matching of the tattooed skin may be achieved at the time of tattooing but it tends to become grayish blue with time. In addition, iron oxide yellow color can be obtained by using cadmium oxide, while white titanium oxide can be used to mix and match various shades required with iron oxide. Cinnabar and mercuric sulfate are red pigments which can also be used to obtain various shades by mixing and matching. The red pigments, however, have more allergenic potential than others, and iron oxide is the most versatile pigment as it can give various shades and has the least sensitizing potential [5].

PROCEDURE

The procedure can be accomplished as an office procedure under strict aseptic conditions using local anesthesia. A pigment paste is generally prepared using distilled water, normal saline, glycerin, or alcohol to obtain a reasonable consistency which does not flow. Inlaying of the pigment can be achieved by using a simple hypodermic needle for a small area of vitiligo like focal vitiligo. Motorized tattoo machines (tattoo guns) are also available commercially, which have a group of needles to inlay pigment into dermis with a back-and-forth motorized movement. These tattoo machines can be sterilized with autoclaving or with chemical sterilization for the needles [3,4]. A watchmaker's pin vise can also be used innovatively to hold multiple sewing needles to tattoo a small area manually [6]. These sewing needles can be used as disposable needles, so the complication of reuse can be avoided [6]. The pigment shows in the tattooed area immediately, and it becomes swollen due to multiple pricks and requires prophylactic systemic and topical antibiotics and analgesics.

Too much bleeding and very close pricks may lead to leaching out of the pigment along with blood and tissue fluids. Normal depth of pigment deposition ranges from 1–2 mm, with an average of 1.5 mm as the best depth. Too superficial pigment, i.e., less than 1 mm in depth, is usually thrown out along with crust at 2–4 weeks, while too deep pigment more than 2 mm usually migrates to lymph nodes and macrophages. The results also depend upon elasticity and laxity of the skin along with blood flow and consistency of pigment paste.

INDICATIONS

Tattooing in vitiligo is most suitable for mucosal and mucocutaneous vitiligo or recalcitrant patches of vitiligo on glabrous skin not responding to or suitable for surgical therapy. Vitiligo limited to mucosal and mucocutaneous areas of lips, visible area of inside of lip, gums or gingiva, etc. are best treated with micropigmentation (Figure 44.1) [7–14]. Genital vitiligo involving the glans penis, shaft of the penis, scrotum, vulva, and perineal and perigenital areas, umbilicus, etc. (Figure 44.2), which are normally darker than the other parts of the skin, are best suited for tattooing for micropigmentation. The present evidence also indicates its use in recalcitrant lesions of vitiligo, especially over the distal digits, lips, umbilicus, hands, wrists, axillae, elbows, perianal areas, lower legs, mucosae, and mucocutaneous junctions. Micropigmentation has also been used for nipple areola reconstruction, enhancement of eyebrows and eyelashes, permanent repigmentation of achromic burn scars, reconstitution of eyebrows following recalcitrant alopecia areata, and aesthetic improvements of scars and skin grafts, especially to camouflage hairless patches. It is useful adjunctive therapy for camouflaging disturbing discolorations and scars of the head and neck, reports of which have included color matching of vermilionplasty after radial forearm free flap reconstruction of the lower lip, cleft lip, and cleft palate scars, senile lip rejuvenation, and an alternative treatment for disturbing corneal scars [15–20]. Until 1984, tattooing was mainly performed as a permanent eyeliner for enhancing eye expression. Micropigmentation or dermatography has been used in the fields of craniomaxillofacial, reconstructive, and cosmetic surgery. Tattooing has also been done with gold salts, such as 20% aurothioglucose in sesame oil for vitiligo. Others have used this procedure for implanting various earthtone color pigments to the base of the eyelash as cosmetic eyeliner. Excellent color matching has been reported in cutaneous, mucosal, and mucocutaneous vitiligo; contact leukoderma; and postinflammatory depigmentation and scarring in various studies, especially in dark individuals [21–24]. The latest Cochrane review on treatment of vitiligo, however, fails to find well-controlled studies on this the subject of micropigmentation as a treatment option for vitiligo [1].

CONTRAINDICATIONS

1. Keloidal tendencies
2. Contact allergy to pigments composition
3. Infections
4. Active vitiligo

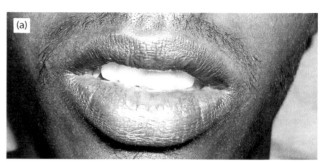
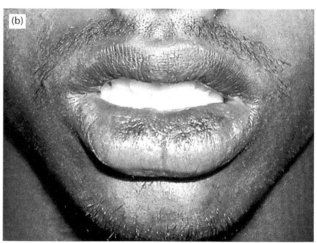
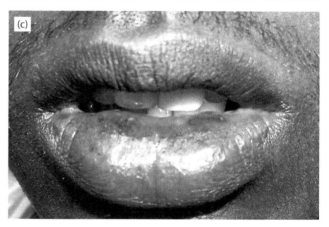

Figure 44.1 (a) Mucosal vitiligo before tattooing. (b) Mucosal vitiligo immediately after procedure. (c) Tattooed pigment 2 months after procedure.

SEQUELAE AND COMPLICATIONS

- Immediate
  - Ecchymosis
  - Crusting
  - Inflammatory edema
  - Reactivation of recurrent herpes simplex
  - Secondary bacterial infections
- Late
  - Pigment extrusion/mismatching of color loss of pigment with crust if it is deposited very superficially
  - Leaching, fading, or washing out of pigment if it is deposited too deeply
  - Tyndall effect—gradual lightening of pigment (blue color) due to migration of pigment into deep dermis

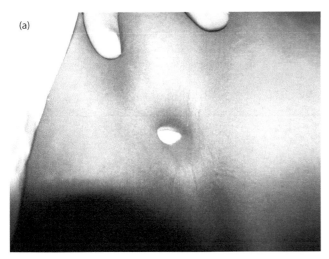

(a)

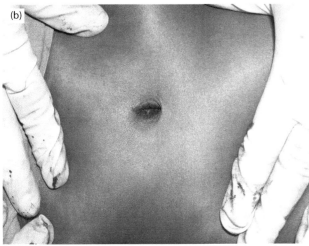

(b)

Figure 44.2 (a) Umbilical vitiligo before tattooing. (b) Umbilical vitiligo immediately after tattooing.

- Reactions to tattoo pigments—contact allergy, foreign body, and granulomatous reactions
- Inoculation of infections if strict precautions of asepsis are not adhered to—syphilis, tuberculosis, leprosy, verruca, hepatitis B and C, HI
- Reactivation of other dermatoses (Koebnerization)—tattoos may act as foci of localized disease such as (especially around mercury dye) psoriasis, lichen planus, sarcoidosis, lupus erythematosus
- Rarely, malignant melanoma, basal cell carcinoma, reticulohistosarcoma

CONCLUSION

Tattooing is a safe, inexpensive, outpatient procedure for certain forms of vitiligo with excellent aesthetic results when it is done with strict adherence to universal precautions of sterilization. Present-day emphasis is to reserve this procedure for therapeutic indications or as an adjunctive to surgical management of vitiligo. It is extremely helpful in coloring and concealing patches of vitiligo which at times may be stigmatic to reveal. The best patients with vitiligo for this procedure are those who do not want white skin spots and any other shade shall be acceptable for them and are looking for instant results. The long-term drawbacks of micropigmentation are its gradual fading requiring retouching, developing a bluish gray hue, and the

lifelong permanency and difficulty in removal of pigment without scarring. The permanency of the procedure must be explained to the patient in no uncertain terms before carrying it out.

SALIENT FEATURES

- Careful selection of patient, counseling of patient regarding outcomes of color matching and its permanency should be done.
- Excellent color matching has been reported on cutaneous, mucosal, and mucocutaneous lesions, especially in dark individuals.
- Underdoing of procedure is preferable to overdoing because of its permanency.
- Initial fading of pigment occurs for 6–8 weeks.
- Touch-up tattooing (if required) should be done after 3 months.

REFERENCES

1. Whitton ME, Pinart M, Batchelor J, Leonardi-Bee J, González U, Jiyad Z, Eleftheriadou V, and Ezzedine K. Interventions for vitiligo. *Cochrane Database Syst Rev* 2015 Feb 24;CD003263.

2. Patel NS, Paghdal KV, and Cohen GF. Advanced treatment modalities for vitiligo. *Dermatol Surg* 2012 Mar;38(3):381–91.

3. Thami GP. Micropigmentation. In: Gupta S, Olsson MJ, Kanwar AJ, Ortonne J, eds. *Surgical Management of Vitiligo*, 1st ed. USA: Blackwell Publishing; 2007, pp. 249–54.

4. Garg G, and Thami GP. Micropigmentation for medical purposes. *Dermatol Surg* 2005;31:928–31.

5. Thami GP. Micropigmentation: A brief reappraisal. *Asian Pigment Bulletin* 2007;2:18–22.

6. Singal A, Thami GP, and Bhalla M. Watchmaker's pin-vise for manual tattooing of vitiligo. *Dermatol Surg* 2004;30:203–4.

7. Mahajan BB, Garg G, and Gupta RR. Evaluation of cosmetic tattooing in localized stable vitiligo. *J Dermatol* 2002;29:726–30.

8. Singh AK, and Karki D. Micropigmentation: Tattooing for the treatment of lip vitiligo. *J Plast Reconstr Aesthet Surg* 2010 Jun;63(6):988–91. Epub 2009 May 28.

9. Malakar S, and Lahiri K. Successful repigmentation of six cases of herpes labialis induced lip leucoderma by micropigmentation. *Dermatology* 2001;203:194.

10. De Cuyper C. Permanent makeup: Indications and complications. *C Clin Dermatol* 2008 Jan-Feb;26(1):30–4.

11. Earley MJ. Basal cell carcinoma arising in tattoos: A clinical report of two cases. *Br J Plast Surg* 1983;36:258–9.

12. Halder RM, Pham HN, Breadon JY, and Johnson BA. Micropigmentation for treatment of vitiligo. *J Dermatol Surg Oncol* 1989;15:1092–8.

13. van der Velden EM, Baruchin AM, Jairath D et al. Dermatography: A method for permanent repigmentation of achromic burn scars. *Burns* 1995;21:304–7.

14. Centre JM, Mancini S, Baker GI et al. Management of gingival vitiligo with use of a tattoo technique. *Br J Dermatol* 1998;138:359–60.

15. Traquina AC. Micropigmentation as an adjuvant in cosmetic surgery of scalp. *Dermatol Surg* 2001;27:123–8.

16. Tsur H, and Kaplan HY. Camouflaging hairless areas on male face by artistic tattoo. *Plast Reconstr Surg* 1993;92:357–60.

17. Angres GG. Angres Permalid: Liner method—a new surgical procedure. *Ann Ophthalmol* 1984;16:145–8.

18. vander Velden EM, Drost Brigitte HIM, Ijsselmuiden OE et al. Dermatograph as a new treatment for alopecia areata of the eyebrows. *Int J Dermatol* 1998;37:617–21.

19. Byars LT. Tattooing of free skin grafts and pedicle flaps. *Ann Surg* 1945;121:644–8.

20. Conway H. Tattooing of nevus flammeus for permanent camouflage. *JAMA* 1953;152:666–9.

21. Fulton JE, Rahimi AD, Helton P et al. Lip rejuvenation. *Dermatol Surg* 2000;26:470–4.

22. Spear SL, Convit R, and Little JW. Intradermal tattoo as an adjunct to nipple-areolar reconstruction. *Plast Reconstr Surg* 1989;83:907–11.

23. Francis A, Criton S, Shojan A, and Philip R. Micropigmentation in vitiligo of lateral lower lip. *J Cutan Aesthet Surg* 2013;6:236–7.

24. Carney MJ, Weissler JM, Sauler M, and Serletti JM. Looking beyond the knife: Establishing a framework for micropigmentation following breast reconstruction. *Plast Reconstr Surg* 2017;140(1):243e–4e.

Chapter 45

MYTHS IN VITILIGO

Sneha Ghunawat and Neha Dubey

CONTENTS

INTRODUCTION

Vitiligo is a common acquired depigmentation disorder affecting around 3%–4% of the general Indian population [1] and 0.5% of the world's population [2]. In this autoimmune condition, depigmentation is caused by the loss of functional melanocytes from the affected area of the epidermis. Although the exact etiology is still obscure, the following hypotheses have been put forward: autoimmune, neural, self-destruct, polygenic, and multifactorial [2–4]. Of all these, the autoimmune etiology seems most plausible.

Vitiligo is classified as segmental, acrofacial, generalized, and universal, or by pattern of involvement as focal, mixed, and mucosal types [5]. Children and adults of both sexes are affected equally, but the number of reports among females is much higher, which may be due to the greater social consequences faced by them [6].

HISTORY

Vitiligo is an ancient contagion. It has been detected in various medical literature from around the world, including the Old Testament, Ayurveda, Eberus Papyrus, and Vinaypitika [7]. The earliest authentic reference dates back to the period of Aushooryan (2200 BC) in the classic *Tarikh-e-Tibe-e-Iran* [8]. Two types of diseases affecting the color of the skin have been described in Pharonic medicine in the Ebers Papyrus: (i) with tumors, probably leprosy, and (ii) with only color change, probably vitiligo. The latter is believed to be treatable [9]. Its presence since antiquity has affected the general understanding of the disease deeply. With passing generations, many myths and misconceptions have crept in related to its cause, complications, and spreadability.

VITILIGO—A PSYCHOPHYSIOLOGIC DISORDER

Rarely accompanied by itching or other somatic symptoms [10], this aesthetically disfiguring ailment is more often than not accompanied by severe psychosocial impairment. People affected with the disease are very sensitive to the way others perceive them and upon the thought of being rejected they tend to withdraw. This makes the patient and their family follow many different types of rituals rather than seeking medical help. The disease is further complicated by the delay in treatment. Because of the huge cosmetic impact of the disease, patients tend to become depressed, which further triggers their disease condition. Vitiligo affects the affected individual's routine activities, emotions, and thinking. A study conducted on the stigmatization experience, coping, and sense of coherence in vitiligo patients supported the notion that treatment of vitiligo patients should address the emotional effects like stress, stigmatization, and depression and also include tools for psychological intervention [10]. This not only can result in better adaptation to the disease but also improved quality of life [11].

The treatment should be aimed at improving the overall quality of life and reduction in feelings of stigmatization caused by this chronic ailment. Hence debunking common myths around vitiligo with actual facts is important to the treating dermatologist as it forms a crucial part of counseling patients. Myths are popular beliefs or stories that have become associated with a person, community, or occurrence, especially when considered to illustrate a cultural ideal [12]. Many myths and misconceptions exist related to the disease and these vary from one part of the world to another. The commons ones are that the disease is not treatable, it is contagious, it is a form of leprosy, it is always hereditary, it is related to specific types of food and drinks, and it may ultimately lead to skin cancers [13].

This chapter deals with some of the most common myths prevalent about vitiligo in the society.

MYTHS RELATED TO THE CAUSE

MYTH 1

It is caused by microorganisms. In a recent study conducted in central India about knowledge and attitudes related to vitiligo, 18.9% of participants believed that it is caused by microorganisms [14].

FACT

Vitiligo is an autoimmune condition. The fact that its exact etiology is elusive and in order to understand the etiopathogenesis, various hypotheses have been put forward over the years points to lack of an infective etiology.

MYTH 2

It is caused by the wrath of God or wrongdoing. In India, unfortunately vitiligo is associated with some religious beliefs. For example, it is believed that a person who did "Guru droh" (an act of offending one's Guru) in his/her previous life suffers from vitiligo.

FACT

If Myth 2 is true, then the incidence should have been much higher than the highest recorded (8.8%) in the general Indian population [1].

MYTH 3

Mixed race parents. It is a popular belief that patients affected with vitiligo are born with uneven patchy skin because they have parents from different races [15].

FACT

Vitiligo is not related to the ethnicity of the parents, and most of the patients affected by it are born with normal skin and only later in life do they develop depigmented patches.

MYTH 4

Only dark-skinned people are affected by vitiligo.

FACT

Vitiligo is disfiguring in all races; however, the depigmentation is more noticeable in dark skin because of the strong contrast [16]. In fact, research in Nigerians described high levels of stigmatization because of the stark difference between normal and affected skin [17].

MYTHS RELATED TO FOOD

MYTH 1

Drinking milk shortly after having fish causes or aggravates vitiligo. In a study conducted by Asati et al., 27.6% of the participants believed that vitiligo is triggered by drinking milk after having fish [14].

MYTH 2

Excessive sour or citrus foods can exacerbate the lesions. The theory behind this myth is the doubtful role of ascorbic acid in vitiligo; it is promoted as an agent to reduce melanin production.

FACTS (1 AND 2)

A study conducted to evaluate the beneficial effects of antioxidant vitamin (A, C, E) and mineral (zinc, selenium) supplementation for vitiligo treatment documented a clear regimentation in 70% of the treated mice [18].

MYTH 3

Non-vegetarian food aggravates vitiligo. Many communities in India who strictly follow a vegetarian diet as per their religious sentiments believe that following a non-vegetarian diet causes or aggravates vitiligo.

FACT

No such correlation is proven.

MYTHS RELATED TO SPREADABILITY

MYTH 1

It is infectious, caused by touch or sharing meals. Many people believe vitiligo to be a type of leprosy and therefore contagious. This confusion can be associated with leprosy being called "Kushtha-rog"

and vitiligo being termed "Shwetkushtha" in the ancient Indian texts [7].

FACT

Vitiligo is an autoimmune condition and is not contagious.

MYTHS IN RELATION TO ITS ASSOCIATION WITH OTHER DISEASES

MYTH 1

Vitiligo is related to skin cancers, leprosy, and albinism.

FACT

The frequently reported associations of vitiligo include premature graying of hair, leukotrichia, halo nevus, lichen planus, and alopecia areata [19]. Occasionally, other skin disorders such as giant congenital melanocytic nevus with neurotization, nevus depigmentosus, and malignant melanoma have been reported in association with vitiligo [20–22]. The presence of any of the aforementioned or other conditions can be a mere coincidence and is not always a rule. Moreover, the pathogenesis of vitiligo is not the same as skin carcinomas, leprosy, or albinism.

MYTH 2

People affected with vitiligo often have other physical and mental disabilities.

FACT

Vitiligo patients are like any other normal individuals with life-altering and not life-threatening skin disorders. It does not produce any physical handicaps. The disease disfigures the patient without producing any physical disabilities. They might suffer from severe psychological and social problems rather than any "mental" problem. The majority of vitiligo patients experience depression, anxiety, frustration, and embarrassment when meeting strangers and have disturbed interpersonal relationships or difficulty in beginning a new sexual relationship [11]. However, the disease may be more common in people with other autoimmune disorders like hyperthyroidism, adrenocortical insufficiency, pernicious anemia, or alopecia areata.

MYTHS RELATED TO TREATMENT

MYTH 1

Treatment of vitiligo is "impossible."

MYTH 2

Allopathy deteriorates the disease. A recent study from central India showed that 18.4% of the participants believed that allopathy worsens the disease and 55.7% believed that AYUSH (Ayurveda, Yoga & Naturopathy, Unani, Siddha & Homeopathy) can cure it completely [14].

MYTH 3

Oral psoralens are toxic to the liver.

MYTH 4

Psoralens plus UVA (PUVA) treatment for vitiligo causes skin cancer.

FACTS (1, 2, 3, AND 4)

Vitiligo is a treatable condition and various treatment modalities are available that can be used depending on the vitiligo type and extent of involvement. There is no evidence in the literature to suggest that allopathy deteriorates the condition; this myth in fact misguides many patients and they are propelled toward various scientifically unproven methods of treatment, thus ultimately worsening the prognosis.

Psoralens are furocoumarins that have photosensitizing properties and are used topically and orally with ultraviolet (UV) irradiation in the treatment of vitiligo. Psoralens have been linked to a low rate of transient serum enzyme elevations during therapy, and on rare instances of clinically apparent acute liver injury. In open-label trials, serum AST or ALT elevations occurred in 2%–12% of subjects treated with methoxsalen and UV light. The elevations were usually mild to moderate in severity, asymptomatic, and self-limiting, and only in isolated case reports clinically apparent acute liver injury has also been reported with oral methoxsalen therapy including one instance attributed to topical therapy. While most cases of acute liver injury due to psoralen have been mild to moderate in severity and have a self-limited in course, there have been reports of fatal instances in patients with preexisting liver disease [23].

Phototherapy forms the cornerstone of treatment of widespread vitiligo. PUVA and PUVAsol therapy are usually preferred for widespread vitiligo in adults that is unresponsive to topical or other modalities of treatment. PUVA induces repigmentation of lesions but has to be given for a prolonged duration, with at least 100–200 sessions at least a day apart, two to three times a week [24]. If there is no response after approximately 50 sessions, PUVA should be discontinued [25], as high cumulative exposure to oral PUVA is associated with a dose-related increase in the risk of nonmelanoma skin cancer, particularly squamous cell carcinoma [26]. Hence it is not the treatment but overtreatment or improper treatment that can in certain cases lead to skin cancer. With proper patient selection and by following the set guidelines, this is does not occur.

CONCLUSION

The magnitude of the social stigma attached to this curable disease can be gauged by the fact that it is considered one of the three major medical problems in India by Pt. Jawaharlal Nehru, next to leprosy and malaria at one of time. Vitiligo has also been referred to as Shwetkushtha or "white leprosy." Multiple factors play a role in the prevailing myths about the disease. These include a lack of awareness about the disease, poor educational status, social misconceptions, and cultural beliefs. People affected with vitiligo are often treated as outcasts mainly because the white patches stand out on dark complexions, especially in India. The negative impact on the psyche of the patients magnified in Indians, as most of the population is colored (Fitzpatrick scale IV or V) [1,16]. Many studies have outlined the psychological trauma caused by vitiligo [27–30]. Most of the dermatological ailments require a lot of counseling; it is needed all the more in vitiligo. Our role as dermatologists should not only be limited to providing a cure in the form of medical and surgical options but also to create awareness among patients and their families about the true nature of the disease and its curability. Analyzing the prevailing myths in our community will also empower us to launch quality health education programs, as these are the reasons why most vitiligo patients opt for complementary and alternative medicine which eventually can do more harm than good. This will also promote the patient to pursue the right kind of treatment.

REFERENCES

1. Dhar S, Dua P, and Malakar R. Pigmentary disorders. In: Valia RG, and Valia AR, eds. *IADVL Textbook of Dermatology.* 3rd ed. Mumbai: Bhalani Publishing House; 2008, pp. 736–98.

2. Njoo MD, and Westerhof W. Vitiligo. Pathogenesis and treatment. *Am J Clin Dermatol* 2001;2:167–81.

3. Mantovani S, Garbelli S, Palermo B et al. Molecular and functional bases of self-antigen recognition in long-term persistent melanocyte-specific CD8+ T cells in one vitiligo patient. *J Invest Dermatol* 2003;121:308–14.

4. Yildirim M, Baysal V, Inaloz HS et al. The role of oxidants and antioxidants in generalized vitiligo at tissue level. *J Eur Acad Dermatol Venereol* 2004;18:683–6.

5. Halder RM, and Taliaferro SJ. Introduction. In: Wolff K, Goldsmith LA, Katz SI, Gilchrest BA, Paller AS, and Leffel DJ, eds. *Fitzpatrick's Dermatology in General Medicine* 7th ed. New York: McGraw Hill; 2008, pp. 617–21.

6. Srivastava G. Vitiligo - Introduction Asian Clinic. *Dermatology* 1994;1:1–5.

7. Prasad PV, and Bhatnagar VK. Medico-historical study of "Kilasa" (vitiligo/leucoderma) a common skin disorder. *Bull Indian Inst Hist Med Hyderabad* 2003;33:113–27.

8. Najamabadi M. *Tarikh-e-Tib-e-Iran.* Vol I. Tehran: Shamsi; 1934.

9. Ebbel B. *The Papyrus Ebess Copenhagen.* Levin and Munksgaard; 1937, p. 45.

10. Schmid-Ott G, Künsebeck HW, Jecht E, Shimshoni R, Lazaroff I, Schallmayer S, Calliess IT, Malewski P, Lamprecht F, and Goetz A. Stigmatization experience, coping and sense of coherence in vitiligo patients. *J Eur Acad Dermatol and Venereol* 2007;21:456–61.

11. Papadopoulos L, Bor R, and Legg C. Coping with the disfiguring effects of vitiligo: A preliminary investigation into the effects of cognitive-behavioural therapy. *Br J Med Psychol* 1999;72:385–96.

12. Farlex. The free dictionary. Available from: http://www.the-freedictionary.com/Myths.online edition

13. Kids Health. Available from: http://kidshealth.org/parent/infections/skin/vitiligo.html

14. Asati DP, Gupta CM, Tiwari S, Kumar S, and Jamra V. A hospital-based study on knowledge and attitude related to vitiligo among adults visiting a tertiary health facility of central India. *J Nat Sc Biol Med* 2016;7:27–32.

15. Mandeep K. Myths about vitiligo. *Get Healthy Stay Healthy.* http://gethealthystayhealthy.com. Published 2016. N.p., 2017.

16. Matto SK, Handa S, Kaur I, Gupta N, and Malhotra R. Psychiatric morbidity in vitiligo: Prevalence and correlates in India. *J Eur Acad Dermatol Venereol* 2002; 16(6):573–8.

17. Onunu AN, and Kubeyinjie EP. Vitiligo in the Nigerian African. A study of 351 patients in Benin City, Nigeria. *Int J Dermatol* 2003;42:800–2.

18. Jalel A, Soumaya GS, and Hamdaoui MH. Vitiligo treatment with vitamins, minerals and polyphenol supplementation. *Indian J Dermatol* 2009;54(4):357–60.

19. Sehgal VN, and Srivastava G. Vitiligo: Compendium of clinico-epidemiological features. *Indian J Dermatol Venereol Leprol* 2007;73:149–56.

20. Shin JH, Kim MJ, Cho S, Whang KK, and Hahm JH. A case of giant congenital nevocytic nevus with necrotization and onset of vitiligo. *J Eur Acad Dermatol Venereol* 2002;16:384–6.

21. Kang IK, and Hann SK. Vitiligo coexistent with nevus depigmentosus. *J Dermatol Tokyo* 1996;23:187–90.

22. Malignant melanoma and vitiligo. *J Invest Dermatol* 1979;73:491–4.

23. Psoralens. *livertox.nlm.nih.gov*. N.p., 2017.

24. Shenoi SD, and Prabhu S. Photochemotherapy (PUVA) in psoriasis and vitiligo. *Indian J Dermatol Venereol Leprol* 2014;80:497–504.

25. Stern RS, Thibodeau LA, Kleinerman RA, Parrish JA, and Fitzpatrick TB. Risk of cutaneous carcinoma in patients treated with oral methoxsalen photochemotherapy for psoriasis. *N Engl J Med* 1979;300:809–13.

26. Stern RS, Laird N, Melski J, Parrish JA, Fitzpatrick TB, and Bliech HL. Cutaneous squamous-cell carcinoma in patients treated with PUVA. *N Engl J Med* 1984;310:1156–61.

27. Pahwa P, Mehta M, Khaitan BK, Sharma VK, and Ramam M. The psychosocial impact of vitiligo in Indian patients. *Indian J Dermatol Venereol Leprol* 2013;79:679–85.

28. Kent G, and al-Abadie M. Factors aff ecting responses on dermatology life quality index items among vitiligo sufferers. *Clin Exp Dermatol* 1996;21:330–3.

29. Parsad D, Pandhi R, Dogra S, Kanwar AJ, and Kumar B. Dermatology life quality index score in vitiligo and its impact on the treatment outcome. *Br J Dermatol* 2003;148:373–4.

30. Kiprono S, Chaula B, Makwaya C, Naafs B, and Masenga J. Quality of life of patients with vitiligo attending the regional dermatology training center in Northern Tanzania. *Int J Dermatol* 2013;52:191–4.

INDEX

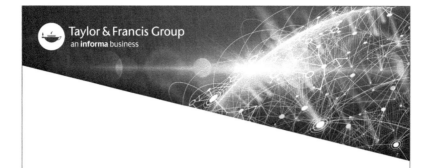

T - #0572 - 071024 - C316 - 280/210/14 - PB - 9780367543723 - Gloss Lamination